ADVANCES IN NEUROLOGY

Volume 59

Advances in Neurology

Advances in Neurology
Volume 59

Neural Injury and Regeneration

Editor

Fredrick J. Seil, M.D.
Director, Office of Regeneration
Research Programs
Veterans Affairs Medical Center;
and Professor, Departments of Neurology
and Cell Biology and Anatomy
Oregon Health Sciences University
Portland, Oregon

Raven Press New York

Raven Press, Ltd., 1185 Avenue of the Americas, New York, New York 10036

Made in the United States of America

Library of Congress Cataloging-in-Publication Data

Neural injury and regeneration/editor, Fredrick J. Seil.
p. cm.—(Advances in neurology; v. 59)
Includes bibliographical references and index.
ISBN 0-88167-948-8
1. Nerves—Regeneration. I. Seil, Fredrick J. II. Series.
[DNLM: 1. Alzheimer's Diseases—physiopathology—congresses.
2. Central Nervous System—physiopathology—congresses. 3. Nerve Regeneration—physiology—congresses. 4. Spinal Cord Injuries—physiopathology—congresses. W1 AD684H v. 59/WL 300 N49373]
RC321.A276 vol. 59
[QP363.5]
616.8 s—dc20
[616.8]
DNLM/DLC
for Library of Congress 92-19861
ISSN 0091-3952

The material contained in this volume was submitted as previously unpublished material, except in the instances in which some of the illustrative material was derived.

Great care has been taken to maintain the accuracy of the information contained in the volume. However, neither Raven Press nor the editor can be held responsible for errors or for any consequences arising from the use of the information contained herein.

Materials appearing in this book prepared by individuals as part of their official duties as U.S. Government employees are not covered by the above-mentioned copyright.

9 8 7 6 5 4 3 2 1

Advances in Neurology Series

Vol. 59: Neural Injury and Regeneration: *F. J. Seil, editor.* 384 pp., 1993.
Vol. 58: Tourette Syndrome: Genetics, Neurobiology, and Treatment: *T. N. Chase, A. J. Friedhoff, and D. J. Cohen, editors.* 400 pp., 1992.
Vol. 57: Frontal Lobe Seizures and Epilepsies: *P. Chauvel, A. V. Delgado-Escueta, E. Halgren, and J. Bancaud, editors.* 752 pp., 1992.
Vol. 56: Amyotrophic Lateral Sclerosis and Other Motor Neuron Diseases: *L. P. Rowland, editor.* 592 pp., 1990.
Vol. 55: Neurobehavioral Problems in Epilepsy: *D. B. Smith, D. Treiman, and M. Trimble, editors.* 512 pp., 1990.
Vol. 54: Magnetoencephalography: *S. Sato, editor.* 284 pp., 1990.
Vol. 53: Parkinson's Disease: Anatomy, Pathology, and Therapy: *M. B. Streifler, A. D. Korczyn, E. Melamed, and M. B. H. Youdim, editors.* 640 pp. 1990.
Vol. 52: Brain Edema: Pathogenesis, Imaging, and Therapy: *D. Long, editor.* 640 pp., 1990.
Vol. 51: Alzheimer's Disease: *R. J. Wurtman, S. Corkin, J. G. Growdon, and E. Ritter-Walker, editors.* 308 pp., 1990.
*Vol. 50: Dystonia 2: *S. Fahn, C. D. Marsden, and D. B. Calne, editors.* 688 pp., 1988.
*Vol. 49: Facial Dyskinesias: *J. Jankovic and E. Tolosa, editors.* 560 pp., 1988.
Vol. 48: Molecular Genetics of Neurological and Neuromuscular Disease: *S. DiDonato, S. DiMauro, A. Mamoli, and L. P. Rowland, editors.* 288 pp., 1987.
Vol. 47: Functional Recovery in Neurological Disease: *S. G. Waxman, editor.* 640 pp., 1987.
Vol. 46: Intensive Neurodiagnostic Monitoring: *R. J. Gumnit, editor.* 336 pp., 1987.
Vol. 45: Parkinson's Disease: *M. D. Yahr and K. J. Bergmann, editors.* 640 pp., 1986.
Vol. 44: Basic Mechanisms of the Epilepsies: Molecular and Cellular Approaches: *A. V. Delgado-Escueta, A. A. Ward, Jr., D. M. Woodbury, and R. J. Porter, editors.* 1,120 pp., 1986.
Vol. 43: Myoclonus: *S. Fahn, C. D. Marsden, and M. H. Van Woert, editors.* 752 pp., 1986.
Vol. 42: Progress in Aphasiology: *F. Clifford Rose, editor.* 384 pp., 1984.
Vol. 41: The Olivopontocerebellar Atrophies: *R. C. Duvoisin and A. Plaitakis, editors.* 304 pp., 1984.
Vol. 40: Parkinson-Specific Motor and Mental Disorders, Role of Pallidum: Pathophysiological, Biochemical, and Therapeutic Aspects: *R. G. Hassler and J. F. Christ, editors.* 601 pp., 1984.
*Vol. 39: Motor Control Mechanisms in Health and Disease: *J. E. Desmedt, editor.* 1,224 pp., 1983.
Vol. 38: The Dementias: *R. Mayeux and W. G. Rosen, editors.* 288 pp., 1983.
Vol. 37: Experimental Therapeutics of Movement Disorders: *S. Fahn, D. B. Calne, and I. Shoulson, editors.* 339 pp., 1983.
Vol. 36: Human Motor Neuron Diseases: *L. P. Rowland, editor.* 592 pp., 1982.
Vol. 35: Gilles de la Tourette Syndrome: *A. J. Friedhoff and T. N. Chase, editors.* 476 pp., 1982.
Vol. 34: Status Epilepticus: Mechanisms of Brain Damage and Treatment: *A. V. Delgado-Escueta, C. G. Wasterlain, D. M. Treiman, and R. J. Porter, editors.* 579 pp., 1983.
*Vol. 33: Headache: Physiopathological and Clinical Concepts: *M. Critchley, A. Friedman, S. Gorini, and F. Sicuteri, editors.* 417 pp., 1982.
*Vol. 32: Clinical Applications of Evoked Potentials in Neurology: *J. Courjon, F. Mauguiere, and M. Revol, editors.* 592 pp., 1982.
Vol. 31: Demyelinating Diseases: Basic and Clinical Electrophysiology: *S. Waxman and J. Murdoch Ritchie, editors.* 544 pp., 1982.
Vol. 30: Diagnosis and Treatment of Brain Ischemia: *A. L. Carney and E. M. Anderson, editors.* 424 pp., 1981.
*Vol. 29: Neurofibromatosis: *V. M. Riccardi and J. J. Mulvihill, editors.* 288 pp., 1981.
Vol. 28: Brain Edema: *J. Cervós-Navarro and R. Ferszt, editors.* 539 pp., 1980.
*Vol. 27: Antiepileptic Drugs: Mechanisms of Action: *G. H. Glaser, J. K. Penry, and D. M. Woodbury, editors.* 728 pp., 1980.
*Vol. 26: Cerebral Hypoxia and Its Consequences: *S. Fahn, J. N. Davis, and L. P. Rowland, editors.* 454 pp., 1979.
*Vol. 25: Cerebrovascular Disorders and Stroke: *M. Goldstein, L. Bolis, C. Fieschi, S. Gorini, and C. H. Millikan, editors.* 412 pp., 1979.

*Vol. 24: The Extrapyramidal System and Its Disorders: *L. J. Poirier, T. L. Sourkes, and P. Bédard, editors.* 552 pp., 1979..
*Vol. 23: Huntington's Chorea: *T. N. Chase, N. S. Wexler, and A. Barbeau, editors.* 864 pp., 1979.
Vol. 22: Complications of Nervous System Trauma: *R. A. Thompson and J. R. Green, editors.* 454 pp., 1979.
*Vol. 21: The Inherited Ataxia: Biochemical, Viral, and Pathological Studies: *R. A. Kark, R. Rosenberg, and L. Schut, editors.* 450 pp., 1978.
Vol. 20: Pathology of Cerebrospinal Microcirculation: *J. Cervós-Navarro, E. Betz, G. Ebhardt, R. Ferszt, and R. Wüllenweber, editors.* 636 pp., 1978.
*Vol. 19: Neurological Epidemiology: Principles and Clinical Applications: *B. S. Schoenberg, editor.* 672 pp., 1978.
*Vol. 18: Hemi-Inattention and Hemisphere Specialization: *E. A. Weinstein and R. P. Friedland, editors.* 176 pp., 1977.
*Vol. 17: Treatment of Neuromuscular Diseases: *R. C. Griggs and R. T. Moxley, editors.* 370 pp., 1977.
Vol. 16: Stroke: *R. A. Thompson and J. R. Green, editors.* 250 pp., 1977.
*Vol. 15: Neoplasia in the Central Nervous System: *R. A. Thompson and J. R. Green, editors.* 394 pp., 1976.
*Vol. 14: Dystonia: *R. Eldridge and S. Fahn, editors.* 510 pp., 1976.
Vol. 13: Current Reviews: *W. J. Friedlander, editor.* 400 pp., 1975.
Vol. 12: Physiology and Pathology of Dendrites: *G. W. Kreutzberg, editor.* 524 pp., 1975.
*Vol. 11: Complex Partial Seizures and Their Treatment: *J. K. Penry and D. D. Daly, editors.* 486 pp., 1975.
*Vol. 10: Private Models of Neurological Disorders: *B. S. Meldrum and C. D. Marsden, editors.* 270 pp., 1975.
*Vol. 9: Dopaminergic Mechanisms: *D. B. Calne, T. N. Chase, and A. Barbeau, editors.* 452 pp., 1975.
*Vol. 8: Neurosurgical Management of Epilepsies: *D. P. Purpura, J. K. Penry, and R. D. Walter, editors.* 370 pp., 1975.
Vol. 7: Current Reviews of Higher Nervous System Dysfunction: *W. J. Friedlander, editor.* 202 pp., 1975.
Vol. 6: Infectious Diseases of the Central Nervous System: *R. A. Thompson and J. R. Green, editors.* 402 pp., 1974.
*Vol. 5: Second Canadian-American Conference on Parkinson's Disease: *F. McDowell and A. Barbeau, editors.* 526 pp., 1974.
*Vol. 4: International Symposium on Pain: *J. J. Bonica, editor.* 858 pp., 1974.
*Vol. 3: Progress in the Treatment of Parkinsonism: *D. B. Calne, editor.* 402 pp., 1973.
*Vol. 2: The Treatment of Parkinsonism—The Role of DOPA Decarboxylase Inhibitors: *M. D. Yahr, editor.* 304 pp., 1973.
Vol. 1: Huntington's Chorea, 1872–1972: *A. Barbeau, T. N. Chase, and G. W. Paulson, editors.* 902 pp., 1973.

* Asterisk books are out of print.

Contents

Contributing Authors

Peter-Brian Andersson, 309
Dennis A. Aquino, 349
M. F. Barbe, 293
Jose L. Becerra, 75
Joan W. Berman, 349
J. A. Black, 135
W. F. Blakemore, 125
Andrew R. Blight, 91
Charles S. Booth, 105
Celia F. Brosnan, 349
I. R. Brown, 293
Michael C. Brown, 309
Wolfgang Brück, 327
Richard P. Bunge, 75
Jonathan S. Carp, 163
Carol A. Colton, 321
Margaret Corpuz, 315
Carl W. Cotman, 35
A. J. Crang, 125
Brian J. Cummings, 35
Tom Curran, 285
C. de Felipe, 263
Alejandro F. De Nicola, 199
Stephen B. Dunnett, 53
R. J. M. Franklin, 125
Reinhard L. Friede, 327
Daniel L. Gilbert, 321
Dana Giulian, 315
Edward D. Hall, 241
William F. Hickey, 337
S. P. Hunt, 263
R. Jenkins, 263
Kathryn J. Jones, 227
Pamela E. Knapp, 105
N. W. Kowall, 5
Christopher C. Lucas, 175
Daniel Luk, 285
Alexander Marcillo, 75
A. C. McKee, 5
A. R. Mihajlov, 185
J. E. Minturn, 135
Michael C. Molleston, 337
S. J. Moorman, 185
Joseph Mora, 113
James I. Morgan, 285
Satoshi Nakashiro, 47
H. O. Nornes, 185
John Oberdick, 285
R. O'Shea, 263
Ronald Parmer, 175
V. Hugh Perry, 309
Christian J. Pike, 35
William R. Puckett, 75
B. E. Pulford, 185
Robert M. Quencer, 75
B. R. Ransom, 135
Paul J. Reier, 175
Norman Robbins, 47
Linda Robertson, 285
W. Z. Rymer, 157
Stephen M. Sagar, 273
Karl Schilling, 285
Bridget Shafit-Zagardo, 349
Frank R. Sharp, 257, 273
Richard B. Simerly, 207
Robert P. Skoff, 105
Richard J. Smeyne, 285
Marion E. Smith, 305
H. Sontheimer, 135
Robert D. Terry, 1
Matthew L. Thomas, 337
Floyd J. Thompson, 175
Michael Tytell, 293
S. G. Waxman, 135
Henry deF. Webster, 67
L. R. Whalen, 185
T. S. C. Williams, 263
Jonathan R. Wolpaw, 163
Patrick M. Wood, 113
Wise Young, 249

Preface

This book explores some of the mechanisms by which the nervous system is injured in disease and trauma, and the possible repair or regenerative responses that may be available, including therapeutic interventions. It is aimed at both clinicians and basic neuroscientists and comprises contributions from clinical and laboratory sectors. The focus is on topics of current interest in neural regeneration research where some new information has become available or some new therapeutic approaches have been suggested. There is an attempt to balance the enthusiasm for the new with the cautious reminder of reality, as is apparent in the opening chapter and reflected in others.

The book has been divided into six major sections, including *Regeneration in Alzheimer Disease and Aging, Myelin Injury and Repair, Spinal Cord Injury: Physiology and Transplantation, Steroid Hormones and Neuronal Regeneration, Regulatory Genes in Regeneration and Plasticity,* and *The Function of Phagocytic Cells in the Nervous System.* Each section begins with an introductory or overview chapter. These introductory chapters were written by the prominent senior investigators who chaired sessions at the Fourth International Symposium on Neural Regeneration (December 11–15, 1991, The Asilomar Conference Center, Pacific Grove, California), upon which this volume is based. Subsequent chapters on specific topics in each of the sections were contributed by invited session speakers and their coworkers. These authors were selected because of their contributions to recent advances in their areas of investigation.

The material contained in this volume represents a cohesive sample of the endeavors in the ever-growing field of research in neural injury and regeneration. Both the difficulties with this work and the bases for optimism are portrayed, with such examples as the painstaking effort required to define the pathological changes in spinal cord trauma and the promise of early steroid treatment in acute spinal cord injury. At the molecular level, the genetic regulation of regeneration and the neural reaction to injury is beginning to be understood. It has become evident that even the aged nervous system can mount a regenerative response, although it may be of no or limited benefit given our present state of knowledge. Remyelination of central nervous system axons has been demonstrated in animal models and provides a basis for further work to encourage remyelination in human demyelinative conditions. Macrophages have proven to be very interesting cells, with key roles in both injury and repair processes. The stage is set for the next series of developments, which we hope will bring us still closer to our goal of clinical application.

Fredrick J. Seil

Acknowledgments

The Fourth International Symposium on Neural Regeneration was cosponsored by the U.S. Department of Veterans Affairs (Medical Research Service), the Paralyzed Veterans of America (Spinal Cord Research Foundation), the National Institutes of Health (National Institute of Neurological Disorders and Stroke, National Institute of Child Health and Development, and National Institute of Aging), the American Paralysis Association, and the Alzheimer's Association.

The Program Planning Committee included Drs. Bruce M. Carlson (University of Michigan), Cheryl Chanaud (Paralyzed Veterans of America), Mary Ellen Michel (National Institute of Neurological Disorders and Stroke), Monica M. Oblinger (The Chicago Medical School), Inder Perkash (Veterans Affairs Medical Center, Palo Alto and Stanford University), Paul J. Reier (University of Florida), Fredrick J. Seil (Veterans Affairs Office of Regeneration Research Programs), Frank R. Sharp (Veterans Affairs Medical Center and University of California, San Francisco), Marion E. Smith (Veterans Affairs Medical Center, Palo Alto and Stanford University), Roy A. Tassava (The Ohio State University), and Stephen G. Waxman (Veterans Affairs Medical Center, West Haven and Yale University).

I would like to thank the symposium keynote speaker, Dr. Bernice Grafstein (Cornell University Medical College), featured speakers Drs. Yehezkel Ben-Ari (INSERM, Paris, France), and Raymond Lund (University of Pittsburgh/University of Cambridge, England), and the many poster presenters whose efforts insured the symposium's success.

Advances in Neurology, Vol. 59, edited by
Fredrick J. Seil. Raven Press, Ltd.,
New York © 1993.

1

Regeneration in Alzheimer Disease and Aging

Robert D. Terry

*Department of Neurosciences, University of California,
San Diego, La Jolla, California 92093-0624*

The first section of this volume has to do with regeneration in Alzheimer disease and in aging. Functional regeneration in the central nervous system is poorly recognized in most respects. Studies on this subject are necessarily complex and slow, requiring an optimistic attitude on the part of the experimentalist. But the editor of this volume has rightly or wrongly chosen a pathologist to introduce the subject. One cannot expect much optimism from a pathologist, for we see too much of the wreckage of disease and death without adequate regeneration. What one can expect is a hard look at the problems, and that is what I propose for this brief survey.

The general problems are numerous. (a) Most commonly, the disease is superimposed on and therefore additive to the changes of normal aging. Prevalence rises exponentially after age 65, and the highest prevalence rate is in the ninth decade of life. (b) The disease is manifest very widely in the brain, although the microscopic lesions are not ubiquitous. The lower brainstem and cord are untouched, and the cerebellum is affected in only a very minor way. On the other hand, most of the neocortex, the limbic areas, the basal forebrain, and the rostral brainstem are quite significantly affected, but variably so from case to case. (c) The disease is progressive. Some of the lesions are old and some are recent in any autopsy specimen. (d) Many transmitter systems are deficient, not just the cholinergic system. (e) The disorder leads to loss of large neurons in many areas and to an even greater proportional loss of presynaptic terminals. (f) Long projection systems seem to be involved more severely than the local connections among small cells. (g) There is prominent formation and deposition of two different abnormal proteins: β-amyloid and phosphorylated tau.

Although normal aging leaves many subjects with good cognitive ability, there are always changes in the brain parenchyma. The brain loses weight, the cortex thins, and the ventricles enlarge mildly. Cell counts in the neocortex have clearly demonstrated a diminished number of large neurons. There is still debate to as to whether these have disappeared totally (1) or whether they have simply shrunken into a smaller size category (2). In either case, however, there is a loss of presynaptic terminals as measured recently by immunocytochemical techniques (3). We have found a fairly steady decline in the dorsal prefrontal cortex beginning in the fourth decade of life with a correlation coefficient of 0.66. There is an approximately 20% difference between specimens from subjects under 60 years of age and those older, and this change is statistically significant at $p < 0.001$. The decrement undoubtedly brings the normal subject closer to that threshold at which symptoms of cognitive loss would be found were there to be further, disease-related loss.

The classical lesions of Alzheimer disease (AD) are found throughout the cerebral cortex in the typical case, with only relative sparing of the primary sensory and motor areas. The entorhinal cortex and the hippocampal pyramids are severely affected, as is the amygdala and usually the basal nucleus of Meynert (4). The rostral locus ceruleus (5) and the dorsal raphe (6) are also involved. Only diffuse plaques are found in the cerebellum, but there seems not to be a specific loss of neurons in the cerebellar cortex unless there is additional change related to secondary factors such as malnutrition. A minority of cases with typical dementing illness have many neocortical plaques but no tangles in that location. Usually in such instances there are frequent tangles in the entorhinal and hippocampal areas. Some of these cases, but not all, have Lewy bodies in the neocortical neurons. We identify those with Lewy bodies plus plaques or plaques and tangles as the Lewy body variant of Alzheimer disease (7), whereas we identify those with neocortical plaques only and tangles elsewhere as Alzheimer disease (8), since all other parameters seem to be equal to cases of typical plaque-and-tangle Alzheimer disease.

In essentially all cases of AD we find diffuse plaques in addition to more mature forms in all the usual areas. These diffuse plaques are widely believed to be an immature form (9). In regard to tangles, there are many neurons with small tangles and others with large aggregates of paired helical filaments. In the entorhinal cortex many of the neurons are lost, leaving behind extraneuronal tangles, but this is unusual in the neocortex. It is important to note that many neurons die in AD without having developed neurofibrillary tangles.

The deficiency of choline acetyltransferase in autopsied AD tissue was first reported in 1976 (10,11), and partly because it was the first abnormal transmitter, as well as because much had been learned in previous years about the cholinergic system, it was almost immediately assumed to be the critical factor in Alzheimer disease. The cholinergic deficiency apparently comes from a loss, shrinkage, or dysfunction of neurons in the basal nucleus of Meynert (4). Many therapeutic trials involving the administration of antiesterase or of cholinomimetic drugs have been instituted on that basis (12). None, however, has been shown to produce more than very minimal slowing of the disease or very slight lessening of symptoms. Subsequently, a number of other transmitters, including norepinephrine (13) related to the locus ceruleus, serotonin (13) arising from the dorsal raphe, and the neuropeptides somatostatin (14) and substance P (15), have been shown to be significantly reduced in the disease. Many susceptible cells are glutamatergic. One must question, therefore, whether stimulation or augmentation of any one of these systems will reverse or arrest the global symptoms of dementia.

Cell counts in the hippocampus have shown major decrements of the pyramids in AD, especially in area CA1, which seems to be particularly sensitive (16). The entorhinal cortex, especially in layer 2, also loses neurons from clusters of those cells that project to the hippocampus by the way of the perforant pathway (17). Cortical counts have revealed major losses of large neurons (18) that are more severe in the younger cases than in the older ones (19). This may well relate to the phenomenon referred to above, where a more severe disease is needed to bring the young intact brain beyond the threshold where symptoms will be revealed than would be the case in an older patient, where large neurons have already been lost or shrunken and the disease produces an additive effect.

Neocortical presynaptic terminals have been quantified by both electron microscopic (20) and immunocytochemical (21) techniques. This decrement is greater than that of neurons. Prefrontal synapse loss correlates strongly with the level of dementia as measured by global tests such as the Blessed Information Memory Concentration Test, the Mini-Mental State Examination, and Dementia Rating Scale (22). The midfrontal synapse density correlates with the number of large neurons in the parietal area, indicating involvement of forward projection systems.

Although population density of synapses correlates with the level of dementia, the concentration of plaques does not correlate, at least in our series and several others (23). This implies that the amyloid load as expressed by the senile plaques is not the critical factor in causing the symptoms of Alzheimer disease.

β-Amyloid (24) is the most popular target of Alzheimer research these days. This protein is expressed in the disease in the form of masses of extracellular filamentous material that are surrounded by dystrophic neurites. Together dystrophic neurites and the amyloid core comprise the mature senile plaque. It is debated whether the dystrophic changes precede (25,26) or follow (27) the deposition of amyloid. β-Amyloid is derived from a much larger precursor protein (28) by means of abnormal processing involving cleavage in the transmembrane area of the precursor molecule. Certain components of the precursor molecule have been shown to be toxic, and others are trophic (29). Transfection studies involving certain of the epitopes of amyloid precursor protein are now in process in several laboratories, with results being published almost monthly (30). Unfortunately, this exciting and promising work is beyond the scope of this brief introduction.

Given this multiplicity and variety of problems in the Alzheimer disease brain, it seems to this author that making available pluripotential maintenance factors rather than neuronal regeneration offers the best hope for successful arrest or prevention of Alzheimer disease.

REFERENCES

1. Brody H. Organization of the cerebral cortex. III. A study of aging in the human cerebral cortex. *J Comp Neurol* 1955;102:511–556.
2. Terry RD, DeTeresa R, Hansen LA. Neocortical cell counts in normal human adult aging. *Ann Neurol* 1987;21:530–539.
3. Masliah E, Mallory M, Hansen LA, DeTeresa R, Terry RD. Quantitative alterations in the human neocortex during normal aging.
4. Whitehouse PJ, Price DL, Clark AW, Coyle JT, DeLong MR. Alzheimer's disease: Evidence for selective loss of cholinergic neurons in the nucleus basalis. *Ann Neurol* 1981;10:122–126.
5. Bondareff W, Mountjoy CQ, Roth M. Selective loss of neurons of origin of adrenergic projection to cerebral cortex (nucleus locus ceruleus) in senile dementia. *Lancet* 1981;1:783–784.
6. Yamamoto T, Hirano A. Nucleus raphe dorsalis in Alzheimer's disease: Neurofibrillary tangles and loss of large neurons. *Ann Neurol* 1985;17:573–577.
7. Hansen L, Salmon D, Galasko D, et al. The Lewy body variant of Alzheimer's disease: A clinical and pathological entity. *Neurology* 1990;40:1–8.
8. Terry RD, Hansen LA, DeTeresa R, Davies P, Tobias H, Katzman R. Senile dementia of the Alzheimer type without neocortical neurofibrillary tangles. *J Neuropathol Exp Neurol* 1987;46:262–268.
9. Tagliavini F, Giaccone G, Frangione B, Bugiani O. Preamyloid deposits in the cerebral cortex of patients with Alzheimer's disease and nondemented individuals. *Neurosci Lett* 1988;93:191–194.
10. Davies P, Maloney AJR. Selective loss of central cholinergic neurons in Alzheimer's disease. *Lancet* 1976;2:1403.
11. Bowen DM, Smith CB, White P, Davison AN. Neurotransmitter-related enzymes and indices of hypoxia in senile dementia and other abiotrophies. *Brain* 1976;99:459–495.
12. Becker R, Giacobini E, eds. *Cholinergic basis for Alzheimer therapy*. Boston: Birkhäuser; 1991.
13. Reinikainen KJ, Paljarvi L, Huuskonen M, Soinen H, Laakso M, Riekkinen P. A post-mortem study of nonadrenergic, serotonergic and GABAergic neurons in Alzheimer's disease. *J Neurol Sci* 1988; 84:101–116.
14. Davies P, Terry RD. Cortical somatostatin-like immunoreactivity in cases of Alzheimer's disease and senile dementia of the Alzheimer type. *Neurobiol Aging* 1981;2:9–14.
15. Crystal HA, Davies P. Cortical substance P-like immunoreactivity in cases of Alzheimer's disease and senile dementia of the Alzheimer type. *J Neurochem* 1982;38:1781.
16. Ball MJ. Neuronal loss, neurofibrillary tangles and granulovacuolar degeneration in the hippocampus with aging and dementia. A quantitative study. *Acta Neuropathol* 1977;37:111–118.
17. Hyman BT, Van HGW, Damasio AR, Barnes CL. Alzheimer's disease: Cell-specific pathology isolates the hippocampal formation. *Science* 1984;225: 1168–1170.
18. Terry RD, Peck A, DeTeresa R, Schechter R, Horoupian DS. Some morphometric aspects of the brain in senile dementia of the Alzheimer type. *Ann Neurol* 1981;10:184–192.
19. Hansen LA, DeTeresa R, Davies P, Terry RD. Neocortical morphometry, lesion counts, and choline acetyltransferase levels in the age spectrum of Alzheimer's disease. *Neurology* 1988;38:48–54.
20. Scheff SW, DeKosky ST, Price DA. Quantitative assessment of cortical synaptic density in Alzheimer's disease. *Neurobiol Aging* 1990;11:29–37.

21. Masliah E, Terry RD, Alford M, DeTeresa R. Quantitative immunohistochemistry of synaptophysin in the human neocortex—an alternative method to quantify synapses in paraffin sections. *J Histochem Cytochem* 1990;38:837–844.
22. Terry RD, Masliah E, Salmon DP, et al. Physical basis of cognitive alterations in Alzheimer disease: synapse loss is the major correlate of cognitive impairment. *Ann Neurol* 1991;30:572–580.
23. Morris JC, Mirra S, Davis P, et al. Correlation of dementia severity with plaque and tangle frequencies in midfrontal cortex in CERAD cases with Alzheimer's disease. *Ann Neurol* 1991;30:249.
24. Glenner GG, Wong CW. Alzheimer's disease and Down's syndrome: Sharing of a unique cerebrovascular amyloid fibril protein. *Biochem Biophys Res Commun* 1984;122:1131–1135.
25. Terry RD, Wisniewski HM. The ultrastructure of the neurofibrillary tangle and the senile plaque. In: Wolstenholme GEW, O'Connor M, eds. *CIBA Foundation symposium on Alzheimer's disease and related conditions.* London: J & A Churchill; 1970:145–168.
26. Cork LC, Masters C, Beyreuther K, Price DL. Development of senile plaques. Relationships of neuronal abnormalities and amyloid deposits. *Am J Pathol* 1990;137:1383–1392.
27. Selkoe DJ. Amyloid β protein deposition as a seminal pathogenetic event in AD: An hypothesis. *Neurobiol Aging* 1990;11:99.
28. Kang J, Lemaire HG, Unterbecka L, et al. The precursor of Alzheimer's disease amyloid A 4 protein resembles a cell surface receptor. *Nature* 1987; 325:733–736.
29. Yankner BA, Duffy LK, Kirschner DA. Neurotrophic and neurotoxic effects of amyloid β protein: Reversal of tachykinin neuropeptides. *Science* 1991;250:279–281.
30. Kawabata S, Higgins GLA, Gordon JW. Amyloid plaques, neurofibrillary tangles, and neuronal loss in brains of transgenic mice overexpressing a C-terminal fragment of human amyloid precursor protein. *Nature* 1991;354:476–478.

Advances in Neurology, Vol. 59, edited by
Fredrick J. Seil. Raven Press, Ltd.,
New York © 1993.

2

The Histopathology of Neuronal Degeneration and Plasticity in Alzheimer Disease

N. W. Kowall and A. C. McKee

Departments of Neurology and Neuropathology, Massachusetts General Hospital and Harvard Medical School, Boston, Massachusetts 02114

In recent years, the fundamental biochemical and pathological processes affecting the neuron and its local environment in Alzheimer disease (AD) have been greatly clarified by use of histopathological techniques. The relationship between these alterations and the clinical expression of dementia is better understood, and novel experimental studies have elucidated potential mechanisms of neuronal degeneration. In this context the damaged nervous system mounts a proliferative and reparative response, illustrating the plasticity and regenerative capacity of the aged nervous system.

Neuronal populations are differentially affected by the degenerative process in AD. Neuronal processes immunoreactive for a wide variety of neurotransmitters are incorporated into senile plaques (SP), but only selected neuronal subsets accumulate neurofibrillary tangles (NFT). Populations of cortical neurons containing neurofilament and substance P immunoreactivity and cholinergic, serotonergic, and adrenergic projections from the brainstem to the cerebral cortex are especially vulnerable to degeneration, while other cortical neuronal populations and brainstem nuclei are largely spared.

The neuronal cytoskeleton is profoundly altered in AD. The microtubule-associated protein (MAP) tau is abnormally phosphorylated and displaced from its normal axonal locale to become an integral component of perikaryal NFT and fibrillary neuritic inclusions called dystrophic neurites, neuropil threads, or curly fibers. Dendritic MAP 2 and neurofilament immunoreactivity are lost; the developmentally regulated MAP, MAP 1B, is reexpressed; and tyrosylated tubulin immunoreactivity is increased. These changes suggest that microtubule stability is reduced in AD. The normal segregation of dendritic and axonal spectrin isoforms, however, is maintained, indicating that the cytoskeletal involvement is selective.

Golgi and immunocytochemical studies show that axonal plasticity and dendritic proliferation occur in AD. Immunoreactivity for laminin, a major growth-promoting protein normally found in the extracellular matrix, is increased in cortical neurons, possibly because of cross-reactivity with intracellular laminin-related peptides. Several growth factors are enriched in surviving neurons and/or glia, including nerve growth factor (NGF), basic fibroblast growth factor (bFGF), and transforming growth factor beta (TGFβ). Growth-related membrane glycoproteins such as neural cell adhesion molecule (NCAM) and Thy-1 are also increased.

The mechanisms responsible for this array of degenerative and proliferative changes in AD are not known, but recent evidence suggests that altered protein phosphorylation and membrane proteolysis are of fundamental importance. Experimental inhibition of protein phosphatases leads to increased cytoskeletal protein phosphorylation and neuronal degeneration *in vivo*. The neuronal distribution of protein kinase immunoreactivity is altered in AD. β-Amyloid, the major constituent of SP, is a product of altered membrane proteolysis that may directly cause neuronal degeneration and NFT formation. Intracerebral injections of β-amyloid in experimental animals produce cytoskeletal alterations that closely resemble those found in AD. The severity of clinical dementia correlates more closely with cytoskeletal changes and synaptic depletion than with β-amyloid deposition. Disruption of the cytoskeleton, perhaps produced by altered protein phosphorylation and the toxic effects of β-amyloid, may lead to synaptic depletion, neuronal degeneration, and aberrant neuritic regeneration in AD.

THE PATHOLOGICAL FEATURES OF AD

The neuropathological hallmarks of AD are the NFT and the SP. The NFT are intraneuronal accumulations of abnormal filamentous proteins first recognized in 1907 by Alois Alzheimer using the Bielschowsky silver stain (1–3). In the 1960s, Kidd and Terry identified paired helical filaments (PHF) as the major ultrastructural component of NFT (4,5). Recent studies have conclusively shown that the microtubule-associated protein, tau, is an integral component of PHF (6–8). Antibodies specific for tau, including ALZ 50, label NFT and a striking array of dystrophic neurites in the cortical neuropil in AD (9–13). Dystrophic neurites are similar to NFT ultrastructurally except for their location in dendritic and axonal processes rather than neuronal perikarya. There is some evidence to suggest that dystrophic neurites develop prior to the formation of perikaryal NFT (14).

Fully developed SP consist of a focal extracellular deposit of amyloid fibrils surrounded by abnormal neuronal and glial processes. A major protein component of SP amyloid was isolated from meningeal blood vessels and senile plaque cores and named beta protein or A4 (15,16). This abnormal protein is widely deposited as diffuse plaques in many brain regions in AD brain (17–20). Beta protein is a 38- to 42-amino-acid proteolytic fragment cleaved from a transmembrane precursor glycoprotein, amyloid precursor protein (APP), synthesized in neurons, nonneuronal cells, and sites outside the nervous system (21). There is one APP gene on chromosome 21, but several isoforms of APP are generated by alternative mRNA splicing (22–25). The beta protein domain of APP extends from within the membrane to the extracellular domain. Altered proteolysis may be required to release the beta fragment from its precursor (26,27).

The relationship between SP and NFT is unknown. β-Amyloid may be an early result of neuronal degeneration; however, because β-amyloid deposition precedes the development of neurofibrillary pathology, β-amyloid may cause neuronal damage. The latter possibility has been greatly strengthened by the finding that solubilized beta protein is toxic to neurons in culture (28–30) and by the definition of three different mutations in APP at codon 717 in several unrelated families with early-onset AD (31–34). Transgenic mice overexpressing the carboxy-terminal fragment of APP (including the entire β-amyloid sequence) in neurons, however, did not develop extracellular β-amyloid deposits or neurofibrillary degeneration (35).

DIFFERENTIAL NEURONAL INVOLVEMENT IN AD

Neuronal subsets are differentially vulnerable to degeneration in AD. Morphological and quantitative changes occur in neurofilament, substance P, somatostatin, neuropeptide Y, and corticotrophin-releasing hormone neurons (36–39). Neurites immunoreactive for diverse peptide neurotransmitters are associated with senile plaques (40). Recently it has been directly shown that glutamatergic neurons develop NFT in AD (41). Neurofilament-containing cortical projection neurons are selectively lost as NFT develop (42,43). These projection neurons are sensitive to degeneration in Huntington disease and to excitotoxic injury (44,45). Substance P neurons are severely depleted despite modest decreases in bulk transmitter content (39). Somatostatin and neuropeptide Y perikarya persist despite morphological distortion and loss of terminals (46). These peptidergic neurons degenerate without NFT formation, suggesting that NFT formation is only one of many possible forms of neuronal involution in AD.

A subset of layer III cortical neurons that contain neurofilament immunoreactivity are especially sensitive to degeneration in AD. These neurons give rise to the corticocortical connections that may play an important role in cognition (42,47–49). These neurons, as identified by the SMI 32 antibody, which labels nonphosphorylated neurofilaments in the neuronal cell body, are profoundly depleted and sensitive to NFT accumulation. How the axonal or synaptic domains of these neurons are specifically altered in AD remains unknown. Axons and synapses are enriched in phosphorylated neurofilaments and can be detected with SMI 31 antibody (50). Given the earlier and more sensitive correlation of dementia with synaptic loss than with neuronal cell body loss, changes in these compartments may be especially relevant to the disease pathogenesis.

CLINICAL–PATHOLOGICAL CORRELATIONS

Initial quantitative studies indicated that SP correlated with the presence and severity of dementia in AD (51,52). However, the majority of subsequent reports demonstrated a weak and inconsistent correlation between the severity of dementia and the density of SP (53–56). Methodological differences hamper the direct comparison of these studies, yet in most, methods that failed to disclose preamyloid beta protein deposition were used. Diffuse deposits of beta protein, which most likely represent an early stage of SP, consist of preamyloid or amyloid without the β-pleated-sheet configuration. Therefore, before the development of specific antibodies against beta protein, investigators generally underestimated the extent of deposition (55,56). It has now become clear that many elderly patients without overt dementia have widespread cortical beta protein deposition. Masters and colleagues found that 80% of 80-year-olds have beta protein, yet only 15% to 20% are demented (57). However, in a prospective cohort of nondemented patients with widespread beta accumulation without other neuropathological abnormalities, Crystal and co-workers found evidence of mild cognitive loss (58). This suggests that beta protein, by itself, exerts some neurotoxic effects without producing recognizable dementia.

Neurofibrillary tangles are clearly and consistently correlated with the severity of dementia (14,53,54,59–61). In our retrospective study of 22 nondemented elderly controls and 34 demented patients with AD pathology, we found that 46% of controls had no beta protein deposition and 54% of controls had widespread beta protein deposition but no neocortical neurofibrillary or neuritic pathology. Of the 34 demented patients, 79% had widespread SP and NFT, and 21% had neocortical SP with rare NFT. All demented patients had widespread neocortical tau-immunoreactive, silver-positive dystrophic neurites as well as extensive beta protein deposits. The neurites were found free in the neuropil and surrounding SP. Quantitative analysis showed that the density of dystrophic neurites correlated significantly with the clinical severity of dementia. Although cerebral beta protein, by itself, is insufficient for the development of dementia, it may induce

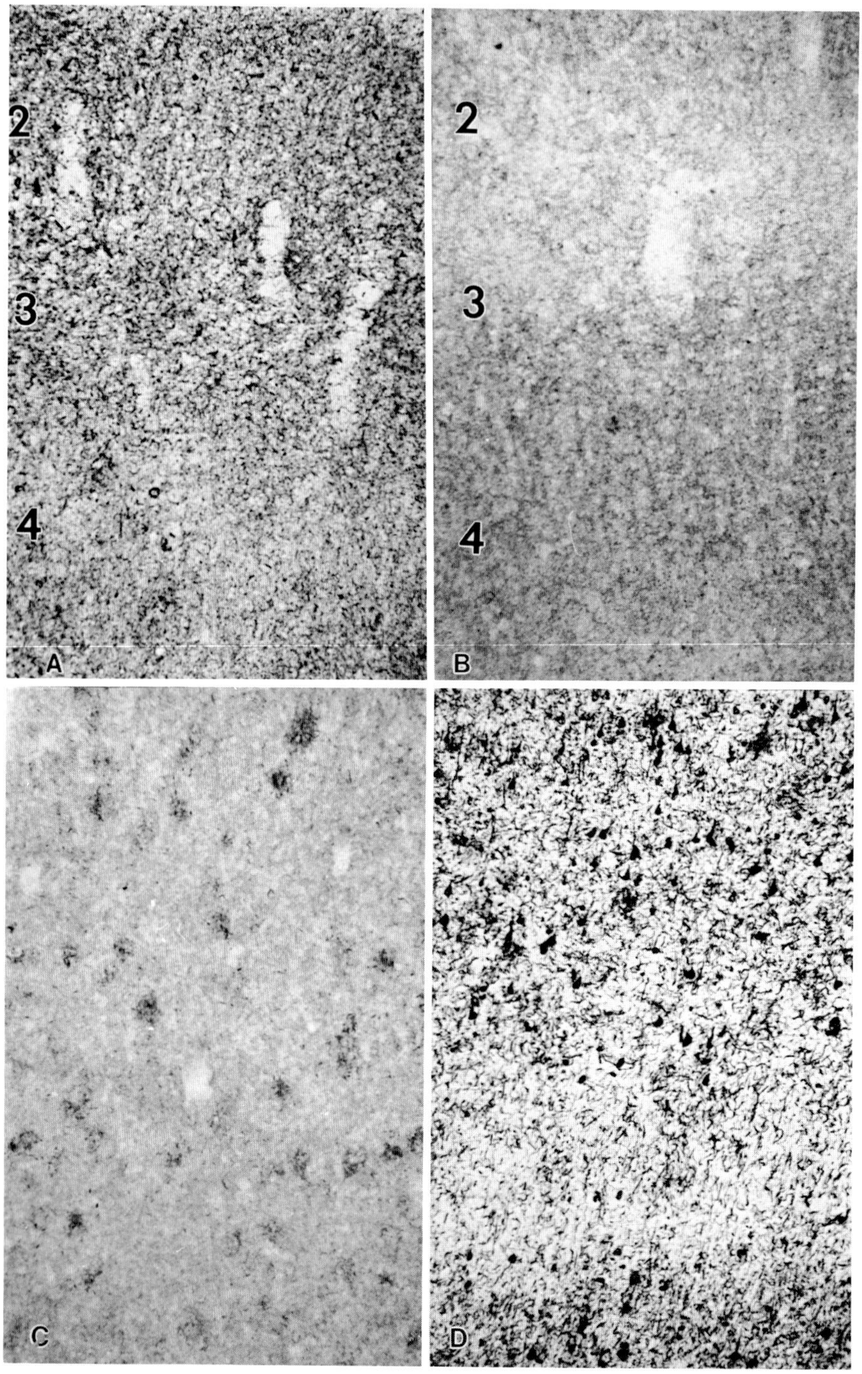

FIG. 1. (**A**) Alz 50 immunoreactivity is prominent in neurites and neurofibrillary tangles that form intense bands in layers 2 and 3 of Alzheimer temporal isocortex. (**B**) An adjacent section stained with synaptophysin monoclonal antibody shows a clear band of decreased immunoreactivity in layers 2 and 3. Quantitative analysis will be needed to define the extent of these changes and their interrelationship. (**C**) Tau 1 immunoreactivity in Alzheimer temporal isocortex without alkaline phosphatase treatment shows some neurites in senile plaques and in the neuropil. (**D**) Tau 1 immunoreactivity after alkaline phosphatase treatment shows greatly enhanced immunoreactivity, suggesting that phosphorylation blocks the site recognized by this antibody in the tau molecule.

neuronal degeneration in the form of dystrophic neurites and NFT, and those changes correlate with the severity of dementia in AD.

SYNAPTIC DEPLETION AND DYSTROPHIC NEURITES IN AD

The severity of dementia in AD also correlates with the loss of synapses and large cortical neurons (62–64). Synaptic loss averaging 45% is found in all cortical layers as determined by synaptophysin immunocytochemistry (65).

In serial sections stained with synaptophysin, Alz 50, and ubiquitin in specimens of temporal isocortex from control and AD patients, we found that synaptophysin immunoreactivity was normally distributed in a specific laminar pattern (66). Layers I to IV contained the most prominent band of immunoreactivity, layer VI somewhat less, and layer V the least (Fig. 1). Qualitatively, there was no clear overall reduction of synaptophysin immunoreactivity in AD, but there was a laminar pattern of loss in cortical layers II, III, and V, corresponding to the cortical layers with intense dystrophic neurite and NFT formation. This suggests that synaptic loss may be associated with the development of laminar neuritic pathology. Preliminary computerized quantitation performed in collaboration with Dr. W. R. Markesbery at the University of Kentucky showed that dystrophic neurites occupied approximately 20% of the neuropil area in layers III and V of superior frontal cortex. Abnormal synaptophysin-positive neurites are also found in SP and in the neuropil in AD (65).

CYTOSKELETAL ALTERATIONS, DEGENERATION, AND PLASTICITY IN AD

The structural stability of the neuron ensures the fidelity of synaptic contacts, axonal trajectories, and long-range transport, whereas the ability of the neuron to alter its shape in response to environmental cues is integral to development, regeneration, and learning. The balance between these two opposing functions, stability and plasticity, is thought to be regulated by MAPs. The MAPs bind to microtubules and promote tubulin polymerization *in vitro* (67); they also play a pivotal role in the initiation and outgrowth of neural processes (68). Neurite sprouting corresponds to a marked rise in concentrations of high-molecular-weight MAPs, including MAP 2, whereas concentrations of tau, a low-molecular-weight MAP, correlate with neurite elongation (69). Dendrites enriched in MAP 2 exhibit enhanced branching ability, suggesting that MAP 2 plays a role in the maintenance of dendritic arborization (70).

The MAPs have distinct regional, cellular, and intracellular distributions. Normally tau immunoreactivity is found in axons in the cerebral cortex (12,71), whereas MAP 2 is concentrated in cell bodies and dendrites (72,73) (Fig. 2A). Tau protein and MAP 2 colocalize in regenerating neurites in culture and in embryonic neurons *in situ;* with maturation these proteins assume their appropriate intracellular distribution (74). The microtubule-bundling characteristics of tau protein change during maturation from a fetal to an adult form (75). These observations show that the composition of the neuronal cytoskeleton is modified during neurite outgrowth and regeneration.

A variety of data indicate that neuritic outgrowth and plasticity occur in Alzheimer disease. Golgi impregnation studies have demonstrated dendritic sprouting with the development of filopodia and growth cone structures, and neuritic sprouting has been identified in the regions of senile plaques (76–81). Histochemical studies have shown evidence of axonal plasticity and reorganization in the molecular layer of the dentate gyrus (82–84). Because of these observations we examined how the neuronal cytoskeleton is altered in AD.

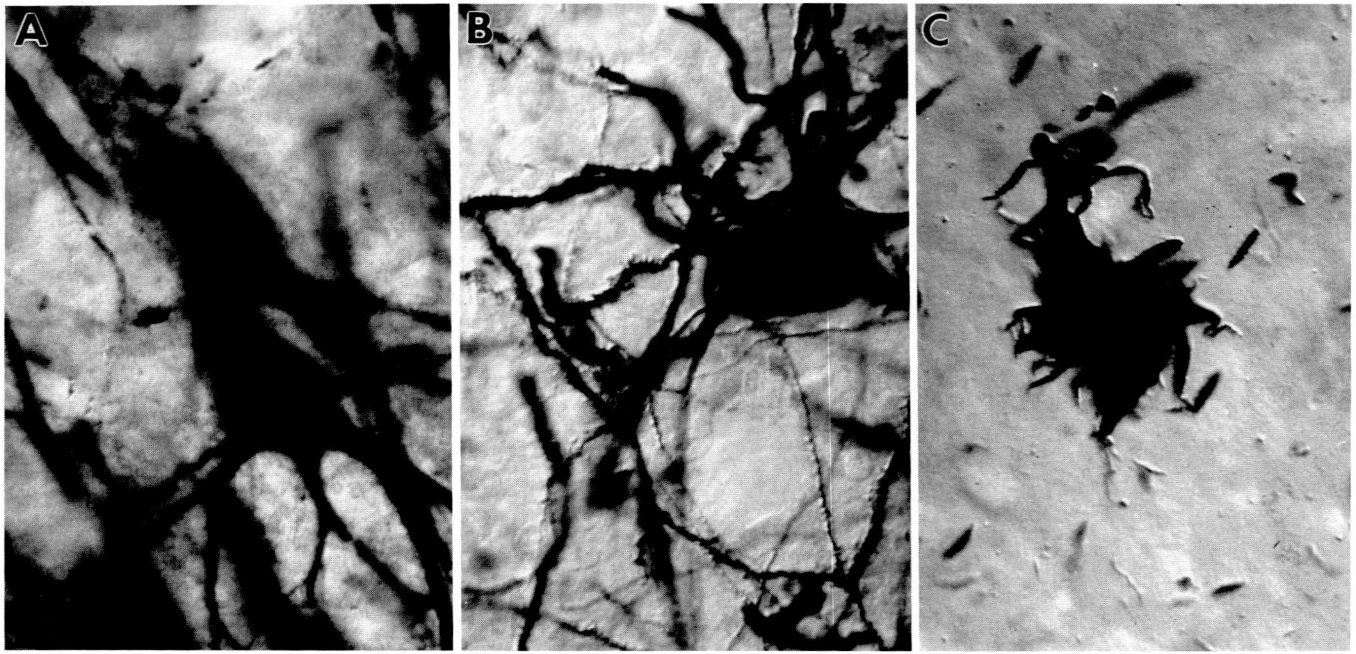

FIG. 2. (**A**) MAP 2 immunoreactivity in normal pyramidal neuron in CA1 field of the hippocampus. Immunoreactivity is confined to the cell body and dendrites, which taper smoothly and ramify. Original magnification ×780. (**B**) MAP 2 immunoreactivity in the CA1 field of the hippocampus in Alzheimer disease. Numerous tortuous dendritic processes lined with spine-like excrescences are clearly visible. Original magnification ×780. (**C**) Tau-immunoreactive neurofibrillary tangle forms a "medusa head" appearance because of immunoreactivity in proximal basal dendrites. Original magnification ×780.

NEUROFILAMENTS, MAP 2, AND TAU PROTEIN

Both MAP 2 and nonphosphorylated neurofilament protein (labeled by the antibody SMI 32) are normally confined to the perikarya and dendrites of specific subsets of cortical neurons. Morphological abnormalities are found in some classes of MAP-2-immunoreactive neurons in AD, including stellate cells of the entorhinal cortex and hippocampal pyramids. In all regions of the entorhinal cortex, a major convergence relay point for cortical input to the hippocampus, layer II star cells and layer III, V, and VI pyramids are stained by MAP 2 and SMI 32 antisera. The cytoarchitectonic features that define the entorhinal subfields are seen well with both antisera, although the density of MAP-2-immunoreactive neurons is greater than that of SMI 32 neurons. In AD, the regular array of apical dendritic bundles of layer V and VI pyramids is disorganized. Individual MAP 2 and SMI 32 neurons are lost and replaced by neurofibrillary tangles, especially in layer II of lateral and intermediate entorhinal cortex. The MAP 2 histochemistry shows distortion and dissolution of apical dendrites, including abrupt truncations, varicose changes, and proliferation of fine proximal branches (Fig. 2B). Immunoreactive perikarya are occasionally enlarged and hyperconvex. In regions severely affected by NFT, remaining neurons exhibit rampant proliferation of basal dendrites (Fig. 2). Fibrillar tau can extend into these MAP-2-positive dendrites, which demonstrate other features reminiscent of regenerating neurons in culture, including lamellipodia and filopodia of growth-cone-like structures (Fig. 2C). Although these proliferative and degenerative changes are found throughout the hippocampal formation and entorhinal cortex, the striking regional and laminar variability suggests that susceptibility to degeneration is determined by specific connectional or biochemical features.

A characteristic sequence of cytoskeletal changes occur in degenerating neurons that acquire NFT. Initially, tau and tubulin form granular deposits in normal-appearing perikarya. As further tau is deposited, tubulin reactivity diminishes, and NFT develop. Mature NFT contain the heat shock protein ubiquitin. Abnormal tau-reactive neurites are evident even in regions with little or no NFT formation. A subset of these neurites is reactive for tubulin and ubiquitin. The distribution of abnormal filamentous tau-positive neurites suggests a dendritic origin. Other dot-like or globular neurites are probably axonal or synaptic in origin. Tubulin and neurofilament immunoreactivity are found in granulovacuolar degeneration, and actin and tau immunoreactivity are located in Hirano bodies (85–89).

MAP 1B

A number of MAPs have been identified and characterized in mammalian brain, including the high-molecular-weight MAPs, MAP 1 and MAP 2, and a group of low-molecular-weight tau proteins (75,90–92). MAP 1B is a 320-kD protein under strong developmental regulation (75,93–95) that has been variously designated MAP 5, MAP 1x, and MAP 1.2 (96,97). Concentrations of MAP 1B are tenfold greater in fetal and neonatal brains and fall to a persistently low level in mature animals (94,98–100). During development, MAP 1B is the first MAP to appear in growing axons (101,102) and is the only MAP present in neurons prior to terminal differentiation (100). In cultured PC 12 cells, MAP 1B concentrations increase tenfold in conjunction with nerve-growth-factor-induced neuritic outgrowth (103). Regions of mature brain that undergo continual neuronal differentiation and remodeling, such as the rodent olfactory system and retina, demonstrate persistent expression of MAP 1B (98,104,105). We examined AD hippocampal formation for evidence of MAP 1B immunoreactivity in proliferating and/or regenerating structures using immunoperoxidase procedures and monoclonal antibodies raised against MAP 1B (Fig. 3). In normal

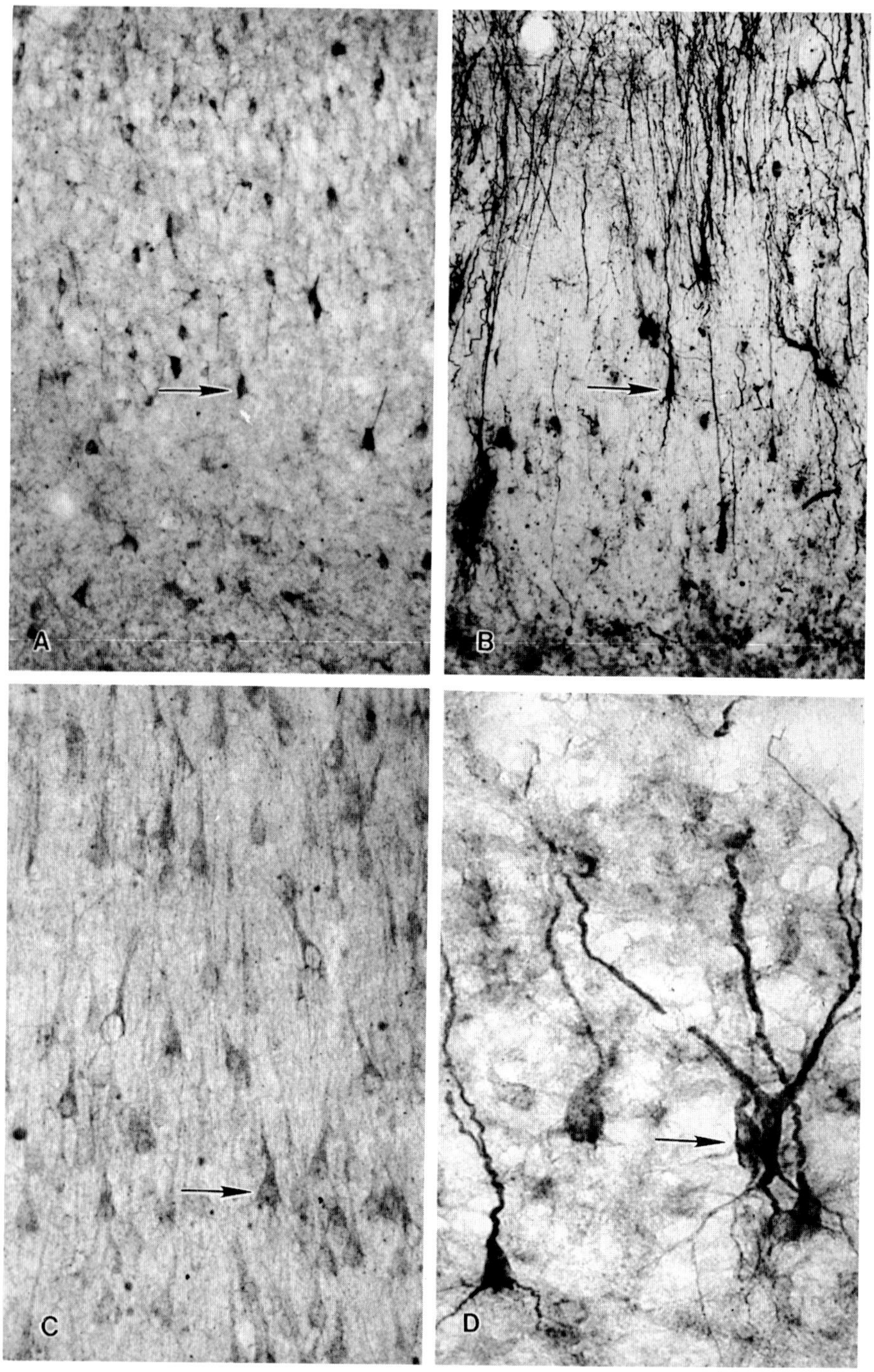

FIG. 3. (**A**) MAP 1B immunoreactivity is confined to scattered neurons in the CA1 field of adult hippocampus but is present in a moderate number of pyramidal neurons in the newborn human shown here. A typical neuron is shown with arrow. ×100. (**B**) In Alzheimer disease the number of MAP 1B immunoreactive neurons in CA1 is increased compared to adult controls, and intense immunoreactivity is present in neurons with abnormal distorted dendrites (*arrow*) and distal dendritic sprouts. ×100. (**C**) Basic fibroblast growth factor immunoreactivity is present in normal pyramidal neurons (*arrow*) in the CA1 and subiculum of adult hippocampus. ×200. (**D**) In Alzheimer disease, subiculum and CA1 neuronal density is reduced, but remaining neurons are often intensely immunoreactive with bizarre dendritic processes (*arrow*). ×320.

aged brain, dentate granule cells and mossy fiber terminals in CA4 and CA3 are positive. Neurons in CA4, CA3, and CA2 are more intensely stained than CA1 neurons. Nonneuronal elements are rarely seen. In AD, the intensity of granule cell staining is increased. Intensely stained CA1 neurons with proliferated basal dendrites are prominent (Fig. 3). Dystrophic neurites and senile plaque neurites, which contain tau but not MAP 2 immunoreactivity, show pronounced MAP 1B immunoreactivity throughout the hippocampus. Neurofibrillary tangles are not immunoreactive. The prominence of MAP 1B staining in abnormal neurites suggests that neuritic proliferation is associated with the reemergence of fetal characteristics in AD. Because MAP 1B less effectively stabilizes microtubules than MAP 2, it is possible that microtubule stability is compromised in the context of neuritic proliferation (75).

Ihara and colleagues produced and screened a series of MAP 1B monoclonal antibodies for NFT and neurite staining. Although most of their antibodies did not stain NFT, two monoclonal antibodies against phosphorylated forms of MAP 1B stained NFT (106). The presence or absence of tau binding domains within the epitopes recognized by MAP 1B antibodies may account for this variability (107). Our antibodies probably recognize nonphosphorylated MAP 1B epitopes (106)

POSTTRANSLATION MODIFICATIONS OF TUBULIN IN AD

The stability of microtubules is regulated in part by posttranslational modification of tubulin monomers. Enzymatic removal of the carboxy-terminal tyrosine residue of α-tubulin results in detyrosinated tubulin, which is enriched in stable subclasses of microtubules, whereas tyrosinated tubulin is incorporated into a more dynamic subset of microtubules (108,109). Polymerized tubulin is also acetylated on a specific lysine residue (110). Thus, recently polymerized microtubules contain tyrosinated tubulin, whereas mature or stabilized microtubules are acetylated. We examined the distribution of tyrosinated and acetylated tubulin in normal aged and AD hippocampal formation to determine if this relatively dynamic form of tubulin is differentially localized in AD (Fig. 4). We used a monoclonal antibody (1A2) raised against a synthetic carboxy-terminal peptide of tyrosinated tubulin. Binding of this antibody to tubulin is significantly reduced after carboxypeptidase treatment, suggesting that 1A2 reacts specifically with epitopes present in tyrosinated tubulin. In normal hippocampus, dentate granule cells are moderately immunoreactive. Pyramidal neurons throughout the CA fields, including their axons, dendrites, and dendritic spines, are immunoreactive. The greatest density of immunoreactive perikarya is found in the subiculum, typically in the deeper laminae. In contrast to tyrosinated tubulin normally present in the distal dendritic tree and axons of normal CA1 pyramids in adult human hippocampus, acetylated and whole polymeric tubulin is primarily confined to the cell body and proximal processes. In AD, the intensity of tyrosinated tubulin staining is generally increased in all regions, particularly in the apical dendrites of CA1 and subicular pyramids. A dense plexus of distorted, irregularly twisted, and swollen dendrites is evident in the molecular layer of Ammon's horn, most notably in CA1. Layer I of subiculum also demonstrates a striking band of distorted apical dendritic tufts. Globular neurites in senile plaques are occasionally immunoreactive. Immunoreactivity is not concentrated in NFT. We show that posttranslational modification of tubulin monomers is altered in AD. Decreased microtubule stability may reflect a primary defect in tubulin detyrosination or represent a secondary decrease in microtubule stability associated with neurite outgrowth and plasticity.

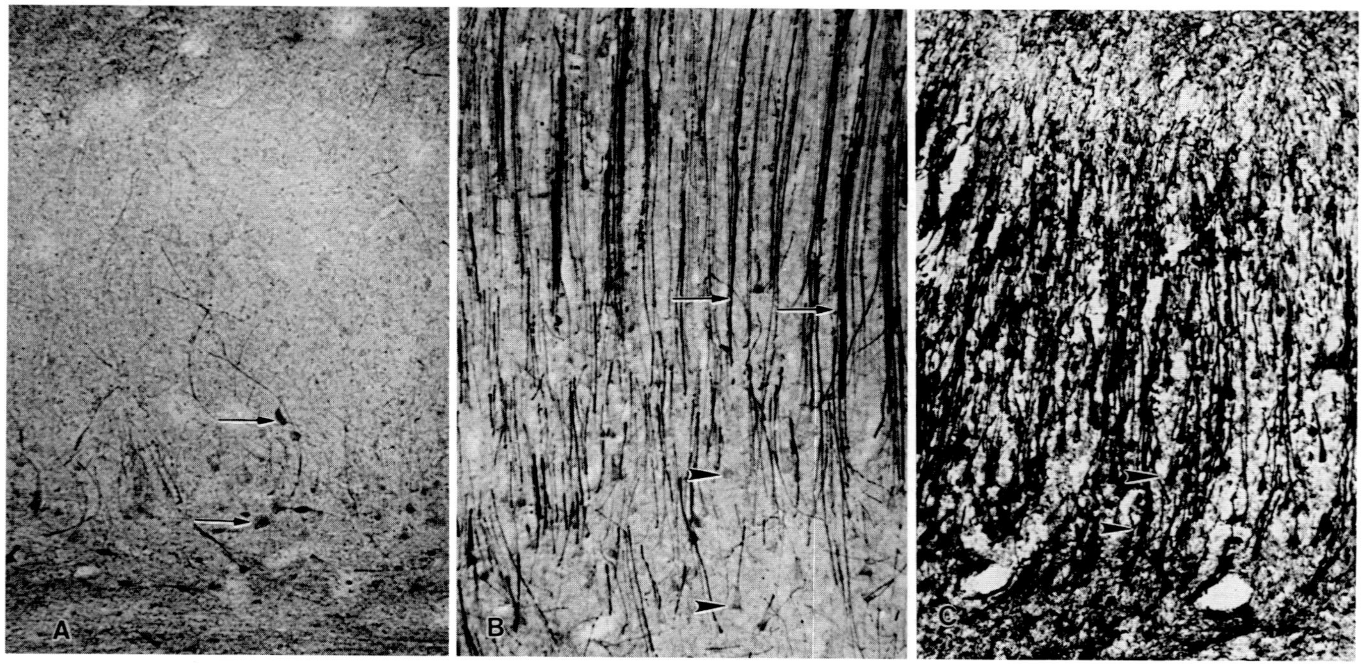

FIG. 4. (**A**) Acetylated tubulin immunoreactivity in normal CA1 is primarily located in proximal dendrites and cell bodies (*arrows*). (**B**) Tyrosylated tubulin is enriched in more distal apical dendrites (*arrows*) and is less prominent in cell bodies (*arrowheads*). (**C**) In Alzheimer disease, tyrosylated tubulin is prominent in cell bodies in CA1 (*arrowheads*) as well as dystrophic dendrites. Original magnification ×80.

NEURONAL SPECTRIN

In normal neurons, subtypes of the major submembranous cytoskeletal protein, spectrin, are differentially distributed in axons and dendrites, suggesting a possible role in the generation and maintenance of neuronal polarity. We examined the distribution of dendritic spectrin in normal and AD hippocampus using a polyclonal antibody that recognizes the dendritic isoform of spectrin (240/235E) to determine whether specific alterations of the somatodendritic compartment occur in AD (111). In normal human hippocampus, red blood cells were prominently stained. A discrete band of immunoreactivity defined the dentate gyrus granule cells and the inner molecular layer. Neurons were prominent in CA1 with occasional intensely reactive granulovacuolar degeneration (GVD). Rare astrocytes were immunoreactive. In AD, immunoreactivity in the dentate gyrus extended into the outer molecular layer, and a band of decreased immunoreactivity was seen in the polymorphic layer. Occasional intensely reactive neurons containing NFT or GVD were found in CA1 and the subiculum. Spectrin (240/235E) retained its normal somatodendritic localization in the dentate gyrus in AD, but its distribution shifted in conjunction with dendritic reorganization. The GVD contained prominent dendritic spectrin immunoreactivity. A small subset of NFT-bearing neurons was intensely immunoreactive, suggesting that the synthesis and/or proteolysis of dendritic spectrin may be altered in AD. In contrast to tau protein, axonal spectrin (235/240) is not shifted to dendrites. This suggests that disruption of neuronal polarity is not a generalized process in AD.

ABNORMAL PHOSPHORYLATION IN AD: KINASES AND PHOSPHATASES

Considerable evidence points to phosphorylation as a key posttranslational modification that profoundly affects protein function. The stability and interaction of the cytoskeletal components are in part determined by their state of phosphorylation (112), which in turn is regulated by specific kinases and phosphatases. Proteins are phosphorylated by two broad categories of kinases: tyrosine kinases and serine/threonine kinases. Tyrosine phosphorylation is implicated in the mediation of growth factor effects (113). Receptors for growth factors such as basic fibroblast growth factor, epidermal growth factor, and platelet-derived growth factor are single-pass transmembrane tyrosine-specific protein kinases with a cytoplasmic catalytic domain. The other major group of tyrosine kinases is associated with the submembranous cytoskeleton and includes the protooncogene products $pp60^{c\text{-}src}$ and $p120^{abl}$. A unique form of the *c-src* gene product, termed $pp60^{c\text{-}src(+)}$, is found in the brain, where it is enriched in growth cones (114). It is the most abundant tyrosine-specific kinase in purified synaptic vesicles, suggesting that it may play a role in signal transduction. We examined $pp60^{c\text{-}src}$ immunoreactivity with two different monoclonal antibodies and found that $pp60^{c\text{-}src}$ immunoreactivity is faintly present in some pyramidal neurons in the normal human hippocampus and cortex (115). In AD, there is intense immunoreactivity associated with neurites in senile plaques and occasional intensely stained neurons (Fig. 5). It is not known if $pp60^{c\text{-}src}$ substrates such as paxillin or the p22 are phosphorylated in AD.

The major serine threonine kinases include cAMP-activated kinase (A kinase), phospholipid-Ca-activated protein kinase (PKC), and calcium/calmodulin-dependent kinases (CaM kinase), which act as second messengers mediating the intracellular response to extracellular signals (116). Receptor–ligand interaction leads to calcium influx or activation of GTP-binding proteins, which in turn activate phospholipase C or adenylate cyclase. Activated kinases phosphorylate substrates including MAPs and neurofilament and transcription-regulating factors (117).

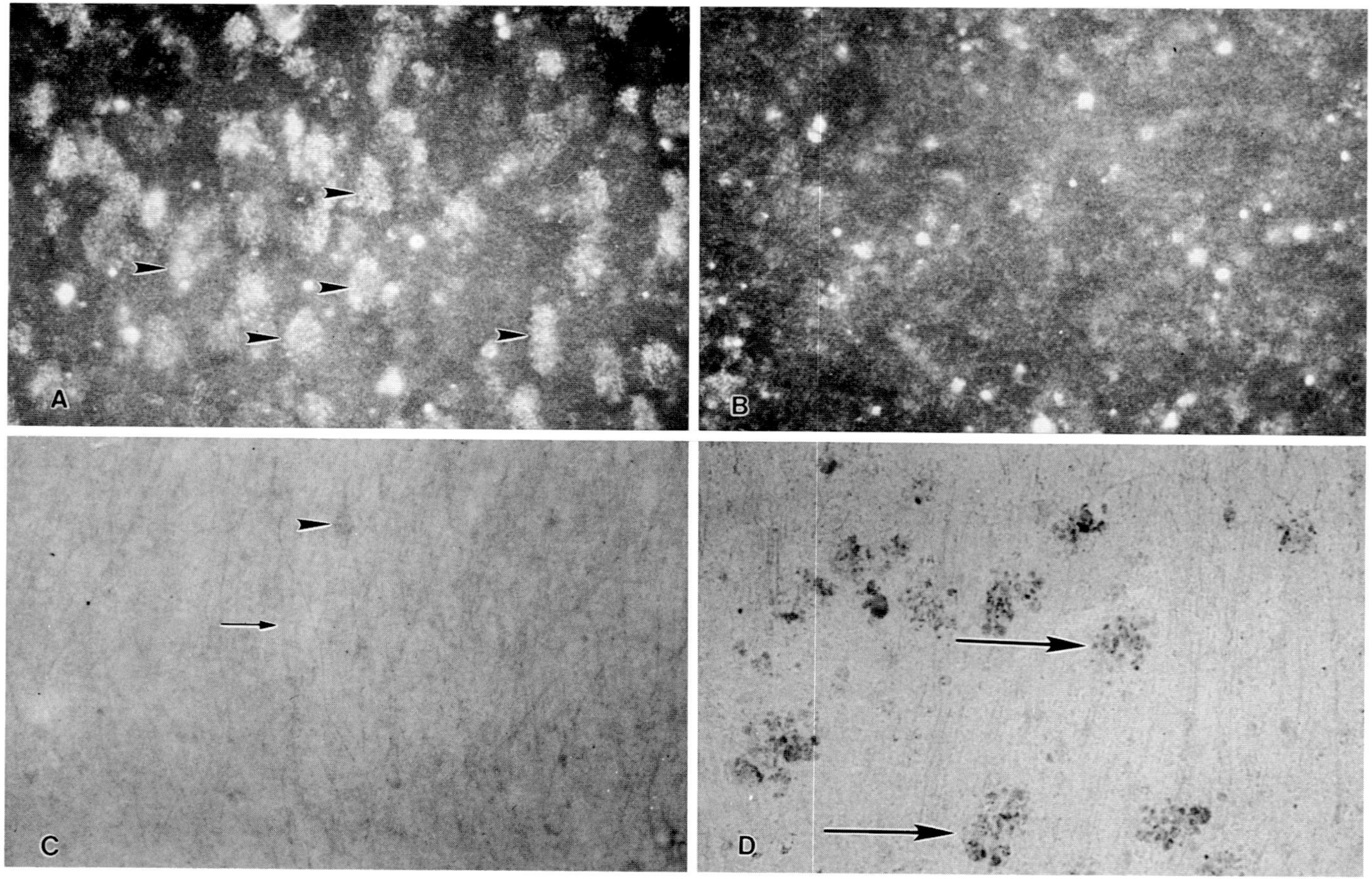

FIG. 5. (**A**) Calcineurin immunoreactivity in normal CA1 seen under darkfield illumination forms granular deposition in pyramidal neurons (*arrowheads*). (**B**) In Alzheimer disease, calcineurin immunoreactivity in CA1 neurons is depleted. (**C**) $pp60^{c\text{-}src}$ immunoreactivity in normal temporal isocortex weakly labels dendrites (*arrow*) and occasional pyramidal cell bodies (*arrowhead*) in layers 3 and 5. (**D**) In Alzheimer disease, globular dystrophic neurites (*arrows*) and occasional neurons are intensely $pp60^{c\text{-}src}$ immunoreactive in the cerebral cortex and subiculum. This result was seen with two different monoclonal antibodies.

Phosphate residues are removed by protein phosphatases (PP) active on either tyrosine or serine/threonine residues (118). There are three main categories of PPs. Neurons are especially enriched in PP2B or calcineurin, which dephosphorylates cytoskeletal proteins (119). Specific inhibitors of protein phosphatases, such as okadaic acid, increase the phosphorylation state of neurons in culture, leading to alterations in the neuronal cytoskeleton. Calcineurin has been localized to subsets of neurons in the human hippocampus and basal ganglia (120). We examined calcineurin immunoreactivity in normal and AD hippocampus and have preliminary data suggesting that calcineurin immunoreactivity may be depleted in AD, although quantitation will be required to verify this observation (Fig. 5). The dinoflagellate toxin okadaic acid is a potent and specific inhibitor of protein phosphatases 2A and 1 in cell-free extracts and cell culture systems. The effects of this toxin *in vivo* are discussed below.

Aberrant phosphorylation of the cytoskeleton may be critically involved in the generation of Alzheimer neurofibrillary lesions. Tau 1 immunoreactivity is dramatically increased in NFT after phosphatase pretreatment, suggesting that additional phosphate molecules alter or mask the tau 1 epitope in AD (121) (Fig. 1). Recently the antibody ALZ 50, which demonstrates early changes in AD, was shown to recognize abnormally phosphorylated tau protein (122). A direct assessment of the phosphorylation state of tau derived from tangle-rich AD tissue shows that tau is hyperphosphorylated (123). A group of hyperphosphorylated proteins derived from fractions of PHF that migrate more slowly than tau have distinct solubility properties. These modified tau proteins, which do not purify with brain microtubules, were initially termed A68 (124). Recently these proteins were definitively identified as tau by antibody cross-reactivity and direct protein sequencing (8,123,125). The phosphate content of these soluble fractions is approximately four times greater than normal tau. This modified tau protein, termed PHF-tau, can be recognized by specific antibodies (7). Rosenblum et al. (126) suggest that serine-396 is a critical site of altered phosphorylation in PHF-tau, but the massive increase in phosphorylation suggests that multiple sites may be involved. It is possible that excessively phosphorylated tau directly aggregates to form PHF. Tau hyperphosphorylation may inhibit its ability to bind microtubules, leading to destabilization of axonal microtubules.

The kinase that phosphorylates PHF tau has not been defined. Reports indicate that CaM kinase immunoreactivity is enriched in NFT-bearing neurons, whereas PKC and casein kinase II activity are reduced in AD (127–129). The CaM kinase type II, a candidate kinase that may phosphorylate tau in NFT (128), is enriched in neurons predisposed to NFT formation in the hippocampus and cerebral cortex. In AD, degenerating neurons with NFT are often intensely CaM kinase immunoreactive. PKCβII immunoreactivity is associated with diffuse amyloid deposits in AD, where it may play a role in the generation of β-amyloid from its precursor (130). The possible contribution of decreased phosphatase activity to increased tau phosphorylation is unknown, but our preliminary observations showing decreased calcineurin immunoreactivity in AD are provocative. Increased kinase activity or decreased phosphatase activity could induce much of the cytoskeletal reorganization found in the AD brain. The dissociation of phosphorylated MAPs from microtubules could lead to their destabilization, and concomitant neurofilament phosphorylation in dendrites could contribute to loss of dendritic identity.

Excess phosphorylation could alter proteolytic processing of APP in AD. A consensus sequence for PKC in APP may, by analogy to other membrane phosphoproteins such as epidermal growth factor receptor, regulate APP internalization and degradation (131). The presence of APP immunoreactivity in lysosomes and lipofuscin in AD suggests that APP may be internalized in human brain

(132,133). Inhibition of phosphatases by okadaic acid in cell culture yields large carboxy-terminal fragments of APP that may contain the entire β-amyloid sequence intact (131). Aberrant phosphorylation of APP may, therefore, lead to altered proteolysis and to the formation of free β-amyloid or a toxic fragment thereof.

Increased phosphorylation of cytoskeletal proteins is produced by experimental axotomy. Transection of the rat fimbria–fornix leads to microtubule dissolution and the appearance of phosphorylated neurofilament immunoreactivity in the somatodendritic compartment (134). In the lamprey, close axotomy results in a similar phenomenon. Ectopic axon-like sprouts grow from dendritic tips, and dendrites are transformated into axon-like structures containing densely packed neurofilaments and presynaptic elements (135). Superior cervical ganglion deafferentation in the rat causes increased PKCβ-like immunoreactivity (136). It is not known specifically if phosphorylation of tau protein is altered by axotomy.

GROWTH FACTORS IN AD

It is unclear if the neuritic sprouting and remodeling that come about in the face of ongoing neuronal degeneration are beneficial or deleterious to cognitive function. This issue is especially important, given the potential therapeutic value of neurotrophic factors. It is possible that enhancing the proliferative response may further exhaust stressed neuronal populations and precipitate cell death. Chaotic reconnections may contribute to the pathogenesis of cognitive dysfunction. Alternatively, plasticity may reestablish effective synaptic connectivity and help maintain mental function. A specific growth factor deficiency, however, has not been demonstrated to date in AD.

Nerve Growth Factor

Atrophy and depletion of NGF-dependent cholinergic basal forebrain neurons that project to the cerebral cortex cause the profound decrease in cortical acetylcholine characteristic of AD (137). In animal models, axotomy induces involution of cholinergic septal neurons that is prevented or reversed by NGF (138). If a similar process occurs in AD, or if there is decreased synthesis of NGF in the cortical targets of the basal forebrain, NGF may rescue and prevent degeneration of cholinergic neurons. We studied the distribution of NGF in postmortem samples of human brain using a polyclonal NGF antibody and two monoclonal antibodies raised against human recombinant NGF (139). Immunocytochemical analysis showed that pyramidal neurons in the neocortex and hippocampus contain NGF immunoreactivity in normal controls. In AD, despite neuronal depletion, NGF immunoreactivity is prominent in both neurons and cortical neuropil and is associated with SP. Our results show that NGF immunoreactivity is not depleted out of proportion to neuronal loss in AD cerebral cortex. Basal forebrain neurons may degenerate despite preserved cortical NGF because of impaired retrograde axonal transport. It remains to be shown whether damaged NFT-bearing magnocellular basal forebrain neurons are able to regenerate in response to exogenously administered NGF. Even if NGF treatment prevents neuronal involution, it may not necessarily lead to the reestablishment of competent cholinergic innervation of the cerebral cortex.

Basic Fibroblastic Growth Factor

The factors responsible for altered microtubular organization and growth response in AD have not been defined. One candidate is bFGF, an agent known to stimulate neuritic sprouting in hippocampal cell culture that binds to a specific receptor–tyrosine kinase (140). The powerful neurite-promoting activity of bFGF is underscored by its 200-fold greater potency than NGF on PC12 cells (141). Like NGF, bFGF prevents death of cholinergic neurons after axotomy (142).

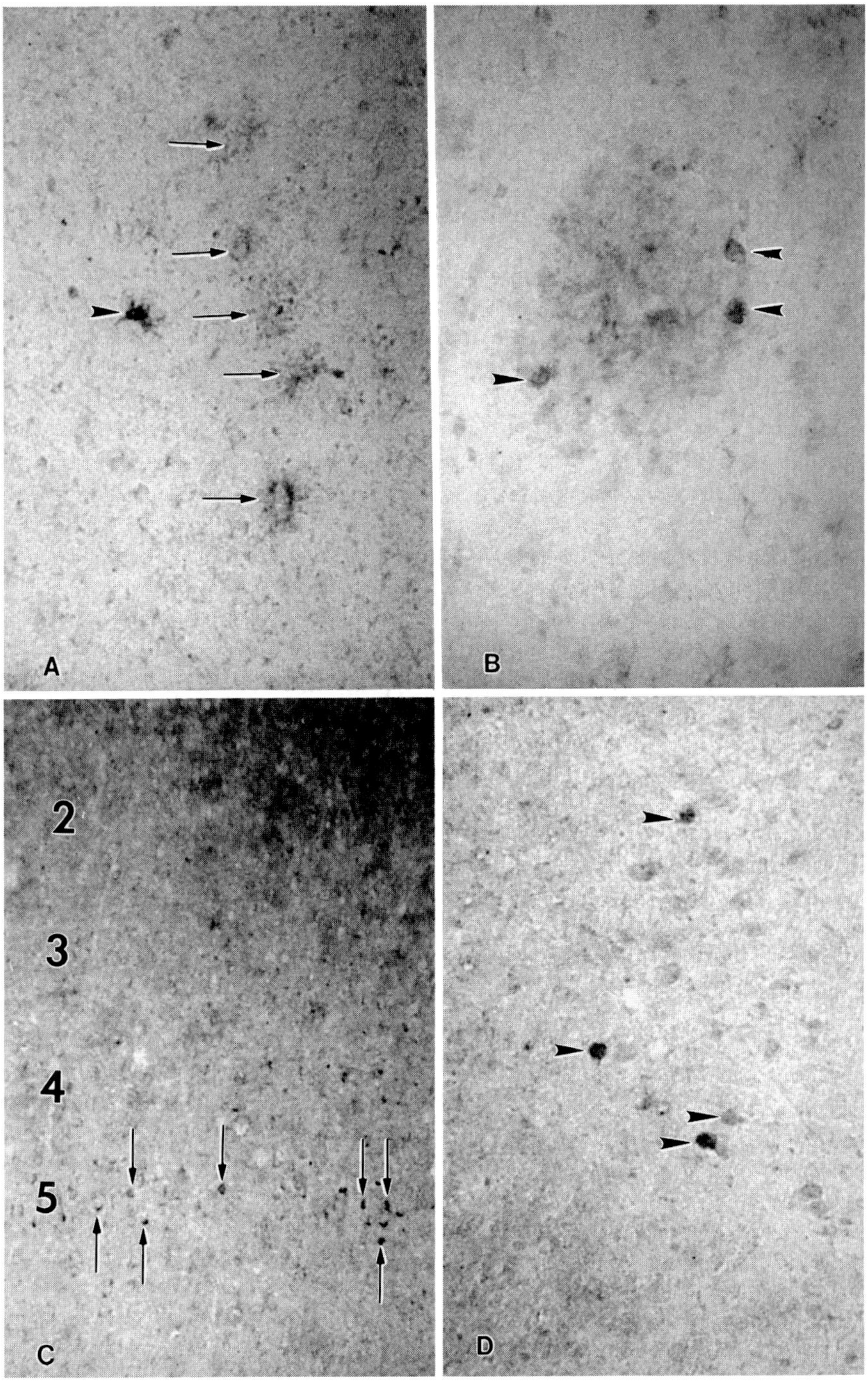

FIG. 6. (**A**) Transforming growth factor β immunoreactivity is present in astrocytes (*arrowhead*) and in microglia and astrocytic processes in senile plaques (*arrows*) in Alzheimer disease brain. (**B**) A higher power view of microglial cells (*arrowheads*) and processes in senile plaques. (**C**) *Fos* immunoreactivity in the temporal isocortex in Alzheimer disease is present in neuronal nuclei, forming a distinct band in layer 5 (*arrows*). (**D**) *Egr-1* immunoreactivity was present in clusters of layer 2 entorhinal stellate neurons (*arrowheads*).

We examined AD and control human hippocampus using several polyclonal affinity-purified antibodies raised against peptide fragments of bFGF and recombinant bFGF (142a) (Fig. 3). These antisera recognize bFGF on Western blots of brain homogenates. Elution of the antisera over a column of bFGF bound to sepharose beads greatly reduces specific staining in tissue sections. Incubation of sections in antiserum preabsorbed with bFGF results in NFT staining from binding of bFGF to heparan sulfate residues in the tissue (143). Throughout normal human hippocampus, bFGF immunoreactivity is present in neurons and rare astrocytes. In AD, neuronal density is reduced in CA1, but occasional neurons and astrocytes are intensely bFGF immunoreactive. Increased tissue bFGF may contribute to neuritic plasticity in AD.

Transforming Growth Factor β

Transforming growth factor β is a family of related peptides (TGFβ1, -1.2, -2) with complex effects on cellular growth and differentiation. *In vitro* studies suggest that TGFβ stimulates mesenchymal cells and inhibits epithelial cells. *In vivo* it generally acts as a potent growth inhibitor yet functions to enhance connective tissue formation and wound healing (143a). TGFβ2 mRNA is present in mouse brain (143b). We examined a small series of AD and control brains with a well-characterized polyclonal antibody that recognizes TGFβ1 and TGFβ2 (R&D systems, Minneapolis, MN) (Fig. 6). TGFβ was not detected in normal brain but was seen in nonneuronal cells that morphologically resemble microglia and in cell processes in the vicinity of SP. Control sections incubated in preimmune serum were not immunoreactive. Examination of nondemented patients with amyloid deposits will be necessary to determine if TGFβ plays an early and specific role in the development of SP or neuronal degeneration in AD.

IMMEDIATE EARLY GENE PRODUCTS IN POSTMORTEM AD BRAIN

Immunoreactivity for the immediate early gene products Fos and Egr-1 protein was detected in postmortem human brain (Fig. 6). Unfortunately, preterminal illness may nonspecifically activate immediate early gene transcription, so immunocytochemical studies of postmortem human brain tissue must be interpreted cautiously. Nevertheless, Fos protein was localized in neuronal nuclei in layer V of temporal cortex in postmortem tissue specimens from AD patients. There was no clear relationship to either SP or NFT. Similarly, the Egr-1 protein (also called the *zif/268* gene product) was localized in the nuclei of layer II stellate neurons in the entorhinal cortex (Fig. 6). No specific pattern correlating with classical neuropathological changes was seen.

MEMBRANE GLYCOPROTEINS AND PLASTICITY IN AD

As mentioned earlier, there is substantial evidence that axonal and dendritic processes are elaborated by viable neurons to fill vacated synaptic sites in response to neuronal degeneration in AD (111,144). The array of tau-positive dystrophic neurites typical of AD (11,12) has been described as "massive dendritic sprouts" that may represent proliferation without typical growth cone formation (145). It is not clear whether these abnormal neurites represent a degenerative or proliferative response within axons or dendrites (144–146). Axonal growth cones are enriched in specific proteins including the growth protein GAP 43, neural cell adhesion molecule (NCAM), and $pp60^{c\text{-}src}$ (147–149). If neurites are proliferating, they may show evidence of growth-cone-related membrane proteins. Abnormal neurites identified with tau antibodies do not contain GAP 43 immunoreactivity (unpublished observations).

Neural Cell Adhesion Molecule

We studied the distribution of NCAM, an integral cell surface glycoprotein found on neurons, glia, and myocytes, in postmortem human hippocampus (150). In cells expressing it on their surface, NCAM is directly involved in the formation of intercellular bonding (for review see 151). The NCAM immunoreactivity is concentrated in axonal growth cone structures of cultured rat hypothalamic and mesencephalic cells and is highly concentrated in growth cone filopodia (148). In AD, neuronal loss and NFT formation in layer II entorhinal stellate cells lead to deafferentation of dentate granule cells. Cholinergic septohippocampal projections proliferate into the outer part of the molecular layer of the dentate gyrus normally occupied by the entorhinal projections. We looked for evidence of plasticity and axonal sprouting in the dentate gyrus in AD using NCAM expression as a marker for axonal growth cone formation (150). In normal dentate gyrus, diffuse terminal-like NCAM immunoreactivity forms a band in the inner third of the dentate molecular layer. In AD, the fraction of the molecular layer containing NCAM immunoreactivity is increased, and abundant fine filiform structures are found in the outer molecular layer. Our findings suggest that neuronal degeneration in the aged brain is associated with axonal proliferation and increased expression of growth-related proteins normally present during neurite outgrowth in the developing brain.

Thy-1

The membrane glycoprotein Thy-1, a member of the immunoglobulin superfamily, is present in high concentrations in the brain. Growing dendrites in rat Purkinje cells are intensely Thy-1 immunoreactive, and antibodies against Thy-1 enhance neuritic regeneration in cell culture. Because of these properties, we examined the distribution of Thy-1 immunoreactivity in normal elderly and AD hippocampus using a well-characterized monoclonal antibody (152). In normal elderly hippocampus, Thy-1 was primarily located in irregular patches on the perikarya and dendrites of pyramidal neurons and their axons. Dentate granule cells were lightly stained. A blush of granular immunoreactivity often surrounded small blood vessels in gray and white matter. In AD brain, immunoreactivity within pyramidal neurons was often collected at the base of the apical dendrite and within the cytoplasm of NFT-bearing neurons. Dendritic spines and filopodial outgrowths were occasionally labeled with Thy-1, but dystrophic neuropil neurites were not identified. Occasional reactive neurites were seen in SP, and a blush of Thy-1 immunoreactivity often surrounded SP amyloid cores. The persistent labeling of neuronal perikarya and blood vessels in the human hippocampus is similar to the transient labeling of developing Purkinje cells and blood vessels in the newborn rat. The enhanced pattern of Thy-1 staining suggests that active dendritic remodeling persists in AD.

Laminin

Laminin, a major glycoprotein component of the basal lamina, is a potent promoter of neurite outgrowth and the principal factor produced by cells promoting neurite extension in culture. It allows NGF-dependent cell lines to survive temporarily without NGF and plays a role in regeneration following injury. Laminin was initially thought to be confined to the basement membranes of blood vessels in the central nervous system (CNS). Subsequent studies showed laminin immunoreactivity in nonneuronal cells in the CNS (153). Recently, laminin mRNA has been localized to neurons in rodent brain, and laminin-immunoreactive neurons have been found in several forebrain structures of the human brain, including the hippocampus (154). We used two monoclonal antilaminin antibodies to study the distribution of laminin immunoreactivity in normal elderly and AD brain (155). One antibody (MAB 1975, Chemicon) was raised against murine laminin and recognizes a conformational epitope on the B1 and B2 heterodimer and P1 fragment of laminin. This antibody does not inhibit laminin-mediated adhesion. The second antibody (LAM-1, ICN) stains basement membranes and smooth muscle in a wide variety of organs in both mouse and human. MAB 1975 stained the basement membrane surrounding blood vessels in both control and AD hippocampus. No cellular or other localized immunoreactivity was visible. Perivascular staining with LAM-1 was present, although weaker, in all cases. In control brains, scattered pyramidal neurons and occasional astrocytes were weakly immunoreactive with LAM-1. In AD, neuronal perikarya were more frequently immunopositive in the CA fields and subiculum. Astrocytes were occasionally seen. Senile plaque cores were often laminin immunoreactive. Increased expression of laminin or laminin-like peptides in AD may play a primary role in neuritic proliferation in the neuropil and around senile plaques. Alternatively, laminin synthesis may be increased in response to neuronal injury and degeneration in AD.

MECHANISMS OF NEURONAL DEGENERATION: ANIMAL MODELS

Cytoskeletal Changes Induced by Aluminum

Intraventricular injections of aluminum cause pyramidal projection neurons in the cerebral cortex of rabbits to accumulate phosphorylated neurofilament immunoreactivity and develop neurofibrillary degeneration. Tau protein and MAP 2 immunoreactivity are not present, in contrast with human NFT (156). NADPH diaphorase and somatostatin neurons do not accumulate neurofilament and are spared. The population of cerebral cortical projection neurons that develop NFT in human AD, therefore, are also selectively affected by cytoskeletal disorganization in the cortex of aluminum-treated rabbits. This animal model does not completely reproduce the histological or neurochemical features of AD; rather, it suggests that projection neurons are uniquely prone to cytoskeletal disruption from disparate causes.

Okadaic Acid Neurotoxicity and Cytoskeletal Phosphorylation

The dinoflagellate toxin okadaic acid is a potent and specific inhibitor of protein phosphatases in cell-free extracts and cell culture systems. We stereotactically injected two doses (100 ng and 10 ng) of okadaic acid into the rat hippocampal formation to define its effects on cytoskeletal protein phosphorylation and neuronal viability *in vivo* (157). Dose-dependent lesions consisting of focal neuronal loss and gliosis were seen surrounding injections in tissue sections examined after 1 week's survival time (Fig. 7).

In normal rat hippocampus and cortex, nonphosphorylated neurofilament (SMI 32) immunoreactivity is confined to neuronal perikarya, in contrast to phosphorylated neurofilament (SMI 31) and tau immunoreactivity, which are located in axons. SMI 32-positive neurons were distorted and depleted around the okadaic acid injections, and occasional cell bodies, dendrites, and distorted cell processes were SMI 31 immunoreactive. The distribution and phosphorylation state of tau protein were examined using tau 1, tau 2, and ALZ 50 monoclonal antibodies. Okadaic acid lesions depleted tau 1 immunoreactivity surrounding the lesion, but ALZ 50 and tau 2 immunoreactivity were increased in the neuropil and in neuronal perikarya. Alkaline phosphatase pretreatment attenuated the decrease in tau 1 immunoreactivity surrounding the lesion.

In AD, the tau 1 epitope is similarly masked by phosphorylation, and ALZ 50, which specifically labels both normal and abnormally phosphorylated tau, is greatly increased in neuronal cell bodies and dendrites. These observations suggest that okadaic acid

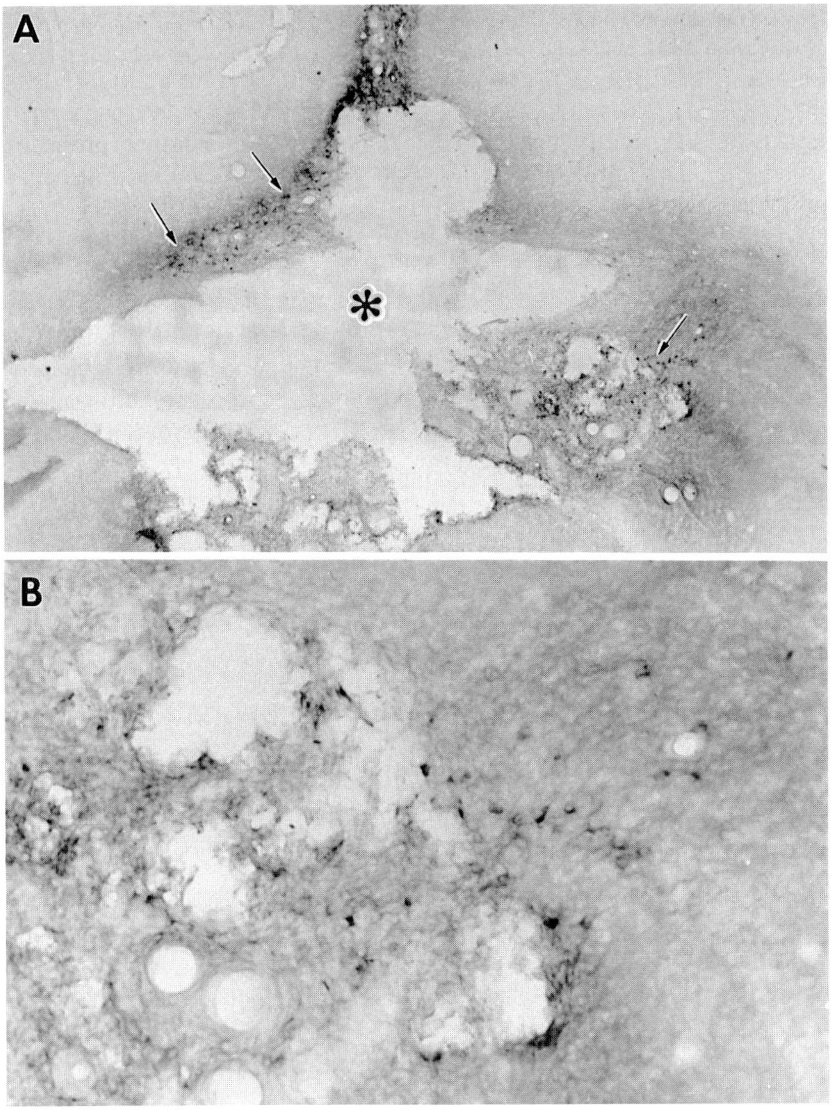

FIG. 7. (**A**) High-dose (100 ng) okadaic acid produces localized necrosis in the rat hippocampus. Custers of ALZ 50-immunoreactive cells (*arrows*) are visible surrounding the injection site (*asterisk*). (**B**) Higher-power view showing ALZ 50-positive cells adjacent to the okadaic acid injection. Perikaryal immunoreactivity is evident, but no neurofibrillary changes are seen.

neurotoxicity *in vivo* disrupts neuronal polarity and produces a pattern of excessive cytoskeletal phosphorylation resembling that found in AD.

β-Amyloid Neurotoxicity *In Vivo*

Solubilized synthetic β-amyloid protein induces degeneration of hippocampal neurons in culture (158). To determine if neurons are differentially sensitive to degeneration *in vivo,* we studied the effects of β-amyloid protein injected into the cortex, hippocampus, striatum, basal forebrain, and cerebellum of the rat (159). To assess the extent of neuronal degeneration and establish if cytoskeletal changes resembling those found in Alzheimer's disease occur, we stained sets of se-

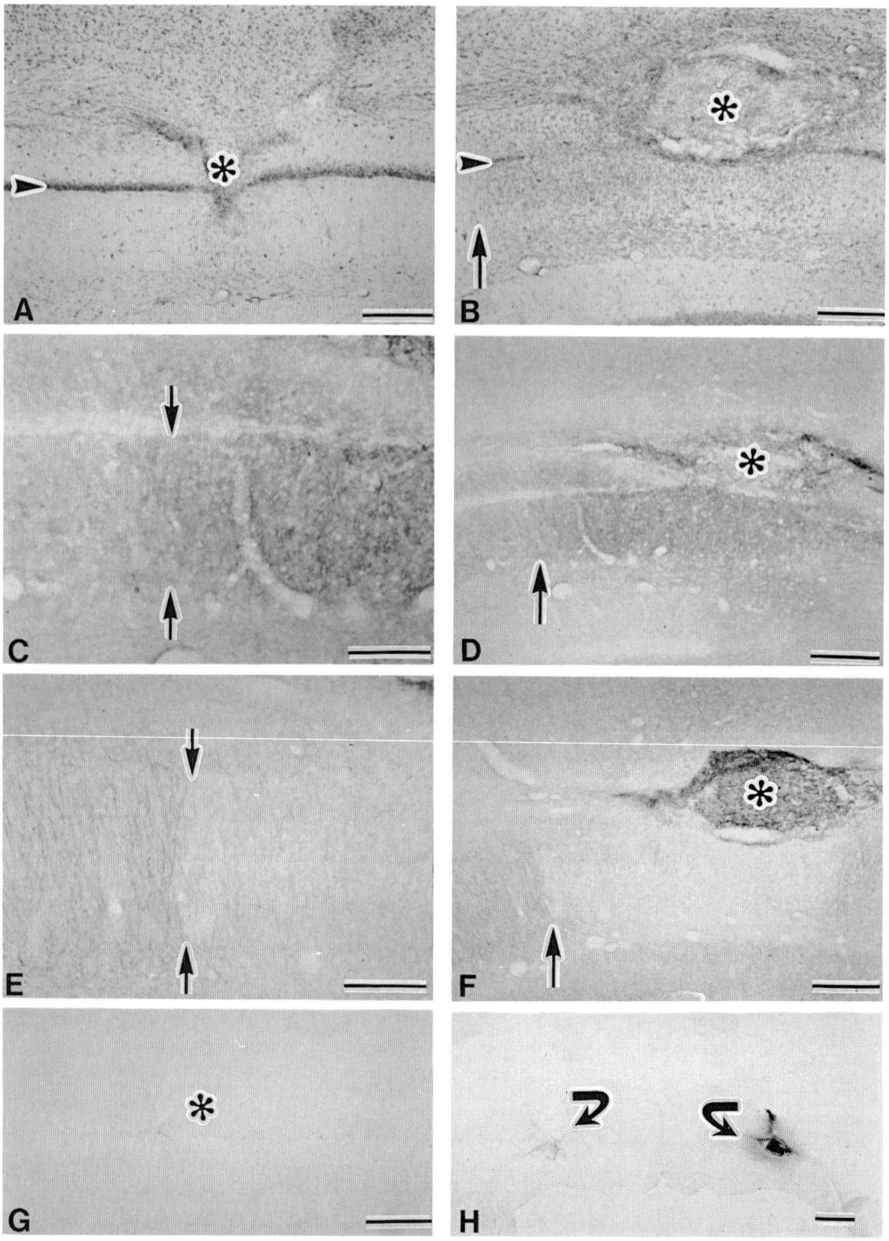

FIG. 8. Patterns of neuronal degeneration produced by high-dose β(1–40) and control peptide (A37) injected into left and right hemispheres, respectively, after 2-week survival. Injection sites are in deep cerebral cortex and the CA1 field of the hippocampus (*asterisks*), and the lateral border of the lesion in CA1 induced by β(1–40) is shown with an *arrow* in **B–F.** (**A**) A37 induces minimal local gliosis and disruption of the CA1 pyramidal cell layer (*arrowhead*). Cresyl violet stain; *bar,* 200 μm. (**B**) The contralateral injection produces a much greater loss of CA1 neurons (*arrowhead*) and gliosis extending into stratum radiatum and lacunosum moleculare. *Bar,* 200 μm. (**C,D**) Pattern of tau 1 immunoreactivity associated with β(1–40). Region of enhanced tau immunoreactivity corresponds to the area of neuronal degeneration seen in **B.** Higher-power view (**C**) shows increased neuropil tau immunoreactivity. *Bar* in **C,** 100 μm; in **D,** 200 μm. (**E,F**) Pattern of MAP 2 immunoreactivity surrounding β(1–40) injection. MAP 2 immunoreactivity is depleted in a pattern complementary to the increased local tau immunoreactivity. *Bar* in **E,** 100 μm; in **D,** 200 μm. (**G**) Tau immunoreactivity is minimal surrounding the contralateral injection of the control peptide (A37). Tau 2 immunocytochemistry. *Bar,* 200 μm. (**H**) Tau 2 immunoreactivity produced by injections of high-dose β(1–40) can be seen grossly, whereas A37 induces minimal changes in the contralateral hemisphere (*curved arrows* indicate injections). *Bar,* 1 mm.

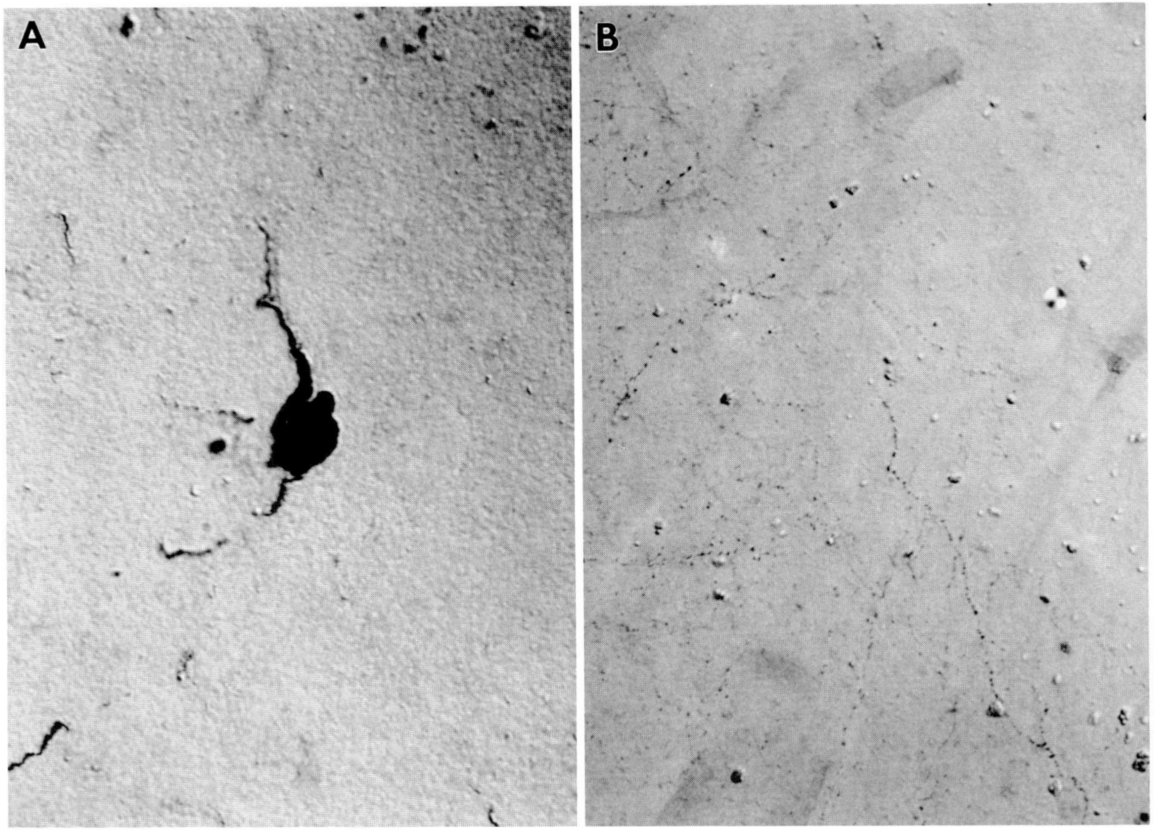

FIG. 9. (**A**) High-power view of an ALZ 50 positive neuron and abnormal thread-like neurites in the vicinity of a β(1–40) injection in cynomolgus monkey cerebral cortex. The morphology of the ALZ 50-positive inclusion bears a striking resemblance to the neurofibrillary tangles (NFT) typically found in Alzheimer disease. ALZ 50-immunoreactive neuronal perikarya are prominent around the β(1–40) injection in monkey cerebral cortex. These are not seen in the vicinity of control injections of reverse peptide solubilized in the same vehicle. Injections in the rat produce diffusely ALZ 50-immunoreactive neurons that do not closely resemble NFT. (**B**) ALZ 50 immunoreactive perikarya are not seen around the reverse peptide β(40–1) injection site in cynomolgus monkey cerebral cortex. Scattered fine beaded axon-like processes are normally seen in primate cerebral cortex.

rial sections through the injected regions with cresyl violet, four monoclonal tau antibodies (tau 1 and tau 2, courtesy of Dr. L. I. Binder; 5E2, courtesy of Dr. K. S. Kosik; and ALZ 50, courtesy of Dr. P. Davies), and a monoclonal MAP 2 antibody (5F9, courtesy of Dr. K. S. Kosik) (Fig. 8). Neuronal degeneration was prominent in the hippocampus, cerebral cortex, and basal forebrain. The striatum and cerebellum were minimally affected. Surrounding the injections in the cerebral cortex, hippocampus, and basal forebrain, MAP

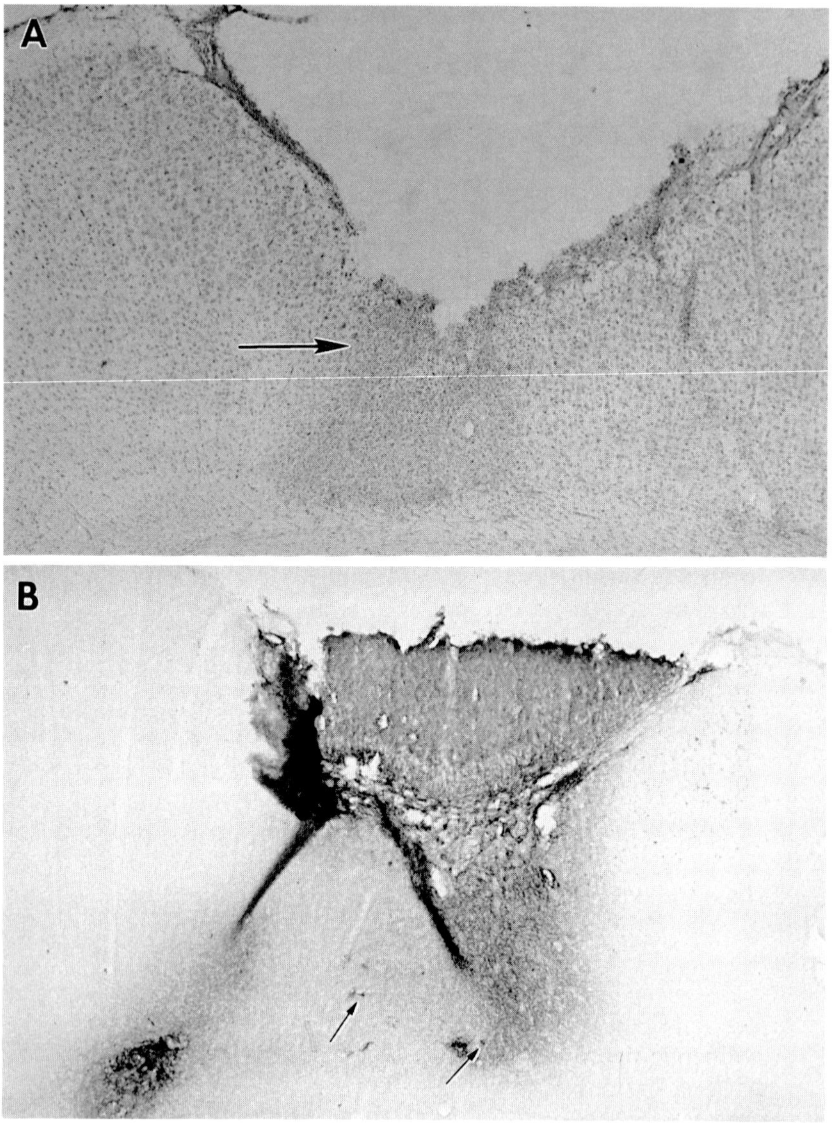

FIG. 10. (**A**) Injections of β(25–35) (synthesized by Bachem, Inc) dissolved as a trifluoroacetate salt in water produce lesions similar to β(1–40) solubilized in acetonitrile. Shown is a cresyl-violet-stained section of the cerebral cortex of a rat sacrificed 7 days after receiving an injection of 3 nmol β(25–35). A focal area of necrosis and neuronal loss was produced (*arrow*). (**B**) Tau immunoreactivity is also increased by β(25–35) injections in rat cerebral cortex. Neuropil immunoreactivity is focally increased and neurons with immunoreactive perikarya are occasionally seen (*arrows*).

2 immunoreactivity was depleted, but tau immunoreactivity was increased in neurites and occasional perikarya. Quantitation of the area of tau immunoreactivity and photodensitometry showed a significant region-specific gradient of tau induction: hippocampus $\geq$ cerebral cortex $\geq$ nucleus basalis $\gg$ striatum = cerebellum. Our results show that neurons are differentially sensitive to β-amyloid protein toxicity *in vivo* and that degenerating neurons develop cytoskeletal changes resembling those seen in AD.

We recently reported that β-amyloid is neurotoxic in the primate (160) (Fig. 9). Injections of solubilized β-amyloid in elderly female cynomolgus monkeys produced dose-dependent cortical lesions and striking NFT-like abnormalities very similar to those found in AD. These NFT were identified with silver stains, thioflavine S fluorescence, and antisera that specifically recognize abnormally phosphorylated tau protein. This effect was not seen in young monkeys (160,161), suggesting that toxicity may be age dependent.

The β(25–35) peptide fragment of β(1–40) dissolved in an aqueous vehicle is also neurotoxic *in vivo* in the rat (162; Lee et al., personal communication) (Fig. 10). This peptide shows sequence homology to the tachykinin family of neuropeptides (163), and substance P antagonists reproduce the neurotoxic effects of β-amyloid in culture (158). Furthermore, substance P can ameliorate β-amyloid toxicity in a dose-dependent manner *in vivo* (164).

If β-amyloid neurotoxicity in AD is mediated by antagonism of substance P effects, the distribution of neuronal degeneration in AD should match the distribution of substance P receptors. Substance P receptors are expressed in cholinergic neurons in the rat and human striatum and basal forebrain (165; Lu et al., personal communication). Substance P neurons, which are normally prominent in human cortex, are depleted in AD (39). The tachykinins have been shown to have neurotrophic and neurotoxic effects (166–169). Substance P expression is stimulated by inflammation, and substance P-positive astrocytes are present in multiple sclerosis lesions (170,171). Peripherally administered substance P has behavioral effects and can cross the blood–brain barrier and modulate central dopamine concentrations (172). These findings are consistent with the observation that systemic administration of substance P can reduce β-amyloid toxicity (159). Even if substance P does not traverse the normal blood–brain barrier, it may gain access to the lesion via a breach in the barrier produced by injection of the β-amyloid.

Recent evidence suggests that β-amyloid does not bind to substance P receptors or inhibit substance P receptor activation (173,174). Joslin et al. recently showed that β-amyloid and substance P both bind to the serpin–enzyme complex (SEC) receptor (175). Although the distribution of the SEC receptor is not known in the nervous system, it has been identified on PC 12 cells (175). The SEC receptor mediates internalization and lysosomal degradation of serine proteases complexed to their inhibitors (serpins) and regulates synthesis of serpins (174). The serpin α_1-antichymotrypsin accumulates as an early and universal component of senile plaques (176). β-Amyloid may therefore block neuronal SEC receptors, leading to altered lysosomal function, cytoskeletal disorganization, and neuronal degeneration in AD. Further investigation into the role of the SEC receptor and proteases may further clarify the mechanisms of neuronal degeneration and plasticity in AD.

ACKNOWLEDGMENTS

We would like to thank Karen Harrington, Alida Evans, Andrew Singer, and Laurence Cherkas for technical assistance. Supported by NIH grants AG 05134 and NS 25588.

REFERENCES

1. Alzheimer A. Über eine eigenartige Erkrankung der Hirnrinde. *Allg Z Psychiat* 1907;64:146–148.

2. Kemper T. *Neuroanatomical and neuropathological changes in normal aging and in dementia.* London: Oxford University Press; 1984.
3. Katzman R. Alzheimer's disease. *N Engl J Med* 1986;314:964–973.
4. Terry RD. The fine structure of neurofibrillary tangles in Alzheimer's disease. *J Neuropathol Exp Neurol* 1963;22:629–642.
5. Kidd M. Alzheimer's disease. An electron microscopical study. *Brain* 1964;87:307–320.
6. Goedert M, Spillantini MG, Potier MC, Ulrich J, Crowther RA. Cloning and sequencing of the cDNA encoding an isoform of microtubule-associated protein tau containing four tandem repeats: differential expression of tau protein mRNAs in human brain. *EMBO J* 1989;8:393–399.
7. Greenberg SG, Davies P. A preparation of Alzheimer paired helical filaments that displays distinct tau proteins by polyacrylamide gel electrophoresis. *Proc Natl Acad Sci USA* 1990;87:5827–5831.
8. Lee VM-Y, Balin BJ, Otvos LJ, Trojanowski JQ. A68: a major subunit of paired helical filaments and derivatized forms of normal tau. *Science* 1991;251:675–678.
9. Tabaton M, Whitehouse PJ, Perry G, Davies P, Autilio GL, Gambetti P. Alz 50 recognizes abnormal filaments in Alzheimer's disease and progressive supranuclear palsy. *Ann Neurol* 1988;24: 407–413.
10. Tabaton M, Mandybur TI, Perry G, Onorato M, Autilio-Gambetti L, Gambetti P. The widespread alteration of neurites in Alzheimer's disease may be unrelated to amyloid deposition. *Ann Neurol* 1989;26:771–778.
11. Braak H, Braak E, Grundke-Iqbal I, Iqbal K. Occurrence of neuropil threads in the senile brain and in Alzheimer's disease. A third location of paired helical filaments outside of neurofibrillary tangles and neuritic plaques. *Neurosci Lett* 1986;65:351–355.
12. Kowall NW, Kosik KS. Axonal disruption and aberrant localization of tau protein characterize the neuropil pathology of Alzheimer's disease. *Ann Neurol* 1987;22:639–643.
13. Delacourte A, Flament S, Dibe EM, et al. Pathological proteins tau 64 and 69 are specifically expressed in the somatodendritic domain of the degenerating cortical neurons during Alzheimer's disease. Demonstration with a panel of antibodies against tau proteins. *Acta Neuropathol* 1990;80:111–117.
14. McKee AC, Kosik KS, Kowall NW. Neuritic pathology and dementia in Alzheimer's disease. *Ann Neurol* 1991;30:156–165.
15. Glenner G, Wong C. Alzheimer's disease: initial report of the purification and characterization of a novel cerebrovascular amyloid protein. *Biochem Biophys Res Commun* 1984;122:885–890.
16. Masters C, Simms G, Weinman N, Multhaup G, McDonald B, Beyreuther K. Amyloid plaque core protein in Alzheimer's disease and Down's syndrome. *Proc Natl Acad Sci USA* 1985;82: 4245–4249.
17. Ikeda S, Allsop D, Glenner GG. A study of the morphology and distribution of amyloid beta protein immunoreactive plaque and related lesions in the brains of Alzheimer's disease and adult Down's syndrome. *Prog Clin Biol Res* 1989;317:313–323.
18. Miyakawa T, Shimoji A, Kuramoto R, Higuchi Y. The relationship between senile plaques and cerebral blood vessels in Alzheimer's disease and senile dementia. Morphological mechanism of senile plaque production. *Virchows Arch B* 1982;40: 121–129.
19. Shoji M, Hirai S, Yamaguchi H, Harigaya Y, Kawarabayashi T. Amyloid beta-protein precursor accumulates in dystrophic neurites of senile plaques in Alzheimer-type dementia. *Brain Res* 1990;512:164–168.
20. Yamaguchi H, Hirai S, Morimatsu M, Shoji M, Harigaya Y. Diffuse type of senile plaques in the brains of Alzheimer-type dementia. *Acta Neuropathol* 1988;77:113–119.
21. Selkoe DJ, Podlisny MB, Joachim CL, et al. β-Amyloid precursor protein of Alzheimer disease occurs as 110- to 135-kilodalton membrane-associated proteins in neural and nonneural tissues. *Proc Natl Acad Sci USA* 1988;85:7341–7345.
22. Higgins GA, Oyler GA, Neve RL, Chen KS, Gage FH. Altered levels of amyloid protein precursor transcripts in the basal forebrain of behaviorally impaired aged rats. *Proc Natl Acad Sci USA* 1990;87:3032–3036.
23. Tanzi RE, Gusella JF, Watkins PC, et al. Amyloid beta-protein gene: cDNA, mRNA distribution, and genetic linkage near Alzheimer locus. *Science* 1987;235:880–884.
24. Kitaguchi N, Takahashi Y, Tokushima Y, Shiojiri S, Ito H. Novel precursor of Alzheimer's disease amyloid protein shows protease activity. *Nature* 1988;331:530–532.
25. De Sauvage F, Octave JN. A novel mRNA of the A4 amyloid precursor gene coding for a possibly secreted protein. *Science* 1989;245:651–653.
26. Selkoe DJ. Review: The molecular pathology of Alzheimer's disease. *Neuron* 1991;6:487–498.
27. Yankner BA, Mesulam M-M. Seminars in medicine of the Beth Israel Hospital: Beta amyloid and the pathogenesis of Alzheimer's disease. *N Engl J Med* 1991;325:1849–1857.
28. Kaelin WGJ, Ewen ME, Livingston DM. Tumor suppressor genes: the p53 and retinoblastoma sensitivity genes and gene products. *Biochim Biophys Acta* 1990;1032:119–136.
29. Koh J-Y, Yang LL, Cotman CW. β-Amyloid protein increases the vulnerability of cultured cortical neurons to excitotoxic damage. *Brain Res* 1990;533:315–320.
30. Roher AE, Ball MJ, Bhave SV, Wakade AR. Beta amyloid from Alzheimer's disease brains inhibits sprouting and survival of sympathetic neurons. *Biochem Biophys Res Commun* 1991;174:572–579.
31. Chartier-Harlin M-C, Crawford F, Houlden H, et al. Early-onset Alzheimer's disease caused by mutations at codon 717 of the β-amyloid precursor protein gene. *Nature* 1991;353:844–846.
32. Goate A, Chartier-Harlin M-C, Mullan M, et al. Segregation of a missense mutation in the amyloid precursor protein gene with familial Alzheimer's disease. *Nature* 1991;349:704–706.
33. Naruse S, Igarashi S, Aoki K, et al. Mis-sense muta-

tion Val→Ile in exon 17 of amyloid precursor protein gene in Japanese familial Alzheimer's disease. *Lancet* 1991;337:978–979.
34. Murrell J, Farlow M, Ghetti B, Benson MD. A mutation in the amyloid precursor protein associated with hereditary Alzheimer's disease. *Science* 1991;254:97–99.
35. Kawabata S, Higgins GA, Gordon JW. Alzheimer retraction. *Nature* 1992;356:23.
36. Hof PR, Cox K, Morrison JH. Quantitative analysis of nonphosphorylated neurofilament-immunoreactive neurons in normal and Alzheimer's disease brain. *Soc Neurosci Abstr* 1988;14:1086.
37. Kelley M, Kowall NW. Corticotrophin-releasing factor immunoreactive neurons persist throughout the brain in Alzheimer's disease. *Brain Res* 1989;501:392–396.
38. Kowall NW, Ferrante RJ, Beal MF, et al. Neuropeptide Y, somatostatin, and NADPH diaphorase in human striatum: a combined immunocytochemical and enzyme histochemical study. *Neuroscience* 1987;20:817–828.
39. Quigley BJ, Kowall NW. Substance P-like immunoreactive neurons are depleted in Alzheimer's disease cerebral cortex. *Neuroscience* 1991;41:41–60.
40. Struble RG, Powers RE, Casanova MF, Kitt CA, Brown EC, Price DL. Neuropeptidergic systems in plaques of Alzheimer's disease. *J Neuropathol Exp Neurol* 1987;46:567–584.
41. Kowall NW, Beal MF. Glutamate-, glutaminase-, and taurine-immunoreactive neurons develop neurofibrillary tangles in Alzheimer's disease. *Ann Neurol* 1991;29:162–167.
42. Hof PR, Cox K, Morrison JH. Quantitative analysis of a vulnerable subset of pyramidal neurons in Alzheimer's disease: I. Superior frontal and inferior temporal cortex. *J Comp Neurol* 1990;301:44–54.
43. Morrison JH, Lewis DA, Campbell MJ, et al. A monoclonal antibody to nonphosphorylated neurofilament protein marks the vulnerable cortical neurons in Alzheimer's disease. *Brain Res* 1987;416:331–336.
44. Cudkowicz M, Kowall NW. Degeneration of pyramidal projection neurons in Huntington's disease cortex. *Ann Neurol* 1990;27:200–204.
45. Beal MF, Swartz KJ, Finn SF, Mazurek MF, Kowall NW. Neurochemical characterization of excitotoxic lesions in the cerebral cortex. *J Neurosci* 1991;11:147–158.
46. Kowall NW, Beal MF. Cortical somatostatin, neuropeptide Y, and NADPH diaphorase neurons: normal anatomy and alterations in Alzheimer's disease. *Ann Neurol* 1988;23:105–114.
47. Hof PR, Morrison JH. Neocortical neuronal subpopulations labeled by a monoclonal antibody to calbindin exhibit differential vulnerability in Alzheimer's disease. *Exp Neurol* 1991;111:293–301.
48. Campbell MJ, Hof PR, Morrison JH. A subpopulation of primate corticocortical neurons is distinguished by somatodendritic distribution of neurofilament protein. *Brain Res* 1991;539:133–136.
49. Campbell MJ, Morrison JH. A monoclonal antibody to neurofilament protein (SMI 32) labels a subpopulation of pyramidal neurons in the human and monkey neocortex. *J Comp Neurol* 1989;282:191–205.
50. Sternberger LA, Sternberger NH. Monoclonal antibodies distinguish phosphorylated and nonphosphorylated forms of neurofilaments *in situ*. *Proc Natl Acad Sci USA* 1983;80:6126–6130.
51. Roth M, Tomlinson BE, Blessed G. Correlation between scores for dementia and counts of senile plaques in cerebral gray matter of elderly subjects. *Nature* 1966;206:109–110.
52. Blessed G, Tomlinson BE, Roth M. The association between quantitative measurements of dementia and of senile changes in the cerebral grey matter of elderly subjects. *Br J Psychiatry* 1968;114:797–811.
53. Dayan AD. Quantitative histological studies on the aged human brain. ii. Senile plaques and neurofibrillary tangles in senile dementia. *Acta Neuropathol* 1970;16:95–102.
54. Wilcock GK, Esiri MM. Plaques, tangles and dementia. A quantitative study. *J Neurol Sci* 1982;56:343–356.
55. Behrouz N, Defossez A, Delacourte A, Mazzuca M. Alzheimer's disease: the beta amyloid protein A4 is also present in the cortical white matter. *J Histochem Cytochem* 1990;38:1201–1207.
56. Kitamato T, Ogomori K, Tateishi J, Prusiner SB. Formic acid pretreatment enhances immunostaining of cerebral and systemic amyloids. *Lab Invest* 1987;57:230–236.
57. Davies L, Wolska B, Hilbich C, et al. A4 amyloid protein deposition and the diagnosis of Alzheimer's disease: Prevalence in aged brains determined by immunocytochemistry compared with conventional neuropathological techniques. *Neurology* 1988;38:1688–1693.
58. Crystal H, Davies P, Dickson D, Scicutella A, Blau A, Masur D. Neuropsychological characteristics of subjects with and without neocortical Alz-50 immunoreactivity. *Prog Clin Biol Res* 1989;317:165–173.
59. Crystal H, Dickson D, Fuld P, et al. Clinico-pathologic studies in dementia: nondemented subjects with pathologically confirmed Alzheimer's disease. *Neurology* 1988;38:1682–1687.
60. Katzman R, Terry R, DeTeresa R, et al. Clinical, pathological, and neurochemical changes in dementia: a subgroup with preserved mental status and numerous neocortical plaques. *Ann Neurol* 1988;23:138–144.
61. Barcikowska M, Wisniewski HM, Bancher C, Grundke-Iqbal I. About the presence of paired helical filaments in dystrophic neurites participating in plaque formation. *Acta Neuropathol* 1989;78:225–231.
62. Masliah E, Terry RD, DeTeresa RM, Hansen LA. Immunohistochemical quantification of the synapse related protein synaptophysin in Alzheimer's disease. *Neurosci Lett* 1989;103:234–239.
63. DeKosky ST, Scheff SW. Synapse loss in frontal cortex biopsies in Alzheimer's disease: correlation with cognitive severity. *Ann Neurol* 1990;27:457–464.
64. Terry RD, Peck A, DeTeresa R, Schechter R, Horoupian DS. Some morphometric aspects of the

brain in senile dementia of the Alzheimer type. *Ann Neurol* 1981;10:184–192.
65. Masliah E, Terry RD, Alford M, DeTeresa R, Hansen LA. Cortical and subcortical patterns of synaptophysin-like immunoreactivity in Alzheimer's disease. *Am J Pathol* 1991;138:235–246.
66. Brunelli MP, Kowall NW, Lee JM, McKee AC. Synaptophysin immunoreactivity is depleted in cortical laminae with dense dystrophic neurites and neurofibrillary tangles. *J Neuropathol Exp Neurol* 1991;50:315.
67. Drubin DG, Kirschner MW. Tau protein function in living cells. *J Cell Biol* 1986;103:2739–2746.
68. Drubin DG, Feinstein SC, Shooter EM, Kirschner MW. Nerve growth factor induced neurite outgrowth in PC12 cells involves the coordinate induction of microtubule assembly and assembly-promoting factors. *J Cell Biol* 1985;101:1799–1807.
69. Couchie D, Faivre-Bauman A, Puymirat J, Guilleminot J, Tixier-Vidal A, Nunez J. Expression of microtubule-associated proteins during the early stages of neurite extension by brain neurons cultured in a defined medium. *J Neurochem* 1987;47:1255–1261.
70. Chamak B, Fellous A, Glowinski J, Prochiantz A. MAP 2 expression and neuritic outgrowth and branching are coregulated through region-specific neuro-astroglial interactions. *J Neurosci* 1987;7:3163–3170.
71. Binder LI, Frankfurter A, Rebhun I. The distribution of tau in the mammalian central nervous system. *J Cell Biol* 1985;101:1371–1378.
72. Matus A, Bernhardt R, Hugh-Jones T. High molecular weight microtubule-associated proteins are preferentially associated with dendritic microtubules in brain. *Proc Natl Acad Sci USA* 1981;78:3010–3014.
73. DeCamelli P, Miller P, Navone F, et al. Distribution of microtubule-associated protein 2 in the nervous system of the rat studied by immunofluorescence. *Neuroscience* 1984;11:819–846.
74. Kosik KS, Finch EA. MAP 2 and tau segregate into dendritic and axonal domains after the elaboration of morphologically distinct neurites: an immunocytochemical study of cultured rat cerebrum. *J Neurosci* 1987;7:3142–3153.
75. Matus A. Microtubule-associated proteins: their potential role in determining neuronal morphology. *Annu Rev Neurosci* 1988;11:29–44.
76. Scheibel AB, Tomiyasu U. Dendritic sprouting in Alzheimer's presenile dementia. *Exp Neurol* 1978;60:1–8.
77. Ferrer I, Aymani A, Rovira A, Grau Veciana JM. Growth of atypical dendrites in atypical Alzheimer's disease. A study with a Golgi method. *Acta Neuropathol* 1983;59:167–170.
78. Buell S, Coleman PD. Dendritic growth in the aged human brain and failure of growth in senile dementia. *Science* 1979;206:854–856.
79. Paula-Barbosa MM, Cardoso RM, Guimares ML, Cruz C. Dendritic degeneration and regrowth in patients with Alzheimer's disease. *J Neurol Sci* 1980;45:129–134.
80. Probst A, Basler V, Bron B, Ulrich J. Neuritic plaques in senile dementia of Alzheimer type: a Golgi analysis in the hippocampal region. *Brain Res* 1983;268:249–254.
81. Arendt T, Zventseva HG, Leontovich TA. Dendritic changes in the basal nucleus of Meynert and in the diagonal band nucleus in Alzheimer's disease—a quantitative investigation. *Neuroscience* 1986;19:1265–1278.
82. Geddes JW, Monaghan DT, Cotman CW, Lott IT, Kim RC, Chui H-C. Plasticity of hippocampal circuitry in Alzheimer's disease. *Science* 1985;230:1179–1181.
83. Busciglio J, Ferreira A, Steward O, Caceres A. An immunocytochemical and biochemical study of the microtubule-associated protein, tau, during post-lesion afferent reorganization in the hippocampus of the adult rat. *Brain Res* 1987;419:244–252.
84. Hyman B, Van Hoesen G, Kromer L, Damasio A. Perforant pathway changes and the memory impairment of Alzheimer's disease. *Ann Neurol* 1986;20:472–481.
85. Price DL, Struble RG, Atschuler RJ, Casanova MF, Cork LC, Murphy DB. Aggregation of tubulin in neurons in Alzheimer's disease. *J Neuropathol Exp Neurol* 1985;44:366.
86. Dickson DW, Ksiezak-Reding H, Davies P, Yen S. A monoclonal antibody that recognizes a phosphorylated epitope in Alzheimer neurofibrillary tangles, neurofilaments and tau proteins immunostains granulovacuolar degeneration. *Acta Neuropathol* 1987;73:254–258.
87. Kahn J, Anderton BH, Probst A, Ulrich J, Esiri MM. Immunohistological study of granulovacuolar degeneration using monoclonal antibodies to neurofilaments. *J Neurol Neurosurg Psychiatry* 1985;48:924–926.
88. Galloway PG, Perry G, Gambetti P. Hirano bodies contain actin and tropomyosin. *Soc Neurosci Abstr* 1985;11:952.
89. Galloway PG, Perry G, Kosik KS, Gambetti P. Hirano bodies contain tau protein. *Brain Res* 1987:403:337–340.
90. Matus A, Riederer B. Microtubule-associated proteins in the developing brain. *Ann NY Acad Sci* 1986;466:167–179.
91. Nunez J. Differential expression of microtubule components during brain development. *Dev Neurosci* 1986;8:125–141.
92. Olmsted JB. Microtubule-associated proteins. *Annu Rev Cell Biol* 1986;2:421–457.
93. Calvert R, Anderton BH. A microtubule associated protein MAP 1 which is expressed at elevated levels during development of rat cerebellum. *EMBO J* 1985;4:1171–1176.
94. Bloom GS, Luca FC, Vallee RB. Microtubule-associated protein 1B: Identification of a major component of the neuronal cytoskeleton. *Proc Natl Acad Sci USA* 1985;82:5404–5408.
95. Riederer B, Cohen R, Matus A. MAP 5: a novel brain microtubule-associated protein under strong developmental regulation. *J Neurocytol* 1986;15:763–775.

96. Garner CC, Matus A, Anderton BH, Calvert R. Microtubule-associated proteins MAP 5 and MAP 1x: closely related components of the neuronal cytoskeleton with different cytoplasmic distributions in the developing brain. *Mol Biol Res* 1989; 5:85–92.
97. Schoenfeld TA, McKerracher L, Obar R, Vallee RB. MAP 1A and MAP 1B are structurally related microtubule associated proteins with distinct developmental patterns in the CNS. *J Neurosci* 1989;9:1712–1730.
98. Tucker RP, Matus AI. Microtubule-associated proteins characteristic of embryonic brain are found in the adult mammalian retina. *Dev Biol* 1988;130:423–434.
99. Tucker RP, Garner CC, Matus AI. *In situ* localization of microtubule-associated protein mRNA in the developing and adult rat brain. *Neuron* 1989;2:1245–1256.
100. Riederer B, Cohen R, Matus A. MAP 5: A novel brain microtubule-associated protein under strong developmental regulation. *J Neurocytol* 1986; 15:763–775.
101. Tucker RP, Binder LI, Matus AI. Neuronal microtubule-associated proteins in the embryonic avian spinal cord. *J Comp Neurol* 1988;271:44–55.
102. Calvert RA, Woodhams PL, Anderton BH. Localization of an epitope of a microtubule-associated protein 1× in outgrowing axons of the developing rat central nervous system. *Neuroscience* 1987; 23:131–141.
103. Brugg B, Matus A. PC12 cells express juvenile microtubule-associated proteins during nerve growth factor-induced neurite outgrowth. *J Cell Biol* 1988;107:643–650.
104. Viereck C, Tucker RP, Matus A. The adult rat olfactory system expresses microtubule-associated proteins found in the developing brain. *J Neurosci* 1989;9:3547–3557.
105. Tucker RP, Matus AI. Developmental regulation of two microtubule-associated proteins (MAP 2 and MAP 5) in the embryonic avian retina. *Development* 1987;101:535–546.
106. Hasegawa M, Arai T, Ihara Y. Immunocytochemical evidence that fragments of phosphorylated MAP 5 (MAP 1B) are bound to neurofibrillary tangles in Alzheimer's disease. *Neuron* 1990; 4:909–918.
107. Wilson DM, Binder LI. Identification of tau binding proteins. *Neurobiol Aging* 1990;11:278.
108. Kreis TE. Microtubules containing detyrosinated tubulin are less dynamic. *EMBO J* 1987; 6:2597–2606.
109. Gundersen GG, Kalnoski MH, Bulinski JC. Distinct populations of microtubules: tyrosinated and nontyrosinated alpha tubulin are distributed differently *in vivo*. *Cell* 1984;38:779–789.
110. Maruta H, Greer K, Rosenbaum JL. The acetylation of α-tubulin and its relationship to the assembly and disassembly of microtubules. *J Cell Biol* 1986;103:2167–2177.
111. Lee A, Kowall NW. Spectrin (240/235E) and dendritic reorganization in Alzheimer's disease. *Soc Neurosci Abstr* 1991;17:1070.
112. Nestler EJ, Greengard P. *Protein phosphorylation in the nervous system*. New York: John Wiley & Sons, 1984.
113. Yardin Y, Ullrich A. Growth factor receptor tyrosine kinases. *Annu Rev Biochem* 1988;57:443–478.
114. Sugrue MM, Brugge JS, Marshak DR, Greengard P, Gustafson EL. Immunocytochemical localization of the neuron-specific form of the *c-src* gene product, $pp60^{c\text{-}src(+)}$, in rat brain. *J Neurosci* 1990;10:2513–2527.
115. Harrington KM, Lu C, McKee AC, Kowall NW. $pp60^{c\text{-}src}$ immunoreactivity is increased in senile plaque neurites in Alzheimer's disease. *J Neuropathol Exp Neurol* 1992;51:328.
116. Hemmings HC, Nairn AC, McGuiness TL, Huganir RL, Greengard P. Role of protein phosphorylation in neuronal signal transduction. *FASEB J* 1989;3:1583–1592.
117. Sheng M, Greenberg ME. The regulation and function of *c-fos* and other immediate early genes in the nervous system. *Neuron* 1990;4:477–485.
118. Cohen P. The structure and regulation of protein phosphatases. *Annu Rev Biochem* 1989;58:453–508.
119. Goto S, Yamamoto H, Fukunaga K, Iwasa T, Matsukado Y, Miyamoto E. Dephosphorylation of microtubule-associated protein 2, tau factor, and tubulin by calcineurin. *J Neurochem* 1985; 45:276–283.
120. Goto S, Matsukado Y, Mihara Y, Inoue N, Miyamoto E. Calcineurin in human brain and its relation to extrapyramidal system. Immunohistochemical study on postmortem human brains. *Acta Neuropathol* 1986;72:150–156.
121. Wood JG, Mira SS, Pollock NJ, Binder LI. Neurofibrillary tangles of Alzheimer's disease share antigenic determinants with the axonal microtubule-associated protein tau. *Proc Natl Acad Sci USA* 1986;83:4040–4043.
122. Ueda K, Masliah E, Saitoh T, Bakalis SL, Scobie H, Kosik KS. Alz-50 recognizes a phosphorylated epitope of tau protein. *J Neurosci* 1990;10: 3295–3303.
123. Ksiesak-Reding H, Liu W-K, Hradsky J, Yen S-H. Phosphate analysis of different tau preparations from normal and Alzheimer disease brains. *J Cell Biol* 1990;111:435a.
124. Wolozin B, Davies P. Alzheimer-related neuronal protein A68: specificity and distribution. *Ann Neurol* 1987;22:521–526.
125. Flament S, Delacourte A, Hemon B, Defossez A. Characterization of two pathological tau protein variants in Alzheimer brain cortices. *J Neurol Sci* 1989;92:133–141.
126. Rosenblum JS, Bramblett GI, Lee VM-Y. The selective phosphorylation of sites near the microtubule binding domain in normal tau may be an initial event leading to the formation of Alzheimer disease paired helical filaments. *J Cell Biol* 1990;111:435a.
127. Cole G, Dobkins KR, Hansen LA, Terry RD, Saitoh T. Decreased levels of protein kinase C in Alzheimer brain. *Brain Res* 1988;452:165–174.
128. McKee AC, Kosik KS, Kennedy MB, Kowall NW. Hippocampal neurons predisposed to neurofibril-

lary tangle formation are enriched in type II calcium/calmodulin-dependent protein kinase. *J Neuropathol Exp Neurol* 1990;49:49–63.
129. Iimoto DS, Masliah E, DeTeresa R, Terry RD, Saitoh T. Aberrant casein kinase II in Alzheimer's disease. *Brain Res* 1990;507:273–280.
130. Masliah E, Cole GM, Hansen LA, et al. Protein kinase C alteration is an early biochemical marker in Alzheimer's disease. *J Neurosci* 1991;11:2759–2767.
131. Buxbaum JD, Gandy SE, Cicchetti P, et al. Processing of Alzheimer beta/A4 amyloid precursor protein: modulation by agents that regulate protein phosphorylation. *Proc Natl Acad Sci USA* 1990;87:6003–6006.
132. Bancher C, Grundke-Iqbal I, Iqbal K, Kim KS, Wisniewski HM. Immunoreactivity of neuronal lipofuscin with monoclonal antibodies to the amyloid beta protein. *Neurobiol Aging* 1989;10:125–132.
133. Benowitz LI, Rodriguez W, Paskevich P, Mufson EJ, Schenk D, Neve RL. The amyloid precursor protein is concentrated in neuronal lysosomes in normal and Alzheimer disease subjects. *Exp Neurol* 1989;106:237–250.
134. Koliatsos VE, Applegate MD, Kitt CA, Walker LC, DeLong MR, Price DL. Abberant phosphorylation of neurofilaments accompanies transmitter-related changes in rat septal neurons following transection of the fimbria–fornix. *Brain Res* 1989;482:205–218.
135. Hall GF, Cohen MJ. The pattern of dendritic sprouting and retraction induced by axotomy of lamprey central neurons. *J Neurosci* 1988;8:3584–3597.
136. Roivainen R, Koistanaho J. Deafferentation increases protein kinase c-β-like immunoreactivity in the rat superior cervical ganglion. *Soc Neurosci Abstr* 1990;16:628.
137. Whitehouse PJ, Price DL, Clark AW, Coyle JT, Delong MR. Alzheimer disease: evidence for selective loss of cholinergic neurons in the nucleus basalis. *Ann Neurol* 1981;10:122–126.
138. Tuszynski MH, Sang H, Yoshida K, Gage FH. Recombinant human nerve growth factor infusions prevent cholinergic neuronal degeneration in the adult primate brain. *Ann Neurol* 1991;30:625–636.
139. Yankner BA, Kowall N, Chen M. Nerve growth factor is increased in Alzheimer's disease. *Neurology* 1991;41(suppl 1):270.
140. Lee PL, Johnson DE, Cousens LS, Fried VA, Williams LT. Purification and complementary DNA cloning of a receptor for fibroblast growth factor. *Science* 1989;245:57–60.
141. Wallicke PA. Novel neurotrophic factors, receptors, and oncogenes. *Annu Rev Neurosci* 1989;12:103–126.
142. Anderson KJ, Dam D, Lee S, Cotman CW. Basic fibroblast growth factor prevents death of lesioned cholinergic neurons. *Nature* 1988;332:360–361.
142a. McKee AC, Kowall NW, Marotta C, et al. Increased basic fibroblastic growth factor immunoreactivity in Alzheimer's disease brain. *Neurology* 1990;40(suppl 1):406.
143. Snow AD, Lara S, Nochlin D, Wight TN. Cationic dyes reveal proteoglycans structurally integrated within the characteristic lesions of Alzheimer's disease. *Acta Neuropathol* 1989;78:113–123.
143a. Moses HL, Yang EY, Pietenpol JA. TGFβ stimulation and inhibition of cell proliferation: new mechanistic insights. *Cell* 1990;63:245–247.
143b. Miller DA, Lee A, Pelton RW, Chen EY, Moses HL, Derynck R. Murine transforming growth factor-β2 cDNA sequence and expression in adult tissues and embryos. *Mol Endocrinol* 1989;3:113–123.
144. McKee AC, Kowall NW, Kosik KS. Microtubular reorganization and dendritic growth response in Alzheimer's disease. *Ann Neurol* 1989;26:652–659.
145. Ihara Y. Massive somatodendritic sprouting of cortical neurons in Alzheimer's disease. *Brain Res* 1988;459:138–144.
146. McKee AC, Kosik KS, Kowall NW. Dendritic neurites are histochemically and morphologically distinct from axonal neurites in Alzheimer's disease. *Soc Neurosci Abstr* 1990;16:461.
147. Maness PF, Shores CG, Ignelzi M. Localization of the normal cellular *src* protein to the growth cone of differentiating neurons in brain and retina. *Adv Exp Med Biol* 1990;265:117–125.
148. Van den Pol AN, Di-Porzio U, Rutishauser U. Growth cone localization of neural cell adhesion molecule on central nervous system neurons *in vitro*. *J Cell Biol* 1986;102:2281–2294.
149. Skene JHP, Jacobson RD, Snipes GJ, McGuire CB, Norder JJ, Freeman JA. A protein induced during nerve growth (GAP-43) is a major component of growth cone membranes. *Science* 1986;233:783–786.
150. Kowall NW, Kosik KS, McKee AC. NCAM immunoreactive axonal sprouting in the outer molecular layer of the dentate gyrus in Alzheimer's disease. *Neurology* 1989;39:397.
151. Walsh FS, Doherty P. Structure and function of the gene for neural cell adhesion molecule. *Semin Neurosci* 1991;3:271–284.
152. Leifer D, Kowall NW. Thy-1 in hippocampus: normal anatomy and neuritic growth in Alzheimer's disease. *J Neuropathol Exp Neurol* 1992;51:133–141.
153. Liesi P, Dahl D, Vaheri A. Laminin is produced by early rat astrocytes in primary culture. *J Cell Biol* 1983;96:920–924.
154. Hagg T, Muir D, Engvall E, Varon S, Manthorpe M. Laminin-like antigen in rat CNS neurons: distribution and changes upon brain injury and nerve growth factor treatment. *Neuron* 1989;3:721–732.
155. Kowall NW, McKee AC. Laminin immunoreactivity is increased in Alzheimer's disease hippocampus. *Soc Neurosci Abstr* 1990;16:461.
156. Kowall NW, Pendlebury WW, Kessler JB, Perl DP, Beal MF. Aluminum-induced neurofibrillary degeneration in rabbit cerebral cortex, basal forebrain, and upper brainstem affects the same population of neurons that degenerate in Alzheimer's disease brain. *Neuroscience* 1989;29:329–337.
157. Kowall NW, Beal MF, McKee AC, Kosik KS. Okadaic acid produces dose-dependent neurotoxic le-

sions and increased phosphorylation of neurofilament and tau proteins *in vivo. J Cell Biol* 1991;115:385a.
158. Yankner B, Duffy L, Kirschner D. Neurotrophic and neurotoxic effects of amyloid β protein: reversal by tachykinin neuropeptides. *Science* 1990; 250:279–282.
159. Kowall NW, Beal MF, Yankner BA. The beta amyloid protein produces region-specific neuronal degeneration and increased tau immunoreactivity *in vivo. Ann Neurol* 1991;30:236.
160. McKee AC, Kowall NW, Beal MF, Shumacher J, Yankner BA. Effects of beta amyloid III: The primate brain. *Soc Neurosci Abstr* 1991;17:1294.
161. Podlisny M, Stephenson D, Frosch M, et al. *In vivo* effects of β-amyloid protein in primates: microinjection study. *Soc Neurosci Abstr* 1991;17:1446.
162. Beal MF, Kowall NW, Busciglio J, Duffy LK, Yankner BA. Effects of beta amyloid II: Protection by substance P. *Soc Neurosci Abstr* 1991;17:1294.
163. Maggio JE. Tachykinins. *Annu Rev Neurosci* 1988;11:13–28.
164. Kowall NW, Beal MF, Busciglio J, Duffy LK, Yankner BA. An *in vivo* model for the neurodegenerative effects of beta amyloid and protection by substance P. *Proc Natl Acad Sci USA* 1991; 88:7247–7251.
165. Gerfen CR. Substance P (neurokinin-1) receptor mRNA is selectively expressed in cholinergic neurons in the striatum and basal forebrain. *Brain Res* 1991;556:165–170.
166. Jonsson G, Hallman H. Substance P modifies the 6-hydroxydopamine induced alteration of postnatal development of central noradrenaline neurons. *Neuroscience* 1982;7:2909–2918.
167. Anand P, McGregor GP, Gibson SJ, Maden M, Polak JM, Bloom SR. Increase of substance P-like immunoreactivity in the peripheral nerve of the axolotl after injury. *Neurosci Lett* 1987;82:241–245.
168. Freedman J, Hökfelt T, Post C, et al. Immunohistochemical and behavioral analysis of spinal lesions induced by a substance P antagonist and protection by thyrotropin releasing hormone. *Exp Brain Res* 1989;74:279–292.
169. Grabow TS, Gaumann DM, Yaksh TL. Electroencephalographic and behavioral assessment of intracerebroventricular somatostain and substance P analogue. *Brain Res* 1989;489:223–230.
170. Freidin M, Kessler JA. Cytokine regulation of substance P expression in sympathetic neurons. *Proc Natl Acad Sci USA* 1991;88:3200–3203.
171. Kostyk S, Kowall NW, Hauser S. Substance P immunoreactive astrocytes are present in multiple sclerosis plaques. *Brain Res* 1989;504:284–288.
172. Boix F, Mattioli R, Adams F, Schwarting RKW, Huston JP. Peripherally administered substance P: effects on functional recovery after nigrostriatal 6-OHDA lesions and on striatal dopamine as measured by *in vivo* microdialysis. *Soc Neurosci Abstr* 1990;16:908.
173. Mitsuhashi M, Akiyata T, Turk CW, Payan DG. Amyloid beta protein substituent peptides do not interact with the substance P receptor expressed in cultured cells. *Mol Brain Res* 1991;11:177–180.
174. Joslin G, Fallon RJ, Bullock J, Adams SP, Perlmutter DH. The SEC receptor recognizes a pentapeptide neodomain of α-antitrypsin-protease complexes. *J Cell Biol* 1991;266:11282–11288.
175. Joslin G, Krause JE, Hershey AD, Adams SP, Fallon RJ, Perlmutter DH. Amyloid-β peptide, substance P, and bombesin bind to the serpin–enzyme complex receptor. *J Biol Chem* 1991;266: 21897–21902.
176. Abraham CR, Selkoe DJ, Potter H. Immunochemical identification of the serine protease inhibitor alpha-1-antichymotrypsin in the brain amyloid deposits of Alzheimer's disease. *Cell* 1988;52: 487–501.

Advances in Neurology, Vol. 59, edited by Fredrick J. Seil. Raven Press, Ltd., New York © 1993.

3

Adaptive Versus Pathological Plasticity

Possible Contributions to Age-Related Dementia

Carl W. Cotman, Christian J. Pike, and Brian J. Cummings

Department of Psychobiology, University of California, Irvine, California 92717

Plasticity processes are involved in normal brain function (e.g., learning and memory) and are critical in recovery of function after injury or disease. However, plasticity processes can not only improve function but also may contribute to dysfunction, depending on the exact changes in the brain's circuitry. As the brain ages, it increasingly depends on its regulatory and plastic capacities. A goal of basic research is to identify critical plasticity processes, to understand what regulates them, and to apply this information to understand normal function better and to treat disease. One plasticity process that seems to be critical is reactive synaptogenesis. Reactive synapogenesis is characterized by the enhanced viability and neuritic sprouting of neurons surviving an insult. The sprouting reaction appears to require two components: growth factors (e.g., basic fibroblast growth factor) and suitable substrates (e.g., heparan sulfate). In this chapter, we discuss *in vitro* data that support roles of basic fibroblast growth factor (bFGF) and heparan sulfate (HS) in plasticity and then describe *in vivo* data concerning their regulation after injury and possible participation in plasticity. These observations are also discussed in terms of accumulating data that indicate that sprouting also occurs in Alzheimer disease (AD). We compare predictions from animal models of sprouting to AD, focusing on the contributions of bFGF, HS, and β-amyloid. We suggest that plasticity processes in the AD brain are initially adaptive but may actually accelerate dysfunction over time. Specifically, events associated with regenerative growth in AD appear to interact with the β-amyloid protein, ultimately increasing the probability of neuronal pathology and degeneration.

IN VITRO NEURONAL GROWTH: SUPPORT FROM GROWTH FACTORS AND SUBSTRATE COMPONENTS

Basic FGF is among the most effective growth factors for supporting the survival and neuritic outgrowth of cultured neurons. Immature, developing neuronal cultures from both hippocampus (1,2) and cerebral cortex (3–5) exhibit greatly enhanced survival in response to treatments with bFGF at concentrations as low as 1 pM.

Cellular microenvironments provide trophic support not only through growth factors but also by containing many different substrate components, including laminin, fibronectin, and glycosaminoglycans. Substrate factors are involved in a variety of processes essential to plastic and regenerative responses. The glycosaminoglycan HS is one substrate factor that has been linked recently to plastic events. For example, neurons grown on an HS substrate show dramatically increased axonal elongation in culture. After 24 hr *in vitro,* the neurites of hippocampal neurons grown on HS-coated tissue culture dishes exhibit approximately a twofold increase in length in comparison to those grown on noncoated dishes (unpublished observations). This effect is concentration dependent and may be specific to HS, since the related glycosaminoglycan, chondroitin sulfate, is ineffective in neurite promotion.

Reciprocal Interactions Between bFGF and HS

Accumulating evidence suggests that bFGF and HS effectively promote plastic changes via independent actions as well as through interactions. These interactions are facilitated in part by the strong binding affinity of bFGF for HS and for the closely related glycosaminoglycan heparin (6,7). As a result of this association, the biological activities of bFGF and HS may be reciprocally influenced. In fact, when bound to HS or heparin, bFGF has a larger effective radius from its source because of increased diffusion (8) and is protected from proteolytic degradation (9). In addition, recent evidence suggests that bFGF is internalized into cells only when it is bound to heparin (10). Thus, the activity of bFGF may require interaction with the substrate factors HS and heparin. Conversely, the activity of HS may require, or at least be enhanced by, association with bFGF. In support of this position, the neurite outgrowth *in vitro* induced by bFGF is potentiated on HS and heparin substrates (11,12).

In Vivo Levels of bFGF Increase Following CNS Injury

Injury to the central nervous system (CNS) evokes a time-dependent increase in neurotrophic factor activity (13). However, the identity of these factors was not determined. Recently, we evaluated the possibility that bFGF might represent one such trophic factor exhibiting an increase following injury.

After a unilateral lesion of entorhinal cortex, the ipsilateral hippocampus shows an enhanced bFGF immunoreactivity in a terminal synaptic region for entorhinal fibers, the dentate gyrus outer molecular layer. The number of bFGF-immunopositive astrocytes increases until 1 week post-lesion but eventually returns to near-normal levels within 2 weeks. The bFGF-immunoreactive astrocytes that surround lesioned areas exhibit strong reactivity in their processes and enlarged, intensely stained cell bodies; together these observations suggest a possible translocation mechanism of bFGF release. There is also an increase in bFGF immunoreactivity within the extracellular matrix surrounding bFGF-positive astrocytes.

This increase in bFGF immunoreactivity detected in the extracellular matrix supports the belief that bFGF is released from astrocytes and then may become available to neurons, possibly by binding to the HS found in the extracellular matrix. Together, these findings suggest that in response to degenerative events, bFGF is made more available to local neurons and, consequently, may aid in cell survival and the reestablishment of synaptic connections. Thus, as predicted by both tissue culture and animal models, bFGF may function in compensatory regenerative processes.

In Vivo HS Levels May Increase After CNS Injury

Considerable *in vitro* data implicate HS as an important element in plastic responses, although *in vivo* corroboration of such a role is only beginning to accumulate. At present, there is little data concerning changes in HS after CNS injury. Giftochristos et al. (14) found that two substrate molecules, laminin and HS proteoglycan, increased proximal to a transection of the optic nerve; however, neither was at its highest level within the immediate sprouting region.

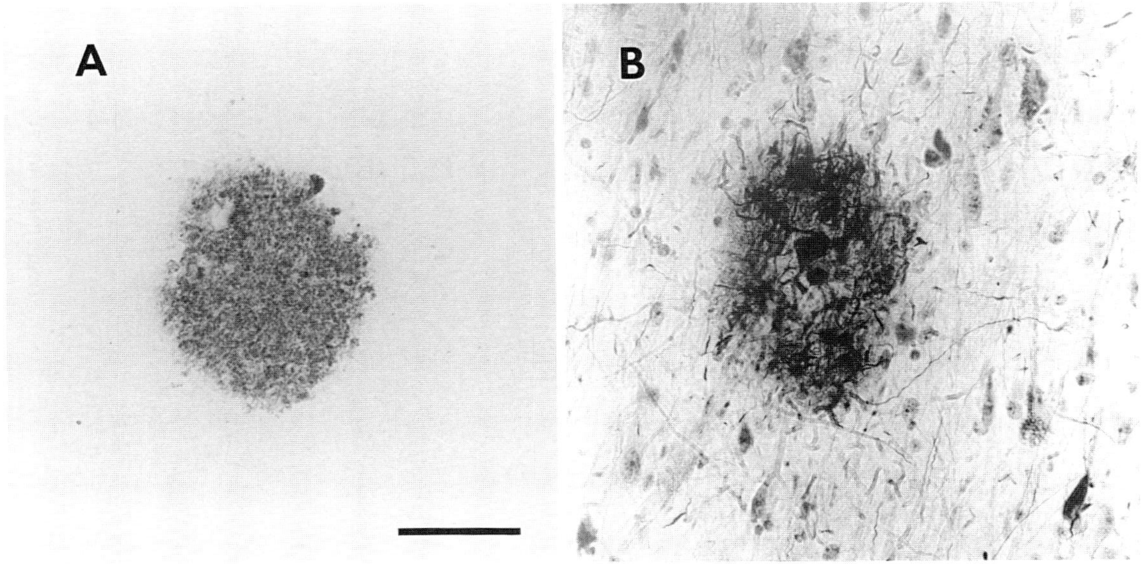

FIG. 1. (**A**) A "primitive" senile plaque stained with an antibody to β-amyloid. This plaque was found in the entorhinal cortex of an 88-year-old AD brain and is approximately 75 μm in diameter. Primitive plaques, as in this example, are often devoid of dystrophic neurites. (**B**) A classical "neuritic" plaque from the same tissue as in **A.** This plaque was stained with the Bielschowsky silver method and clearly demonstrates numerous dystrophic neurites within and entering the plaque. Scale bar, 50 μm for both A and B.

We have begun to examine the changes in HS, HS proteoglycan (HSPG), and laminin after transection of the perforant path from entorhinal cortex to the dentate gyrus. In agreement with Giftochristos and coworkers, we have observed increases in laminin, HS, and HSPG immunoreactivity proximal to the lesion. In the region of the deafferented dentate gyrus, there appears to be a slight increase in HS immunoreactivity in comparison to the nonlesioned contralateral side; however, the change may not be quantitatively significant. Although there is little net change in HS levels, this does not necessarily indicate that target and supporting cells have not increased their expression of HS. In fact, since many input fibers have degenerated at the time points examined (7 and 14 days), there may actually be an underlying compensation by other elements (e.g., target neurons or glia) that maintains substrate levels in the absence of input. In any event, it appears that following CNS injury, HS is available as a substrate to support sprouting neurites.

PLASTIC RESPONSES ARE OBSERVED IN NORMAL AGING AND IN ALZHEIMER DISEASE

The aged human brain appears capable of compensatory dendritic sprouting and synaptic reestablishment, perhaps in response to declines in neuronal number with increasing age (15,16). In addition to normal age-related sprouting, regenerative responses can also occur in response to brain injuries resulting from disease conditions such as AD. In AD, major neuronal loss occurs in the temporal lobe, particularly in layers II and III of the entorhinal cortex (17–19).

Based on findings in rodents after entorhinal lesions, we predicted and found enhanced acetylcholinesterase (AChE) staining in the dentate gyrus of AD brains indicative of regenerative sprouting (20). Thus, we have suggested that following initial cell loss during the early course of the disease, the remaining cells sprout new connections in a compensatory fashion in order to maintain some state of circuitry completion (21). In addition to the intense AChE staining within the molecular layer of the dentate gyrus in AD brains, we noticed structures that were not predicted from animal models: small, round, cholinesterase-positive material usually surrounded by astrocytes. These cholinesterase-rich deposits corresponded to senile plaques, as revealed by positive thioflavin staining indicative of amyloid plaques. The AChE-positive plaques appeared to form along the areas of interface between degeneration and neuronal sprouting and thus appear to be foci of these opposing processes.

We suggested that the sprouting reactions might both be stimulated by and contribute to plaque formation (20,22). As the sprouting reaction progresses, it appears to be directed at senile plaques rather than at functional targets (see Fig. 1). At this time, however, it was unknown whether senile plaques contained trophic molecules in conjunction with suitable substrate factors.

THE MICROENVIRONMENT OF SENILE PLAQUES MAY BE CONDUCIVE TO NEURONAL SPROUTING

Basic FGF is Associated with Senile Plaques in AD

Neurite growth and degeneration coexist in AD. If sprouting is misdirected into plaques, a key issue becomes the identification of the specific molecules driving such growth. It would be predicted that the trophic and substrate elements detailed above play a critical role. Accordingly, we evaluated the possibility that bFGF is present in or around senile plaques. Using AD brain tissue, we found immunocytochemically that many plaques contain bFGF immunoreactivity (23). These bFGF-positive plaques are found both in the entorhinal cortex and along the middle of the dentate gyrus molecular layer in a linear organization.

Others have also demonstrated bFGF-immunopositive plaques and suggested that whole-brain levels of bFGF are elevated in AD compared to normal aged brains (24). Recently, Kato and colleagues demonstrated that exogenous bFGF can bind to plaques and neurofibrillary tangles in sectioned AD tissue (25). Perry and co-workers have shown that bFGF binding to neurofibrillary tangles is HS mediated (26). Recently, we have observed that bFGF-positive plaques are heavily infiltrated with tau-1-immunopositive neurites, thereby supporting a relationship between bFGF and regenerative sprouting (unpublished observations).

Thus, observations within AD brains parallel those from animal studies and support the hypothesis that in response to degenerative events, astrocytes and possibly select neurons produce and release bFGF, stimulating neuronal plasticity. In the case of AD, however, bFGF appears to concentrate within senile plaques and may misdirect plastic responses toward these structures rather than denervated targets.

Heparan Sulfate Is Associated with Senile Plaques in AD

In addition to trophic factors like bFGF, substrate components might also contribute to the AD regenerative response. Previous work has shown that glycosaminoglycans not only are elevated in AD (27) but also are associated with plaques (28). More specifically, using monoclonal antibodies to HS and HSPG, we and others have shown positive HS immunoreactivity within plaques as well as in selected neurons and tangles (29–31). Thus, HS, as well as bFGF, may accumulate in concentrated areas associated with senile plaques, providing a microenvironment that could divert sprouting and plasticity processes away from potentially beneficial functions.

βA4 Peptide May Stimulate Aberrant Plasticity and Enhance Susceptibility to Cell Death

Although bFGF, HS, and numerous other minor components are associated with senile plaques, the primary component of plaques is β-amyloid. β-Amyloid protein (βAP) is a 40- to 42-amino-acid polypeptide derived from abnormal processing of the amyloid precursor protein (APP). Since senile plaques appear to be centers of both degeneration and regeneration, knowledge of β-amyloid's potential contribution to these events is vital.

We treated neuronal cultures with synthetic homologs of βAP in order to investigate how β-amyloid may affect the degenerative and/or regenerative responses seen in the AD brain. Using a low density culture system optimized for measurement of trophic effects, we reported that soluble β-amyloid peptides corresponding to both the initial 28 residues [β(1–28)] and the full-length protein [β(1–42)] increased the survival of developing hippocampal neurons (32,33). Also, β(1–42) caused significant axonal elongation and dendritic arborization in these cultures (32,34).

In addition to trophic activities, βAP has neurotoxic properties. Yankner and colleagues reported that βAP directly caused neurotoxicity in older hippocampal cultures, an effect reported to be potentiated by nerve growth factor (NGF) (35,36). Further, it was reported that *in vivo* injections of βAP caused focal toxicity (37). Thus, β-amyloid may participate in the delicate balance between regenerative and degenerative processes. Clearly, it is important to determine the basis for this apparent opposing activity.

Aggregated β-Amyloid Is More Damaging to Neurons Than Soluble β-Amyloid

In the brain, βAP assembles into insoluble aggregates to form plaques or plaque-like structures. We have previously suggested that

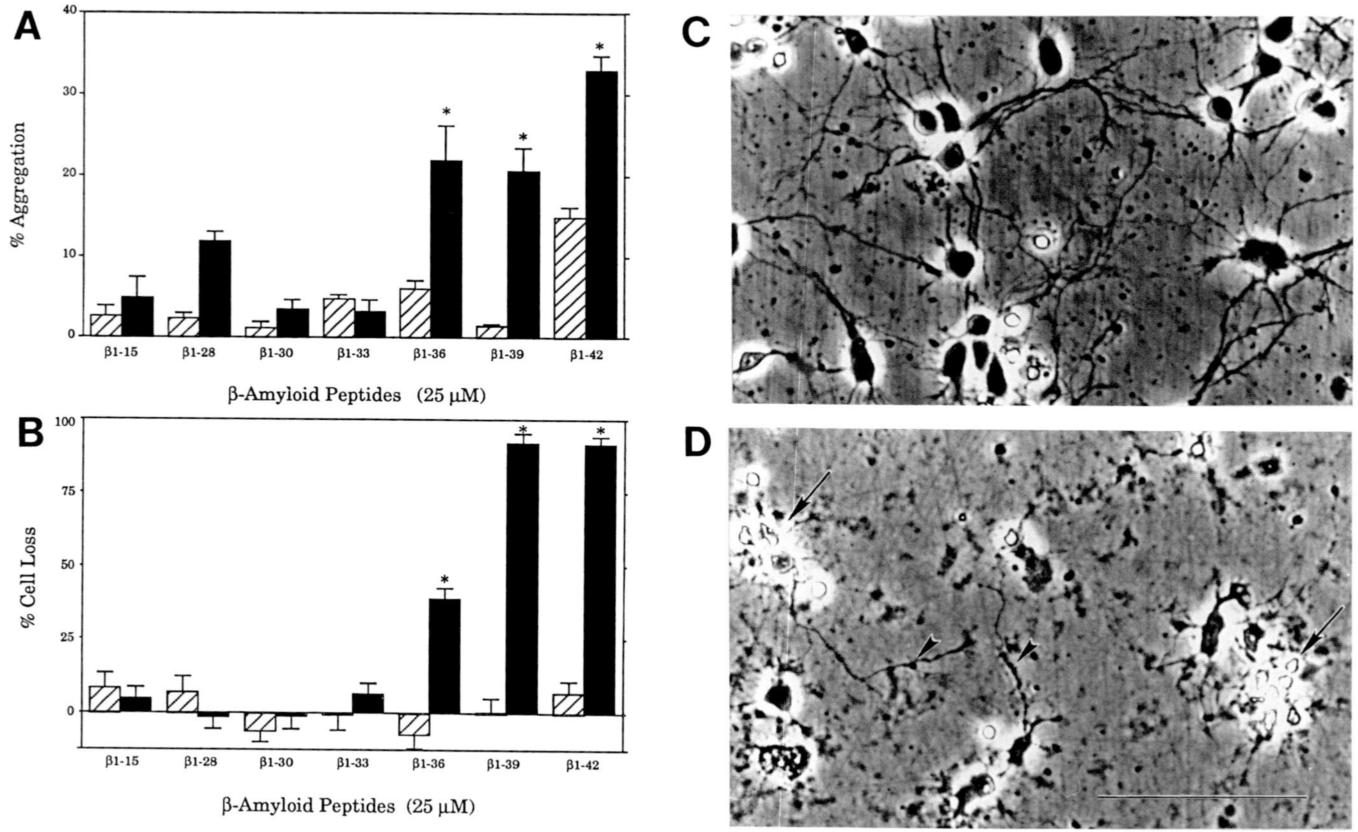

FIG. 2. (A) The state of aggregation of several βAPs was assessed following both initial peptide solubilization *(hatched bars)* and 7-day incubation of these solutions *(solid bars)*. Aggregation was quantified as the percentage of sedimentable peptide resulting from ultracentrifugation (100,000 x *g*, 1 hr) of 25 μM βAP solutions. $^*p < 0.05$ relative to nonaggregating peptide. **(B)** Significant cell loss in hippocampal cultures was induced only by those βAPs that also exhibited significant aggregation. Cell viability was determined 24 hr after addition of newly solubilized *(hatched bars)* and preincubated *(solid bars)* βAP solutions (25 μM). $^*p \leq 0.05$ relative to untreated controls. **(C)** Neurons from untreated control hippocampal cultures appear healthy and extend extensive, fine neuritic processes. **(D)** However, cultures treated with aggregated βAPs [incubated β(1-42) here] exhibit extensive cell loss *(arrows)* and degenerated neurites *(arrowheads)*; aggregated β-peptide is visible throughout the field. Scale bar, 100 μm.

the neurotoxic effects of β-amyloid may be related to an aggregated form of the protein, perhaps in conjunction with the age and health of the neurons. The βAP has an inherent ability to spontaneously form insoluble aggregations *in vitro,* which may parallel the self-assembly of βAP hypothesized to occur in AD following its aberrant processing from APP (38–40).

The *in vitro* formation of β(1–42) aggregates is maximized by incubation of concentrated, slightly acidic peptide solutions (39). Following such an incubation, sheet-like aggregates are visible at the light microscope level. Also, β(1–42) shows an altered electrophoresis profile following incubation. In addition to a band at the predicted monomeric molecular weight, reducing gels also show higher-order bands indicative of aggregated, insoluble peptides (34,39). A similar electrophoresis pattern has been reported for β-amyloid isolated from AD tissue (41,42). Further, these aggregations show positive Congo red and thioflavin staining, which is characteristic of senile plaques (39). Interestingly, stable SDS-resistant aggregates are not found following incubation of β-amyloid peptides such as β(1–28) that lack a substantial hydrophobic domain (39,43).

To examine the possibility that the biological properties of βAP vary as a function of its state of aggregation, we studied the actions of several βAP peptides both in newly solubilized states and following incubation. In studies of cultured neurons, trophic influences are best examined with low-density cultures (less than 7,000 cells/cm^2) in defined media, which regularly degenerate unless a trophic factor is added; toxic effects are identified using higher-density cultures, which survive longer, probably because of autocrine support. In a higher-density defined medium culture system (approximately 16,000 cells/cm^2), immature hippocampal neurons treated with newly solubilized, nonaggregated β(1–42) showed greatly enhanced neurite outgrowth and no toxicity. However, sister cultures treated with the incubated or aged β(1–42) exhibited a dose-dependent toxicity that approached 100% at a concentration of 100 μg/ml (34). We also treated cultures with aged β(1–28) but found this treatment to lack toxicity (44). In addition, we found that β(1–28), unlike β(1–42), did not form peptide aggregates that were stable under tissue culture conditions. The structure–activity relationships of several βAPs support the hypothesis that aggregated βAPs contribute to the degeneration of cultured neurons (see Fig. 2).

Thus, it appears that both the self-aggregation and toxic-promoting properties of βAP require β-amyloid fragments that include significant portions of the transmembrane region [β(29–42)] (43). Although βAP appears capable of enhancing neuritic growth and survival, it may also promote and even cause degeneration.

Aggregated β-Amyloid May Cause Neurites to Become Dystrophic

As a plaque forms in AD, it is believed to progress from a diffuse amyloid plaque to the "classical" neuritic plaque. Developed plaques show a prominent involvement of neurites, many of which appear bulbous or dystrophic (Fig. 1B). Select neurites in and around these plaques typically have enlarged endings and swellings along their lengths and frequently bifurcate on entering the plaque.

Recently we have begun to examine the response of neurites to the presence of aggregated βAP derivatives in cultured hippocampal neurons. In these cultures, neuritic processes that encounter aggregated β-amyloid peptides undergo morphological changes similar to those seen in neuritic plaques. Responsive processes, which morphologically appear to be axons, become thickened and swollen and often exhibit retraction and/or fragmentation. Interestingly, other neurites from affected neurons that are not in contact with the aggregated βAP appear morphologically normal (55).

β-Amyloid Makes Neurons More Vulnerable to Excitotoxic Injury

Our data and those of others discussed above suggest that β-amyloid can contribute to the degeneration of cultured neurons. Neurons in the brain that are exposed to β-amyloid not only may be directly compromised but may also be rendered more susceptible to other types or combinations of insults that may exist in the aged brain. Known risk factors include conditions associated with excitotoxicity. In order to evaluate experimentally the possibility that βAP potentiates excitotoxic risk factors, high-density cortical cultures were grown approximately 14 days *in vitro* and then treated with soluble β(1–42). One- to 4-day exposures to this peptide alone did not result in neuronal degeneration. However, following such β-amyloid exposure, the addition of sublethal doses of glutamate caused massive cell death (45). At present, we have not examined the effect of aggregated βAP in this excitotoxicity paradigm.

We further examined βAP-mediated enhanced vulnerability by studying the combination of βAP with another excitotoxic risk factor, glucose deprivation. When these same cortical cultures are exposed to a brief episode of glucose deprivation, which normally causes only mild injury, in conjunction with soluble β(1–42), severe cell loss results (46). These findings may be especially relevant to understanding the progression of AD, since senile plaque distribution often corresponds to the terminals of glutamate pathways (47).

PLAQUE FORMATION AND GROWTH

The Tendency of β-Amyloid to Aggregate May Contribute to Plaque Formation

One of the early stages in plaque formation is likely the aggregation of β-amyloid peptides into microplaques, small diffuse plaques scattered throughout the neuropil. Some of these deposits may accumulate other available substances, based on selective interactions and affinities. For example, bFGF will bind to HS and form a macromolecular complex. In turn, HS will bind to β-amyloid aggregates (unpublished observations). The small aggregate may continue to grow, accumulating material as it becomes available in the extracellular space. Local neurites may then enter the plaque, attracted in part by bFGF and HS, but eventually become dystrophic in response to β-amyloid influences (Fig. 1). Degeneration, in turn, is predicted to cause an injury-induced expression of bFGF, which would bind to the plaques, stimulate misdirected neuritic sprouting, and so on. Once initiated, any reaction that drives the synthesis of APP and βAP would ultimately accelerate plaque growth.

Misregulation of Growth Factor Cascades May Stimulate Plaque Growth

A number of interwoven molecular cascades exist within the neuronal microenvironment, several of which may contribute to the formation of plaques. Each of the components we have discussed above, bFGF, HS, and APP, is implicated in regulatory pathways that are relevant to AD. For example, bFGF stimulates the production of APP mRNA in cultured glial cells (48). Thus, increases in bFGF may indirectly stimulate production of βAP.

Recently we demonstrated that the addition of βAP to purified astrocyte cultures increases the release of bFGF from these cells (49). The addition of β(1–42) at concentrations as low as 1 μg/ml caused an increase in the release of bFGF into the cell culture medium within 3 hr. In addition, bFGF, when added to culture medium, elevated astrocytic secretion of the potent trophic substance NGF twofold (50); NGF has been reported to potentiate βAP toxicity (35). Additionally, it has been shown that NGF can increase APP secretion (51), illustrating another complex interwoven pathway. Thus, if bFGF enhances the production of APP, a cycle is cre-

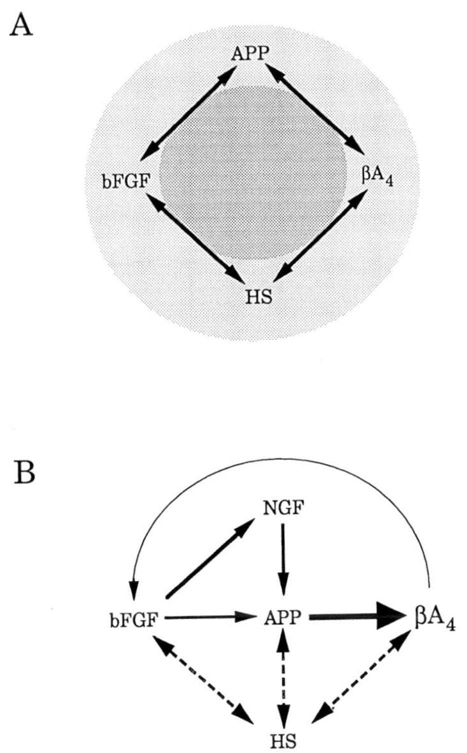

FIG. 3. (**A**) Pictorial representation of the major components found within plaques. The amyloid precursor protein (APP), basic fibroblast growth factor (bFGF), heparan sulfate (HS), and the β-amyloid peptide (βA4) are each found within plaques. An accumulation of any one of them may initiate plaque formation. (**B**) Some of the possible positive feedback cascades and interactions among primary plaque components. For example, a focal injury or infarct could initiate an increase in bFGF, which in turn increases the production of both NGF and APP. Accumulations of APP are processed to form βA4, which in turn feeds back and increases bFGF production. Concurrently, NGF is capable of increasing the production of APP as well. The *dashed arrows* indicate mutual binding interactions between several plaque components and HS, resulting in further growth of a plaque. As diagrammed in **A,** this type of plaque growth cycle could be initiated at several entry points, illustrating routes by which plasticity mechanisms can drive pathology.

ated that could accelerate the production of βAP. Conversely, if APP or β-amyloid accumulation results in injury, bFGF levels would be predicted to increase. Both bFGF and APP show a high affinity for binding HS (7,52–54). The relationship among HS, bFGF, NGF, and APP in AD may represent another example of a shift toward toxicity in the delicate degenerative–regenerative balance. These responses are likely to be complementary, resulting in positive feedback cycles (Fig. 3).

CONCLUSION

In summary, there appears to be a fine balance between adaptive and pathological plasticity in the AD brain. Sprouting, though an initially adaptive response, may become misdirected and contribute to pathogenesis. With the demonstration of bFGF, HS, and β-amyloid in senile plaques, one can speculate that the environment may support a potential recursive cycle of plaque formation: β-amyloid accumulations stimulate bFGF production and bind to HS; elevated bFGF levels, possibly made resistant to degradation by binding to HS, increase APP levels; increases in APP may yield higher βAP levels; βAP feeds back by increasing bFGF. These positive feedback cascades have the potential to accelerate senile plaque formation and potentiate the associated neurodegenerative responses.

In conclusion, the neurodegeneration of AD may be instigated by a misdirected plasticity cycle and ultimately concluded by various mechanisms related to glutamate receptors. In addition to β-amyloid's role as a risk factor, normally supportive molecules such as bFGF ironically may contribute to pathology in AD. It may be that the overall balance and availability of supportive factors to the proper targets are critical. In this way, trophic imbalances in combination with increases in risk factors, including glutamate, glucose deficits, and β-amyloid, may converge on a final common pathway that causes degeneration.

REFERENCES

1. Mattson MP, Murrain M, Guthrie PB, Kater SB. Fibroblast growth factor and glutamate: opposing

roles in the generation and degeneration of hippocampal neuroarchitecture. *J Neurosci* 1989;9: 3728–3740.
2. Walicke P, Cowan W, Ueno N, Baird A, Guillemin R. Fibroblast growth factor promotes survival of dissociated hippocampal neurons and enhances neurite extension. *Proc Natl Acad Sci USA* 1986;83: 3012–3016.
3. Mattson MP, Rychlik B. Glia protect hippocampal neurons against excitatory amino acid-induced degeneration: involvement of fibroblast growth factor. *Int J Dev Neurosci* 1990;8:399–415.
4. Morrison RS, Sharma A, de Vellis J, Bradshaw RA. Basic fibroblast growth factor supports the survival of cerebral cortical neurons in primary culture. *Proc Natl Acad Sci USA* 1986;83:7537–7541.
5. Walicke PA. Basic and acidic fibroblast growth factors have trophic effects on neurons from multiple CNS regions. *J Neurosci* 1988;8:2618–2627.
6. Baird A, Schubert D, Ling N, Guillemin R. Receptor and heparin binding domains of basic fibroblast growth factor. *Proc Natl Acad Sci USA* 1988;85: 2324–2328.
7. Gospodarowicz D, Cheng J, Lui G, Baird A, Bohlent P. Isolation of brain fibroblast growth factor by heparin-sepharose affinity chromatography: identity with pituitary fibroblast growth factor. *Proc Natl Acad Sci USA* 1984;81:6963–6967.
8. Flaumenhaft R, Moscatelli D, Rifkin DB. Heparin and heparan sulfate increase the radius of diffusion and action of basic fibroblast growth factor. *J Cell Biol* 1990;111:1651–1659.
9. Saksela O, Moscatelli D, Sommer A, Rifkin D. Endothelial cell-derived heparan sulfate binds basic fibroblast growth factor and protects it from proteolytic degradation. *J Cell Biol* 1988;107:743–751.
10. Ruoslahti E, Yamaguchi Y. Proteoglycans as modulators of growth factor activities. *Cell* 1991;64: 867–869.
11. Neufeld G, Gospodarowicz D, Dodge L, Fujii DK. Heparin modulation of the neurotropic effects of acidic and basic fibroblast growth factors and nerve growth factor on PC12 cells. *J Cell Physiol* 1987;131:131–140.
12. Walicke P. Interactions between basic fibroblast growth factor (FGF) and glycosoaminoglycans in promoting neurite outgrowth. *Exp Neurol* 1988; 102:144–148.
13. Nieto-Sampedro M, Lewis ER, Cotman CW, et al. Brain injury causes a time-dependent increase in neurotrophic activity at the lesion site. *Science* 1982;217:860–861.
14. Giftochristos N, David S. Laminin and heparan sulphate proteoglycan in the lesioned adult mammalian central nervous system and their possible relationship to axonal sprouting. *J Neurocytol* 1988; 17:385–397.
15. Buell SJ, Coleman PD. Dendritic growth in the aged human brain and failure of growth in senile dementia. *Science* 1979;206:854–856.
16. Buell SJ, Coleman PD. Quantitative evidence for selective dendritic growth in normal human aging but not in senile dementia. *Brain Res* 1981; 214:23–41.
17. Coleman PD, Flood DG. Neuron numbers and dendritic extent in normal aging and Alzheimer's disease. *Neurobiol Aging* 1987;8:521–545.
18. Hyman BT, Kromer LJ, Van Hoesen GW. Reinnervation of the hippocampal perforant pathway zone in Alzheimer's disease. *Ann Neurol* 1987;21: 259–267.
19. Hyman BT, Van Hoesen GW, Kromer LJ, Damasio AR. Perforant pathway changes and the memory impairment of Alzheimer's disease. *Ann Neurol* 1986;20:472–481.
20. Geddes JW, Anderson KJ, Cotman CW. Senile plaques as aberrant sprout-stimulating structures. *Exp Neurol* 1986;94:767–776.
21. Cotman CW, Anderson KJ. Synaptic plasticity and functional stabilization in the hippocampal formation: possible role in Alzheimer's disease. *Adv Neurol* 1988;47:313–335.
22. Cotman CW, Cummings BJ, Whitson JS. The role of misdirected plasticity in plaque biogenesis and Alzheimer's disease pathology. In: Hefti F, Brachet P, Will B, Christen Y, eds. *Growth factors and Alzheimer's disease*. Berlin: Springer-Verlag; 1991: 222–233.
23. Gomez-Pinilla F, Cummings BJ, Cotman CW. Induction of basic fibroblast growth factor in Alzheimer's disease pathology. *NeuroReport* 1990;1: 211–214.
24. Stopa EG, Gonzalez A, Chorsky R, et al. Basic fibroblast growth factor in Alzheimer's disease. *Biochem Biophys Res Commun* 1990;171:690–696.
25. Kato T, Sasaki H, Katagiri T, et al. The binding of basic fibroblast growth factor to Alzheimer's neurofibrillary tangles and senile plaques. *Neurosci Lett* 1991;122:33–36.
26. Perry G, Siedlak BL, Richey P, et al. Association of heparan sulfate proteoglycan with the neurofibrillary tangles of Alzheimer disease. *J Neurosci* 1991;11:3679–3683.
27. Suzuki K, Katzman R, Korey S. Chemical studies on Alzheimer's disease. *J Neuropathol Exp Neurol* 1955;14:211–222.
28. Snow AD, Wight TN. Proteoglycans in the pathogenesis of Alzheimer's disease and other amyloidoses. *Neurobiol Aging* 1989;10:481–497.
29. Snow AD, Kisilevsky R. Temporal relationship between glycosaminoglycan accumulation and amyloid deposition during experimental amyloidosis: a histochemical study. *Lab Invest* 1985;53:37–44.
30. Snow AD, Mar H, Nochlin D, et al. Early accumulation of heparan sulfate in neurons and in the beta-amyloid protein containing lesions of Alzheimer's disease and Down's Syndrome. *Am J Pathol* 1990;137:1253–1270.
31. Su JH, Cummings BJ, Cotman CW. Localization of heparan sulfate glycosaminoglycan and proteoglycan core protein in aged brain and Alzheimer's disease. [submitted].
32. Whitson JS, Glabe CG, Shintani E, Abcar A, Cotman CW. β-Amyloid protein promotes neuritic branching in hippocampal cultures. *Neurosci Lett* 1990;110:319–324.
33. Whitson JS, Selkoe DJ, Cotman CW. Amyloid beta protein enhances the survival of hippocampal neurons in vitro. *Science* 1989;243:1488–1490.
34. Pike CJ, Walencewicz AJ, Glabe CG, Cotman CW.

In vitro aging of β-amyloid protein causes peptide aggregation and neurotoxicity. *Brain Res* 1991; 563:311–314.
35. Yankner BA, Caceres A, Duffy LK. Nerve growth factor potentiates the neurotoxicity of β-amyloid. *Proc Natl Acad Sci USA* 1990;87:9020–9023.
36. Yankner BA, Duffy LK, Kirschner DA. Neurotrophic and neurotoxic effects of amyloid β-protein: reversal by tachykinin neuropeptides. *Science* 1990; 250:279–282.
37. Kowall NW, Boal MF, Busciglio J, Duffy LK, Yankner BA. An *in vivo* model for the neurodegenerative effect of β amyloid and protection by substance P. *Proc Natl Acad Sci USA* 1991;88: 7247–7251.
38. Barrow CJ, Zagorski MG. Solution structures of β peptide and its constituent fragments: relation to amyloid deposition. *Science* 1991;253:179–182.
39. Burdick D, Soreghan B, Kwon M, et al. Assembly and aggregation properties of synthetic Alzheimer's A4/β amyloid peptide analogs. *J Biol Chem* 1992;267:546–554.
40. Hilbich C, Kisters-Woike B, Reed J, Masters CL, Beyreuther K. Aggregation and secondary structure of synthetic amyloid βA4 peptides of Alzheimer's disease. *J Mol Biol* 1991;218:149–163.
41. Masters CL, Multhaup G, Simms G, Rottgiesser J, Martins RN, Beyreuther K. Neuronal origin of a cerebral amyloid: neurofibrillary tangles of Alzheimer's disease contain the same protein as the amyloid of plaque cores and blood vessels. *EMBO J* 1985;4:2757–2763.
42. Selkoe DJ, Abraham CR, Podlisny MB, Duffy LD. Isolation of low molecular-weight proteins from amyloid plaque fibers in Alzheimer's disease. *J Neurochem* 1986;46:1820–1834.
43. Pike CJ, Burdick D, Walencewicz A, Glabe CG, Cotman CW. Neurodegeneration induced by β-amyloid peptides *in vitro:* evidence for a role of peptide aggregation. [submitted].
44. Pike CJ, Walencewicz AJ, Glabe CG, Cotman CW. Aggregation-related toxicity of synthetic β-amyloid protein in hippocampal cultures. *Eur J Pharmacol* 1991;207:367–368.
45. Koh JY, Yang LL, Cotman CW. β-Amyloid protein increases the vulnerability of cultured cortical neurons to excitotoxic damage. *Brain Res* 1990; 533:315–320.
46. Copani A, Koh J, Cotman CW. β-amyloid increases neuronal susceptibility to injury by glucose deprivation. *NeuroReport* 1991;2:763–765.
47. Maragos WF, Greenamyre JT, Penney JB, Young AB. Glutamate dysfunction in Alzheimer's disease: an hypothesis. *Trends Neurosci* 1987;10:65–68.
48. Quon D, Catalano R, Cordell B. Fibroblast growth factor induces beta-amyloid precursor mRNA in glial but not neuronal cultured cells. *Biochem Biophys Res Commun* 1990;167:96–102.
49. Araujo DM, Cotman CW. β-Amyloid stimulates glial cells *in vitro* to produce growth factors that accumulate in senile plaques in Alzheimer's disease. *Brain Res* 1992;569:141–145.
50. Yoshida K, Gage FH. Fibroblast growth factors stimulate nerve growth factor synthesis and secretion by astrocytes. *Brain Res* 1991;538:118–126.
51. Schubert D, Jin L, Saitoh T, Cole G. The regulation of amyloid beta protein precursor secretion and its modulatory role in cell adhesion. *Neuron* 1989; 3:689–694.
52. Klier FG, Cole G, Stallcup W, Schubert D. Amyloid beta-protein precursor is associated with extracellular matrix. *Brain Res* 1990;515:336–342.
53. Schubert D, LaCorbiere M, Saitoh T, Cole G. Characterization of an amyloid beta-precursor protein that binds heparin and contains tyrosine sulfate. *Proc Natl Acad Sci USA* 1989;86:2066–2069.
54. Van Nostrand WE, Wagner SL, Farrow JS, Cunningham DD. Immunopurification and protease inhibitory properties of protease nexin-2/amyloid beta-protein precursor. *J Biol Chem* 1990;265: 9591–9594.
55. Pike CJ, Cummings BJ, Cotman CW. β-amyloid induces neuritic dystrophy *in vitro:* similarities with Alzheimer pathology. [submitted].

Advances in Neurology, Vol. 59, edited by Fredrick J. Seil. Raven Press, Ltd., New York © 1993.

4

Connections Among Plasticity, Regeneration, and Aging at the Neuromuscular Junction

Norman Robbins and Satoshi Nakashiro

Department of Neurosciences, Case Western Reserve University School of Medicine, Cleveland, Ohio 44106

After denervation, regeneration of functional or morphologically intact neuromuscular junctions (NMJs) is altered in old animals. In this chapter, we explore the premise that these alterations, as well as the "spontaneous" morphological instability in nondenervated NMJs, reflect similar cellular and molecular mechanisms. All the work from our laboratory involved use of the CBF-1 mouse, in which locomotor activity does not decline substantially with age (1) and in which there is no evidence for spontaneous loss of motor neurons with age (2,3).

AGE CHANGES IN NEUROMUSCULAR REGENERATION

Many years ago, Gutmann and colleagues (4) found that recovery of motor function after nerve section was delayed in old rats, even though final recovery of function was complete. Later, it was shown that a reduced rate of axonal regeneration might partly or completely account for these findings (5). Another possibility was that reoccupation of the former endplate by the regenerating nerve changed with age. In order to analyze this factor, we carried out a "terminal denervation" by applying black widow spider venom (BWSV) or its purified component, α-latrotoxin, to mouse muscle, thereby rapidly destroying nerve terminals while leaving most preterminal axons intact and minimizing the requirement for axonal regeneration (6). Morphological reoccupation of the nerve terminal and recovery of the indirect muscle twitch was no slower in old than in adult animals and, in fact, in some circumstances, was actually faster. Thus, the reported age-related delay in regeneration after more proximal nerve section, which we also found in the mouse, was caused primarily by slowing of axonal regeneration rather than by a deficit in reoccupation of the endplate by regenerating nerve terminals.

Nonetheless, nerve terminal reoccupation of the denervated endplate in old mice differed in a more subtle way. Because of the short 3- to 5-day interval between terminal destruction and reoccupation, postsynaptic acetylcholine receptors remained to provide an image of the predenervated area of the NMJ. Thus, by use of simultaneous fluorescence staining of regenerating nerve terminals and acetylcholine receptors, we were able to detect sites where the reoccupying nerve grew beyond its original borders (Fig. 1). There were more instances of nerve terminals greatly overshooting the original borders

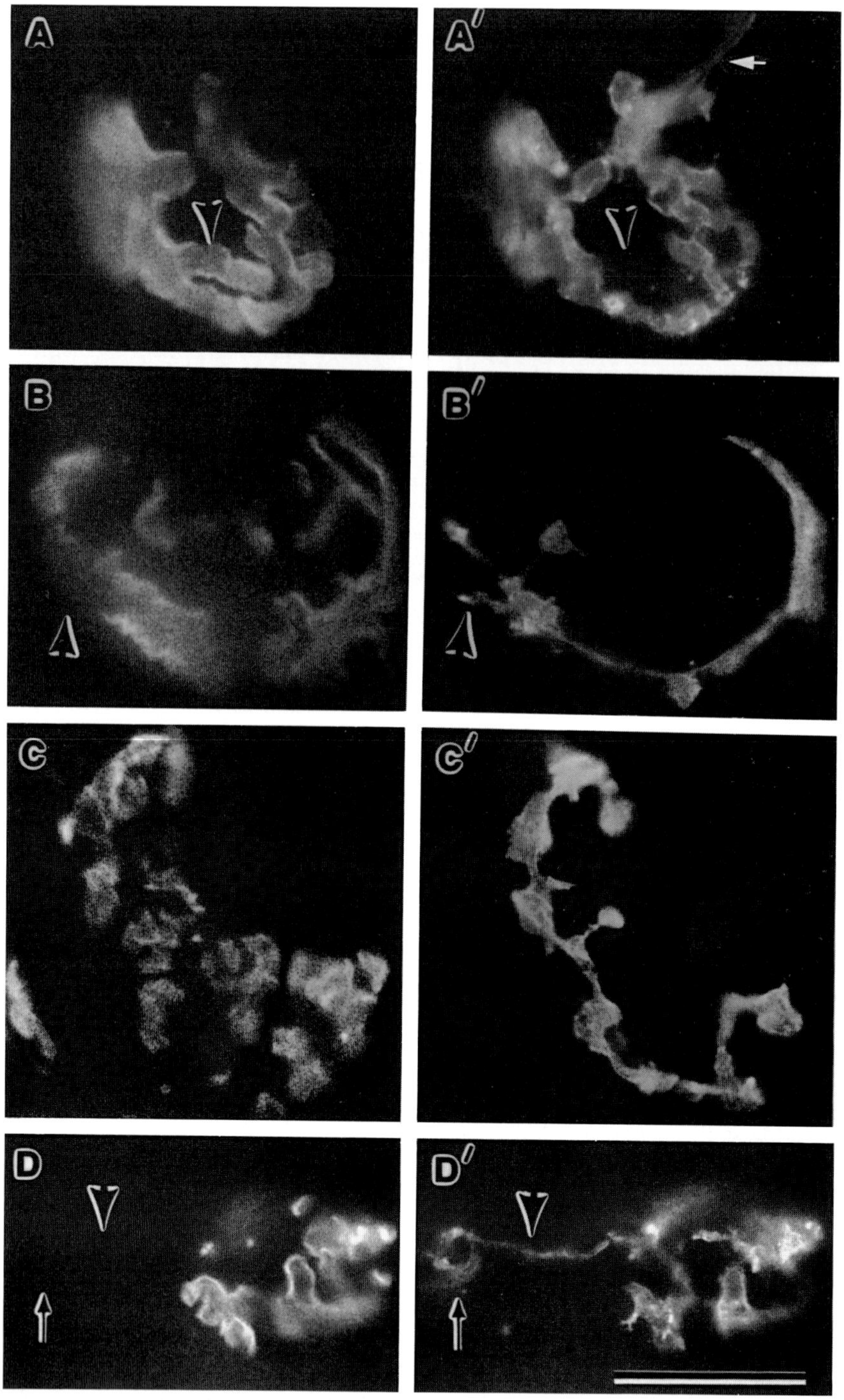

FIG. 1. Soleus neuromuscular junctions of adult (**A, A′, B, B′**) and old (**C, C′, D, D′**) mice showing regeneration of nerve terminals 3 days after destruction by α-latrotoxin or black widow spider venom. Postsynaptic receptors are stained with FITC-α-bungarotoxin (A–D) and corresponding presynaptic terminals with Texas Red-labeled tetanus toxin C-fragment (A′–D′). In A, A′, an almost fully regenerated terminal shows a preterminal axon entering the junction (*arrow*) and also a postsynaptic region lacking reinnervation (*arrowheads*). In other figures, *arrowheads* indicate sites where regenerating nerve terminals grew beyond the previous junctional borders. In D, D′, a long outgrowth (*arrowhead*) forms an elaborate excrescence (*arrow*) with no corresponding postsynaptic sites visible. *Calibration bar,* 25 μm. (Reproduced from Robbins et al., ref. 6, with permission from Pergamon Press.)

in old than in adult mice, and the total number of small and large overshooting sites per junction in old mice was significantly greater than in adults (1.9 sites/100 μm^2 versus 1.1 sites/100 μm^2). Parenthetically, this relative inaccuracy of reinnervation, although not functionally significant at the NMJ, could introduce serious functional disability if the same were true in the central nervous system (CNS). These findings at the NMJ could reflect several age-dependent mechanisms: weaker bonds restraining regenerating nerve terminals to the synaptic matrix, greater adhesion of nerve terminals to perisynaptic structures, or overexpression of sprouting factors or their receptors.

The tendency in old animals toward overgrowth in the process of regeneration was also noted in a study of partial denervation (7). In this case, nodal sprouts of nondenervated motor units in old animals gave rise to exuberant axonal growth and tortuous axonal pathways leading to the reinnervated junctions (Fig. 2). Again, an excess of growth-promoting factors and increased adhesion to nonjunctional surfaces are possible mechanisms.

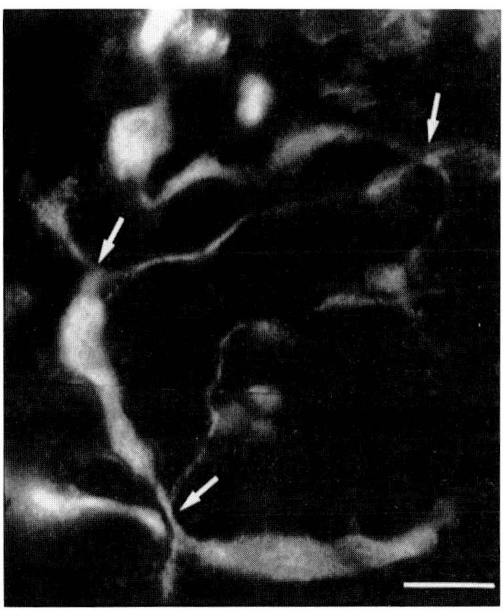

FIG. 2. An example of the tortuous pathways and complex arborizations of presumably regenerated motor axons 60 days after partial denervation of the soleus muscle in an old mouse. Nerve fibers are stained with antibody to neurofilament. *Arrows* indicate presumed nodes of Ranvier. *Calibration bar,* 10 μm. (Reproduced from Jacob and Robbins, ref. 7, with permission from Oxford University Press.)

The partial denervation experiment also revealed that when the motor unit was forced to expand by a factor of 2 to 2.5 through collateral sprouting of remaining neurons to denervated endplates, nerve terminal volume per motor neuron was expanded about 100% in adults but only about 40% in old mice (at 60 days after the partial denervation). The latter was because of the presence of nonreinnervated or incompletely reinnervated endplates. In addition, in old mice the reinnervating axons were often unmyelinated, and correspondingly there was a persistent increase in latency between nerve stimulation and synaptic response (3). These phenomena were attributed to diminished axonal transport in the aged animals.

SYNAPTIC INSTABILITY IN OLD ANIMALS

Are the changes in regeneration observed in old animals totally unexpected, emerging only as sequelae of denervation, or are there similar characteristics in nondenervated NMJs? Several features of the spontaneous structural instability of the NMJ in old mice bear a resemblance to findings during regeneration.

Evidence for instability of NMJ morphology in old animals first emerged from morphological studies that showed, in many species, a reorganization of junctional structure giving rise to a "regionalization" of the nerve terminals [1 (mouse), 8 (rat), 9 (human)] or an altered branch pattern (10,11). Also, electron micrographs of NMJ in old mice showed evidence for nerve terminal outgrowth and retraction within the synaptic groove with no sign of total denervation (12,13). In order to determine whether these changes in structure reflect a slow monotonic process or, alternatively, an ongoing outgrowth and retraction of nerve terminals, we developed fluorescence techniques to follow the structure of individual junctions over time *in vivo* (14).

The most striking findings in identified endplates followed at intervals of 7 or 30 days were a greater incidence in old mice of focal constriction and expansion of nerve terminals, i.e., radial retraction of nerve terminals from synaptic matrix, denuding acetylcholine receptors, or the reverse process of reoccupation of these small denuded sites (15). Recent electron microscopic work using serial sectioning (16) has shown that in both adults and old mice, constrictions actually present a variety of nerve/Schwann/muscle cellular arrangements, even along the length of an individual constriction. These range from a "normal" but small-diameter synapse to probable transitional forms, e.g., reduction in nerve terminal caliber with or without Schwann cell engulfment and with or without reduction in height of postsynaptic folds (a probable sign of longer-term terminal–muscle dissociation). We infer that some sites progress to a morphological situation resembling that of an unmyelinated axon, i.e., complete Schwann cell engulfment, mainly axonal cross-sectional appearance of the nerve terminal, and totally absent postsynaptic folds. At least part of the process involves detachment of the terminal from the synaptic matrix. The same process at other sites in the nerve terminal probably contributes to another major finding in the study of identified NMJs *in vivo,* namely, that nerve terminals in old mice showed greater swings in outgrowth or retraction beyond the synaptic borders between observations.

Thus, nerve terminals in nondenervated, nonregenerating NMJs of old mice behave in ways similar to those found during regeneration: a tendency to overgrowth of nerve terminals to perisynaptic regions, possibly coupled with decreased bonding of the nerve terminals to the synaptic matrix and inability to maintain nerve terminal volume.

POSSIBLE CELLULAR OR MOLECULAR MECHANISMS OF ALTERED REGENERATION AND SYNAPTIC INSTABILITY IN OLD ANIMALS

Neural Cell Adhesion Molecules

Increased adhesiveness of nonsynaptic muscle surface might account both for tortuous exuberant extrajunctional growth of regenerating nerve fibers and also for increased perisynaptic outgrowth of nondenervated nerve terminals. One molecule associated with NMJ adhesion is neural cell adhesion molecule (N-CAM). Elevated levels of N-CAM were found in embryonic and denervated muscle (17), and antibodies to N-CAM interfere with regeneration in the adult (18,19). Recently, we analyzed relative N-CAM abundance in adult and old muscles, comparing age changes in two muscles with histological evidence of synaptic instability (sternomastoid, soleus) and one, the diaphragm, showing no substantial morphological change with age (20). The abundant 140-kD form of muscle N-CAM increased two- to fourfold in old sternomastoid and soleus muscles but stayed unchanged in diaphragm. In the sternomastoid, the most prominent changes were in the endplate region. Possibly because the increase in N-CAM was distributed across all the N-CAM-containing cellular elements, a single cellular locus of increased N-CAM was not detectable by immunohistochemistry. In any event, altered regulation of N-CAM expression in old animals may be one important mechanism affecting both synaptic instability and regeneration. It remains to be determined whether many other adhesion molecules are also overexpressed and whether altered N-CAM expression is primary or secondary to increased NMJ remodelling.

Sprouting Factors

Elevated release of soluble factors stimulating nerve outgrowth in old animals may also account for some of the observations. For instance, it was reported that there was a small but significant increase in cells with neurites in cultures of embryonic chick motor neurons when the cells were exposed to extracts of rat muscle from old rather than adult animals (21). The molecular nature of the growth factors is unknown.

Altered Bonding of Nerve Terminals to Synaptic Matrix

We recently discovered that sites of maximal nerve–matrix adhesion are localized specifically over secondary folds (22). This was demonstrated by subjecting NMJs to hypertonic solutions during fixation, thus shrinking the terminals away from the matrix except at the points of greatest adhesion. These points proved to be long regions of adherence, including but not confined to active zones. A few other specialized sites of adherence were also found at the sides and tips of the terminal branches and at the lateral junctions with Schwann cells. At the nerve–matrix attachment sites over secondary folds, there were small accumulations of actin (detected by ultrastructural immunocytochemistry). However, in old mice, the number of these accumulations and the amount per site were significantly less than in adults. These results raise the possibility that the synaptic and regenerative instability of nerve terminals in old mice may result in part from weakening of these adhesive bonds, whether from altered matrix or instrinsic neuronal factors.

Axonal Transport

As noted above, reduced axonal transport, as described in the rat, might explain incomplete expansion of the motor unit after partial denervation in old mice. The same deficit in a "resting" NMJ, by reducing maintenance of nerve terminal volume, could give rise to the observed greater tendency for withdrawal of terminals at focal sites. Since it is technically difficult to use conventional radioactive injection and timed studies to analyze transport in the mouse, we turned to some less conventional approaches. One, modeled after the work of Dahlstrom and colleagues (e.g., ref. 23), was to mechanically constrict nerves and follow the buildup of a synaptic vesicle protein, synaptophysin (24), proximal to the constriction sites 3 hr later. Using the length of pileup of immunopositive material as an index, we found that synaptophysin accumulation was about 40% less in old than in adult mouse soleus nerve (unpublished observations). The soleus motor nerve was also used for *in vitro* differential interference contrast studies of movement of particles traveling at the average speed of fast transport. Again, the net number of particles moving in a distal direction per unit time was significantly reduced in old mice (unpublished observations). These studies are consistent with the hypothesis that reduced fast axonal transport in old mice may play a role both in the observed tendency to "spontaneous" withdrawal of nerve terminals and in the incomplete reinnervation found after partial denervation.

CONCLUSION

Phenomenological observations of nerve–muscle regeneration and "resting" instability of nerve terminals in old animals show a number of resemblances. It is suggested that these stem from similar cellular or molecular mechanisms. Thus, the increased tendency for nerve outgrowth may result from increased N-CAM (or other adhesive molecule) expression or from greater release of sprouting factors. Incomplete regeneration and tendency to withdrawal from the synaptic matrix may depend on reduced number or strength of intrasynaptic adhesive sites and/or diminished fast axonal transport. The experimental data presented here demonstrate the plausibility of these suggestions. The next, more difficult phase is to provide experimental support.

ACKNOWLEDGMENTS

Supported by grants AG08886 and AG06641 from the National Institute of Aging.

REFERENCES

1. Robbins N, Fahim MA. Progression of age changes in mature mouse motor nerve terminals and its relation to locomotor activity. *J Neurocytol* 1985;14:1019–1036.
2. Banker BQ, Kelly SS, Robbins N. Neuromuscular transmission and correlative morphology in young and old mice. *J Physiol* 1983;239:355–375.
3. Jacob JM, Robbins N. Differential effects of age on neuromuscular transmission in partially denervated mouse muscle. *J Neurosci* 1990;10:1522–1529.
4. Drahota Z, Gutmann E. The influence of age on the course of reinnervation of muscle. *Gerontologia* 1961;5:88–109.
5. Pestronk A, Drachman DB, Griffin JW. Effects of aging on nerve sprouting and regeneration. *Exp Neurol* 1980;70:65–82.
6. Robbins N, Kuchynski M, Polak J, Grasso A. Motor nerve terminal restoration after focal destruction in young and old mice. *Int J Dev Neurosci* 1990;8:667–678.
7. Jacob JM, Robbins N. Age differences in morphology of reinnervation of partially denervated mouse muscle. *J Neurosci* 1990;10:1530–1540.
8. Courtney J, Steinbach JH. Age changes in neuromuscular junction morphology and acetylcholine receptor distribution on rat skeletal muscle fibres. *J Physiol* 1981;320:435–447.
9. Oda K. Age changes of motor innervation and acetylcholine receptor distribution on human skeletal muscle fibers. *J Neurol Sci* 1984;66:327–338.
10. Wernig A, Herrera AA. Sprouting and remodelling at the nerve–muscle junction. *Prog Neurobiol* 1986;27:251–291.
11. Fahim MA, Holley JA, Robbins N. Scanning and light microscopic study of age changes at a neuromuscular junction in the mouse. *J Neurocytol* 1983;12:13–25.
12. Fahim MA, Robbins N. Ultrastructural studies of young and old mouse neuromuscular junction. *J Neurocytol* 1982;11:641–656.
13. Cardasis CA. Ultrastructural evidence of continued reorganization at the aging (11–26 months) rat soleus neuromuscular junction. *Anat Rec* 1983;207:395–415.
14. Hill RR, Robbins N, Fang Zi-P. Plasticity of presynaptic and postsynaptic elements of neuromuscular junctions repeatedly observed in living adult mice. *J Neurocytol* 1991;20:165–182.
15. Robbins N, Hill J, Hill R. Increased plasticity of aging mouse pectineus neuromuscular junctions observed *in vivo*. *Soc Neurosci Abstr* 1990;16:1162.
16. Nakashiro S, Robbins N. New forms of neuromuscular plasticity in adult and old mice revealed by EM serial sectioning. *Soc Neurosci Abstr* 1991;17:876.
17. Sanes JR, Schachner M, Covault J. Expression of several adhesive macromolecules (N-CAM, L1, J1, NILE, uvomorulin, fibronectin, laminin and HSPG) in embryonic, adult and denervated muscle. *J Cell Biol* 1986;102:420–431.
18. Rieger F, Nicolet M, Pincon-Raymond M, Murawsky M, Levi G, Edelman GM. Distribution and role in regeneration of N-CAM in the basal laminae of muscle and Schwann cell. *J Cell Biol* 1988;107:707–719.
19. Booth CM, Kemplay SK, Brown, MC. An antibody to neural cell adhesion molecule impairs motor nerve terminal sprouting in a mouse muscle locally paralyzed with botulinum toxin. *Neuroscience* 1990;35:85–91.
20. Kobayashi H, Robbins N, Rutishauser U. Neural cell adhesion molecule (N-CAM) in aged mouse muscle. *Neuroscience* 1992;48:237–248.
21. Rosenheimer JL, Smith DO. Age-related increase in soluble and cell surface-associated neurite-outgrowth factors from rat muscle. *Brain Res* 1990;509:309–320.
22. Robbins N, Polak J. Focal adhesions of nerve terminal to synaptic matrix and Schwann cell at mouse neuromuscular junctions. *Soc Neurosci Abstr* 1989;15:258.
23. Booj S, Larsson P-A, Dahllof A-G, Dahlstrom A. Axonal transport of synapsin 1- and cholinergic synaptic vesicle-like material; further immunohistochemical evidence for transport of axonal cholinergic transmitter vesicles in motor neurons. *Acta Physiol Scand* 1986;128:155–165.
24. Wiedenmann B, Franke WW. Identification and localization of synaptophysin, an integral membrane glycoprotein of M_r 38,000 characteristic of presynaptic vesicles. *Cell* 1985;41:1017–1028.

Advances in Neurology, Vol. 59, edited by
Fredrick J. Seil. Raven Press, Ltd.,
New York © 1993.

5

The Role and Repair of Forebrain Cholinergic Systems in Short-Term Memory

Studies Using the Delayed Matching-to-Position Task in Rats

Stephen B. Dunnett

Department of Experimental Psychology, University of Cambridge, Cambridge CB2 3EB, England

A variety of experimental manipulations have been employed over the last decade in the search for valid and suitable animal models of dementia, including lesions, toxins, drugs, and the process of aging itself (1). In particular, considerable attention has been given over the last decade to the role of forebrain cholinergic systems in normal learning and memory processes and to their involvement when dysfunctional in the cognitive deficits of dementia, leading to the so-called cholinergic hypothesis of geriatric memory dysfunction (1–7).

The most common research strategy has been to characterize the behavioral deficits resulting within a particular model and relate these to the profile of deficits observed in aged or demented patients. For example, Drachman and Sahakian have drawn systematic comparisons between the profile of functional deficits induced by the anticholinergic drug scopolamine in young subjects and the deficits that develop within the aged population (4). Similar comparisons have been drawn between the behavioral effects in animals of lesions in the basal forebrain that disrupt the cholinergic innervation of the cortex and the cognitive deficits manifested by human patients with dementia (1–3,5–7). These animal studies have typically employed a range of tasks that provide simple challenges of learning and memory function, in particular tasks involving either avoidance or spatial maze-learning paradigms.

Of greater theoretical interest may be the alternative strategy of developing selective behavioral tests that enable specific aspects of an animal's functional capacity to be analyzed in greater detail. This can then be used to evaluate and compare the extent to which different animal models provide valid representations of the human condition. Indeed, several of the maze paradigms, including the Olton radial maze and the Morris water maze, were initially developed to provide detailed analyses of the psychological and neuroanatomical organization of spatial functions in the rat (8,9). However, in subsequent dementia research, these tasks have been used primarily in a screening capacity, to provide simple and convenient indices of behavioral dysfunction following various experimental manipulations, rather than for their powerful analytical features to analyze the functional nature of resulting deficits.

BEHAVIORAL DEFICITS AFTER BASAL FOREBRAIN LESIONS

The analysis of various maze-learning tasks has recently come under particular scrutiny in experimental studies arising from the cholinergic hypothesis of geriatric memory dysfunction. In particular, the issue of whether basal forebrain lesions disturb learning and memory function has been challenged from two distinct perspectives. First, it appears increasingly likely that most neurotoxic lesions of the basal forebrain destroy noncholinergic as well as cholinergic neurons and that the maze-learning deficits induced by such lesions are independent of specific cholinergic damage (10–12). Second, a subset of the deficits may be attributable to cholinergic dysfunction, but these involve impairments in, e.g., conditional discrimination tasks and most probably reflect an attentional deficit, whereas memory and new learning can be completely spared by relatively specific lesions of the cortical cholinergic projection (11,13,14).

The present chapter addresses the second of these two issues, related to functional specificity. In particular, can the development of improved behavioral test paradigms identify more precisely a specific role of central cholinergic systems, and especially the cortical innervation, in memory processes? The first issue, relating to the neurochemical specificity of various basal forebrain lesions, is alluded to here but has been reviewed in detail elsewhere (11).

DMTP/DNMTP: A TASK TO ASSESS RATS' SHORT-TERM MEMORY

In order to address the issue of functional specificity, a number of laboratories have sought to develop better behavioral tests that enable specific aspects of the functional deficit, in particular memory impairments, to be analyzed in greater detail. The most powerful strategy presently available for the characterization of an animal's memory capacity comes from the range of delayed-response tasks that have been most fully developed in the primate literature (15–18). Of these, delayed matching and delayed nonmatching to sample are the most flexible and lend themselves to automated operant test procedures in addition to the conventional hand testing approach in the Wisconsin general test apparatus.

All delayed-response tasks involve presenting an item or items of information to the subject (whether human or animal) at an identified time for recall at some later time. The information may be the location of hidden food (as in conventional delayed-response tests in animals), a list of to-be-remembered words (for human subjects only), or a visually presented object or other nonverbal stimulus (to either humans or other animals) to be subsequently tested for remembrance. In the human literature, a distinction has been made between probing retention of the sample information by recall or by recognition (19). Similarly, recall can be tested in animals' delayed-response tasks by their return to the critical location, but, in the absence of a verbal response, recognition paradigms are more common. In this case, the animal indicates retention of the sample information by choosing from a number of presented alternatives and is rewarded for selecting the same stimulus/object as had been presented as the sample earlier in the trial (in delayed matching to sample) or for selecting the stimulus/object that differs from the sample (in delayed nonmatching to sample) (Fig. 1A and B, respectively).

The essential feature of an effective delayed-response task is that performance accuracy can be evaluated over different delay intervals separating the sample and choice stages of each trial. The decline in performance at increasing delays then indicates the loss or decay of the relevant information from memory. This can be represented graph-

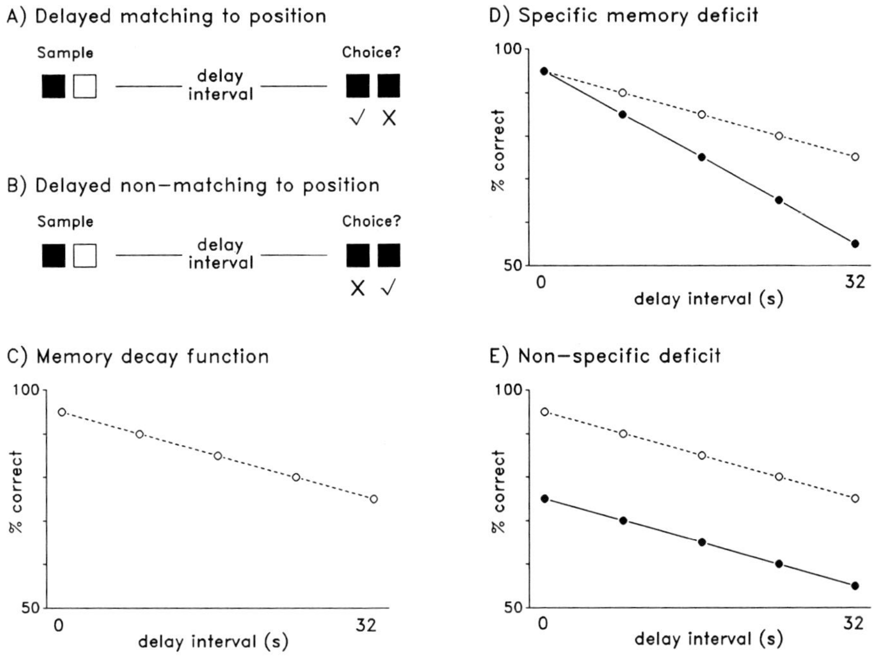

FIG. 1. Schematic representation of the design and alternative outcomes in delayed matching- and nonmatching-to-position tasks. **A:** In the DMTP task for rats, one of two levers is extended into the test chamber (*black*) to denote the sample. When the rat responds, the lever is removed for a variable delay interval, and then both levers are presented. The correct response is to choose the sample lever (*check*), whereas pressing the other lever is punished with time out (*cross*). **B:** In DNMTP, the converse contingencies apply. **C:** Theoretical outcome in a control experiment, in which the memory trace weakens so that the accuracy of performance declines as the delay interval is increased. The slope of the curve indicates the rate of forgetting. **D:** A specific impairment in short-term memory is manifested by an absence of impairment at the shortest delay, but performance declines more rapidly, and the slope of the function is greater, than in the control condition. **E:** A nonspecific impairment is manifested by a disruption of performance at all delays equally. The delayed matching and nonmatching to sample are conceptually similar, other than that the sample is one of two discrete objects rather than one of two positions.

ically in a delay–performance function, the slope of which indicates the rate of forgetting (Fig. 1C). The importance of the memory decay function is that it enables experimental treatments that enhance or disrupt memory specifically to be distinguished from the plethora of manipulations that disturb other nonspecific aspects of performance. Thus, an increase in the slope of the forgetting function indicates a specific impairment in the animal's short-term memory as information is lost more rapidly (Fig. 1D). In this situation, the experimental animal shows normal performance at the shortest delays when the memory load is minimal, which indicates that it has learned the discrimination rule, it can distinguish and is attending to the relevant stimuli, it is motivated to respond, and it has no marked motor impairment or bias that inhibits making the correct response. Conversely, a generalized delay-independent disturbance of performance at all delays (Fig. 1E) indicates a nonspecific impairment, i.e., one that cannot be attributed to a dysfunction in memory *per se,* although, of course, alternative interpretations of the precise nature of the deficit in terms of attention, discrimination learning, motivation, or sensory/motor function cannot be resolved from these results alone. Not surprisingly, most treatments that disturb performance of delayed matching and nonmatching tasks induce delay-independent deficits.

It has proved extremely difficult to train rats in operant versions of delayed matching- and nonmatching-to-sample tasks using visual stimuli, perhaps because of their relative inattention to the visual modality. Therefore, different laboratories have either used maze versions of delayed response and delayed matching tasks with highly distinctive three-dimensional junk objects or goal boxes as the samples (20–22) or modified the operant tasks to produce conditional discrimination tasks with a built in delay component (23), or utilized spatial information as the sample information in delayed matching- and nonmatching-to-position tasks (DMTP/DNMTP) (24,25). The present chapter focuses on the latter task, as developed in the author's laboratory (24,26).

Rats are trained on the DMTP and DNMTP tasks in conventional operant chambers with two retractable levers and central food collection panel (24,26). The essence of the task is that one lever is extended into the chamber as the sample and is then retracted as soon as the rat presses it. After a variable delay (typically between 0 and 64 sec in duration), during which the rat is required to remain in a central position between the two levers, both levers are extended again into the test chamber, and the rat must make a choice response. The rat is rewarded with a food pellet delivered to the central food well if it makes a correct choice by pressing the

TABLE 1. *Delay-dependent and delay-independent effects in the DMTP/DNMTP task*

Delay-dependent effects on STM	Delay-independent effects	No effects on accuracy of task performance
Aging[a]		
Aging[31–33,62]		
Septal grafts in aged HPC[62]	Arecoline in aged rats[31]	Atipamezole in aged rats[33]
Septal grafts in aged PFC[62]	Physostigmine in aged rats[31]	
Lesions[b]		
FF Lesion[24,56,66]	NBM lesion (ibo)[24,26]	NBM lesion (quis)[13,58 c]
Rostral PFC aspiration[66]	Caudal PFC aspiration[66]	Motor cortex aspiration[66]
Nucleus accumbens lesion[66,69]	Caudate-putamen lesion[66]	Parietal cortex aspiration[66]
Anterior thalamus[56]		Mamillary bodies[56]
Trimethyl tin[70]		Dorsal noradrenergic bundle[58]
Drugs		
Clonidine i.p.[34]	Nicotine[47]	Nicotine[34 c]
	Scopolamine[13,24,43–47,55]	Oxotremorine[47]
	Physostigmine[24,34,43]	Physostigmine[24,34,43,46]
	Tacrine[43]	Tacrine[43,46,47]
	Diisopropylfluorophosphate[45]	
Scopolamine in HPC[48]	Scopolamine in PFC[48]	
Arginine-vasopressin[49,50]	Arginine-vasopressin[50]	
Ethanol[52]	Amphetamine[24,53]	
Chlordiazepoxide[52]	Phencyclidine[55 d]	
	Tetrahydrocannabinol[55 d]	
	MK-801[55 d]	
Other		
Cold exposure[71]	Sex differences[44]	Sex differences[25,44]
Intertrial interval[34,70]		
Proactive interference[34]		

[a] Superscript numbers indicate the source reference.
[b] Abbreviations: FF, fimbria-fornix; HPC, hippocampus; ibo, ibotenic acid; NBM, nucleus basalis magnocellularis; PFC, prefrontal cortex; quis, quisqualic acid; STM, short-term memory.
[c] Although these treatments did not influence basic task performance, they did have effects on task acquisition or susceptibility to interference.
[d] The study by Yamamoto et al. (55) reports dose-related deficits but does not indicate whether the deficits are delay-dependent or delay-independent.

sample lever (in DMTP) or the opposite lever (in DNMTP), whereas the converse response is punished by a "time-out" period during which the chamber lights are switched off.

Rats are trained on either the DMTP or the DNMTP version of the task. They first learn the discrimination rule without delays, which is generally achieved within 1 to 2 weeks of daily training sessions. They are then switched to a range of random delay intervals and trained until they reach an asymptotic level of performance, which generally requires a further 4 to 6 weeks of training. Although the rate of acquisition of the task is informative about the animals' general learning abilities (13), the most valuable data are provided by the memory decay functions obtained once the animals have reached asymptote. These provide the data both for evaluating changes in short-term memory and forgetting and for testing the effects of drugs or other manipulations against a stable base line.

COMPARISON OF ALTERNATIVE ANIMAL MODELS

Delayed matching-to-sample tasks have been found to provide sensitive measures of the onset of memory problems in human aging and dementia. Thus, old humans and monkeys show mild deficits even in the absence of overt neuropathology or dementia (27,28), and more profound deficits are apparent in patients newly diagnosed for dementia of the Alzheimer type (28–30). It is notable that in each case the deficits were found to be delay dependent, indicating that the impairments in aging and the early stages of dementia are caused by a relatively selective problem with short-term memory as distinct from a more generalized cognitive impairment.

Such deficits in the human condition provide good face validity for the use in animals of the DMTP and DNMTP tasks to evaluate and compare different models of aging and dementia. The results of such experiments provide the primary topic of the present chapter and are summarized in Table 1.

Aging Effects on DMTP/DNMTP

The simplest test of validity of the DMTP/DNMTP task is: do old rats show comparable delay-dependent deficits to those seen in old primates and humans? They do. In the first test of this question, separate groups of rats of three different ages—6 months, 15 months, and 24 months—were compared on both DMTP and DNMTP (31). The 24-month groups were impaired with respect to 6-month groups on both versions of the task, whereas the 15-month groups were impaired only when tested on DMTP but not when tested on DNMTP. Thus, the DMTP task appeared to be more sensitive to early deficits. However, the DNMTP task was found to be more reliable, to show more consistent gradients of acquisition between rats, and to have the lower variance at asymptotic levels of performance within each group (31). Therefore, the DNMTP task may be considered to be the more reliable test for further studies of aging effects. The delay-dependent deficit in aged rats has been replicated several times (32,33).

The delay-dependent effects of old animals are akin to the delay-dependent decline in performance that results from proactive interference from previous trials when the intertrial intervals are short (34). It is therefore plausible to ask: is the deficit in old rats attributable to an increased susceptibility to interference from previous trials? Old rats do show proactive interference effects, and the decline in performance from interference is greater in absolute magnitude at long delays than is seen in young rats (32). However, this difference turns out to be caused by scaling effects resulting from measuring the changes in performance of young and old rats on interference trials against different baselines. Conversely, when the baseline levels of performance of the young and old rats are equated by testing the two groups over different ranges of delay intervals, then the susceptibility of the two groups to interference from the previous trials is found to be directly comparable (32). Thus, old animals are susceptible to proactive interference, but to the same degree as young animals. Consequently, interference processes cannot readily account for the more rapid forgetting of old rats in standard versions of the task. Having experimentally excluded an explanation in terms of interference effects, it appears more plausible that the deficit in aging is indeed attributable directly to a more rapid decay of the hypothesized short-term trace.

The next issue is to ask whether the delay-dependent deficits in aged rats have a cholinergic substrate. As a first approach to this issue, we can ask: can cholinergic drugs alleviate the deficit in old rats? Such a possibility is suggested by the report of Bartus and colleagues that the deficits of old rats in simple avoidance tasks can be alleviated by various cholinomimetic treatments, including the muscarinic agonist arecoline and the cholinesterase inhibitor physostigmine (35). However, the efficacy of such treatments on delayed-matching tasks is more controversial. Bartus has reported that physostigmine can alleviate delayed response deficits in monkeys (36). However, in patients, the cholinesterase inhibitor tacrine was found to benefit simpler rule learning but not delayed matching-to-sample performance, and the effects were attributed to changes in attentional rather than mnemonic function (37). In agreement with these latter results, it was not possible to identify any dose of either arecoline or physostigmine that would improve the performance of either young, middle-aged, or old rats in either the DMTP task or the DNMTP task, whereas higher doses of arecoline further impaired performance below the untreated or saline-treated levels (31). Similarly, Sirvio et al. (33) reported that another cholinesterase inhibitor, atipamezole, also had no effect on the delay-dependent deficit of aged rats.

Drug Effects on DMTP/DNMTP

Until recently, relatively few drugs had been evaluated in the DMTP/DNMTP task, but the range is increasing rapidly (see Table 1), in particular now that the task is being adopted in a number of pharmaceutical screening programs.

It is well established that anticholinergic drugs can disrupt performance on a wide range of learning and memory tests (2–4, 38–40), although it appears likely that the deficits are attributable to disturbances of discrimination or attentional function as opposed to a specifically mnemonic impairment (40–42). In agreement with this perspective, the muscarinic antagonist scopolamine produces a generalized disruption of both DMTP and DNMTP (13,24,43,44) that can be as great at short delays when the memory load is minimal as at long delays. Administration of various cholinomimetic drugs has generally either been found to be without effect or to further impair performance when administered at higher doses (24,43,45–47). Although one study has reported that moderate doses of physostigmine or of the newer cholinesterase inhibitor tacrine can block the delay-independent deficits induced by scopolamine (43), a second group has failed to find any benefit with these same compounds (46; D. C. Rogers, personal communication).

Nevertheless, since any anticholinergic drug will influence all forebrain cholinergic systems, the observation of delay-independent deficits following scopolamine treatment cannot rule out the possibility that some central cholinergic neurons are involved in the modulation of memory functions. Rather, it may be that specific delay-dependent effects are masked by additional nonspecific actions of the drugs on other systems. Indeed, in a number of studies, it has appeared that the deficits in choice accuracy under scopolamine become greater at the longer delay intervals, even if a significant deficit is also observed at the shorter delays (13).

In order to test this hypothesis, cannulae were implanted directly into the anterior cingulate cortex and hippocampus of pretrained rats. Injections of scopolamine into the hippocampus produced a dose- and delay-independent deficit in short-term memory, suggesting that this system is indeed involved in the regulation of short-term memory function, although the response to cingulate injections was more ambiguous (48).

The matching task has proved particularly powerful for disentangling the influence of proposed memory-enhancing drugs such as vasopressin on actual memory performance in rats. In a detailed series of analyses, Sahgal and colleagues (49,50) have confirmed an apparent improvement of delay-dependent performance on the delayed-matching version of the task. However, the counterintuitive result was that the same drug treatments impaired performance on the nonmatching contingency (50). The discrepancy was resolved by observing that arginine-vasopressin induced a marked shift in animals' response biases in the task, which interacted with the limited hold design employed in this series of studies. The effect of a side bias in the drugged rats on DMTP was that they had an increased chance of a correct guess on the side to which the drug induced a bias, whereas they failed to respond on the other side, which, although registered as an increased number of omissions, was not included in the percentage correct analysis. Conversely, the drug-induced bias worked against correct responding in the DNMTP task. This study revealed the utility of a variety of additional parameters based on signal detection theory in the analysis of DMTP/DNMTP performance and cautions against exclusive reliance on a percentage correct analysis (51). Related developments based on signal detection analysis have been proposed by Melia et al. (52) and by Kirk et al. (23).

The influence of other classes of drugs on DMTP/DNMTP is as yet still largely unexplored in any detail. Several studies have indicated that amphetamine induces a generalized delay-independent disruption of performance by virtue of changes in response bias (24,53). Conversely, one report suggests that both the anxiolytic drug chlordiazepoxide and low doses of ethanol can enhance choice accuracy (52). This study used a negative exponential decay analysis to model the forgetting function (54) and confirmed that the enhancement in performance by both drugs was attributable to a reduction in the decay constant rather than to any change in response bias (52). A further study has investigated the effects of other rewarding drugs on DMTP performance, including drugs of abuse such as phencyclidine and tetrahydrocannabinol, but although these were both found to disrupt performance, the results were not reported in sufficient detail to determine whether the impairments were specific or nonspecific (55).

Lesion Effects on DMTP/DNMTP

As with the pharmacological studies, the first studies of the effects of circumscribed central nervous system lesions on DMTP/DNMTP evaluated the effects of damage in the central cholinergic systems projecting to the hippocampus and neocortex (24). Whereas damage in both systems produced deficits in the performance by pretrained rats on the DMTP task, the memory decay function of the deficit was quite different in the two cases. The fimbria–fornix lesions, which transected the cholinergic projections to the hippocampus, produced a delay-dependent deficit in short-term memory. This pattern of deficit is compatible with the long-established human and primate literature on the effects of temporal lobe damage (17,18,57), indicating a role for the hippocampus in learning and memory, including delayed matching-to-sample performance. By contrast, ibotenic acid lesions of the basal forebrain, which destroyed the cortically projecting cholinergic neurons of the nucleus basalis magnocellularis (NBM), induced an initial delay-independent deficit that recovered over a period of approximately 2 weeks' further training (24). Thus, the contribution of neocortical cholinergic systems suggested by the cholinergic hypothesis in its simplest form appeared to be relatively nonspecific rather than subserving short-term memory function *per se.*

Nevertheless, neither of these lesion paradigms is neuroanatomically specific. In the case of the fimbria–fornix lesion, this destroys all subcortical afferents to the hippocampus, including noradrenergic, serotoninergic, and GABAergic projections in addition to the cholinergic projections, as well as the main subcortical efferent projections back to the septum, diencephalon, and midbrain. A contribution of this latter component to the deficit is suggested by the fact that lesions in the anterior thalamus, a major subcortical target of the hippocampus, produce similar delay-dependent deficits in DNMTP to those induced by fimbria lesions themselves (58). However, the particular involvement of the cholinergic innervation in modulating short-term memory function in the hippocampus is suggested by the duplication of the delay-dependent deficit by selective cholinergic blockade following central injection of scopolamine directly into this target structure (48).

The situation with regard to the NBM cholinergic projections to the neocortex is more confused. Following the initial demonstration of delay-independent deficits caused by ibotenic acid lesions of the NBM, two subsequent studies have used a more selective toxin, quisqualic acid. Although this latter toxin produces greater depletions of cholinergic activity in the neocortex, it induces less widespread cell damage than ibotenic acid and fewer general neurological impairments in the lesioned animals (10,11). Quisqualic acid lesions of the basal forebrain were found to produce either small or no detectable deficit in performance of both the DMTP and DNMTP tasks, indicating that the large deficit induced by ibotenic acid lesions was probably not attributable to disturbance of cholinergic systems at all (13,58). However, although quisqualic acid lesions produced no deficit in pretrained rats, they did induce a pronounced but circumscribed deficit in the animals' abilities to learn the nonmatching discrimination rule, both during acquisition learning and during reversal of the task contingencies from matching to nonmatching (13). This suggests that the animals' deficits do not involve a specific impairment in mnemonic function but rather reflect a difficulty in conditional discrimination learning, perhaps resulting from an underlying impairment in selective attention (11).

REPAIR OF CORTICAL CHOLINERGIC SYSTEMS

A major motivation for the development of the cholinergic hypothesis lay in the possibility of providing a rational basis for the development of novel therapeutic strategies based on selective neurotransmitter replacement. This has been developed most extensively in terms of the active search for novel pharmaceutical compounds with more selective cholinomimetic activity. The limited efficacy of various cholinomimetic treatments to reverse deficits induced by aging or antimuscarinic drugs in the DMTP/DNMTP task has already been referred to above.

Graft Effects in Lesioned Rats

There is now an extensive literature indicating that grafts rich in cholinergic neurons, derived from the embryonic septum, can alleviate functional deficits on a range of simple avoidance and maze-learning tasks that are sensitive to central cholinergic lesions (59). Thus, for example, ibotenic acid lesions of the basal forebrain impair passive avoidance learning and retention and spatial navigation in the Morris water maze (60) in addition to the deficits in DMTP described above. Cholinergic-rich septal grafts (but not control grafts of hippocampal tissue) implanted into the neocortex of the basal-forebrain-lesioned rats ameliorate both the retention deficits and the precision of the animals' search for the escape platform determined on probe trials in the water maze (60).

Although several experiments have been conducted to evaluate the efficacy of similar grafts in the DMTP and DNMTP tasks (26; S. B. Dunnett, unpublished data), the results have so far been disappointing. Thus, significant delay-independent deficits induced by basal forebrain lesions can be reversed by cholinergic grafts implanted in multiple cortical sites (26). However, in the NBM-cortical model system, the deficits made by quisqualic acid lesions are small, and they are not specifically mnemonic. Of more interest in any model investigating the role of central cholinergic systems in memory deficits would be restitution of the fimbria–fornix lesion deficit, in view of the delay-dependent nature of the deficit involved in this latter lesion model. However, in three separate studies of the effects of cholinergic and noncholinergic grafts implanted in the hippocampus of such animals, the delay-dependent deficits that are observed in the DMTP/DNMTP task when tested immediately after making fimbria–fornix lesions have been found to recover over a period of 2 to 4 months. Since this length of time is necessary to allow the grafts to become established and form extensive connections with the host brain, there have been no residual deficits when the grafted animals come to testing, even though the lesioned animals remain impaired on other operant tasks that are responsive to the same graft treatments (61).

Graft Effects in Aged Rats

The efficacy of grafts in aged rats has been more encouraging. Thus, the delay-dependent deficit in aged rats in the DNMTP task has been replicated and can be reduced significantly following implantation of cholinergic-rich grafts in either the neocortex or in the hippocampus (62). Although the benefit was somewhat greater following implantation in the hippocampus, the effects in the cortical implantation site were also found to be significant.

However, the benefit was only partial in either site. Several alternative strategies may be possible to increase the level of benefit. First, a more extensive recovery may be achieved by combining the cortical and hippocampal placements in the same animal, a strategy that has been found to benefit radial maze learning in rats with cholinergic cell damage from alcohol intoxication (63). Second, it may be that the efficacy of cholinergic grafts is promoted by cotransplantation with serotoninergic tissues, which has proved an effective way of enhancing recovery in the Morris water maze task by rats with septal lesions (64). Third, it is likely that other cortical/hippocampal systems are also implicated in the maintenance of normal learning and memory function and might also be susceptible to graft-derived ameliorations in aged animals. In particular, the involvement of noradrenergic systems in age-related deficits has been suggested by the demonstration that embryonic locus coeruleus grafts in the hippocampus can alleviate passive avoidance deficits in aged rats (65). In fact, it is likely that each of these alternative strategies will be found to contribute to the profile of deficits manifested by different individual aged animals.

ROLE OF CORTICAL CHOLINERGIC SYSTEMS IN SHORT-TERM MEMORY

There is an apparent contradiction in the studies of the effects of grafts on the DNMTP performance of aged animals. How can a graft of cholinergic tissues implanted in the neocortex ameliorate delay-dependent deficits in the DNMTP task if selective (i.e., quisqualate) lesions of the cortical cholinergic innervation arising in the NBM do not produce deficits in this same task? The resolution appears to relate to a mismatch between the cortical areas into which the grafts are placed and the topography of the denervation induced by basal forebrain lesions (66). It turns out that the studies in which a good functional response was observed in the old animals (62) included grafts implanted into the prefrontal/cingulate areas in the medial wall of the neocortex as well as implants in the frontoparietal areas of the dorsolateral neocortex. By contrast, basal forebrain lesions destroy the cholinergic innervation of the whole dorsolateral neocortical mantle but spare the innervation of the medial and orbital prefrontal and cingulate areas. It is just these prefrontal zones that might be predicted *a priori* to be critical in the performance of complex learning and memory tasks (67,68).

Thus, the apparent contradiction can be resolved by proposing the following multistage hypothesis (66):

1. The medial prefrontal cortex is the critical cortical area involved in normal short-term memory performance, as assessed by DMTP/DNMTP and related tasks.
2. The functional decline of cholinergic innervation of the medial prefrontal cortex contributes to the age-related deficit in short-term memory performance.
3. The alleviation of short-term memory deficits by cholinergic grafts is attributable to reinnervation in the medial prefrontal cortex rather than of other dorsolateral cortical areas.
4. Basal forebrain lesions that remove the cholinergic innervation of the neocortex relatively selectively (e.g., using quisqualic acid) fail to induce short-term memory deficits because they fail to destroy the circumscribed cholinergic projection to the critical medial prefrontal area.
5. The deficits induced by nonspecific basal forebrain lesions (e.g., ibotenic acid), if not caused by destruction of cortical cholinergic projections, may instead be attributable to collateral damage of the descending efferent projections of the prefrontal cortex passing via the nucleus accumbens and ventral pallidum/substantia innominata area in the basal forebrain.

Several lesion experiments have been conducted to test this hypothesis. First, aspirative lesions of the medial frontal cortex, like transection lesions of the fimbria–fornix, do disrupt rats' performance of the DNMTP task. In particular, the medial wall area of the frontal cortex can be subdivided into a prefrontal zone, in which damage induces a selective delay-dependent deficit in short-term memory, and an anterior cingulate zone, in which damage induces a more generalized delay-independent deficit (66). Second, aspirative lesions of the frontoparietal motor cortex or of the parietal cortex, which are both in the dorsolateral areas influenced by basal forebrain lesions, are each without any detectable effect on DNMTP performance (66). Third, the cholinergic selectivity of this involvement of the medial frontal cortex was confirmed by reproduction of the deficits following injection of the muscarinic antagonist scopolamine directly into this area, although the separation of two distinct subdivisions was not replicated in this preliminary central injection study (48). Finally, the involvement of the ventral pallidal outflow system in the deficits associated with nonspecific basal forebrain lesions was corroborated by the demonstration that lesions in the first stages of the prefrontal and anterior cingulate cortical outputs to the nucleus accumbens and medial caudate nucleus resulted in delay-dependent and delay-independent deficits in DNMTP, respectively (66,69).

CONCLUSION

Our understanding of the role and the possibilities of repair of cortical cholinergic systems in dementia have progressed through several stages. The hypothesis was initially greeted with great optimism, opening the way for developing novel therapies based on rational principles. However, this new theoretical framework was not followed by dramatic breakthroughs in treatment, and the pendulum swung the other way toward a period of marked scepticism. It seemed that the cholinergic hypothesis was based on secondary or nonspecific phenomena at both the neuropathological and functional levels, and the only way forward would be through the new advances in the molecular biological analysis of the classical cortical neuropathology—the plaques and tangles of Alzheimer disease. However, it now appears that when subjected to a more careful analysis, the cholinergic systems do appear to contribute to the regulation of complex cortical function, and that cholinergic dysfunction can result in circumscribed impairments in cognition, learning, and memory. Although, it is unlikely that cholinergic deterioration is the primary neuropathological event, nor is it central to the neuropsychological deficit, in most cases of dementia, including dementia of the Alzheimer type, it may nevertheless contribute to the more modest deficits in normal aging. Moreover, cholinergic decline may contribute to the dementia in certain diseases, such as parkinsonism, where the degenerative neuropathology in the basal forebrain cholinergic neurons takes place in the absence of apparent widespread cortical degeneration.

ACKNOWLEDGMENTS

I thank Linda Hoag, Fran Martel, Anne Wareham, TracyAnn Perry, Derek Rogers, and Eduardo Torres, who have all provided skilled research assistance in the experimental studies using the DMTP/DNMTP task. The studies have been funded by the Mental Health Foundation and the Medical Research Council.

REFERENCES

1. Dunnett SB, Barth TM. Animal models of Alzheimer's disease and dementia (with an emphasis on cortical cholinergic systems). In: Willner P, ed. *Behavioural models in psychopharmacology.* London: Cambridge University Press, 1991:359–418.
2. Bartus RT, Dean RL, Beer B, Lippa AS. The cholinergic hypothesis of geriatric memory dysfunction. *Science* 1982;217:408–417.
3. Coyle JT, Price DL, DeLong MR. Alzheimer's disease: a disorder of cortical cholinergic innervation. *Science* 1983;219:1184–1190.
4. Drachman DA, Sahakian BJ. Memory, aging and pharmacosystems. In: Stein D, ed. *The psychobiology of aging: problems and perspectives.* Amsterdam: Elsevier; 1980;347–368.
5. Smith G. Animal models of Alzheimer's disease: experimental cholinergic denervation. *Brain Res Rev* 1988;13:103–118.
6. Wenk GL, Olton DS. Basal forebrain cholinergic neurons and Alzheimer's disease. In: Coyle JT, ed. *Animal models of dementia: a synaptic neurochemical perspective.* New York: Alan R Liss; 1987: 81–101.
7. Collerton D. Cholinergic function and intellectual decline in Alzheimer's disease. *Neuroscience* 1986;19:1–28.
8. Morris RGM. Spatial localisation does not require the presence of local cues. *Learn Motiv* 1981; 12:239–260.
9. Olton DS, Becker JT, Handelmann GE. Hippocampus, space and memory. *Behav Brain Sci* 1979; 2:313–365.
10. Dunnett SB, Whishaw IQ, Jones GH, Bunch ST. Behavioural, biochemical and histochemical effects of different neurotoxic amino acids injected into nucleus basalis magnocellularis of rats. *Neuroscience* 1987;20:653–669.
11. Dunnett SB, Everitt BJ, Robbins TW. The basal forebrain–cortical cholinergic system: interpreting the functional consequences of excitotoxic lesions. *Trends Neurosci* 1991;14:494–501.
12. Everitt BJ, Robbins TW, Evenden JL, Marston HM, Jones GH, Sirkiä TE. The effects of excitotoxic lesions of the substantia innominata, ventral and dorsal globus pallidus on the acquisition and retention of a conditional visual discrimination: implications for cholinergic hypotheses of learning and memory. *Neuroscience* 1987;22:441–469.
13. Dunnett SB, Rogers DC, Jones GH. Effects of nucleus basalis magnocellularis lesions on delayed matching and non-matching to position tasks: disruption of conditional discrimination learning but not of short-term memory. *Eur J Neurosci* 1989;1:395–406.
14. Robbins TW, Everitt BJ, Marston HM, Wilkinson J, Jones GH, Page KJ. Comparative effects of ibotenic acid- and quisqualic acid-induced lesions of the substantia innominata on attentional function in the rat: further implications for the role of the cholinergic neurons of the nucleus basalis in cognitive processes. *Behav Brain Res* 1989;35:221–241.
15. D'Amato MR. Delayed matching and short-term memory in monkeys. *Psychol Learn Motiv* 1973;7:227–269.
16. Jarrard LE, Moise SL. Short-term memory in the monkey. In: Jarrard LE, ed. *Cognitive processes of nonhuman primates.* New York: Academic Press; 1971:1–24.

17. Mishkin M. A memory system in the monkey. *Phil Trans R Soc Lond B* 1982;298:85–95.
18. Zola-Morgan S, Squire LR, Mishkin M. The neuroanatomy of amnesia: amygdala–hippocampus vs temporal stem. *Science* 1982;218:1337–1339.
19. Warrington EK. Neurological disorders of memory. *Br Med Bull* 1971;27:243–247.
20. Aggleton JP. One-trial object recognition by rats. *Q J Exp Psychol* 1985;37B:279–294.
21. Roitblat HL, Harley HE. Spatial delayed matching-to-sample performance in rats: learning, memory and proactive interference. *J Exp Psychol Anim Behav Proc* 1988;14:71–82.
22. Rothblat LA, Hayes LL. Short-term object recognition memory in the rat: nonmatching with trial—unique junk objects. *Behav Neurosci* 1987;101: 587–590.
23. Kirk RC, White KG, McNaughton N. Low dose scopolamine affects discriminability but not rate of forgetting in delayed conditional discrimination. *Psychopharmacology* 1988;96:541–546.
24. Dunnett SB. Comparative effects of cholinergic drugs and lesions of nucleus basalis or fimbria–fornix on delayed matching in rats. *Psychopharmacology* 1985;87:357–363.
25. van Haaren F, van Hest A. Spatial matching and non-matching in male and female Wistar rats: effects of delay-interval duration. *Anim Learn Behav* 1989;17:355–360.
26. Dunnett SB. Anatomical and behavioural consequences of cholinergic-rich grafts to the neocortex of rats with lesions of the nucleus basalis magnocellularis. *Ann NY Acad Sci* 1987;495:415–430.
27. Bartus RT, Fleming D, Johnson HR. Aging in the rhesus monkey: debilitating effects on short-term memory. *J Gerontol* 1978;33:858–871.
28. Flicker C, Ferris SF, Bartus RT, Crook T. Effects of aging and dementia upon recent visuo-spatial memory. *Neurobiol Aging* 1984;5:75–83.
29. Irle E, Kessler J, Markowitsch HJ. Primate learning tasks reveal strong impairments in patients with presenile or senile dementia of the Alzheimer type. *Brain Cognition* 1987;6:429–449.
30. Sahakian BJ, Morris RG, Evenden JL, et al. A comparative study of visuospatial memory and learning in Alzheimer-type dementia and Parkinson's disease. *Brain* 1988;111:695–718.
31. Dunnett SB, Evenden JL, Iversen SD. Delay-dependent short-term memory impairments in aged rats. *Psychopharmacology* 1988;96:174–180.
32. Dunnett SB, Martel F, Iversen SD. Proactive interference effects on short-term memory in rats. II. Effects in young and aged rats. *Behav Neurosci* 1990;104:666–670.
33. Sirvio J, Lukkarinen K, Riekkinen P, et al. The effects of atipamezole, an alpha-2 antagonist, on the performance of young and aged rats in the delayed non-matching to position task. *Pharmacol Biochem Behav* 39:1991;1015–1019.
34. Dunnett SB, Martel FL. Proactive interference effects on short-term memory in rats. I. Basic parameters and drug effects. *Behav Neurosci* 1990; 104:655–665.
35. Bartus RT, Flicker C, Dean RL. Logical principles for the development of animal models of age-related memory impairments. In: Crook T, Ferris S, Bartus R, eds. *Assessment in geriatric psychopharmacology.* New Canaan: Mark Powley Associates; 1983: 263–299.
36. Bartus RT. Physostigmine and recent memory: effects in young and aged nonhuman primates. *Science* 1979;206:1087–1089.
37. Eagger SA, Levy R, Sahakian BJ. Tacrine in Alzheimer's disease. *Lancet* 1991;337:989–992.
38. Deutsch JA. The cholinergic synapse and the site of memory. *Science* 1971;174:788–794.
39. Hagan JJ, Morris RGM. The cholinergic hypothesis of memory: a review of animal experiments. In: Iversen LL, Iversen SD, Snyder SH, eds. *Handbook of psychopharmacology, Vol 20, Psychopharmacology of the aging nervous system.* New York: Plenum Press; 1988:237–323.
40. Sahakian BJ. Cholinergic drugs and human cognitive performance. In: Iversen LL, Iversen SD, Snyder SH, eds. *Handbook of psychopharmacology, Vol 20, Psychopharmacology of the aging nervous system.* New York: Plenum Press; 1988:393–424.
41. Heise GA. Discrete trial analysis of drug action. *Fed Proc* 1975;34:1898–1903.
42. Warburton DM. The effects of scopolamine on a two-cue discrimination. *Q J Exp Psychol* 1974; 26:395–404.
43. Murray TK, Cross AJ, Green AR. Reversal by tetrahydroaminoacridine of scopolamine-induced memory and performance deficits in rats. *Psychopharmacology* 1991;105:134–136.
44. van Hest A, Stroet J, van Haaren F, Feenstra M. Scopolamine differentially disrupts the behavior of male and female Wistar rats in a delayed non-matching to position procedure. *Pharmacol Biochem Behav* 1990;35:903–909.
45. Bushnell PJ, Padilla SS, Ward T, Pape CN, Olszyk VB. Behavioral and neurochemical changes in rats dosed repeatedly with diisopropylfluorophosphate. *J Pharmacol Exp Ther* 1991;256:741–750.
46. Rogers DC, Ballard TM, Hunter AJ, Hill RG. Comparison of the effects of scopolamine and tacrine in the Morris water maze and delayed non-matching to sample task. *Psychopharmacology* 1990;101:186.
47. Sahgal A, Keith AB, Lloyd S. Effects of nicotine, oxotremorine and 9-amino 1,2,3,4-tetrahydroacridine (tacrine) on matching and non-matching to position in rats: no evidence for mnemonic enhancement. *J Psychopharmacol* 1990;4:210–218.
48. Dunnett SB, Wareham AT, Torres EM. Cholinergic blockade in prefrontal cortex and hippocampus disrupts short-term memory in rats. *NeuroReport* 1990;1:61–64.
49. Sahgal A. Contrasting effects of vasopressin, desglycinamide-vasopressin and amphetamine on a delayed matching to position task in rats. *Psychopharmacology* 1987;93:243–249.
50. Sahgal A, Keith AB, Lloyd S. Opposing effects of vasopressin on matching versus nonmatching to position: further evidence for response, not memory, modulation. *Psychopharmacology* 1990;102:130–135.
51. Sahgal A. Some limitations of indices derived from signal detection theory: evaluation of an alternative index for measuring bias in memory tasks. *Psychopharmacology* 1987;91:517–520.

52. Melia KF, Koob GF, Ehlers CL. Ethanol effects on delayed spatial matching as modeled by a negative exponential forgetting function. *Psychopharmacology* 1990;102:391–398.
53. Reading PJ, Dunnett SB. Response disinhibition on a delayed matching to position task induced by amphetamine, nicotine and age. *Psychopharmacology* 1991;104:137–139.
54. White KG. Characteristics of forgetting functions in delayed matching to sample. *J Exp Anal Behav* 1985;44:15–34.
55. Yamamoto T, Hironaka K, Ueki S. Learning and memory in rats with delayed matching to lever location procedures. *Eur J Pharmacol* 1990;183: 2359–2360.
56. Aggleton JP, Keith AB, Sahgal A. Both fornix and anterior thalamic, but not mammillary, lesions disrupt delayed non-matching to position memory in rats. *Behav Brain Res* 1991;44:151–161.
57. Milner B. Memory and the medial temporal regions of the brain. In Pribram KH, Broadbent DE, eds. *Biology of memory*. New York: Academic Press; 1970:29–50.
58. Sahgal A, Keith AB, Lloyd S, Kerwin JM, Perry EK, Edwardson JA. Memory following cholinergic (NBM) and noradrenergic (DNAB) lesions made singly or in combination—potentiation of disruption by scopolamine. *Pharmacol Biochem Behav* 1990; 37:597–605.
59. Dunnett SB. Cholinergic grafts, aging and memory in rats. *Trends Neurosci* 1991;14:371–376.
60. Dunnett SB, Toniolo G, Fine A, Ryan CN, Björklund A, Iversen SD. Transplantation of embryonic ventral forebrain neurons to the neocortex of rats with lesions of nucleus basalis magnocellularis. II. Sensorimotor and learning impairments. *Neuroscience* 1985;16:787–797.
61. Dunnett SB, Martel FL, Rogers DC, Finger S. Factors affecting septal graft amelioration of differential reinforcement of low rates (DRL) and activity deficits after fimbria–fornix lesions. *Restor Neurol Neurosci* 1989;1:83–92.
62. Dunnett SB, Badman F, Rogers DC, Evenden JL, Iversen SD. Cholinergic grafts in the neocortex or hippocampus of aged rats: reduction of delay-dependent deficits in the delayed non-matching to position task. *Exp Neurol* 1988;102:57–64.
63. Arendt T, Allen Y, Sinden J, et al. Cholinergic-rich brain transplants reverse alcohol-induced memory deficits. *Nature* 1988;332:448–450.
64. Nilsson OG, Brundin P, Björklund A. Amelioration of spatial memory impairment by intrahippocampal grafts of mixed septal and raphe tissue in rats with combined cholinergic and serotonergic denervation of the forebrain. *Brain Res* 1990;515:193–206.
65. Collier TJ, Gash DM, Sladek JR. Transplantation of norepinephrine neurons into aged rats improves performance of a learned task. *Brain Res* 1988; 448:77–87.
66. Dunnett SB. Role of prefrontal cortex and striatal output systems in short-term memory deficits associated with ageing, basal forebrain lesions, and cholinergic-rich grafts. *Can J Psychol* 1990;44:210–232.
67. Goldman-Rakic PS. Circuitry of primate prefrontal cortex and regulation of behavior by representational memory. *Handbook of physiology, Vol 5. The nervous system.* Washington: American Physiological Association; 1986:373–417.
68. Kolb B. Functions of the prefrontal cortex of the rat: a comparative review. *Brain Res Rev* 1984;8:65–98.
69. Reading PJ, Dunnett SB. The effects of excitotoxic lesions of the nucleus accumbens on a matching to position task. *Behav Brain Res* 1991;46:17–29.
70. Bushnell PJ. Effects of delay, intertrial interval, delay behavior and trimethyltin on spatial delayed response in rats. *Neurotoxicol Teratol* 1988;10: 237–244.
71. Thomas JR, Ahlers ST, Schrot J. Cold-induced impairment of delayed matching in rats. *Behav Neural Biol* 1991;55:19–30.

Advances in Neurology, Vol. 59, edited by
Fredrick J. Seil. Raven Press, Ltd.,
New York, 1993.

6
Myelin Injury and Repair

Henry deF. Webster

Laboratory of Experimental Neuropathology, National Institute of Neurological Disorders and Stroke, National Institutes of Health, Bethesda, Maryland 20892

Myelin injury and repair are important areas of research, especially for those interested in regeneration of the central nervous system (CNS). In the spinal cord and brain, oligodendroglia are the myelin-forming and myelin-maintaining cells (1). During development, an oligodendrocyte forms processes that ensheath and myelinate many nearby axons. The lipids and proteins needed for myelin growth, maintenance, and regeneration are synthesized in the perikaryon and are transported along microtubules in thin oligodendroglial processes that terminate at the outer, inner, and paranodal margins of each myelin segment (Fig. 1). These myelin segments are compact membrane spirals, and their dimensions are regulated by the axons they surround (2–4). Also, the outer surfaces of myelin sheaths are not covered by glial cell cytoplasm as they are in the peripheral nervous system (PNS) (Fig. 2). Instead, they contact other myelin sheaths, surface membranes of other glial cells and neurons, or the extracellular compartment. Thus, CNS myelin sheaths are more vulnerable to severe injury than those in the PNS because (a) oxygen metabolites, lipid mediators, toxins, viruses, inflammatory cells, cytokines, and other injurious substances can interact directly with myelin sheath surfaces; (b) the amount of myelin membrane maintained by each oligodendrocyte is large; and (c) the thin oligodendroglial processes that transport substances required for sheath maintenance probably also are easily damaged; their injury may interrupt transport and produce myelin breakdown. Demyelination also occurs when axons are injured or transected, a process called Wallerian degeneration.

MYELIN INJURY

Important types of myelin injury are listed in Table 1 along with their targets, main causes, and a few disease examples. Mild hexachlorophene intoxication, electrolyte imbalance, and other types of minor injury may produce reversible separation of myelin lamellae and formation of edematous vacuoles that disappear during recovery. Ion channel distribution may also be affected (Waxman et al., this volume). When myelin sheaths or oligodendroglia sustain more severe injury, entire segments of myelin degenerate, and their remnants are phagocytosed by macrophages and to a much lesser degree by astrocytes. This process is called primary demyelination if most axons remain uninjured and is characteristic of the myelin breakdown seen in multiple sclerosis, experimental autoimmune encephalomyelitis (EAE), and progressive multifocal leukoencephalopathy.

Primary demyelinative lesions may also occur after viral infection of neurons. Martin found multifocal demyelinative lesions in the optic nerves, brain, and spinal cord during experimental infection with herpes virus type 2 (HSV-2) (5,6). Remyelination occurred, and the topographic distribution of spinal

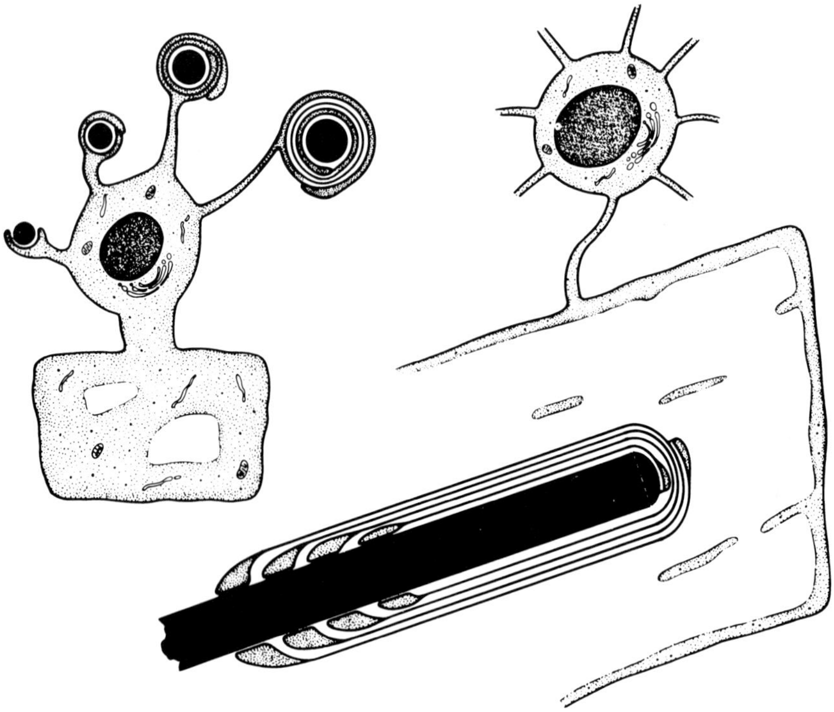

FIG. 1. Developing (**left**) and mature (**right**) oligodendroglia shown with their processes and myelin sheaths, which are compact, spiral extensions of their surface membranes. In the developing and remyelinating cell (**left**), relatively small areas of the spiral are compact. Processes of the mature oligodendrocyte (**right**) extend to many myelin sheaths and are continuous with the thin belt of cytoplasm that surrounds the large area of compact adult myelin. This cytoplasmic belt includes an oligodendrocyte's outer tongue processes, its paranodal (lateral) loops, and its inner (periaxonal) tongue processes. (Reprinted from Webster et al., ref. 52, with permission from Cambridge University Press.)

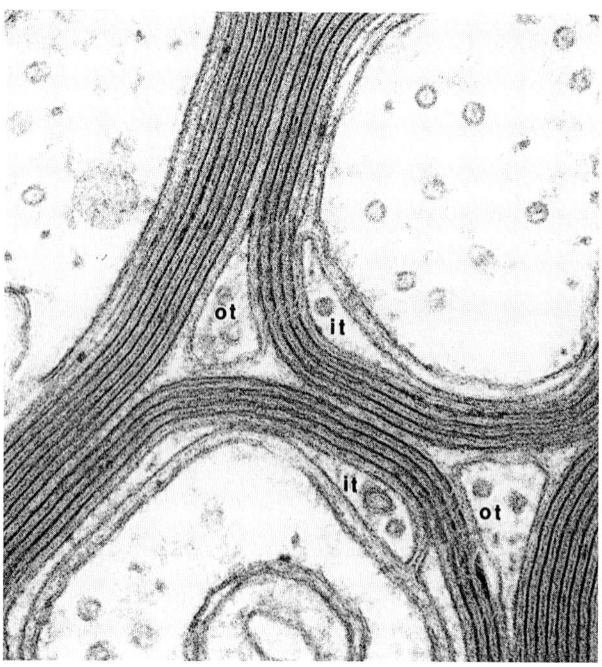

FIG. 2. Electron micrograph of transversely sectioned myelinated CNS axons. Alternating dense and less-dense lines of compact myelin are shown with inner (it) and outer (ot) tongue processes of oligodendroglia. ×180,000.

TABLE 1. *Types of myelin injury*

	Target	Cause	Disease examples
Mild, reversible	Myelin	Chemical	Hexachlorophene
	Myelin	Physical	Concussion, mild compression
Primary demyelination	Myelin	Immunologic	Experimental allergic encephalomyelitis
	Myelin	Chemical	Lysolecithin
	Myelin	Physical	CSF barbotage
	Oligodendrocyte	Viral	PML,[a] JHM mouse hepatitis, HSV[b]
	Oligodendrocyte	Chemical	Cuprizone, cyanide
	Oligodendrocyte and/or myelin	?	Multiple sclerosis
Wallerian degeneration	Axon and myelin	Physical	Axon transection; spinal cord and brain injury

[a] Progressive multifocal leukoencephalopathy.
[b] Herpes simplex virus, type 2.

cord lesions was not tract associated. Instead it resembled that seen in some cases of multiple sclerosis (7). Martin found that axons in early demyelinating lesions contained a few nucleocapsids and viral particles, and he proposed that neuronal infection and axonal transport of virus could lead to foci of oligodendroglial infection and primary demyelination remote from sites of neuronal infection (Fig. 3) (8,9).

In contrast to the findings in primary demyelination, axon injury or transection precedes and causes the myelin breakdown seen in Wallerian degeneration. Recent studies of this process in rat optic nerves have shown that most of the axonal and myelin debris is

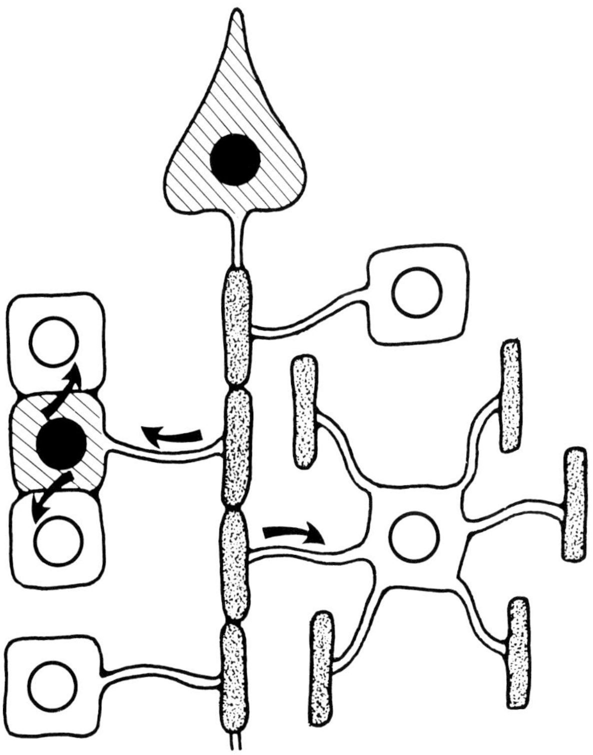

FIG. 3. Model for amplification of white matter infection and demyelination by cell to cell virus spread from infected neurons to oligodendrocytes. Proposed amplification factors are (a) multiplicity of oligodendrocytes providing myelin internodes to each axon (center arrow), (b) secondary spread between oligodendrocytes in glial columns (left arrows), and (c) loss of several internodes for each oligodendrocyte destroyed (right arrow). Reprinted with permission from Plenum Publishing Company from Martin, et al., ref. 9.

removed by macrophages and that oligodendroglia are able to survive in an axon-free environment for many months (10,11).

Early Biochemical Changes

Early biochemical events that produce myelin injury are important because appropriate treatment might prevent a cascade of later changes that lead to myelin breakdown and severe neurological dysfunction. In the presence of iron or other initiators, oxygen metabolites are known to rapidly injure cell membranes and organelles, including those affected by brain ischemia and spinal cord injury (12–16). Important sources of oxygen metabolite release are microglia, invading leukocytes, phagocytic cells, and aggregating platelets in venules and capillaries (17,18; Colton and Gilbert, this volume). Myelin and myelin-related membranes are vulnerable targets, and changes in their constituents have been demonstrated in studies of fractions and brain slices (19–21).

In vivo studies have also shown that lipid peroxidation is an important early event in many types of myelin injury. Peroxidation of ω-6 fatty acids and large myelin lesions have been described in gerbils treated with 100% oxygen after global brain ischemia (22,23). Also, myelinolysis and increased oxidation of soluble brain proteins occur after rapid correction of hyponatremia (24). Superoxide dismutase, which protects cells from damage by superoxide radicals, is reduced by the administration of cuprizone (biscyclohexanone oxalyldihydrazone) (25). This substance is toxic to oligodendrocytes and produces primary demyelination (26–30). In EAE, which is an autoimmune demyelinating disease and a model for multiple sclerosis, early lesions contain lymphocytes, activated macrophages, and other inflammatory cells which produce superoxide and other free radicals (18). When an iron-chelating agent, desferrioxamine, was given to Lewis rats before the onset of EAE, the clinical deficits, inflammatory infiltrates, and demyelination were greatly diminished (31). The beneficial effect was attributed to reduced formation of toxic hydroxyl radicals from superoxide and other reactive oxygen metabolites (31).

Lipid Peroxidation and Multiple Sclerosis

The importance of lipid peroxidation in the breakdown of myelin seen in multiple sclerosis was pointed out first in an hypothesis by Mickel (32,33). The inflammatory infiltrates seen in early lesions contain T lymphocytes, mononuclear cells, and phagocytes (34). Because these cells are major sources of toxic oxygen radicals, Halliwell (18) suggested that they have an important pathogenetic role in autoimmune diseases. Toshniwal and Zarling's (35) recent evidence is strong support for Mickel's hypothesis. They found that levels of ethane and pentane in expired breath samples of patients were abnormally high during an acute attack of multiple sclerosis. Since these alkanes are degradation products of unsaturated fatty acids, their levels have been used as *in vivo* indices of lipid peroxidation (36,37).

Spinal Cord Injury, Peroxidation, and Lipid Mediators

Traumatic spinal cord injury and brain ischemia are often associated with extensive white matter damage that includes necrosis, cavity formation, hemorrhage, and Wallerian degeneration (sometimes called secondary demyelination) (Bunge et al., this volume; Blight, this volume). Reactions of oxygen radicals and lipid mediators have been shown to be important in lesion pathogenesis, and treatment with antioxidants and gangliosides has reduced mortality, neurological disability, and lesion severity (14,16,38). Presumably, these agents inhibit a cascade of toxic reactions, thereby reducing injury to myelinated tracts and gray matter.

MYELIN REGENERATION

Regeneration of myelin in the CNS is a large area of research; it is the subject of several chapters in this volume and has been reviewed recently (39,40).

Remyelination in Experimental Models

Species variation in the capacity to repair and regenerate CNS myelin is well known, but the reasons for these differences remain poorly understood. In fish and amphibia, axons regenerate after they are transected, and oligodendroglia produce new myelin segments. An early study in optic nerves of *Xenopus* (41) as well as observations by Blakemore and co-workers (Franklin, Crang, and Blakemore, this volume) have shown that astrocytes have an important supportive role in the regeneration of myelin. After transection of tracts in the mammalian CNS, there is relatively little regeneration of either axons or myelin. However, in an interesting model of spinal cord injury produced by focal freezing, lesion margins contain regenerated myelin produced by oligodendrocytes and Schwann cells (42).

When axons remain unaffected and primary demyelination is produced immunologically, by viruses, or by toxic agents, oligodendroglia and/or their resident precursors will divide and ensheath and remyelinate most of the demyelinated axons in experimental animal models (26–28,43–45). In these studies, interphase and premitotic oligodendroglial precursors, as well as oligodendrocytes synthesizing myelin sheath constituents and generating new myelin sheaths, have been identified by using immunocytochemistry, autoradiography, *in situ* hybridization, and electron microscopy. Developmental and tissue culture studies have defined other important features of myelin formation (Knapp, Skoff, and Booth, this volume; Wood and Mora, this volume).

Insulin-like Growth Factor I and Remyelination

To learn more about astrocytes and their role in myelin regeneration, Komoly and his collaborators reexamined cuprizone-induced demyelination and found that hypertrophic astrocytes in lesions produced insulin-like growth factor I (IGF-I) mRNA and peptide (30). Regeneration of myelin began when cuprizone treatment stopped, and early in recovery oligodendroglial precursors expressed the receptor for IGF-I, a finding that strongly suggests that IGF-I functions in the metabolism of oligodendroglia and myelin *in vivo* (30). Astrocytic production of IGF-I in other demyelinating diseases is being examined in current experiments.

Remyelination in Multiple Sclerosis

Examination of fresh multiple sclerosis lesions has shown that there are numerous oligodendroglia-like cells and possible precursors with immunoreactivity for myelin-related enzymes, proteins, and glycolipids along with thin newly formed myelin sheaths (46). In more chronic active and in inactive lesions, similar cells and regenerating sheaths are much less frequent, suggesting that the capacity for oligodendroglia to proliferate, ensheath demyelinated axons, and regenerate myelin is reduced during progression of demyelination. In subacute and chronic spinal cord lesions, there may be substantial numbers of regenerated sheaths produced by Schwann cells (47,48), and, as Blakemore and co-workers have shown, astrocytes have an important role in the remyelination process.

CONCLUSION

Myelin is essential for normal nervous system function and is easily injured. Lipid peroxidation and toxic reactions involving oxygen metabolites and lipid mediators may produce a cascade of events in demyelinating diseases and spinal cord injury that lead to myelin breakdown and severe disability. Antioxidants, gangliosides, and inhibitors of platelet-activating factor are among the therapeutic agents that have been tried in brain ischemia (49–51) and may be useful in reducing the severity of toxic reactions associated with many types of myelin injury.

Myelin regeneration in the CNS is a challenging area of research. There has been substantial recent progress that we hope will lead to new therapies for patients with demyelinating diseases and spinal cord injuries.

ACKNOWLEDGMENTS

The author thanks Ms. Yoong Chang for excellent technical assistance.

REFERENCES

1. Peters A, Palay SL, Webster HdeF. *The fine structure of the nervous system: neurons and their supporting cells,* 3rd ed. New York: Oxford University Press; 1990.
2. Blakemore WF. Observations on myelination and remyelination in the central nervous system. In: Garrod DR, Feldman JD, eds. *Development in the nervous system.* Cambridge: Cambridge University Press; 1981:289–308.
3. Friedrich VL, Mugnaini E. Myelin sheath thickness is regulated near the axon. *Brain Res* 1983; 274:329–331.
4. Waxman SG, Sims TJ. Specificity in central myelination: evidence for local regulation of myelin thickness. *Brain Res* 1984;292:179–185.
5. Martin JR. Spinal cord and optic nerve demyelination in experimental herpes simplex virus type 2 infection. *J Neuropathol Exp Neurol* 1982;41:253–266.
6. Martin JR, Stoner GL, Webster HdeF. Lethal encephalitis and non-lethal multifocal central nervous system demyelination in herpes simplex virus type 2 infections in mice. *Br J Exp Pathol* 1982;63: 651–666.
7. Flynn TE, Martin JR. Topography of remyelinated chronic spinal cord lesions in herpes simplex virus type 2 infections of mice. *J Neurol Sci* 1983;61:327–339.
8. Martin JR. Intra-axonal virus in demyelinative lesions of experimental herpes simplex type 2 infection. *J Neurol Sci* 1984;63:63–74.
9. Martin JR, Suzuki S, Webster HdeF. Central nervous system demyelination in herpes simplex virus type 2 infection. In: Crescenzi GS, ed. *A multidisciplinary approach to myelin disease.* New York: Plenum Press; 1988:329–340.
10. Ludwin SK. Oligodendrocyte survival in Wallerian degeneration. *Acta Neuropathol* 1990;80:184–191.
11. Ludwin SK. Phagocytosis in the rat optic nerve following Wallerian degeneration. *Acta Neuropathol* 1990;80:266–273.
12. Freeman BA, Crapo JD. Biology of disease: free radicals and tissue injury. *Lab Invest* 1982;47:412–426.
13. Floyd RA. Oxygen radical-mediated damage to brain tissue. In: Simic MG, Taylor KA, Ward JF, Von Sonntag C, eds. *Basic life sciences, Vol 49: Oxygen radicals in biology and medicine.* New York: Plenum Press; 1988:1015–1023.
14. Hall ED Free radicals and CNS injury. *Crit Care Clin* 1989;5:793–805.
15. Hall ED, Braughler JM. Central nervous system trauma and stroke. II. Physiological and pharmacological evidence for involvement of oxygen radicals and lipid peroxidation. *Free Radic Biol Med* 1989;6:303–313.
16. Hall ED, Yonkers PA, Horan KL, et al. Correlation between attenuation of posttraumatic spinal cord ischemia and preservation of tissue vitamin E by the 21-aminosteroid U74006F: evidence for an *in vivo* antioxidant mechanism. *J Neurotrauma* 1989;6: 169–176.
17. Mickel HS. Peroxidized arachidonic acid effects on human platelets and its proposed role in the induction of damage to white matter. In: Kabara JJ, ed. *Symposium on the pharmacological effects of lipids, AOCS Monograph No. 5.* Champaign: American Oil Chemists' Society; 1978:179–190.
18. Halliwell B. Production of superoxide, hydrogen peroxide and hydroxyl radicals by phagocytic cells: a cause of chronic inflammatory disease? *Cell Biol Int Rep* 1982;6:529–542.
19. Konat GW, Wiggins RC. Effect of reactive oxygen species on myelin membrane proteins. *J Neurochem* 1985;45:1113–1118.
20. Konat G, Gantt G, Gorman A, et al. Peroxidative aggregation of myelin membrane proteins. *Metab Brain Dis* 1986;1:177–185.
21. Domanska-Janik K, Bourre JM. Effect of mercury on rabbit myelin CNP-ase *in vitro. Neurotoxicology* 1987;8:23–32.
22. Mickel HS, Vaishnav YN, Kempski O, et al. Breathing 100% oxygen after global brain ischemia results in increased lipid peroxidation and increased mortality. *Stroke* 1987;18:426–430.
23. Mickel HS, Kempski O, Feuerstein G, et al. Prominent white matter lesions develop in Mongolian gerbils treated with 100% normobaric oxygen after global brain ischemia. *Acta Neuropathol* 1990;79:465–472.
24. Mickel HS, Oliver CN, Starke-Reed PE. Protein oxidation and myelinolysis occur in brain following rapid correction of hyponatremia. *Biochem Biophys Res Commun* 1990;172:92–97.
25. Russanov EM, Ljutakova SG. Effect of cuprizone on copper exchange and superoxide dismutase activity in rat liver. *Gen Pharmacol* 1980;11:535–538.
26. Blakemore WF. Observations on oligodendrocyte degeneration, the resolution of status spongiosus and remyelination in cuprizone intoxication in mice. *J Neurocytol* 1972;1:413–426.
27. Blakemore WF. Demyelination of the superior cerebellar peduncle in the mouse induced by cuprizone. *J Neurol Sci* 1973;20:63–72.
28. Ludwin SK. Central nervous system demyelination and remyelination in the mouse. *Lab Invest* 1978;39:597–612.
29. Komoly S, Jeyasingham MD, Pratt OE, et al. Decrease in oligodendrocyte carbonic anhydrase activity preceding myelin degeneration in cuprizone-induced demyelination. *J Neurol Sci* 1987;79: 141–148.
30. Komoly S, Hudson LD, Webster HdeF, et al. Insulin-like growth factor I (IGF-I) gene expression is

induced in astrocytes during experimental demyelination. *Proc Natl Acad Sci USA* 1992;89: 1894–1898.
31. Bowern N, Ramshaw IA, Clark IA, et al. Inhibition of autoimmune neuropathological process by treatment with an iron-chelating agent. *J Exp Med* 1984;160:1532–1543.
32. Mickel HS. Multiple sclerosis: a new hypothesis. *Perspectives Biol Med* 1975;18:363–374.
33. Mickel HS. Biological effects of lipid peroxides: lipid peroxidation hypothesis of the etiology of multiple sclerosis. In: Kabera JJ, ed. *The pharmacological effect of lipids II.* Champaign: Americal Oil Chemists' Society; 1985:215–246.
34. Raine CS. Multiple sclerosis: a pivotal role for the T cell in lesion development. *Neuropathol Appl Neurobiol* 1991;17:265–274.
35. Toshniwal PK, Zarling EJ. Evidence for increased lipid peroxidation in multiple sclerosis. *Neurochem Res* 1992;17:205–207.
36. Riely CA, Cohen G, Lieberman M. Ethane evolution: a new index of lipid peroxidation. *Science* 1974;183:208–210.
37. Dillard CJ, Tappel AL. Volatile hydrocarbon and carbonyl products of lipid peroxidation: a comparison of pentane, ethane, hexanal and acetone as *in vivo* indices. *Lipids* 1914;14:989–995.
38. Hogan EL, Hsu CY, Liu T-H, Leskawa KC, Xu J, Dasgupta S. Ganglioside modification of nervous system disease. In: Ledeen RW, Hogan EL, Tettamanti G, Yates AJ, Yu RK, eds. *New trends in ganglioside research: neurochemical and neuroregenerative aspects.* Padova: Liviana Press; 1988:647–654.
39. Ludwin SK. Evolving concepts and issues in remyelination. *Dev Neurosci* 1989;11:140–148.
40. Dubois-Dalcq M, Armstrong R. The cellular and molecular events of central nervous system remyelination. *BioEssays* 1990;12:569–576.
41. Reier PJ, Webster HdeF. Regeneration and remyelination of *Xenopus* tadpole optic nerve fibres following transection or crush. *J Neurocytol* 1974;3: 591–618.
42. Collins GH, West NR, Parmely JD. The histopathology of freezing injury to the rat spinal cord. II. Repair and regeneration. *J Neuropathol Exp Neurol* 1986;45:742–757.
43. Ludwin SK. An autoradiographic study of cellular proliferation in remyelination of the central nervous system. *Am J Pathol* 1979;95:683–696.
44. Webster HdeF, Shii H, Lassmann H. Immunocytochemical study of myelin-associated glycoprotein (MAG), basic protein (BP), and glial fibrillary acidic protein (GFAP) in chronic relapsing experimental allergic encephalomyelitis (EAE). *Acta Neuropathol* 1985;65:177–189.
45. Raine CS, Moore GRW, Hintzen R, et al. Induction of oligodendrocyte proliferation and remyelination after chronic demyelination: Relevance to multiple sclerosis. *Lab Invest* 1988;59:467–476.
46. Prineas JW, Kwon EE, Goldenberg PZ, et al. Multiple sclerosis. Oligodendrocyte proliferation and differentiation in fresh lesions. *Lab Invest* 1989; 61:489–503.
47. Itoyama Y, Webster HdeF, Richardson EP Jr, et al. Schwann cell remyelination of demyelinated axons in spinal cord multiple sclerosis lesions. *Ann Neurol* 1983;14:339–346.
48. Itoyama Y, Ohnishi A, Tateishi J, et al. Spinal cord multiple sclerosis lesions in Japanese patients: Schwann cell remyelination occurs in areas that lack glial fibrillary acidic protein (GFAP). *Acta Neuropathol* 1985;65:217–223.
49. Skaper SD, Leon A, Toffano G. Ganglioside function in the development and repair of the nervous system: from basic science to clinical application. *Mol Neurobiol* 1989;3:173–199.
50. Oberpichler H, Sauer D, Rossberg C, et al. PAF antagonist ginkgolide B reduces postischemic neuronal damage in rat brain hippocampus. *J Cereb Blood Flow Metab* 1990;10:133–135.
51. Gilboe DD, Kintner D, Fitzpatrick JH, et al. Recovery of postischemic brain metabolism and function following treatment with a free radical scavenger and platelet-activating factor antagonists. *J Neurochem* 1991;56:311–319.
52. Webster HdeF, Trapp BD, Sternberger NH, Quarles RH. Myelin-forming glial cells: morphological and immunocytochemical observations. In: Garrod DR, Feldman JD, eds. *Development in the nervous system.* Cambridge: Cambridge University Press; 1981:265–288.

Advances in Neurology, Vol. 59, edited by
Fredrick J. Seil. Raven Press, Ltd.,
New York © 1993.

7

Observations on the Pathology of Human Spinal Cord Injury

A Review and Classification of 22 New Cases with Details from a Case of Chronic Cord Compression with Extensive Focal Demyelination

Richard P. Bunge, William R. Puckett, Jose L. Becerra, Alexander Marcillo, and Robert M. Quencer

The Miami Project to Cure Paralysis and the Departments of Neurological Surgery and Radiology, University of Miami School of Medicine, Miami, Florida 33136

Devising new strategies to influence recovery after spinal cord injury (SCI) must be guided by a thorough understanding of both the acute and chronic changes that occur in human spinal cord tissue after injury. This need becomes more urgent as new magnetic resonance (MR) imaging techniques allow increasing resolution of changes in spinal cord tissue in the living state. In many of these instances the histopathological basis of these MR changes is not known. For example, it has been suggested that the extent of increased intramedullary intensity of T2-weighted MR images after cervical cord injury (without evidence of hematoma) may be useful in predicting long-term neurological outcome and the likelihood of some degree of recovery (1). The nature of the tissue change responsible for this altered signal and how certain of these changes may be conducive to functional recovery are not known.

The precedent literature on the pathology of SCI is substantial, but much of this literature was published more than five decades ago, and the more recent literature provides quite limited observations. For example, the chapter on cord trauma in Hughes' *Pathology of the Spinal Cord* (2) contains 11 brief pages of text. Pathological changes in traumatized cord tissue occupy only 14 pages in Brock's *Injuries of the Brain and Spinal Cord* (3). Guttmann's classical text (4) on SCI contains a short chapter on cord pathology with illustrations from only six cases of traumatic injury. More recent reviews have centered on gross pathology (5,6) or on tissue changes common to a number of kinds of injury (7–9). Our present study is aimed at characterizing by imaging and histology the full extent of pathology in each available individual case of SCI. We hope thus to correlate pathological changes as directly as possible with MR images of cord tissue and with the neurological status of the patient at the time of death. We here report an overall summary of 22 cases, with detailed analysis of a unique case showing substantial focal demyelination subsequent to chronic compression of the cervical spinal cord. In examining the patterns of pathology in these 22 cases, we found that the tissue changes could be grouped under four categories. We propose these four categories as a useful classification of the major types of tissue damage after SCI, introducing a new classification, "solid cord injury," for those cases in which no hematoma, central cord softening, or cord laceration is found.

METHODS

During the past 2 years The Miami Project of the University of Miami School of Medicine, with the cooperation of the Department of Neurological Surgery and the medical examiners from several cities in the state of Florida, has obtained over 38 new specimens of spinal cords taken at autopsy from persons who had suffered SCI prior to death. Nine new specimens of uninjured cords have been obtained as controls. Twenty-two of the specimens (taken after SCI) have been subjected to detailed pathological analysis, many after study by MR techniques.

Cords were removed, generally by an anterior approach, within 24 hr of death either by the medical examiner or by a member of the staff of the Department of Neurological Surgery. The cords were placed immediately in 10% buffered formalin for a period of at least 2 weeks, after which they were stored in buffer (0.1 M phosphate buffer; pH 7.2) at 4°C. Most cords were available in their entirety and were subjected to MR after fixation and prior to removal of the dura and cutting into segments for microscopic examination. The gross specimen was photographed after removal of the dura and then sampled at selected segmental levels, depending on the kind and level of injury. In all cases the epicenter of the lesion (when obvious) was sampled, as were adjacent segments. In some cervical injuries in which the epicenter of the lesion was not apparent (as in central cord syndrome), each available cervical and upper thoracic segment was sampled. Segmental levels were determined by specific root identification, and references are, in all cases, to cord, not bony, spinal levels. The cord was also sampled at several regions remote from the lesion to search for unexpected additional lesions and for remote effects of the primary lesion.

Routinely, we used stains for general histology (hematoxylin–eosin), myelin (Solochrome–cyanine), axons (Sevier–Munger), and a stain for connective tissue components (trichrome). In most cases the tissue was examined in transverse (axial) sections, but frontal longitudinal sections were also prepared where indicated, as in the present featured case. We also sometimes embedded 1-mm slices in plastic (as used routinely in electron microscopy), with sectioning at 1 μm and staining with toluidine blue for finer histological detail. Histological findings were documented by extensive photography of the whole specimen, of the separated segments before embedding, and of the stained sections (see figures). An average of approximately 100 photographs documented changes in each specimen.

RESULTS

The age of patients at death ranged from 16 to 80 years (Table 1). Time from injury to death varied from 3 hr to 22 years. As shown in Table 1, 16 of the 22 cases had primary lesions in the cervical region. It has frequently been stated that in approximately 90% of cases of SCI, tissue continuity is retained across the site of maximum lesion (5). Although this may be true if one considers all types of tissue, including meninges and nerve roots, as evidence of continuity, this figure is high if one considers as significant continuity only that tissue that clearly contains central nervous system (CNS) parenchyma, including central axonal elements. We examined each specimen at the epicenter of the lesion by histological analysis and found a complete lack of continuity of CNS parenchyma in

TABLE 1. *Summary of 22 cases[a]*

MP number	Clinical level	Age	Sex	Cause of injury	Injury–death interval	Function: complete/ incomplete	Anatomic: complete/ incomplete	Kind of injury
15	C-1	34	M	MVA	5 wk	Complete	Incomplete	Massive compression
19	C-2	80	M	Fall	4 wk	Complete	Complete	Massive compression
37	C-4	57	M	MVA	6 mo	Complete	Incomplete	Massive compression
17	C4-5	62	M	MVA	22 yr	Complete	Incomplete	Contusion/cyst
43	C4-5	78	M	MVA	4 mo	Incomplete	Incomplete	Solid cord injury
18	C-5	69	F	MVA/ surgery	13 yr	Incomplete	Incomplete	Contusion/cyst
20	C-5	20	F	GSW	8 days	Complete	Incomplete	Laceration
27	C5-6	75	M	MVA	1 yr	Complete	?[b]	Massive compression
29	C5-6	45	F	MVA	1 yr	Complete	Incomplete	Contusion/cyst
3	C-6	67	M	Fall	3 days	Incomplete	Incomplete	Solid cord injury
2	C-6	74	M	MVA	6 days	Complete	Complete	Massive compression
8	C-6	59	M	MVA	12 days	Complete	Incomplete	Contusion/cyst
12	C-6	70	M	MVA	17 days	Complete	Incomplete	Contusion/cyst
13	C-6	64	M	MVA	6 mo	Incomplete	Incomplete	Solid cord injury
6	C-6	29	M	MVA	11 yr	Complete	Complete	Massive compression
7	C-7	60	M	MVA	5 wk	Incomplete	Incomplete	Solid cord injury
16	T-1	26	F	GSW	8.5 yr	Complete	Complete	Laceration
10	T2-3	37	F	GSW	8 yr	Complete	Complete	Laceration
9	T-5	49	F	MVA	7 wk	Complete	Incomplete	Massive compression
5	T-12	19	M	GSW	3 hr	Complete	Complete	Laceration
32	L-2	16	F	GSW	2 wk	Complete	Complete	Laceration
11	L-2	38	M	GSW	18 yr	Complete	Complete	Laceration

[a] Twenty-two new cases studied over the past 2 years at The Miami Project to Cure Paralysis are summarized. These are listed by cord level affected. The clinical level indicates the lowest functioning cord segment. The cause of injury is listed as MVA (motor vehicle accident), GSW (gunshot wound), or fall. The time from injury to death is indicated in hours (hr), days, weeks (wk), months (mo), or years (yr). Each injury is listed as functionally complete (no motor or sensory functions below the lesion) or incomplete; similarly, each lesion was categorized as anatomically complete or incomplete depending on whether any nerve fibers clearly of central type were found to traverse the epicenter of the lesion. The kinds of injury are listed as *massive compression* (closed injuries where most or all of the cord tissue is destroyed by massive compressive forces), *contusion/cyst* (closed injuries where moderate contusive forces leave the continuity of the cord largely intact but result in a centrally located hematomyelia, which evolves to become a stable cyst), *laceration* (open wounds in which cord substance is directly torn by a projectile or by fragments of bone displaced by a projectile), and *solid cord injury* (in which the overall form of the cord is retained and no central hematomyelia or cyst is found; instead the damage is largely to white matter tracts). For greater details of these classifications see text. The case listed as indeterminate in regard to anatomic continuity of fibers at the lesion site was from a patient who died 1 year post-injury. Nerve fibers were found in the connective tissue scar of this lesion, but the origin of these fibers was not clear.

[b] Indeterminate.

eight of 21 cases (38%); in one case, continuity was uncertain. Thus, in our series only 62% of specimens had demonstrated central neural tissue continuity through the epicenter of the lesion.

On the other hand, a substantial proportion of cases judged functionally complete on premortem neurological examination had some parenchymal continuity across the epicenter of the lesion. Thus, of 16 cases judged functionally complete, eight were found to have nerve fibers traversing the lesion site. This is in accordance with clinical physiological studies reported by Demetrijevic (10), who has suggested the term "discomplete" for that large number of patients who have no demonstrable voluntary motor function or detectable sensation below the site of lesion but in whom evoked potentials (sensory or motor) or other testing methods clearly indicate signals traversing the lesion site.

Utilizing histological techniques as well as MR analysis, we found secondary lesions (e.g., remote cysts, results of previous surgical procedures, and congenital abnormalities) in nine of the 22 cases (Table 2). Thus, second-

TABLE 2. *Complications in 22 cases of spinal cord injury*[a]

Cystic changes in cord adjacent to lesion	3
Remote cyst above lesion	1
Remote cauda equina lesion	1
Superimposed root avulsion	2
Residual compressive mass from previous surgery	1
Congenital diastematomyelia	1
Cord atrophy secondary to ischemia	1

[a] Changes in the cord tissue apart from the primary lesion site are listed. Complications were seen in 40% of cases.

ary changes were present in 40% of our cases. Most common were cystic changes extending from the lesion epicenter for substantial distances into adjacent cord segments; in one case the MR imaging revealed a cyst developing in the cervical cord that was remote from the lumbar lesion in this patient. This small cyst was apparently a dilation of the central canal because it was lined in a portion of its wall by ependymal cells (in contrast to the unlined cysts developing as extensions from the primary lesion area). We studied one case with a lesion from a gunshot wound to cord level L-2 that had, in addition to the tissue laceration at L-2, a massive fibrotic knot binding up essentially all roots of the cauda equina about 1 inch below the conus medullaris. Additional complications in other cases included surgically imposed root avulsion and an instance of the spinal parenchyma being split into two parts for a distance of several lumbar segments (diastematomyelia) (11). Two patients had had root avulsion for pain or spasticity, which was reflected in changes in internal cord structure secondary to the Wallerian degeneration induced. In one case of gunshot wound there was dramatic cord atrophy throughout the thoracic levels, possibly resulting from concomitant vascular injury.

Classification of Lesion Type

We found it useful to classify our lesions on the basis of the type of tissue injury sustained. This allows what we think is a useful distinction between those lesions in which the overall configuration and constituents of the cord remain intact and those in which a more severe contusion leads to intramedullary bleeding and tissue softening. In these two instances the pial surface of the cord is not breached, and changes at the epicenter of the lesion involve relatively little connective tissue response. By contrast, in lacerating injuries, such as gunshot wounds and in cases where the cord has been macerated by a massive compression, the pial surface is breached, and the meninges are rent; in these cases a substantial connective tissue response invades the cord and becomes a part of the scar formed at the lesion epicenter. In these two latter cases connective tissue becomes part of a scarring process at the lesion epicenter, whereas in the former two cases it does not. A general description of each of these categories of injury follows.

Contusion/Cyst

The standard animal model of SCI (12,13) involves a contusive injury to the thoracic cord leading to a central hematomyelia that evolves in time (weeks) to become a fluid-filled cyst. This lesion often leaves intact a peripheral rim of white matter and the surrounding pia. Axons retain continuity in this peripheral white matter, although the axon–myelin units may be damaged to the point of malfunction (14). A similar type of lesion has been described in the human (e.g., ref. 7) and was seen in our series as well under the designation "contusion/cyst" to indicate the evolution of tissue changes over time. Five of our 22 lesions (23%) showed this pattern. Thus, the most commonly used animal model of cord injury applies to only 23% of the cases in this series in addition to being located in the more infrequently injured midthoracic region.

Cord Maceration

Seven of our cases suffered massive cord compression after closed injury. In these cases the cord structure is macerated and severely distorted so that the topography of the tissue is lost. Surprisingly, in three of these cases a fragment of remaining CNS parenchyma was found, suggesting that a few fibers may sometimes maintain their continuity across even a region of severe damage. The epicenters of these massive compression lesions were dominated by connective tissue scarring and fragments of nerve roots. All of these patients had been diagnosed as functionally "complete."

Cord Laceration

Six of the 22 cases were open injuries caused by gunshot wounds. All but one of our noncervical-level lesions were of this type. We have classified these as cord lacerations, indicating that cord parenchyma has been directly torn by the injury. Cord parenchyma in the region of laceration is, over time, replaced by dense scar tissue, which often becomes adherent to the overlying dura. Five of these six injuries were functionally and anatomically complete. In one case the dorsal columns were spared by the bullet's course. This patient died 8 days after injury, and it is difficult to be certain if, over the long term, fiber continuity would have been maintained over this tenuous bridge.

Solid Cord Injury

Of particular interest to our present discussion are the four cases we have classified as solid cord injuries. In each of these cases the cord retained its continuity, and there was no focus of central cord softening as is found in the contusion/cyst type of lesion. We did not expect to find this kind of lesion; there is at present no animal model for this type of injury. Furthermore, each of these patients had been diagnosed clinically as "central cord syndrome," where the expected pathology, following from the work of Schneider et al. (15), is a loss of tissue in the area around the central canal. These four cases are discussed in detail below, with special emphasis on the fourth case, who died after both acute injury and chronic compression. Histological analysis in this case indicated changes similar to those we have found in the three previously reported cases of "central cord syndrome" (16), i.e., axonal disruption focused in the lateral white matter with preservation of the gray matter. In the fourth case of "solid cord injury," which we describe below, there was also dramatic focal demyelination of the dorsal columns (without concomitant major axon loss) and substantial motor neuron loss in the anterior gray matter at the epicenter of the compression.

Solid Cord Lesions and Central Cord Syndrome

Elsewhere we report MR/pathological correlations in acute traumatic central cord syndrome (16). Eleven patients were examined by MR, and three patients were available for pathological analysis. All patients examined with MR had hyperintense signal within the parenchyma of the cervical spinal cord on T2-weighted MR, but none demonstrated the characteristic MR features of hemorrhage on either T1 or gradient-echo MR. Pathological studies of the three cords available at autopsy showed no evidence of blood or blood products within the cord parenchyma. This was an unexpected finding inasmuch as it has generally been held that central cord syndrome results from a loss of central cord tissue secondary to hematomyelia (15). This was thought to evolve to a central necrosis, primarily affecting the central gray matter along with the motor fibers of the corticospinal tract directed to the upper extremities. Instead, we found these cords to be grossly intact; on microscopic examination each showed diffuse axonal disruption in the deeper white matter of the lateral columns. This axonal disruption was present to a modest extent in both dorsal and ventral columns but was focused in the lateral columns, particularly in the region of the corticospinal tract. The focal point of the lesion was in the midcervical region, with axonal loss evident in the two cases that survived for longer than several weeks. This axonal loss was dramatic in the dorsal part of the lateral columns. In these three cases we did not demonstrate changes in the gray matter of the cord in the cervical region and saw no evidence of hemorrhage into the cord, confirming the MR findings.

These findings suggest that in a subset of human cord injury the cord lesion present is primarily a focal damage to axon–myelin units, largely confined to white matter regions of the cord. This may be considered a focal axonal loss from white matter damage and may be similar, except in distribution, to the disseminated axonal loss seen in head injury, which has been characterized in the work of Povlishok and his colleagues (17). It remains unclear whether some axon myelin units are damaged rather than destroyed by the initial injury and undergo some degree of repair in this lesion, possibly explaining the recovery seen after injury leading to central cord syndrome. We observed that it was primarily the very large axons that were damaged, with some smaller axons surviving in the lateral columns even at the epicenter of these lesions.

Demyelination After Chronic Cord Compression in the Human

In our fourth case of "solid cord injury," additional changes were found. In addition to the axon loss centered in the lateral white matter that characterized our first three cases of central cord syndrome, this case also showed extensive demyelination.

The patient was a 78-year-old male who suffered paresis after an automobile accident. His medical history prior to this incident was pertinent in that he had undergone a cervical laminectomy approximately 12 years previously because of severe numbness and weakness in his hands. At the time of the accident his vehicle struck a stopped car; he was not wearing a seat belt, and his head struck the visor. He did not lose consciousness but subsequently could not move his arms or legs and had pain in the back of his neck radiating into both shoulders as well as abnormal sensations in his hands. On examination he was found to have weakness in all extremities, most pronounced in his arms, where it was more pronounced distally. Radiological examination showed a laminectomy site at C-3,4,5 with hypertrophic osteoarthritis of the cervical spine. There was severe spinal stenosis with compression of the thecal sac and cervical spinal cord at C3-4 because of a large central posterior bony spur; this stenosis also involved C4-5 and C5-6. Stenosis of the intervertebral foramina was noted at several cervical levels. Spondylitic and facet arthrosis changes were also noted. An MR supported these findings. His clinical diagnosis was central cord syndrome. Three months after his automobile accident he developed a urinary tract infection and pneumonia and died 4 months post-injury.

Autopsy revealed pneumonia and unexpected melanoma metastatic to the brain (occipital lobe) and liver. The disk between cervical vertebral bodies 3 and 4 was fractured, with fragmentation and overlying fibrosis. There was a fracture callus anteriorly. On removal of the spinal cord there was an extradural fibrous mass attached to the dura and overlying cervical cord levels 4, 5, and 6, apparently the result of scarring from the earlier laminectomy. There was no dural–cord adhesion at this point, but the underlying cord was manifestly compressed (Fig. 1A,B). MR-imaging of the cord showed narrowing of the cord centered at C-5, increased signal intensity at this level, and loss of internal cord detail (Fig. 2). Increased signal was also noted at C-4, in this instance confined to the lateral columns. The cord was reduced in diameter at this point (Fig. 1A,C). The internal structure of the cord appeared normal above (C-3) and below (C-6) the lesion. On sectioning the cervical cord, no hemorrhage or softening of cord tissue was seen, but the cord diameter was reduced by about one-third (Fig. 1C) at the area of compression.

Microscopic examination at the epicenter of this narrowing (C-5) showed a cord with

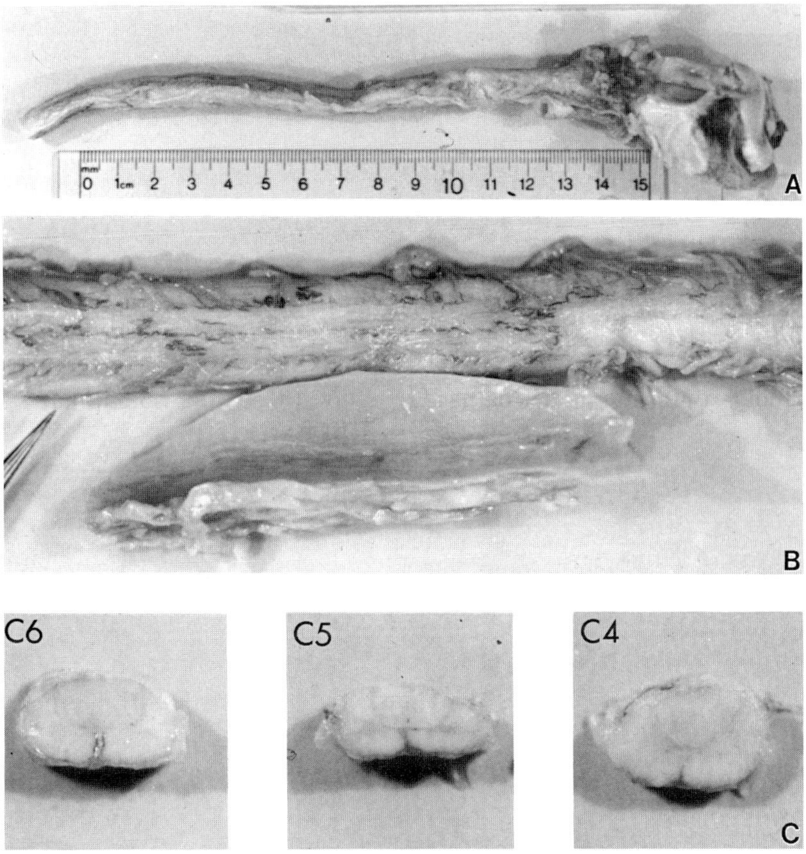

FIG. 1. Gross pathology from a case of cervical spinal cord injury that suffered both chronic compression and acute trauma. (**A**) The brainstem and cervical spinal cord are shown in a lateral view. There is a clearly visible narrowing of the cord, particularly in the anterior–posterior dimension, centered at cervical level 5. (**B**) The portion of the dura is shown that overlies the narrowed cord region with the attached dorsal scar, which had resulted from earlier laminectomy. The continuity of all portions of the cord is retained throughout the area of narrowing without manifest hemorrhage or disruption of the normal cord architecture. (**C**) The cord is shown in cross section at cervical levels 4, 5, and 6 prior to histological sectioning to illustrate the degree of overall narrowing of the cord tissue at C-5.

decreased width and height, decreased gray matter volume, and compression of all white matter regions, especially the dorsal columns. We sought and found the indication of axon damage centered in the lateral columns, as expected from our previous observations on central cord injury (16), but we also noted extensive myelin loss in all white matter regions.

Both white and gray matter appeared to be decreased in area at the center of the lesion, though there was no apparent hemorrhage or areas of softening in the cord. The myelin stain at the level of C-5 indicated substantial loss of myelin in dorsal, lateral, and ventral columns (Fig. 3A). In each of these areas the number of definitive myelin rings present appeared to be in the range of 10% of the normal number (Fig. 3A,C), and degenerating myelin was present. Considering this massive loss of myelin, we were surprised to note that at cervical levels above the lesion the dorsal columns appeared remarkably normal, and the expected Wallerian degeneration, which

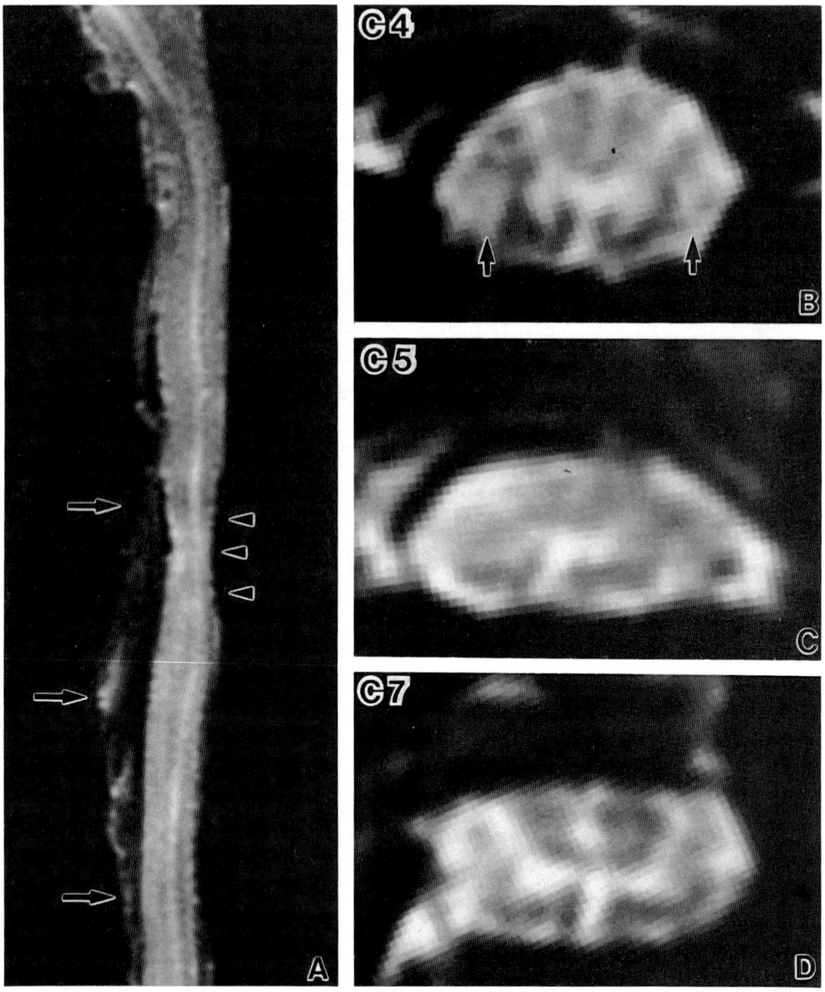

FIG. 2. (**A**) Sagittal T2-weighted MR image (2,000/80/2) (TR/TE/NEX) of the cervical cord shows thickened dura (*arrows*) causing cord compression with increased signal intensity (*arrowheads*). (**B**) Axial T2-weighted MR image (2,000/80/2) at the C-4 level shows increased signal intensity in the lateral columns corresponding to the corticospinal tracts (*arrows*). (**C**) Axial T2-weighted MR image (2,000/80/2) at the C-5 level shows flattening of the cord with loss of a well-defined distinction between central gray and white matter. (**D**) Axial T2-weighted MR image (2,000/80/2) at the C-7 level shows restoration of the gray–white matter distinction.

would have occurred secondary to dorsal column axon loss, was not present (Fig. 3C,D). Examination of axons in the dorsal columns in longitudinal sections (Fig. 4) indicated that there was substantially less axonal damage in the dorsal columns than was seen in the central portions of the lateral columns. Because axonal breakdown in the human extends over a period of many months (18), one would expect to see in this case the characteristic neurofilamentous margination around swollen axons or solid neurofilamentous nodules characteristic of axonal degeneration (as in Fig. 5A) as the hallmark of axonal loss. In order to better study the condition of the axons in the dorsal columns, we prepared longitudinal sections from the dorsal columns at the site of maximum injury. These allowed visualization of both axons and myelin in the frontal plane (Fig. 4). These sec-

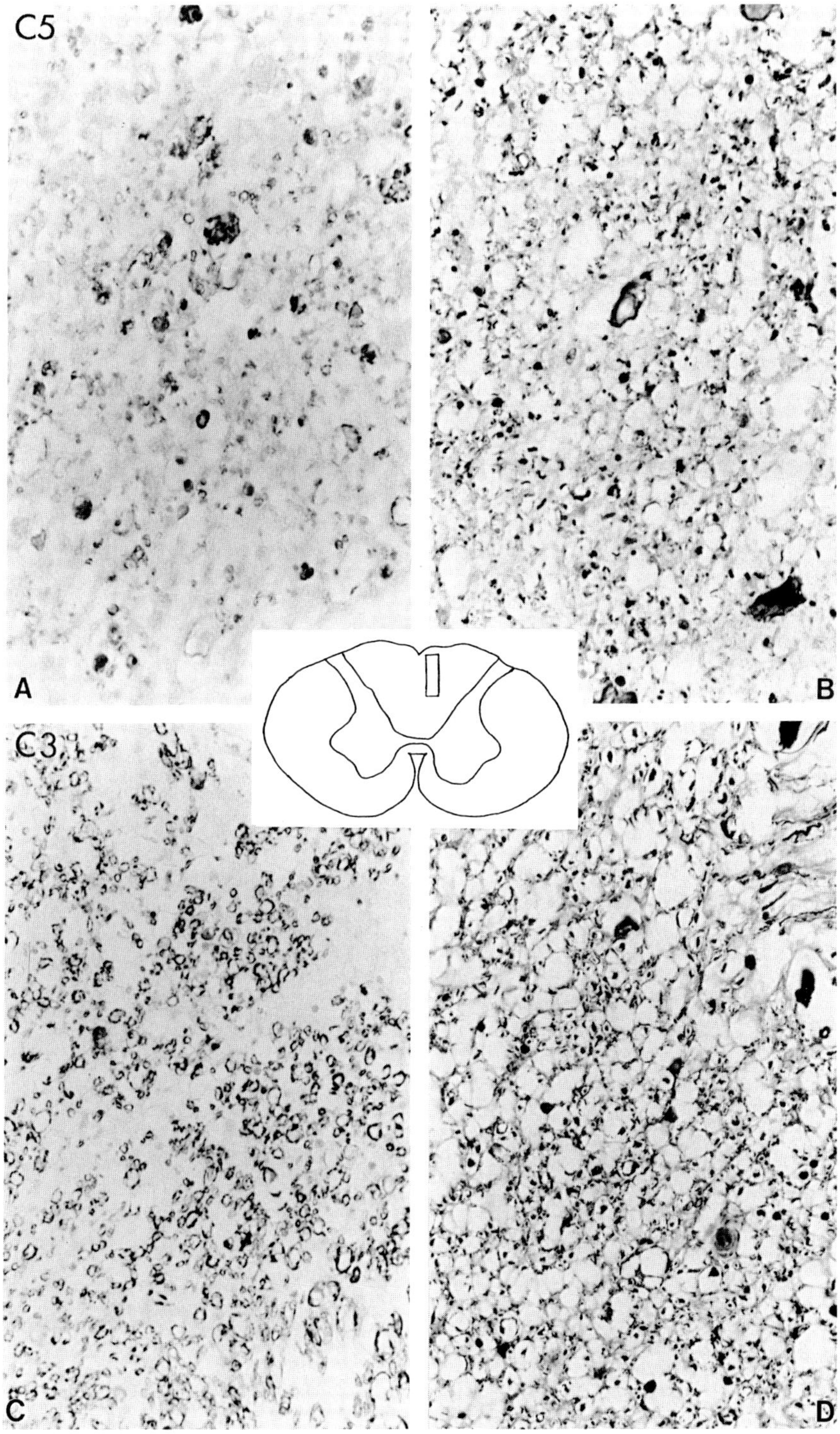

FIG. 3. Photomicrographs of sections stained for myelin (**A, C**) or axons (**B, D**) taken at cervical level 5 (near the epicenter of the lesion) (**A, B**) and cervical level 3 above the epicenter of the lesion (**C, D**). The region of the cord sampled is shown in this and subsequent figures in the inset. These photomicrographs illustrate that at the epicenter of the lesion the amount of myelin is substantially decreased, whereas there is good preservation of the axon population. The axons are not normally spaced, as they are when separated by their attendant myelin sheaths, but are aggregated between spaces occupied by macrophages digesting myelin debris. The preservation of axons in the region of the lesion explains why the dorsal columns above the region show relatively little axon and myelin loss, as shown in **C** and **D.** ×400.

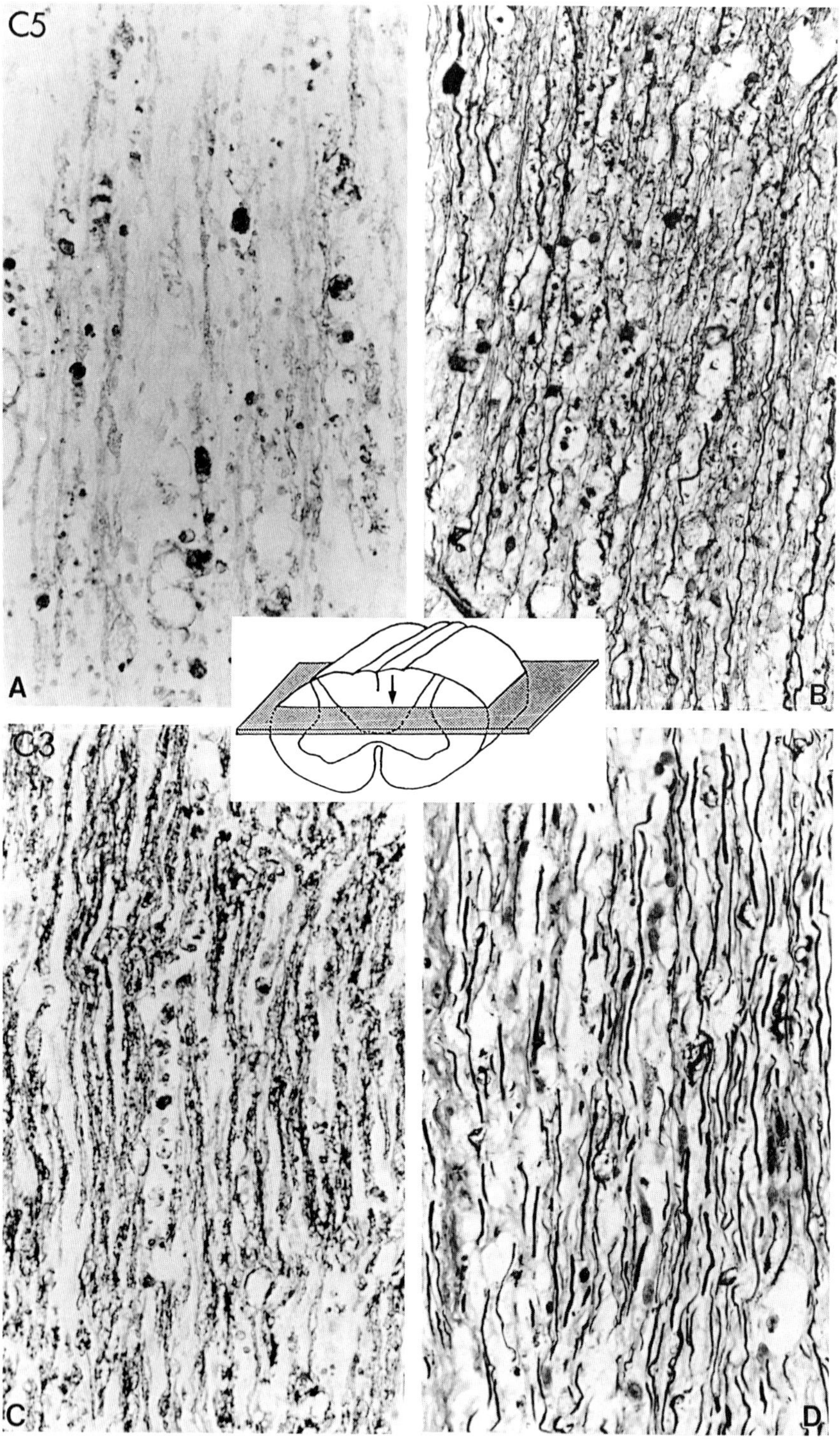

FIG. 4. These photomicrographs illustrate the relative preservation of myelin and axons as viewed in blocks prepared for longitudinal sectioning. Myelin stains are shown in **A** and **C,** and axon stains in **B** and **D. A** and **B** are taken from the epicenter of the lesion at C-5 and show the relative loss of myelin compared to the preservation of axons, which are well shown in this silver stain. The fragmented dark-staining material indicates that there has been some axonal loss in the dorsal columns. **C** and **D** illustrate that at cervical level 3, above the epicenter of the lesion, dorsal columns contain a substantial number of intact axons that retain their myelin sheaths. These longitudinal sections indicate that the demyelination observed in this case is focal, indicating the preservation of the axons traversing the lesion site.

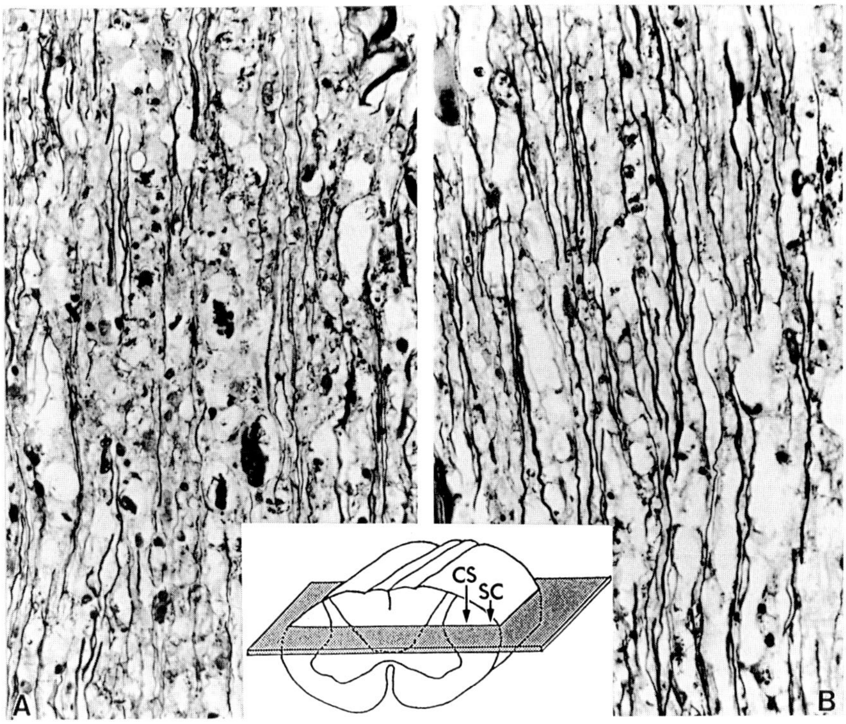

FIG. 5. These two photomicrographs are taken from the lateral column at the epicenter of the lesion to illustrate that there is substantial axonal loss, particularly of the larger axons in the corticospinal tract, as seen in **A,** as compared to the relative preservations of axons seen in the spinocerebellar tract, as seen in **B.** Degenerating axons are marked by aggregates of stained debris sometimes seen in linear arrays ("Wallerian trails"). Axons preserved in this area are generally the smaller-diameter fibers. This is similar to the pattern of lateral column axon loss that has been described in our previous report on the pathology of central cord syndrome (16). This finding would indicate that this case may be considered a variant of central cord syndrome in which substantial myelin loss in the dorsal (and ventral) columns is seen, as well as the loss of both axons and myelin sheaths in the central portion of the lateral columns. The **inset** illustrates the region of the cords sampled in longitudinal section to include the axons of both the corticospinal (CS) and the spinocerebellar (SC) tracts. ×400.

tions confirmed that a substantial number of axons lacking myelin were traversing the epicenter of the lesion in the dorsal columns.

These observations in the dorsal columns were in contrast to the pattern of damage in the lateral columns. Here there was substantial myelin loss (as was noted elsewhere in the white matter at the site of maximum lesion) and also substantial axonal damage (Fig. 5A). This damage was centered in the lateral columns in the portion of the cord containing the corticospinal tract. As we had previously reported in central cord syndrome (16), the spinocerebellar axons (at the cord surface in the lateral columns) were largely spared (Fig. 5B). This axonal change in the lateral columns was observed from the epicenter of the lesion at C-5 and below, as would be expected in Wallerian degeneration of these descending tracts. In the lower cervical levels below the lesion, the cord architecture was not greatly different from normal except for the loss of some myelin and axonal damage in the central portion of the lateral columns.

At the epicenter of the lesion, the gray matter was reduced in volume, and there appeared to be a loss of motor neurons at this level. In the cervical segments immediately above and below the epicenter of the lesion, the gray matter appeared normal.

Thus, this cord, which appeared to have suffered from both chronic compression and an acute contusive episode, had three clear-cut abnormalities at the epicenter of the lesion. These were (a) focal demyelination in the dorsal and ventral columns with preservation of the axonal population, (b) a combination of axon and myelin loss in the central portion of the lateral white matter [as seen in central cord syndrome, as discussed above and in more detail elsewhere (16)], and (c) damage to the gray matter with reduction in overall volume and substantial loss of motor neurons at the lesion epicenter.

Unique to this cord was the remarkable focal loss of myelin in the dorsal columns with preservation of the axon population (established by the staining of myelin-free axons within the epicenter of the lesion) and the presence of large numbers of myelinated axons in the dorsal columns above the lesion.

DISCUSSION

The morphology of silver-stained axons in human autopsy material gives reliable information on their status: degenerating axons are distinctive and therefore identifiable over several months' time (18). Thus, certain conclusions can be drawn from comparing axon and myelin stains after SCI. We feel confident that the distinction between surviving axons that have been demyelinated and those undergoing Wallerian degeneration can be made in tissue harvested 4 months after the acute aspect of this injury. At the lesion epicenter in the distinctive case described above, the dorsal columns showed little axon breakdown but substantial demyelination, whereas the lateral columns revealed substantial axon loss.

Thus, there are certain similarities between the pathology in our case of focal demyelination and the three other cases of central cord syndrome that we have reported elsewhere (16). The onset of a partial paralysis (focused particularly in the upper limbs) occurred subsequent to a motor vehicle accident in which a patient with a history of a narrowed cervical canal suffered an extension injury of the neck. It has been suggested that under these circumstances a buckling of the ligamenta flavae further compromises the vertebral canal, and, as these ligaments project forward, they particularly exert pressure on the lateral columns of the spinal cord (discussed in ref. 16). This is offered as an explanation of why the white matter damage that involves axonal injury seems to be focused in the central portion of the lateral columns bilaterally. If axons were severed in this region, one would expect (4 months after injury) axonal swelling with neurofilamentous margination as well as aggregates of neurofilaments that have been described as marking the degenerating axon (18). These axonal changes are known to begin within 9 days of injury and to continue for a period of several months. We have elsewhere (16) discussed how we believe this kind of axonal damage could explain the clinical symptoms present in classical cases of central cord syndrome.

In addition to this lateral white matter injury, the present patient had a focal zone of demyelination in a region of the cord that was chronically compressed by a connective tissue mass. This mass apparently resulted from the laminectomy performed some 12 years earlier. At the point where this mass compressed the cord, the cord was manifestly thinner, and we expected to see substantial axonal damage throughout the cord. The fact that little axonal interruption had occurred in the dorsal and ventral columns at the site of injury was attested to by the fact that these columns above the injury appeared remarkably normal. Further, at the epicenter of the lesion, there were many axons in the dorsal and ventral columns that did not show signs of degeneration; these were seen in large numbers in portions of white matter that showed very little staining for myelin. The intactness of the axon–myelin units above and below an injury, with loss of myelin and the retention of axon continuity at the site of injury, indicate a focal demyelination.

The fact that chronic compression may

lead to demyelination with axonal preservation has been well documented in a number of animal models (for review, see ref. 19). Chronic compression of peripheral nerve has been demonstrated to cause demyelination with preservation of axon continuity (20). In addition, in experimental animals it has been shown that a number of compressive injuries can lead to focal demyelination in spinal cord white matter (19). It has also been demonstrated that this demyelination can be reversed by remyelination if the compression is removed (21,22). The mechanism by which compression alters the myelin sheaths and yet allows preservation of axonal continuity is not clear.

We believe that our featured case is a variant of central cord injury with the addition of focal demyelination in the dorsal and central columns as well as motor neuron loss at the lesion epicenter. In examining the literature, we have not been able to find any illustrated case of clear-cut demyelination after traumatic injury to the spinal cord of the human. Previous observations on the pathology seen in longstanding cases of spondylitic myelopathy of the cervical spinal cord of the human have described lesions with ascending degeneration in the dorsal columns rostrally and the posterolateral columns caudally, indicating axonal loss at the lesion epicenter rather than demyelination (23). There is some question in our mind, however, whether demyelination may have been a component of the injury in certain of these cases; this is especially suggested by the presence of Schwann cell invasion into the dorsal columns in their Case 9 (23).

Perhaps the best description of human pathology that suggests that chronic compression can cause demyelination in the human spinal cord was given by Holmes in 1906. He described four cases in which he believed there was chronic compression of cord tissue. Three of these were cases of Potts' disease (tuberculosis of the spine), each of which resulted in compression of the spinal cord from vertebral body disease. He described damage to the cord as focal and felt that, despite myelin loss, axons must be traversing the region of lesion because he failed to find Wallerian degeneration above and below the lesion epicenter. Unfortunately, this interesting paper is not illustrated. He writes: "The truth of the Wallerian law . . . is incontestable. Whether destruction . . . of fibers is complete or not is determined by the presence or absence of secondary degeneration in the portions of the fibers separated from the trophic cells by the lesion" (24). Thus, Holmes came to the conclusion that he was observing demyelination on the basis of the fact that the long tracts were not degenerating as expected above and below the epicenter of a lesion where myelin was found to be essentially absent. He surmised that the axons were therefore surviving. The same type of observation caused us to examine in detail the case described above; we were astonished to find the upper cervical segments to appear essentially normal above a midcervical zone that contained little myelin in any part of the white matter. Thus, it appears that almost a century has passed between the observation by Holmes and an opportunity to demonstrate directly that chronic compression of the human spinal cord can lead to focal demyelination. We emphasize the urgent need for additional neuropathological observations on the nature of human spinal cord after trauma to guide the growing number of efforts directed at improving cord function after serious injury (for discussion, see refs. 25,26).

CONCLUSION

Initiation of an aggressive procurement policy by The Miami Project has resulted in obtaining 38 new spinal cord specimens taken at autopsy from patients who died 3 hr to 22 years after suffering spinal cord injury. Detailed magnetic resonance and histological analysis have been completed on 22 of these specimens. The patients were from 16 to 80 years of age at death; 14 were injured in motor vehicle accidents, six by gunshot wounds, and two in falls. We found it useful to classify these cases into four overall categories: two categories in which the cord is lacerated or massively compressed and the injury invokes a prominent connective tissue response and two categories in which the overall cord configuration is retained, the spinal cord surface is not substantially breached, and the connective tissue component of the response is minimal. These latter cases involve those in which contusion leads to damage in the central region of the cord (with tissue softening and hemorrhage evolving to formation of a central fluid-filled cyst) and cases in which the substance of the cord is not softened and intramedullary hemorrhage is not present.

We have termed this latter type of injury (for which, at present, there is no animal model) "solid cord injury." Each of these cases had been classified clinically as central cord syndrome; three are described in detail elsewhere (16). In each case the main focus of injury appeared to be in the dorsal part of the lateral white matter in the midcervical level, where a focus of substantial axon loss was seen. In a fourth case of "solid cord injury," this axon loss in the lateral white matter was present, but in addition there was a focal area at the midcervical level where loss of myelin with axonal preservation indicated a substantial demyelination over one to two cord segments. This myelin loss affected all white matter columns, occurring immediately subsequent to a large epidural connective tissue mass that had visibly compressed (but not disrupted the continuity of) the underlying cord. This compressive mass apparently resulted from a laminectomy done some years earlier. Whereas demyelination after cord compression is well known in experimental lesions in animals, this appears to be the first illustrated case of substantial demyelination following chronic spinal cord compression in humans. The paucity of well-documented descriptions of histological changes after cord injury in man compromises the development of cord injury models relevant to all of the kinds of injury that result from trauma to the human spinal cord.

ACKNOWLEDGMENTS

We are particularly appreciative of the cooperation of the Medical Examiners of several Florida counties in providing specimens for our study. This work was supported by PO1-NS28059 from NIH, NINDS and The Miami Project to Cure Paralysis (Miami, FL).

REFERENCES

1. Schaefer SM, Flanders AE, Osterholm VL, Northrup BE. Prognostic significance of magnetic resonance imaging in the acute phase of cervical spine injury. *J Neurosurg* 1992;76:218–223.
2. Hughes JT. Trauma to the spinal cord. In: Hughes JT, ed. *Pathology of the spinal cord.* London: WB Saunders; 1978:91–104.
3. Hughes JT. Pathology of spinal cord damage in spinal injuries. In: Feiring EH, ed. *Brock's injuries of the brain and spinal cord,* 5th ed. New York: Springer; 1974.
4. Guttmann L. *Spinal cord injuries.* Oxford: Blackwell; 1973.
5. Kakulas BA. Pathology of spinal injuries. *CNS Trauma* 1985;1:117–129.
6. Kakulas BA, Bedbrook GM. Pathology of injuries of the vertebral column. In: Vinken PJ, Bruyn GW, Braakman R, eds. *Handbook of clinical neurology. Injuries of the spine and spinal cord,* Vol 25, Part 1. Amsterdam: Elsevier/North-Holland; 1976:27–42.
7. Balentine JD. Impact injuries of the spine and spinal cord. In: Leestma JE, Kirkpatrick JB, eds. *Forensic neuropathology.* New York: Raven Press; 1988: 254–275.
8. Jellinger K. Neuropathology of cord injuries. In: Vinken PJ, Bruyn GW, Braakman R, eds. *Handbook of clinical neurology. Injuries of the spine and spinal cord,* Vol. 25, Part 1. Amsterdam: Elsevier/North-Holland; 1976:43–121.
9. Wolman L. The neuropathology of traumatic paraplegia. A critical historical review. *Int J Paraplegia* 1964;1:233–251.
10. Dimitrijevic MR. Residual motor functions in spinal cord injury. In: Waxman SG, ed. *Functional recovery in neurological disease.* New York: Raven Press; 1988:139–155.
11. Naidich TP, Harwood-Nash DC. Diastematomyelia: hemicord and meningeal sheaths; single and double arachnoid and dural tubes. *Am J Neuroradiol* 1983;4:633–636.
12. Blight AR. Cellular morphology of chronic SCI in the cat: analysis of myelinated axons by line sampling. *Neuroscience* 1983;10:521–543.
13. Blight AR, DeCrescito V. Morphometric analysis of experimental SCI in the cat: the relationship of in-

jury intensity to survival of myelinated axons. *Neuroscience* 1987;19:321–341.
14. Blight AR, Gruner JA. Augmentation by 4-aminopyridine of vestibulospinal free fall responses in chronic spinal-injured cats. *J Neurol Sci* 1987;82:145–159.
15. Schneider RC, Thompson JM, Bebin J. The syndrome of the acute central cervical spinal cord injury. *J Neurol Neurosurg Psychiatr* 1958;21:216–227.
16. Quencer RM, Bunge RP, Egnor M, Green BA, Puckett W, Post MJD. MR/pathological correlations in acute traumatic central cervical spinal cord syndrome. *Neuroradiology* 1992;34:85–94.
17. Povlishock JT, Becker DP. Fate of reactive axonal swellings induced by head injury. *Lab Invest* 1985;52:540–552.
18. Miklossy J, Clarke S, Van der Loos H. The long distance effects of brain lesions: visualization of axonal pathways and their terminations in the human brain by the Nauta method. *J Neuropathol Exp Neurol* 1991;50:595–614.
19. Waxman SG. Demyelination in spinal cord injury. *J Neurol Sci* 1989;91:1–14.
20. Ochoa J, Fowler TJ, Gilliatt RW. Anatomical changes in peripheral nerves compressed by a pneumatic tourniquet. *J Anat (Lond)* 1972;113:443–455.
21. Gledhill RF, Harrison BM, McDonald WI. Demyelination and remyelination after acute spinal cord compression. *Exp Neurol* 1973;38:472–487.
22. Gledhill RF, McDonald WI. Morphological characteristics of central demyelination and remyelination: a single-fiber study. *Ann Neurol* 1977; 1:552–560.
23. Ogino H, Tada K, Okada K, *et al.* Canal diameter, anteroposterior compression ratio, and spondylotic myelopathy of the cervical spine. *Spine* 1983; 8:1–15.
24. Holmes G. On the relation between loss of function and structural change in focal lesions of the central nervous system, with special reference to secondary degeneration. *Brain* 1906;29:514–523.
25. Young W. Spinal cord injury. *Curr Opin Neurol Neurosurg* 1988;1:611–622.
26. Young W. Recovery mechanisms in spinal cord injury: implications for regenerative therapy. In: Seil FJ, ed. *Neural regeneration and transplantation.* New York: Alan R Liss; 1989:157–169.

Advances in Neurology, Vol. 59, edited by
Fredrick J. Seil. Raven Press, Ltd.,
New York © 1993.

8

Remyelination, Revascularization, and Recovery of Function in Experimental Spinal Cord Injury

Andrew R. Blight

Center for Paralysis Research, School of Veterinary Medicine, Purdue University, West Lafayette, Indiana 47907

Recovery of function following injury to the central nervous system (CNS) is a complex and poorly understood process. Adaptive behavior of neural circuits and synaptic plasticity remote from the lesion site may be the most important elements in some types of injury, especially where there has been discrete interruption of particular pathways. Some of the rules of hierarchy characteristic of such reorganization in the cat spinal cord following hemisection or deafferentation have been documented by Goldberger and Murray (1,2). In traumatic injuries of the spinal cord where damage is less focused and selective, including most clinical cases, cellular reactions at and around the lesion site itself may contribute significantly to both functional loss and recovery (Table 1). Much of our knowledge of the cellular reaction to trauma has been derived from animal models. Clinical histopathology has provided only relatively gross information on the distribution of tissue damage and on the variety of types of injury that may be found (3–5).

Experimental spinal cord injury in animal models typically produces central hemorrhagic necrosis over a length of at least one and sometimes several spinal cord segments, involving at the lesion center all or most of the gray matter and a variable proportion of the surrounding white matter (6–11). Subsequent loss and recovery of function below such a lesion will depend principally on the extent and distribution of loss of axonal tracts. However, it will also depend on the physiological effectiveness of the outer rim of surviving white matter, namely, its ability to conduct action potentials (12–14). The conduction properties of axons are affected by myelination and by vascular supply. They may also be affected by local abnormalities in astrocyte (15,16) and microglial (17) physiology, though there is as yet no detailed understanding of how this might occur. The subject of this review is the role in loss and recovery of function of changes taking place at the lesion site, with particular emphasis on myelination and vasculature.

THE ISSUE OF SECONDARY PATHOLOGICAL MECHANISMS

Part of the difficulty of interpreting mechanisms of recovery of function in spinal cord trauma is that the mechanisms of tissue damage remain undefined. It is a widely held belief that some of the damage results from "secondary" pathological events occurring over at least several hours from the time of the mechanical insult (Table 1). Numerous potential mechanisms exist, and most of these

TABLE 1. *Summary of the sequence of events following spinal cord contusion or compression*

Primary damage
Mechanical disruption of nerve fibers, neuronal and glial cell membranes, and blood vessels
Secondary damage
Further loss of nerve fibers, neurons, and glia, involving hemorrhage, vascular occlusion, and ischemia; ionic disruption, edema; excitotoxicity; lipid peroxidation; energy depletion, lactate formation; inflammatory responses; demyelination
Repair and recovery
Proximal and distal to the lesion: synaptic plasticity. Sprouting.
At the lesion site:
Resolution of edema and inflammation
Reformation of glial parenchyma
Revascularization; remyelination

are interdependent and additive. Ischemia is one of the most thoroughly examined secondary problems in the injured tissue (18–21), though the question is not entirely resolved whether the hypoperfusion that is recorded in various injury models is responsible for, rather than a reflection of, further tissue necrosis. Similarly, the causative role of edema is difficult to evaluate, since it occurs irrespective of injury severity (22). The onset of deleterious free radical reactions, the activation of arachidonate metabolism, and the consumption of endogenous antioxidants are all reflections of a tissue environment that rapidly becomes unfavorable for cell survival (23–26), though the extent to which these changes are compartmentalized within the necrotic part of the tissue rather than affecting otherwise viable cells is not clearly established. The release of excitatory neurotransmitters, particularly amino acids, into the extracellular space is a potential source of secondary damage in a range of insults to the CNS (27). This may include spinal cord trauma (28,29), though the mechanism of effect on survival of axons projecting through the white matter is not clear.

Whatever the precise mechanisms may be, the initial injury appears to be followed by two opposing sets of processes, one tending to cause further tissue damage and functional deterioration and the other producing tissue repair and behavioral recovery. We have to deal with three classes of overlapping variables associated with primary injury, secondary damage, and repair processes. There is no reason to suggest *a priori* that these classes should vary proportionately with each other. The experimenter exercises some control over the input variables of primary mechanical damage, and the attempt to control these variables more directly has received much attention in recent years (10,30–35). However, the usual measured variables of outcome—histopathology, behavioral function, or electrophysiology—are compound products of all three classes of variables. There are currently no readily accessible means of measuring any of the underlying variables in isolation. This makes interpretation of mechanism uncomfortably speculative.

MYELINATION

Abnormalities of myelination are qualitatively obvious in histological sections through chronic experimental lesions. There are usually some completely demyelinated axons in such lesions, but the more common finding is of uneven, thin myelination and abnormally short internodes (8,36–38) typical of incomplete remyelination in the CNS (39,40). In more severe injuries, there is a tendency for widespread remyelination of central axons by peripheral Schwann cells (41). The functional significance of these morphological changes has not been defined in detail. Theoretical analyses have suggested that even minimal reformation of the myelin sheath with a few lamellae may be enough to restore conduction of action potentials (42). Though this interpretation is based on assumptions that considerably simplify axonal structure and biophysics (43), there is clear evidence of restored conduction with thin myelin sheaths following chemical demyelination in cat spinal cord (44). Experimental observations in traumatically injured cat spinal cord indicate that action potential conduction may be blocked at physiological temperatures in a significant proportion of nerve fibers (12,45). This kind of injury differs from chemical demyelination, since trauma induces more extensive degeneration, inflammation, and disruption of the parenchyma. The relative effectiveness of Schwann cell remyelination of central nerve fibers is still to be established, though local remyelination of surviving axons in injured cat spinal cord by Schwann cells can be associated with recovery of action potential propagation in some cases (41).

VASCULATURE

The capillary network in the injured cord is increased in density, and many small vessels are marked by an extensive perivascular space (46). The functional significance of this histopathological picture is not readily assessable. Hypervascularity is a common finding in a wide range of experimental pathological conditions in the CNS (47–50) as it is in equivalent clinical situations. Increased vascular density is often associated with a degree of fibrosis of small vessels (51). Little is known about the physiological significance of these long-term changes in vascularity. Few measurements are available to indicate the metabolic demand or the metabolite supply in chronically injured CNS. Normal oxygen tension in the white matter of adult mammalian spinal cord is high (52) despite the low capillary density relative to gray matter (46,53). Following injury, particularly in fibrotic areas, oxygen tensions may be elevated above normal levels (54). However, we do not know whether oxygen tension in hypervascular regions may become sufficiently abnormal to affect neuronal function.

Chronic hypervascularity and fibrosis are probably the result of inflammation that occurs in response to central hemorrhagic necrosis, particularly the activity of macrophages (55,56). Mononuclear phagocytes invade the necrotic region in large numbers a few days after injury (57), and in the case of traumatic injury to the CNS, most of these are probably derived from circulating monocytes rather than transformed microglia (17) (see also Giulian and Corpuz, this volume; Perry et al., this volume). Macrophages secrete a variety of angiogenic factors, including tumor necrosis factor α (58), the cytokine interleukin 1 (59), and basic fibroblast growth factor (60,61). The extent of stimulation of angiogenesis may depend on the degree or duration of hypoxia occurring during the subacute inflammatory phase (62).

TIME COURSE OF LOSS AND RECOVERY OF FUNCTION

Recovery of function in a wide variety of spinal cord injury models occurs over a similar time course, with most of the improvement occurring between 1 and 4 weeks from the time of injury. This is largely independent of species and functional measure used, at least with regard to the mean response of groups of subjects, as shown in Fig. 1. This graph shows a collation of data from six different injury models using rats, cats, and guinea pigs and measuring function with various combined behavioral scores (9,34, 63), with the cutaneus trunci muscle reflex receptive field and toe-spread response (64) or with somatosensory evoked potentials (65). Individual animals can show widely different histories of recovery around these mean values (35,64). Only with mild injuries does there appear to be significant recovery of function within the first week (9). Overall, the recovery of function in these animals is significantly slower than the recovery of locomotion and accurate beam walking in cats with discrete spinal cord hemisection or deafferentation (1,66,67). In the latter case, it may be assumed that the recovery process is dominated by plasticity of the nervous system remote from the site of lesion. This kind of recovery is extensive within 1 week and appears to be practically complete within 2 weeks of injury.

If recovery of function in traumatic spinal cord injury is determined principally by pro-

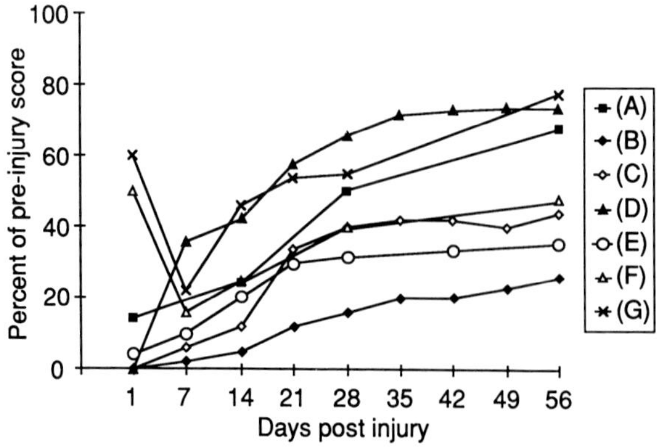

FIG. 1. A graph comparing the average rates of recovery of function recorded in a variety of animal models and species using widely different measures. The data are normalized to a percentage of the preinjury score in each study. The functional measures include a modified Tarlov locomotory behavior score in cats with compression injuries (A), a more complex combined behavioral score in rats with weight-drop contusion injuries of graded intensity (B–D), the receptive field area of the cutaneus trunci muscle reflex below the lesion (E), the toe-spread response (F) in guinea pigs with compression injuries, and the somatosensory evoked potential in cats with weight-drop contusion injuries (G). The data quoted in this figure are estimated from information presented in the following references: (A) 63; (B–D) 84 (where 2 is a severe, 3 a moderate, and 4 a mild injury level); (E–F) 64; (G) 65.

cesses occurring at the injury site itself, such as remyelination, then it should be possible to relate chronic histopathological evidence of those processes to the extent of recovery. In most injury models, it is impossible to distinguish, for individual animals, differences in the extent of recovery from variations in the severity of injury, since even relatively mild injuries produce initially severe behavioral deficits (Fig. 1). However, moderately severe compression of the lower thoracic spinal cord in guinea pigs produces relatively mild behavioral deficits up to 24 hr after injury (64). Subsequently, spontaneous and reflex function below the level of the lesion declines rapidly, usually to complete hindlimb paralysis and sensory loss by 7 days. Recovery from this secondary loss of function can vary from minimal to complete over the course of 2 to 4 weeks. As can be seen in Fig. 1, the average time course of this recovery is consistent with that occurring in other models, where a delayed loss is not seen. This does not appear to be a grossly different kind of injury from that produced by other types of contusion or compression. The morphometric characteristics of the focal spinal cord lesion are remarkably similar to those seen in weight-drop contusion of the cat spinal cord (10).

Delayed onset of functional deficits has also been recorded in cat spinal cord contusion injury using somatosensory evoked potentials (41,65). In this case, the secondary onset of loss of action potential conduction occurred between 6 and 24 hr rather than 1 to 2 days. This loss was clearly distinct from the primary loss of action potential conduction in the spinal cord, which is practically immediate in onset but often reverses within 1 hr. This primary loss and recovery correlate with the immediate disruption of the ionic environment, particularly the elevation and subsequent normalization of extracellular potassium ion activity (68,69). The onset of functional deficits is likely to be a complex function of a number of overlapping pathological processes. The ability to detect early functional changes also depends on the combination of an intermediate level of injury intensity, a rapidly reversible anesthetic, the avoidance of surgical procedures that may in themselves temporarily affect function, and the use of behavioral or electrophysiological measurements that allow functional changes to be observed.

SECONDARY DAMAGE AND RECOVERY IN GUINEA PIGS

It is important to understand the relationship between the various known pathological changes that occur following spinal cord injury and the secondary loss and recovery of function. To what extent do functional losses depend on transient displacement of the tissue ion and water balance, myelination deficits, deficiency of blood flow, or direct loss of neuronal connections? To what degree is recovery of function the result of resolution of the secondary disturbances, or does it depend on adaptation of the surviving part of the nervous system to the primary and secondary loss of connections? The guinea pig spinal cord injury model can be used to address some of these questions by examining the time course of changes in function and by correlating differences in quantitative morphometry of the lesion with differences in secondary functional changes. This comparison benefits from the unusual prominence of delayed secondary loss. This means that variability in secondary loss and recovery can be separated from variation in the primary disturbance.

The methods used in these studies have been described in previous reports. The injury model itself (64) consisted of a brief (15-sec) lateral compression of the thoracic (T-13) spinal cord of adult guinea pig to a thickness of 1.2 mm over a length of 5 mm. This procedure was carried out, following a single-segment laminectomy, under ketamine/xylazine/acepromazine anesthesia. The technique of line sampling of axonal morphometry from 1-μm plastic sections through the center of the lesion has been described in a series of papers (8,10,64). Briefly, 24 sample lines perpendicular to the pial surface were spaced evenly around the section (12 on each side of the midline). All axons intercepted by these lines were measured with the aid of a camera lucida and digitizing pad at a magnification of ×1,000. The depth of each axon from the pial surface, the longest and shortest axes, the width perpendicular to the sample line, and the thickness of the myelin sheath (where present) were all recorded and stored on the computer. A simple formula was then used to calculate the total number of axons and their size distribution, based on the total area of tissue surrounding each sample line (64).

Analysis of vasculature was based on measurements of all the blood vessels in complete transverse sections through the center of the lesion and at 10 and 20 mm rostral and caudal to the lesion center. All the vessels identified in 1-μm toluidine-blue-stained sections were drawn with camera lucida at a magnification of ×400, and the cross-sectional area and luminal width of each vessel were measured on a digitizing pad (46). To analyze the distribution of blood vessels in the presence of considerable loss of tissue at the lesion center, the cord cross section was divided into 200-μm-thick layers from the pial surface and also divided into ventral and dorsal halves. This allowed separation of the changes in white and gray matter vascular densities.

A number of simple behavioral tests were used to monitor function for periods of months post-injury. The most useful of these tests were the cutaneus trunci muscle (CTM) reflex receptive field measurement (64,70), which allows analysis of a specific ventrolateral ascending pathway, and the toe-spread response (64), which provides evaluation of a descending system, probably a form of reticulospinal startle response (71). In addition to these, a more generalized motor score for the hindlimbs was recorded, which provided a measurement of lumbar spinal cord function, including segmental elements—the flexor withdrawal reflex and proprioceptive placing—as well as less-specific effects of descending input, including weight support and locomotion. The CTM reflex receptive field

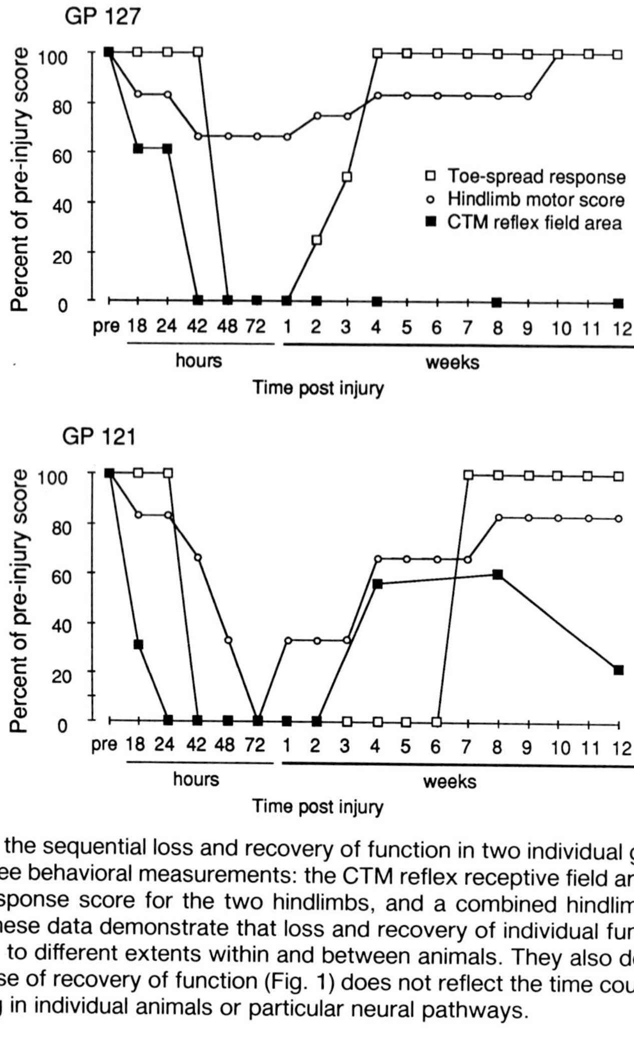

FIG. 2. Graphs of the sequential loss and recovery of function in two individual guinea pigs (GP 127 and 121) using three behavioral measurements: the CTM reflex receptive field area below the lesion, the toe-spread response score for the two hindlimbs, and a combined hindlimb motor score (explained in text). These data demonstrate that loss and recovery of individual functions can occur at different rates and to different extents within and between animals. They also demonstrate that the *average* time course of recovery of function (Fig. 1) does not reflect the time course of processes of recovery occurring in individual animals or particular neural pathways.

area provided a quantitative measurement, whereas the toe-spread response and hindlimb motor control were evaluated as motor scores, based on the sum of the two hindlimb scores assessed separately. An overall combined neurological score was derived by adding the CTM field, toe-spread, and hindlimb motor control values together, weighting them equally, since they appear to measure quite separate functional subsystems within the spinal cord (Fig. 2). Such combined scores are necessarily arbitrary combinations, though they remain useful for characterizing overall deficit, since any single measure, relying on a particular neural pathway, may be selectively affected by the spatial distribution of a given lesion, irrespective of the overall injury severity.

TIME COURSE OF CHANGES IN INDIVIDUAL ANIMALS

Figure 2 shows two examples of guinea pigs in which the three behavioral measurements are plotted against time post-injury. Several striking properties of the loss and recovery of function are seen only by observing the time course of such changes in individual animals rather than the averaged data. (a)

Changes in the three types of function are remarkably independent of each other, which indicates that the mechanisms of both loss and recovery of function are localized to particular tracts within the spinal cord and are not attributable to generalized depression of activity. (b) It is also clear that the average time course of recovery, as seen in Fig. 1, does not reflect the time course in individual animals, where recovery occurs more rapidly but at widely variable times post-injury. (c) Though, on average, the long-term recovery of function tends to approximate the degree of sparing of function seen in the first few hours after injury, individual functions may or may not recover within a 3-month period of observation. Again, the extent to which secondary loss is reversed in the months post-injury appears to be a property of individual subsystems within the spinal cord and is not a generalized phenomenon in each animal. (d) In some animals, such as GP 121 in Fig. 2, secondary deficits in the first week after injury can extend to segmental as well as long-tract function.

CORRELATION BETWEEN HISTOPATHOLOGY AND FUNCTION

The morphometry of these chronic lesions has been described in recent publications (46,64). The principal point of interest here lies in the implications of these data for the interpretation of loss and recovery mechanisms. Some of these implications can be summarized in terms of the correlation observed between widely different measures of outcome from injury. Figure 3 shows the interrelations among six measures of outcome in a group of 11 injured animals, with lines connecting those variables that were significantly ($p < 0.05$) correlated with each other, either positively (+) or negatively (−).

The central measurement is the cross-sectional area of the spinal cord lesion, which correlated with four of the other parameters. The spinal cord typically shrinks at the site of a chronic contusion or compression lesion, at least over the length of one or two spinal segments (10,64). This shrinkage is associated with the loss of central necrotic tissue and the

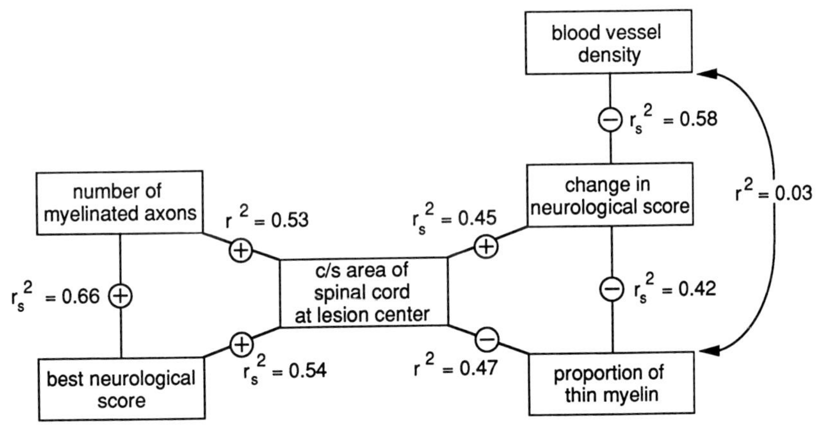

FIG. 3. A diagram to illustrate the significant correlations ($p < 0.05$) among six different measurements of outcome in the guinea pig injury model. Note that the change in combined neurological score between days 1 and 56 post-injury did not correlate with the best score measured in that time period. The best score correlated with the total number of myelinated axons surviving at the lesion center and with the cross-sectional area of the spinal cord at the center of the chronic lesion. The proportion of axons (>2 μm diameter) with thin myelin sheaths (myelination index or *g* ratio > 0.8) correlated negatively with the cross-sectional area and the change in neurological score. The density of small blood vessels in the white matter also correlated negatively with the change in score but with none of the other measurements. The numerical values quoted are the squares of Spearman coefficient of rank correlation (r_{s^2}) for scores or the Pearson product–moment coefficients of correlation (r^2) for continuous measurements.

limited amount of space filling by gliosis. In this case, the cross-sectional area of the lesion was normalized with respect to the cord cross section 10 mm rostral and caudal to the center of the lesion, to allow for variations in the size of the cord before injury. As might be expected, the cross-sectional area correlated with the number of myelinated axons surviving in the outer rim of the tissue at the center of the lesion and with the best combined neurological score recorded in the 8 weeks following injury. The left half of the diagram is therefore straightforward and consistent with a simple relationship in which the combined primary and secondary total loss of tissue is proportional to the survival of axons in the white matter, which in turn is proportional to the sparing of overall function.

The right half of the diagram shows a less predictable set of relations. The change in combined neurological score between 1 and 56 days post-injury correlated with the cross-sectional area of the lesion. It also correlated negatively with the density of blood vessels and with the proportion of surviving axons with thin myelin sheaths in the outer rim of white matter. The striking correlation here was with blood vessel density, since this parameter of the chronic lesion did not correlate with any of the other measurements, including reduced myelin thickness and cord cross-sectional area. Since the chronic lesion shows varying degrees of hypervascularity, this correlation indicates that the more normal the vascular density the better the recovery from injury. The most extreme hypervascularity was associated with lack of recovery from secondary loss of function. Figure 4 shows the relations among delayed functional change, hypervascularity, and thin myelination in a three-dimensional scattergram.

The set of correlations on the right of Fig. 3 and in Fig. 4 indicates that at least two separate processes are involved in secondary loss and recovery of function, one reflected in hypervascularity and the other in incomplete remyelination. Additionally, both of these processes appear to be relatively independent of the overall severity of the injury, as measured by the best neurological score or the number of myelinated axons surviving in the white matter. A possible interpretation of these variables and their interrelations might be that the overall survival of axons and the best neurological score predominantly indicate the extent of primary mechanical damage, with perhaps a small contribution from secondary losses. The change in neurological score, blood vessel density, and the proportion of thinly myelinated axons may then largely represent the outcome of the counteracting influences of secondary damage and reparative mechanisms. On this schema, the cross-sectional area of the lesion would logi-

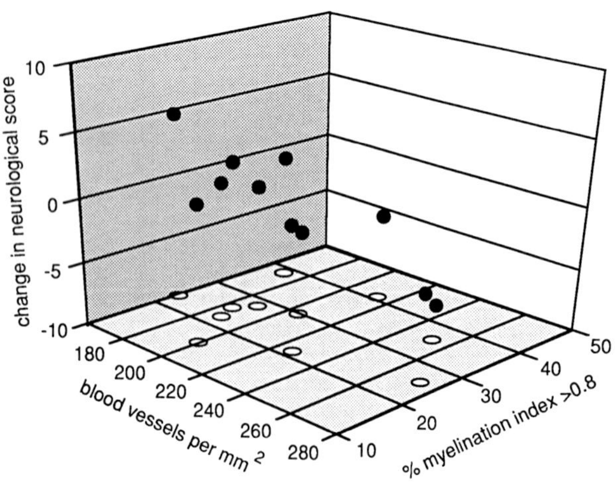

FIG. 4. A three-dimensional scatterplot to illustrate the relations (outlined in Fig. 3) among the change in combined neurological score from 1 to 56 days post-injury, the density of small blood vessels in the outer 400 μm of white matter, and the proportion of axons with myelination index > 0.8 (i.e., thinly myelinated). The experiments underlying these data are presented in more detail elsewhere (46).

cally be related to summation of the effects of primary damage, secondary degeneration, and repair processes, since it is correlated with both sets of variables. Correlation does not signify causation, but causal mechanisms or shared causality would be expected to be marked by correlation, so the absence of correlation between some of these parameters is as important as its presence between others.

Again, this evaluation of correlation deals with the characteristics of a group of animals. Unfortunately, the histopathology of individual animals can be examined at only one time post-injury, but some of the properties of particular lesions are important to relate to the functional changes. Figure 5 shows a transverse section through a small portion of the center of the lesion in a guinea pig spinal cord at 75 days after injury. Segregated areas of apparent demyelination and remyelination of this kind are seen from the first few days after injury, as in the photomicrographs of Fig. 6. This lesion was chosen because it showed a similar asymmetry of demyelination around the ventral fissure, where the demarcation of the demyelination is particularly sharp. Demyelination, like the loss of function following injury, is localized to different subdivisions of the spinal cord cross section. It is also likely that it develops with a different time course within separate subdivisions, but this is not easily demonstrated histopathologically.

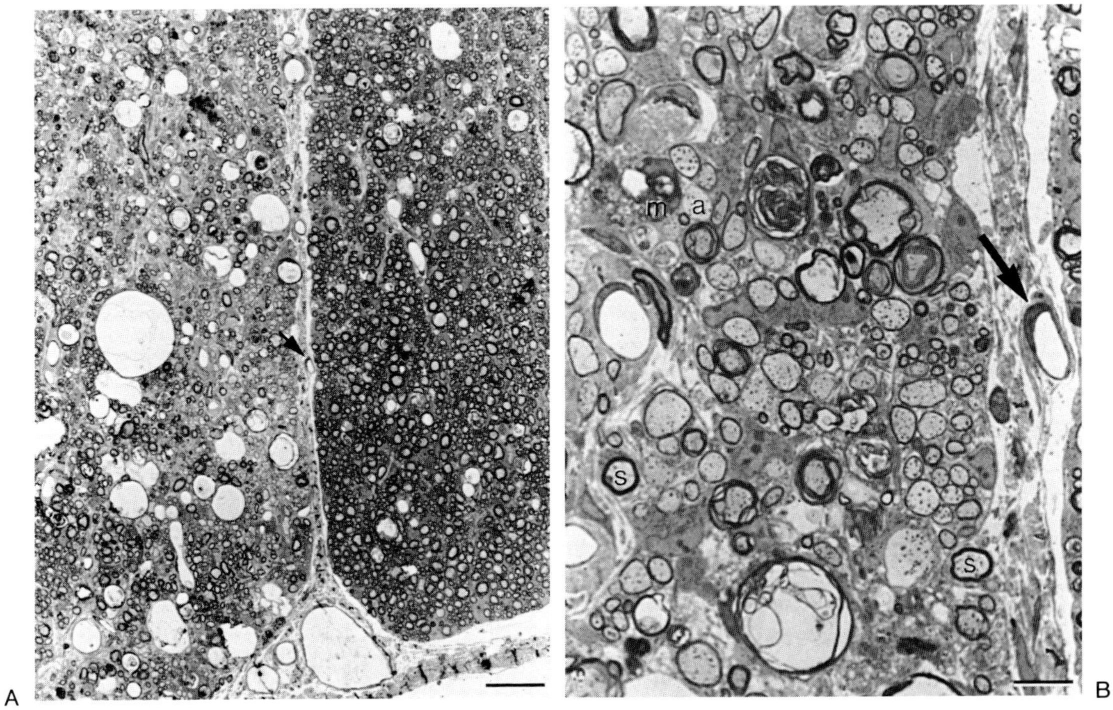

FIG. 5. Photomicrographs to illustrate incomplete remyelination of the spinal cord seen at 2.5 months following injury. (**A**) A toluidine-blue-stained 1-μm plastic transverse section through the ventromedial portion of the spinal cord at the center of the injury. In this case, the extent of degeneration to the left of the ventral median fissure was much greater than that on the right, though the quantitative difference in axonal survival on the two sides was not striking. (**B**) At higher magnification, to the left of the ventral median fissure (*arrow* in **A** and **B**), large numbers of axons were thinly myelinated, a few (a) were without myelin sheaths, and some were myelinated by Schwann cells (s). Macrophages (m) and myelin debris were still present within the tissue. This area of incomplete remyelination included much of the left ventromedial sector of the white matter. Scale bar, 50 μm in **A,** 10 μm in **B.**

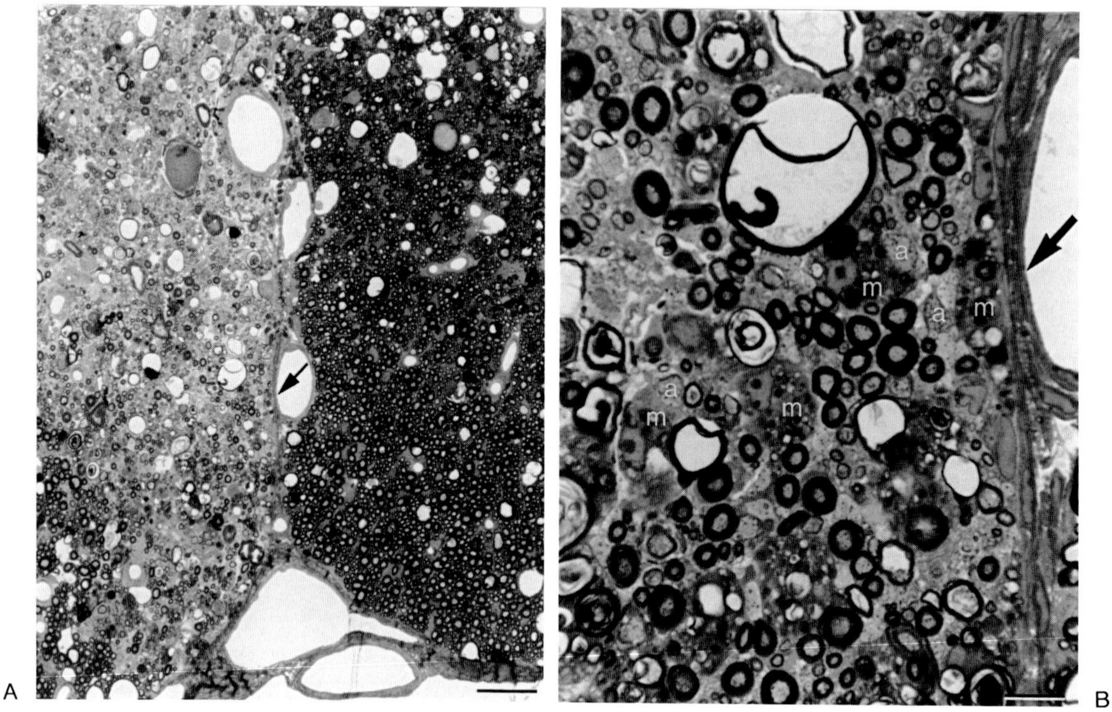

FIG. 6. Photomicrographs, similar to those in Fig. 5, of a similar case of asymmetric demyelination either side of the ventral median fissure (*arrows*), in this case at 4 days post-injury. (**A**) At low magnification, the normal gradient of demyelination with depth from the pia could be seen on the right, whereas extensive demyelination was present at all depths on the left. (**B**) At higher magnification, the axons to the left of the midline were either still myelinated at relatively normal thickness or completely demyelinated (a). The tissue was densely infiltrated with phagocytic cells (m) having the characteristics of macrophages or activated microglia. Many of these were closely associated with, or completely surrounding, demyelinated axons. Scale bar, 50 μm in **A,** 10 μm in **B.**

THE POTENTIAL ROLE OF INFLAMMATORY RESPONSES

Inflammatory responses appear to be the most significant contributors to secondary tissue damage that have particular relevance to demyelination and vascular changes. The close association between demyelination and the invasion of the tissue by large numbers of phagocytic cells can be seen in Fig. 6B and has been described in more detail for the cat spinal cord contusion model (57). Other secondary pathological processes tend to develop more rapidly following injury than the secondary loss of function seen in the guinea pig or the secondary decline of somatosensory evoked potentials in cat. Dramatic changes in the ionic milieu, including the initial stages of edema, begin within the first few minutes (19,22,68). High-energy phosphate depletion and increases in tissue lactic acid occur within minutes (72,73). Release of excitatory neurotransmitters develops immediately, presumably with direct membrane breakdown and with the elevation of extracellular potassium (28,29,74). Evidence of potentially damaging free radical reactions and significant loss of endogenous antioxidants occurs within minutes or a few hours (23–26). Reduction in blood flow usually occurs within 1 hr in the cat and rat (18–20), though the duration and pathophysiological significance of this hypoperfusion have not been established (75).

The role of macrophage activity in post-traumatic damage to the spinal cord has been discussed in more detail in a recent review (17). The potential clearly exists for "bystander damage" (76) to otherwise viable tissue in the presence of intense phagocytic activity. The degree to which it actually occurs in any given situation must be established independently. As is the case with the issue of early free radical damage, the reality of macrophage-induced degeneration depends not only on the existence of the agent of destruction but also on breakdown of endogenous protective systems and failure to compartmentalize a variety of biochemical processes (including free radical reactions) that are potentially extremely dangerous. The question of the practical significance of bystander damage is best addressed experimentally by attempting to interfere directly with the cellular response or with its biochemical consequences.

Recent experiments have taken the former approach by examining the effect of the macrophage toxin silica on the outcome from injury in the guinea pig model (77). A suspension of silica dust, injected intraperitoneally, reduces the numbers of circulating monocytes for a few days and reduces the intensity of the monocytic response to other inflammatory stimuli. Such an approach has been shown to delay the onset and reduce the severity of experimental allergic neuritis (78,79), experimental allergic encephalomyelitis (80), and experimental myasthenia gravis (81). In spinal cord injury, the effects of silica were somewhat surprising in that there was no effect on myelination index, although there was an increased delay in onset of functional deficits and a significant reduction in the hypervascularity of the lesion. The details of these experiments will be examined in a subsequent paper, but, for the purpose of this discussion, it appears that the activity of macrophages in the lesion at early stages may indeed be responsible for the onset of secondary functional losses and for the chronic hypervascularity of the lesion. However, the mechanism of these effects appears, both from the data outlined in Figs. 3 and 4 and from the results of the silica experiments, to be independent of demyelination and remyelination.

Although we are beginning to unravel the various strands of the secondary pathophysiology of spinal cord trauma, many questions remain, and most of the conclusions that can be drawn are tentative. What is the mechanism of demyelination in the traumatized cord? What role is played by the relatively small number of polymorphonuclear leukocytes that enter the lesion at early stages as a result of either hemorrhage or diapedesis (82,83)? What is the functional significance of hypervascularity? How might the activity of macrophages affect function in the injured spinal cord if not through myelination deficits? What proportion of functional recovery is attributable to remyelination? To what extent is chronic incomplete remyelination associated with permanent functional deficits? All these questions are open to investigation in animal models, though few of them are simple to answer. And even when they are answered in animal models, they may have to be asked again in the context of human spinal cord injury. The importance of answering them is clearly determined by the impetus that such knowledge might give to the development and application of acute and chronic therapy.

CONCLUSION

Long-term functional outcome from spinal cord injury depends on a succession of factors—primary mechanical damage, secondary pathological processes, and mechanisms of tissue repair and recovery. These recovery mechanisms include changes occurring at the injury site as well as in remote parts of the nervous system. The average rate of recovery of function appears to be broadly consistent across widely different models of blunt traumatic injury, including compression and contusion, in different laboratories and mammalian species. Recovery in individual animals and neural pathways can occur with widely differing time courses. The extent to which secondary damage and subsequent recovery mechanisms vary independently of the primary injury intensity has not been determined.

Posttraumatic changes in behavioral function in a guinea pig model of spinal cord injury correlated only weakly with a single measure of overall injury intensity, the gross cross-sectional area of the lesion site. Delayed behavioral changes correlated more strongly, but negatively, with the extent of hypervascularity in the chronic lesion and with the proportion of surviving axons having relatively thin myelin sheaths. These two morphometric features of the lesion did not correlate with each other. This set of relationships indicates that the secondary mechanisms of damage vary in intensity independently of the primary mechanical insult. It also indicates that at least two separate mechanisms are responsible for secondary changes. One of these is related to the development of hypervascularity and may be associated with the inflammatory activity of macrophages. The other is related to the sequence of demyelination and remyelination. This may be independent of the macrophage response, since it appears to be unaffected by the macrophage toxin silica under conditions where hypervascularity is reduced and secondary functional deficits are delayed.

ACKNOWLEDGMENT

The original work presented here was supported largely by grant NS-21122 from NIH/NINDS.

REFERENCES

1. Goldberger ME, Murray M. Recovery of movement and axonal sprouting may obey some of the same laws. In: Cotman C, ed. *Neuronal plasticity*. New York: Raven Press; 1978:73–96.
2. Goldberger ME, Murray M. Patterns of sprouting and implications for recovery of function. In: Waxman SG, ed. *Advances in neurology, Vol 47: Functional recovery from neurological disease*. New York: Raven Press; 1988:361–385.
3. Kakulas BA, Bedbrook GM. Pathology of injuries of the vertebral column. In: Vincken PJ, Bruyn GW, Braakman R, eds. *Handbook of clinical neurology, Vol 25, Part 1, Injuries of the spine and spinal cord*. Amsterdam: North-Holland; 1976:27–42.
4. Jellinger K. Neuropathology of cord injuries. In: Vincken PJ, Bruyn GW, Braakman R, eds. *Handbook of clinical neurology, Vol 25, Part 1, Injuries of the spine and spinal cord*. Amsterdam: North-Holland; 1976:43–121.
5. Kakulas BA. Pathology of spinal injuries. *Cent Nerv Syst Trauma* 1984;1:117–129.
6. Allen AR. Surgery of experimental lesion of spinal cord equivalent to crush injury of fracture dislocation of spinal column: a preliminary report. *JAMA* 1911;57:878–880.
7. Bresnahan JC, King JS, Martin GF, Yashon D. A neuroanatomical analysis of spinal cord injury in the rhesus monkey (*Macaca mulatta*). *J Neurol Sci* 1976;28:521–542.
8. Blight AR. Cellular morphology of chronic spinal cord injury in the cat: analysis of myelinated axons by line-sampling. *Neuroscience* 1983;10:521–543.
9. Noble L, Wrathall J. Spinal cord contusion in the rat: morphometric analyses of alterations in the spinal cord. *Exp Neurol* 1985;88:135–149.
10. Blight AR, DeCrescito V. Morphometric analysis of experimental spinal cord injury in the cat: the relation of injury intensity to survival of myelinated axons. *Neuroscience* 1986;19:321–341.
11. Bresnahan JC, Beattie MS, Stokes BT, Conway KM. Three-dimensional computer-assisted analysis of graded contusion lesions in the spinal cord of the rat. *J Neurotrauma* 1991;8:91–101.
12. Blight AR. Axonal physiology of chronic spinal cord injury in the cat: intracellular recording *in vitro*. *Neuroscience* 1983;10:1471–1486.
13. Blight AR, Gruner JA. Augmentation by 4-aminopyridine of vestibulospinal free fall responses in chronic spinal-injured cats. *J Neurol Sci* 1987; 82:145–159.
14. Blight AR, Toombs JP, Bauer MS, Widmer WR. The effects of 4-aminopyridine on neurological deficits in chronic cases of traumatic spinal cord injury in dogs: a phase I clinical trial. *J Neurotrauma* 1991;8:103–119.
15. Black JA, Felts P, Smith KJ, Kocsis JD, Waxman SG. Distribution of sodium channels in chronically demyelinated spinal cord axons: immuno-ultrastructural localization and electrophysiological observations. *Brain Res* 1991;544:59–70.
16. Franklin RJM, Crang AJ, Blakemore WF. Transplanted type-1 astrocytes facilitate repair of demyelinating lesions by host oligodendrocytes in adult rat spinal cord. *J Neurocytol* 1991;20:420–430.
17. Blight AR. Macrophages and inflammatory damage in spinal cord injury. *J Neurotrauma* 1991;8(Suppl 2):S83–S91.
18. Senter HJ, Venes JL. Altered blood flow and secondary injury in experimental spinal cord trauma. *J Neurosurg* 1978;49:569–578.
19. Young W, Flamm ES. Effect of high-dose corticosteroid therapy on blood flow, evoked potentials, and extracellular calcium in experimental spinal cord injury. *J Neurosurg* 1982;57:667–673.
20. Hall ED, Yonkers PA, Horan KL, Braughler JM.

Correlation between attenuation of posttraumatic spinal cord ischemia and preservation of tissue vitamin E by the 21-aminosteroid U74006F. *J Neurotrauma* 1989;6:169–176.
21. Tator CH, Fehlings MG. Review of the secondary injury theory of acute spinal cord trauma with emphasis on vascular mechanisms. *J Neurosurg* 1991;75:15–26.
22. Kwo S, Young W, DeCrescito V. Spinal cord sodium, potassium, calcium and water concentration changes in rats after graded contusion injury. *J Neurotrauma* 1989;6:13–24.
23. Pietronigro DD, Housepian M, Demopoulos HB, Flamm ES. Loss of ascorbic acid from injured feline spinal cord. *J Neurochem* 1983;41:1072–1076.
24. Saunders RD, Dugan LL, Demediuk P, Means ED, Horrocks LA, Anderson DK. Effects of methylprednisolone and the combination of alpha tocopherol and selenium on arachidonic acid metabolism and lipid peroxidation in traumatized spinal cord tissue. *J Neurochem* 1987;49:24–31.
25. Hsu CY, Halushka PV, Spicer KM, Hogan EL, Martin HF. Temporal profile of thromboxane–prostacyclin imbalance in experimental spinal cord injury. *J Neurol Sci* 1988;83:55–62.
26. Hall ED, Braughler JM. Central nervous system trauma and stroke. II. Physiological and pharmacological evidence for involvement of oxygen radicals and lipid peroxidation. *Free Radical Biol Med* 1989;6:303–313.
27. Meldrum B. Possible therapeutic applications of antagonists of excitatory amino acid neurotransmitters. *Clin Sci* 1985;68:113–122.
28. Faden AI, Lemke M, Simon RP, Noble L. N-Methyl-D-aspartate antagonist MK801 improves outcome following traumatic spinal cord injury in rats: behavioral, anatomic and neurochemical studies. *J Neurotrauma* 1988;5:33–45.
29. Liu D, McAdoo DJ. Neurotransmitter release following impact injury and glutamate neurotoxicity in the rat spinal cord. *Soc Neurosci Abstr* 1990; 16:1339.
30. Anderson TE. A controlled pneumatic technique for experimental spinal cord contusion. *J Neurosci Methods* 1982;6:327–333.
31. Ford RWJ. A reproducible spinal cord injury model in the cat. *J Neurosurg* 1983;59:268–275.
32. Wrathall JR, Pettigrew RK, Harvey F. Spinal cord contusion in the rat: production of graded, reproducible injury groups. *Exp Neurol* 1985;88:108–122.
33. Anderson TE. Spinal cord contusion injury: experimental dissociation of hemorrhagic necrosis and subacute loss of axonal conduction. *J Neurosurg* 1985;62:115–119.
34. Somerton SK, Stokes BT. Functional analysis of an electromechanical spinal cord injury device. *Exp Neurol* 1987;96:82–96.
35. Bresnahan JC, Beattie MS, Todd FD III, Noyes DH. A behavioral and anatomical analysis of spinal cord injury produced by a feedback-controlled impation device. *Exp Neurol* 1987;95:548–570.
36. Gledhill RF, Harrison BM, McDonald WI. Demyelination and remyelination after acute spinal cord compression. *Exp Neurol* 1973;38:472–487.
37. Wakefield CL, Eidelberg E. Electron microscopic observations of the delayed effects of spinal cord compression. *Exp Neurol* 1975;48:637–646.
38. Griffiths IR, McCulloch MC. Nerve fibers in spinal cord impact injuries. Part 1. Changes in the myelin sheath during the initial 5 weeks. *J Neurol Sci* 1983;58:335–349.
39. Bunge MB, Bunge RP, Ris H. Ultrastructural study of remyelination in an experimental lesion in adult cat spinal cord. *J Biophys Biochem Cytol* 1961; 10:67–94.
40. Ludwin SK: Remyelination in the central nervous system and the peripheral nervous system. In: Waxman SG, ed. *Advances in neurology, Vol 47: Functional recovery in neurological disease.* New York: Raven Press; 1988:215–254.
41. Blight AR, Young W. Central axons in injured cat spinal cord recover electrophysiological function following remyelination by Schwann cells. *J Neurol Sci* 1989;91:15–34.
42. Koles ZJ, Rasminsky M. A computer simulation of conduction in demyelinated nerve fibers. *J Physiol* 1972;227:351–364.
43. Halter JA, Clark JW Jr. A distributed-parameter model of the myelinated nerve fiber. *J Theor Biol* 1991;148:345–382.
44. Smith KJ, Blakemore WF, McDonald WI. The restoration of conduction by central remyelination. *Brain* 1981;104:383–404.
45. Blight AR. Effect of 4-aminopyridine on axonal conduction-block in chronic spinal cord injury. *Brain Res Bull* 1989;22:47–52.
46. Blight AR. Morphometric analysis of blood vessels in chronic experimental spinal cord injury: hypervascularity and recovery of function. *J Neurol Sci* 1991;106:158–174.
47. Franson P. Quantitative electron microscopic observations on the non-neuronal cells and lipid droplets in the posterior funiculus of the cat after dorsal rhizotomy. *J Comp Neurol* 1985;231:490–499.
48. Eriksdotter-Nilsson M, Björklund H, Dahl D, Olson L, Ingvar M. Sustained seizures cause circumscribed cerebral changes in glial fibrillary acidic protein, neurofilament and laminin immunofluorescence. *Exp Brain Res* 1987;69:155–166.
49. Iadecola C, Arneric SP, Reis DJ. Local and remote microvascular changes in excitotoxin-induced focal brain lesions. *Brain Res* 1989;501:188–193.
50. Trimmer PA, Wunderlich RE. Changes in astroglial scar formation in rat optic nerve as a function of development. *J Comp Neurol* 1990;296:359–378.
51. Lassmann H. *Comparative neuropathology of chronic experimental allergic encephalomyelitis and multiple sclerosis.* Berlin: Springer-Verlag; 1983.
52. Stokes BT, Garwood M, Walters P. Oxygen fields in specific loci of the canine spinal cord. *Am J Physiol* 1981;240:H761–H766.
53. Ireland WP, Fletcher TF, Bingham C. Quantification of microvasculature in the canine spinal cord. *Anat Rec* 1981;200:103–113.
54. Stokes BT, Reier PJ. Oxygen transport in intraspinal fetal grafts: graft–host relations. *Exp Neurol* 1991;111:312–323.
55. Polverini PJ, Cotran RS, Gimbrone MA Jr, Unanue ER. Activated macrophages induce vascular proliferation. *Nature* 1977;269:804–805.

56. Beck DW, Hart MN, Cancilla PA. The role of macrophages in microvascular regeneration following brain injury. *J Neuropathol Exp Neurol* 1983; 42:601–614.
57. Blight AR. Delayed demyelination and macrophage invasion: a candidate for secondary cell damage in spinal cord injury. *Cent Nerv Syst Trauma* 1985;2:299–315.
58. Leibovich SJ, Polverini PJ, Shepard HM, Wiseman DM, Shively V, Nuseir N. Macrophage-induced angiogenesis is mediated by tumour necrosis factor-α. *Nature* 1987;329:630–632.
59. Giulian D, Woodward J, Young DG, Krebs JF, Lachman LB. Interleukin-1 injected into mammalian brain stimulates astrogliosis and neovascularization. *J Neurosci* 1988;8:2485–2490.
60. Baird A, Mormède P, Böhlen P. Immunoreactive fibroblast growth factor in cells of peritoneal exudate suggests its identity with macrophage-derived growth factor. *Biochem Biophys Res Commun* 1985;126:358–364.
61. Knighton DR, Phillips GD, Fiegel VD. Wound healing angiogenesis: indirect stimulation by basic fibroblast growth factor. *J Trauma* 1990;30:S134–S144.
62. Knighton DR, Hunt TK, Scheuentstuhl H, Halliday BJ, Werb Z, Banda MJ. Oxygen tension regulates the expression of angiogenesis factor by macrophages. *Science* 1983;221:1283–1285.
63. Means ED, Anderson DK, Waters TR, Kalaf L. Effect of methylprednisolone in compression trauma to the feline spinal cord. *J Neurosurg* 1981; 55:200–208.
64. Blight AR. Morphometric analysis of a model of spinal cord injury in guinea pigs, with behavioral evidence of delayed secondary pathology. *J Neurol Sci* 1991;103:156–171.
65. Blight AR, Young W. Axonal morphometric correlates of evoked potential in experimental spinal cord injury. In: Salzman S, ed. *Neural monitoring.* Clifton, NJ: Humana Press; 1990:87–113.
66. Goldberger ME, Murray M. Locomotor recovery after deafferentation of one side of the cat's trunk. *Exp Neurol* 1980;67:103–117.
67. Goldberger ME: The role sprouting might play during the recovery of motor function. In: Flohr H, Precht W, eds. *Lesion-induced neuronal plasticity in sensorimotor systems.* Berlin: Springer; 1981: 130–140.
68. Young W, Koreh I. Potassium and calcium changes in injured spinal cords. *Brain Res* 1986;365:42–53.
69. Young W, Rosenbluth J, Wojak JC, Sakatani K, Kim H. Extracellular potassium activity and axonal conduction in spinal cord of the myelin deficient mutant rat. *Exp Neurol* 1989;106:41–51.
70. Blight AR, McGinnis ME, Borgens RB. Cutaneous trunci muscle reflex of the guinea pig. *J Comp Neurol* 1990;296:614–633.
71. Gruner JA. Comparison of vestibular and auditory startle responses in the rat and cat. *J Neurosci Methods* 1989;27:13–23.
72. Anderson DK, Means ED, Waters TR, Spears CJ. Spinal cord energy metabolism following compression trauma to the feline spinal cord. *J Neurosurg* 1980;53:375–380.
73. Braughler JM, Hall ED. Lactate and pyruvate metabolism in injured cat spinal cord before and after a single large intravenous dose of methylprednisolone. *J Neurosurg* 1983;59:256–261.
74. Liu D, Valadez V, Sorkin LS, McAdoo DJ. Norepinephrine and serotonin release upon impact injury to rat spinal cord. *J Neurotrauma* 1990;7:219–227.
75. Young W. Blood flow, metabolic and neurophysiological mechanisms in spinal cord injury. In: Becker DP, Povlishock JT, eds. *Central nervous system trauma status report.* Bethesda, MD: NIH, NINCDS; 1985:463–473.
76. Wisniewski HM, Bloom BR. Primary demyelination as a nonspecific consequence of a cell-mediated immune reaction. *J Exp Med* 1975;141:346–359.
77. Blight AR. Effects of the macrophage toxin silica on secondary damage in spinal cord injury. *Soc Neurosci Abstr* 1991;17:162.
78. Tansey FA, Brosnan CF. Protection against experimental allergic neuritis with silica quartz dust. *J Neuroimmunol* 1982;3:169–179.
79. Craggs RI, King RHI, Thomas PK. The effect of suppression of macrophage activity on the development of experimental allergic neuritis. *Acta Neuropathol* 1984;62:316–323.
80. Brosnan CF, Bornstein MB, Bloom BR. Effects of macrophage depletion on the clinical and pathologic expression of experimental allergic encephalomyelitis. *J Immunol* 1981;126:614–620.
81. Kinoshita I, Nakamura T, Satoh A, et al. Role of the macrophage in the pathogenesis of experimental autoimmune myasthenia gravis. *J Neurol Sci* 1988; 87:49–59.
82. Means ED, Anderson DK. Neuronophagia by leukocytes in experimental spinal cord injury. *J Neuropathol Exp Neurol* 1983;42:707–719.
83. Hsu CY, Dimitrijevic MR. Methylprednisolone in spinal cord injury: the possible mechanism of action. *J Neurotrauma* 1990;7:115–119.
84. Noble LJ, Wrathall JR. Correlative analyses of lesion development and functional status after graded spinal cord contusive injuries in the rat. *Exp Neurol* 1989;103:34–40.

Advances in Neurology, Vol. 59, edited by
Fredrick J. Seil. Raven Press, Ltd.,
New York © 1993.

9

Essential Prerequisites for Remyelination of Oligodendrocytes

Division, Motility, and Structural Rearrangement

Pamela E. Knapp, Robert P. Skoff, and Charles S. Booth

Department of Anatomy and Cell Biology, Wayne State University School of Medicine, Detroit, Michigan 48201

Oligodendrocytes (OLs) are the myelinating cells of the central nervous system (CNS). Unlike their peripheral nervous system counterparts, the Schwann cells, OLs are generally perceived as incapable of mounting a significant remyelinating effort after injury to the CNS. This deficiency is thought to stem, in part, from the inability of OLs to divide and form a population of new OLs that would be available for remyelination. Further, the extensive network of processes established by the mature OL would seem to limit its mobility, a necessary prerequisite for a cell to invade a demyelinated zone. Consequently, it is much easier to envision remyelination as being carried out by an undifferentiated, proliferating cell that possesses migratory capacity rather than by a differentiated cell that has an elaborate cytoarchitecture. To the contrary, a number of lines of evidence from classical studies *in vivo* strongly hint that OLs can function as remyelinating cells. However, the demonstration of such a dynamic role for OLs *in vivo* is difficult and, at best, can only be extrapolated from a series of static images. We have thus developed a tissue culture system that permits us to track an individual OL to determine whether it can divide, how it divides, its mobility, and its potential to recover following injury.

In previous work we have addressed the lineage of glial cells within the CNS *in situ* (e.g., refs. 1–3). Directly relevant to the issue of remyelination is the question of whether OLs have the potential to divide. Our recent studies show that many glia that express glycolipid antigens specific for OLs are proliferating during normal development *in situ* (3). Although these OLs have not yet made myelin sheaths, they nevertheless have an elaborate network of fine processes that extend into the neuropil for considerable distances. Furthermore, these glycolipid$^+$ OLs constitute a majority of the dividing cells around the time of myelination in certain white matter zones (3). The fact that these OLs continue to divide even after expressing markers of differentiated OLs argues that commitment to the OL lineage does not preclude glial cells from further division. This property of OLs is much the same *in vitro,* where young glia from neonatal CNS tissues divide, probably more than once, after expression of specific OL antigenic markers (4). Like their counterparts *in situ,* the OLs proliferating in culture frequently have an elaborate set of processes. Both of these studies show that relatively immature OLs are able to incorporate ^{3}H-thymidine and proliferate, and we have recently begun a series of experiments *in vitro*

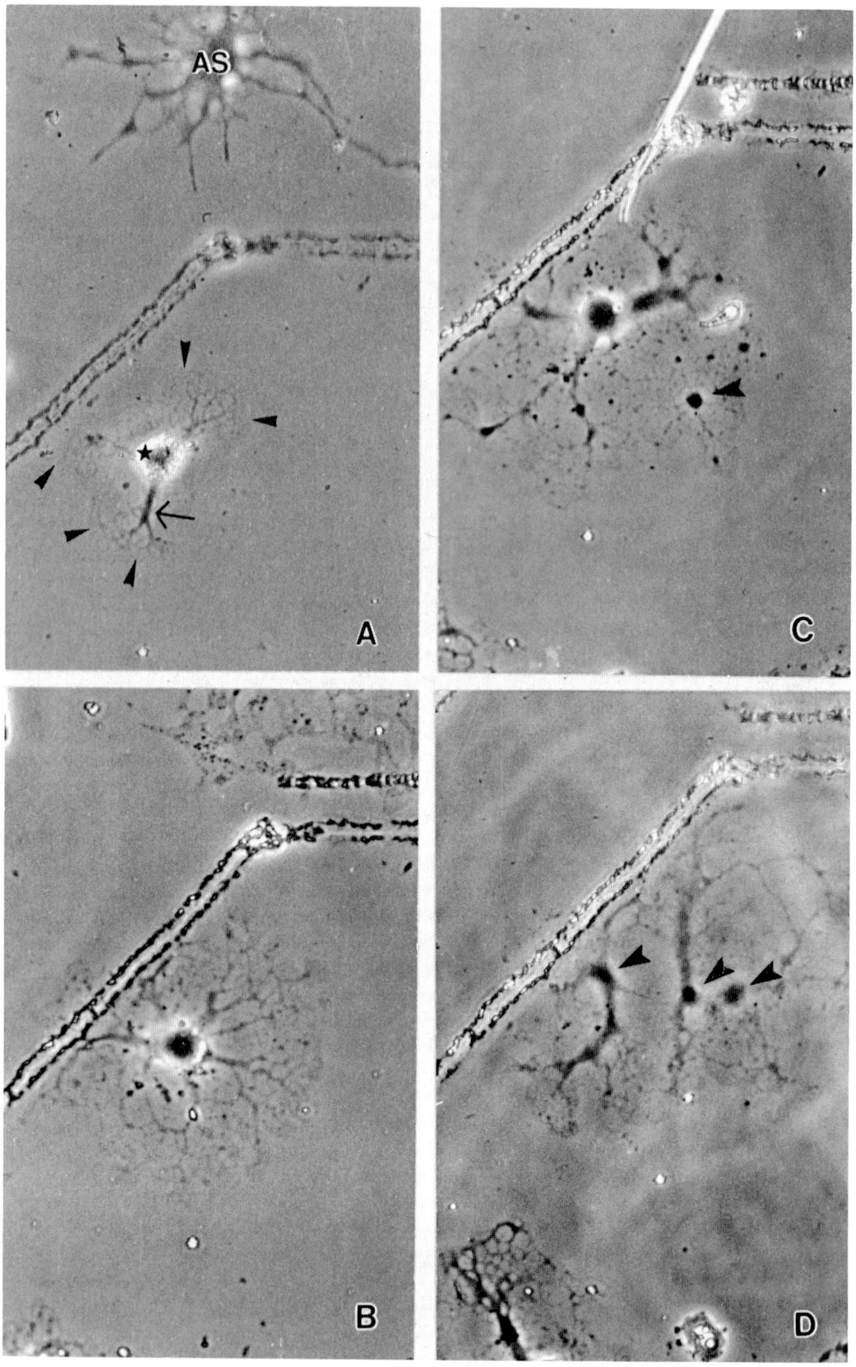

FIG. 1. An OL in an enriched culture undergoes division. These photographs were printed at a relatively high magnification (×750) to show the fine details of this cell's processes. Low magnification pictures show no other cell has migrated into the territory of the OL. **A:** Day 1. The OL has one large process (*arrow*) within a network of smaller processes and membranes. The margins of the membrane sheets (*arrowheads*) surround the cell body (*asterisk*). An astrocyte (AS) is located outside the hexagon. **B:** Day 2. The OL has considerably more cytoplasm and an increased number of processes and membranous areas. The astrocyte has been killed, and only remnants are visible. **C:** Day 3. A second, much smaller cell body (*arrowhead*) appears within the membranous expansion of the original OL. The parent cell has undergone an asymmetric division. **D:** Day 4. It appears that there are now three cell bodies (*arrowheads*) within the area of the parent cell. It is unclear whether the parent or the smaller daughter cell has divided to form the third cell. Note that all of the cell bodies are now roughly of equivalent size.

designed to observe isolated OLs as they proceed through division and differentiation. By following individual OLs in long-term cultures, we have observed that mature OLs with thick, tortuous processes and myelin-like membrane sheets are able to undergo a remarkable degree of structural reorganization involving both processes and membrane sheets. The OLs with these elaborate networks of processes undergo mitosis (Fig. 1), as predicted from the ^{3}H-thymidine experiments. When such OLs are injured by laser ablation of one or more processes, the cells usually survive. In some instances the cut process reforms, but in others it is retracted and/or replaced. These findings suggest that, at least *in vitro,* OLs have a significant capacity for regrowth and remyelination after injury.

IN VITRO METHODS

Primary cultures were established as previously described from 2-day postnatal mouse cerebral cortex and grown in medium containing 10% fetal calf serum (4,5). For some experiments, enriched cultures of OLs were prepared from primary cultures by gently syringing medium over the culture surface to dislodge the superficial layer of cells that contains OLs. These cells were replated at very low density onto glass coverslips coated with poly-L-lysine and maintained in a defined medium containing 1% fetal calf serum. For laser injury studies, cells were plated onto special carbon coated glass coverslips supplied by the laser manufacturer (Meridian Instruments, Okemos, MI). These coverslips absorb and focus the heat generated by the laser within a small area, permitting finely localized ablation. In studies of OL development, OLs were physically isolated and then identified in two ways to permit easy relocation. The position coordinates of selected cells were stored in the computer, and then a hexagonal ring was burned in the carbon surface around the cell with the laser. Because of the known motility of glial progenitors and astrocytes, nearby non-OLs were killed by laser ablation to ensure that only a single cell was followed. Cells were killed by several full-power laser blasts. In regeneration studies, the processes of OLs were injured by a single laser cut at 30–40% laser strength. Approximately 75% of injured cells survived and were followed for 1 week. Some OLs were identified after development or regeneration by fluorescent immunostaining with a monoclonal antibody (RmAb) that recognizes galactocerebroside, a specific OL glycolipid (3,5). Immunostaining was detected by laser scanning at the fluorescein excitation wavelength (488 nm).

RESULTS AND DISCUSSION

Oligodendrocytes Are Able to Divide *in Vitro*

In studies combining ^{3}H-thymidine or bromodeoxyuridine with immunocytochemistry to identify dividing cells, we found that young OLs that express OL-specific glycolipid antigens recognized by the monoclonal antibodies RmAb and 007 constituted 30% to 50% of the dividing, process-bearing cells in primary cultures after 1 to 4 days *in vitro* (DIV) (4). These young, committed OLs were sometimes able to divide several times during a 4-DIV period (4). Typically, these cells had multiple fine processes radiating in several directions, but they did not usually have membrane sheets. Some process-bearing astrocytes, identified with antibodies to glial fibrillary acidic protein (GFAP), were also found to divide during this period. Cells that reacted with the 007 antibody were followed for 4 days in culture and never expressed GFAP. This series of experiments showed that many OLs that express specific markers are able to divide, and that even proliferating OLs could not be switched into the astrocyte lineage by growth in 10% fetal calf serum. These results parallel those seen *in vivo,* where oligodendroblasts and astroblasts have been shown to be in separate lineages (3,6). We used our *in vitro* system to assess the potential of individual OLs to divide and

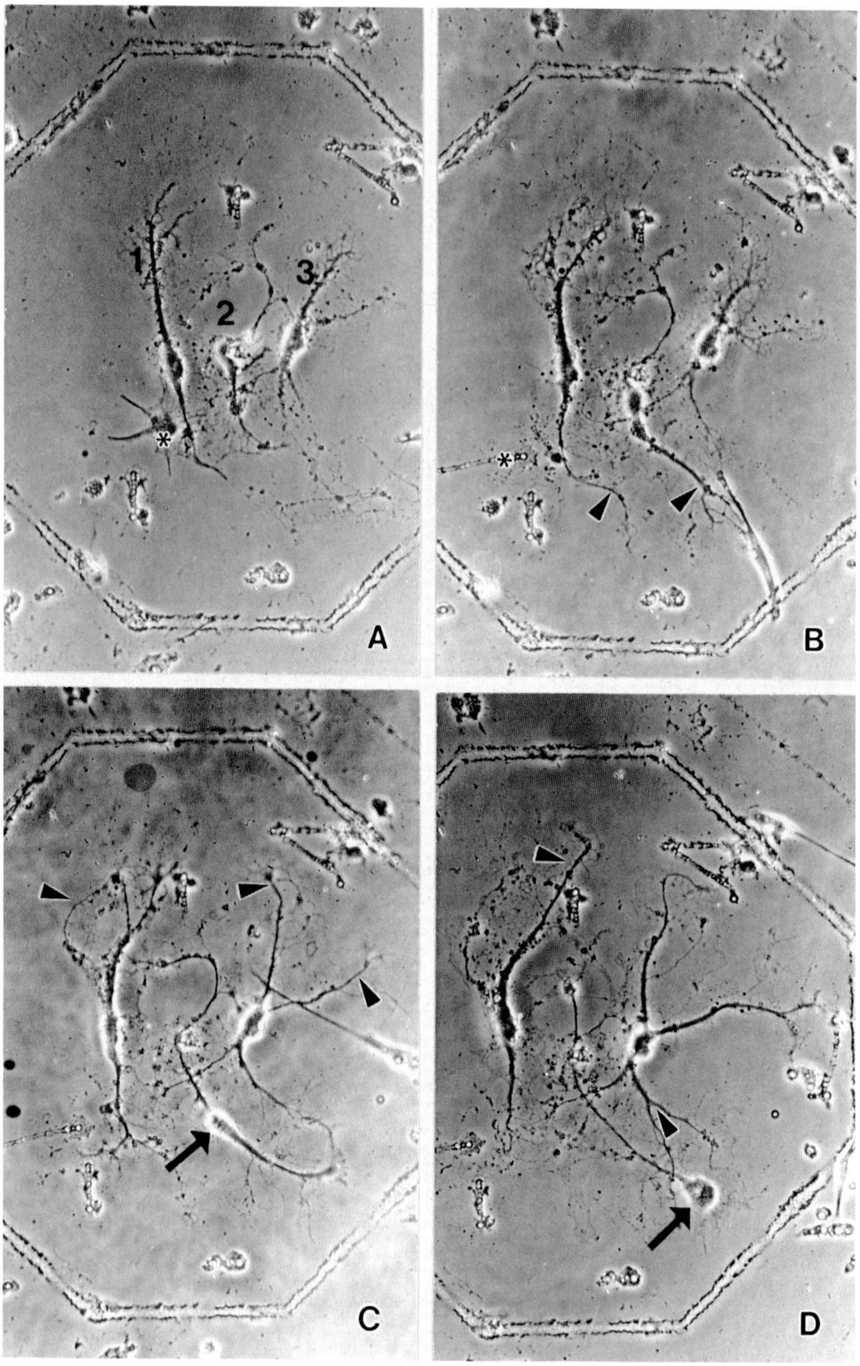

FIG. 2. Three OLs in an enriched culture illustrate the motility and structural reorganization that can occur in these morphologically well-developed cells over time. **A:** Day 1. Three OLs (1–3), each with a network of processes and membrane sheets, and an astrocyte (*asterisk*) are located in the hexagon. **B:** Day 2. The processes of OLs 1 and 2, which are at the bottom of the picture, have elongated (*arrowheads*). The nuclei of OLs 1 and 3 remain in the same position while the cell body of OL 2 begins to shift downward. An encroaching astrocyte has been killed by laser ablation (asterisk indicates a burn mark in the area where the astrocyte was killed). **C:** Day 3. The cell body (*arrow*) of OL 2 has

to describe how division occurs. Isolated cells were followed for periods of up to 10 days in enriched OL preparations. These OLs were at least 13 days *in vitro* at the time that they were selected for observation. The OLs were photographed at least once a day. To ensure that nearby cells were not migrating into our viewing field, non-OLs near the area of interest were killed by laser ablation. Results showed that a small percentage of OLs with large process networks underwent division within the period of observation. The division was usually asymmetric, with the new cell receiving a lesser amount of cytoplasm. Figure 1 shows an example of a dividing OL with an extensive process network. This particular cell increased its cytoplasmic volume and the length and number of its processes in the 2 days preceding division.

The evidence for both *in vivo* and *in vitro* development now indicates that immature OLs are capable of division even after they express markers indicating commitment to the OL lineage. The decision to commit to a particular glial lineage does not seem, *a priori,* to exclude the subsequent division of committed cells. Although the *in vivo* evidence suggests that OL proliferation in the mature CNS is a rare event except in some models of CNS injury (7–9), this does not mean that OLs are inherently unable to divide. It may simply indicate that there are factors or conditions in the mature CNS that inhibit division. Recent evidence from another study indicates that OLs isolated from mature rat CNS have a higher capacity for remyelination than do immature cells (10). These mature OLs may actually have to undergo dedifferentiation and then division before they remyelinate. Such results, when viewed in conjunction with our studies, suggest that it is not necessary to postulate the existence of an undifferentiated "adult 02A progenitor cell" (11) in order to explain remyelination in the mature CNS.

Oligodendrocytes Undergo Continuous Structural Change *in Vitro*

When OLs are grown *in vitro,* they produce large membranous expansions along the lengths and tips of their processes (5). These membrane sheets immunostain for both myelin glycolipids and proteins and are reminiscent of unfurled myelin sheaths. It might be assumed that these myelin-like membranes limit the motility of OLs *in vitro.* In other systems, even very young OLs have been thought to be nonmotile (12). Our long-term studies of isolated OLs *in vitro* now show that this is not the case. Surprisingly, OLs with elaborate processes and membrane sheets are capable of a wide spectrum of structural changes and movements. In some OLs these movements are limited to the processes (Figs. 2, 3). Existing processes can be partially or entirely retracted, and new processes may be formed, or small processes may be extended. The caliber of existing processes may increase or decrease. When a process is attached to a membrane sheet, the sheet appears to grow or to be drawn back in the direction of process movement. In some OLs the cell body moves, usually appearing to migrate along the length of a process (Fig. 2). Very occasionally an entire cell relocates, sometimes several hundred micrometers from its original position over the course of an experiment. Under our culture condi-

←

shifted further along the lower process as indicated by the change in its position from the side of the hexagon. Note that the upper process of OL 2 is still near its original position. The upper branches of OL 3 have undergone considerable elongation (*arrowheads*), and a new process has started to form in OL 1 (*arrowhead*). **D:** Day 4. The cell body (*arrow*) of OL 2 is now at the extreme far end of the lower process. The distance traveled in 2 days by the cell body of OL 2 is approximately 100 to 130 μm. One of the lower processes of OL 3 has developed a thick fork (*arrowhead*), while its upper two processes have thickened and lengthened. The major process in OL 1 has elongated and is also much thicker (*arrowhead*).

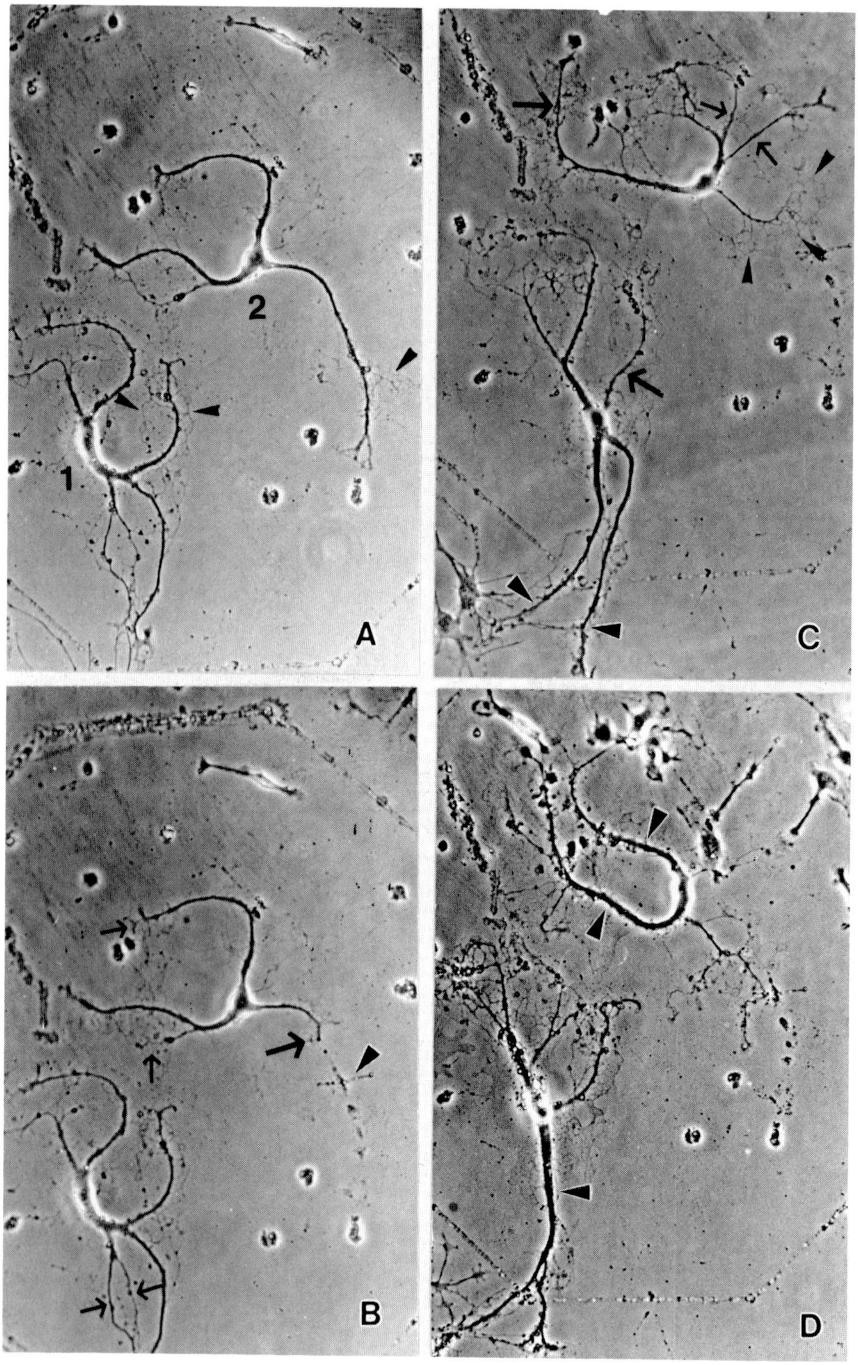

FIG. 3. Two OLs in an enriched culture exhibit striking cytoarchitectural changes. A process of one of the OLs has been severed by the laser. **A:** Day 1. Two OLs (1,2) have several thick, tortuous processes with membranous areas (margins indicated by *arrowheads*). **B:** At 2.5 hr after the lower process of cell 2 was injured (*arrowhead* indicates burn mark left by laser). The cut process is dying back toward the cell body (*large arrow*). There are also subtle differences in other areas of both cells (compare areas at small arrows with the same areas in A). **C:** Day 3. Two days after the cut, both cells show structural changes. In OL 2 the cut process has partially died back, become thinner, and formed

tions, these movements are calculated to be in the range of 3 to 4 μm/hr. This is slower than the rate of movement of perinatal glial progenitors (20 μm/hr), but comparable to the rate of movement of adult glial progenitors (4 μm/hr) (11). Our results show that OLs, even those with extensive processes and membrane sheets, exhibit a surprising degree of motility *in vitro.*

Oligodendrocytes are Able to Regrow Processes after Injury

The ability of OLs to survive and repair after injury was evaluated using the laser cytometer to ablate process(es) of an OL. The great majority of OLs survive this severe physical trauma and respond in one of several ways (Fig. 3). In some cells the severed process is able to regrow. When this happens, the tip of the growing process almost never follows the original pathway. Regrowth may be in roughly the original direction, or it may be in a completely different direction. We do not have any information that suggests what cues may be guiding the path of regrowth. Other cells respond to the injury by entirely retracting the cut process. In these cells new processes are sometimes formed, or existing ones are thickened and/or lengthened. The structural changes seen after injury are not qualitatively different from those seen in the uninjured cells. These observations on the behavior of OLs after mechanical injury suggest that OLs are able to mount effective repair mechanisms, at least *in vitro,* and that these efforts can result in regrowth, new growth, and perhaps even division.

CONCLUSION

To effectively remyelinate an unmyelinated or demyelinated zone, OLs must possess certain attributes. These include one or more of the following: (a) the capacity to proliferate, thereby creating a pool of cells available for remyelination; (b) an ability to migrate into an injured area; and (c) the capacity to reorganize their cytoplasm so that myelinating processes can grow into damaged areas. Our studies show that cells in the OL lineage have the potential to divide during *in situ* development. Although OLs that have established myelin sheaths normally do not proliferate during development, those that do often have an elaborate network of processes. Division of these cells (at least *in vitro*) often appears to be asymmetric, with one of the daughter cells keeping the majority of the cytoplasm and processes and the other daughter cell being smaller with shorter processes. This tissue culture observation is intriguing because OLs *in situ* which are about to undergo division have a nucleus located at one end of the cell and the processes usually located at the opposite end (1). The implication is that OL cell division in the animal is also asymmetric.

A demonstration of OL motility and structural reorganization is more easily made in an *in vitro* environment where individual cells can be followed over time. We have assessed the potential of OLs to move and to recover following injury in an environment in which the OLs are unimpeded by neurons and astrocytes. In this situation, OLs with large membrane sheets are capable of both motility and a high degree of structural rear-

←

a lacy network of fine process outgrowth (*arrowheads*). There are two new processes in OL 2 (*small arrows*), and a horizontal process has taken a turn and is now growing vertically (*large arrow*). The downward processes in OL 1 are much longer (*arrowheads*). A third process (*large arrow*) has thinned out and now emanates from the area of the cell body which has shifted slightly downward and to the right. **D:** Day 7. Six days after the cut both cells are still alive. Only one downward growing process is present in OL 1 (*arrowhead*); it is quite thick, which may indicate fusion of the two earlier processes. OL 2 has now only two very large, thick processes. One of them has reoriented its direction of growth so that both are directed toward the left of the picture (*arrowheads*).

rangement. Even after injury or complete severance, processes are often repaired, and new growth is established from the injured area. This finding argues that OLs have the intrinsic potential to remyelinate tissue. The injury of an OL with an elaborate cytoarchitecture does not impair its capacity to move or to form new processes or myelin-like membranes, at least *in vitro.* These results suggest that the remyelination observed in earlier *in situ* models of CNS injury (7,8) might well have been accomplished by OLs, as originally suggested by those authors. The studies also raise the issue that cellular and molecular interactions between OLs and astrocytes, microglia, macrophages, and neurons may interfere with an OL's capacity to remyelinate in certain disorders.

ACKNOWLEDGMENTS

This work was supported by NIH grant NS15338 and a grant from Meridian Instruments to R.P.S.

REFERENCES

1. Skoff RP, Price DL, Stocks A. Electron microscopic studies of gliogenesis in rat optic nerve. I. Cell proliferation. *J Comp Neurol* 1976;169:291–312.
2. Skoff RP, Price DL, Stocks A. Electron microscopic studies of gliogenesis in rat optic nerve. II. Time of origin. *J Comp Neurol* 1976;169:313–334.
3. Skoff RP, Knapp PE. Division of astroblasts and oligodendroblasts in postnatal rodent brain: evidence for separate astrocyte and oligodendrocyte lineages. *Glia* 1991;4:165–174.
4. Knapp PE. Studies of glial lineage and proliferation *in vitro* using an early marker for committed oligodendrocytes. *J Neurosci Res* 1991;30:336–345.
5. Knapp PE, Bartlett WP, Skoff RP. Cultured oligodendrocytes mimic *in vivo* characteristics: cell shape, expression of myelin specific antigens, and membrane production. *Dev Biol* 1987;120:356–365.
6. Skoff RP. Gliogenesis in rat optic nerve: astrocytes are generated in a single wave before oligodendrocytes. *Dev Biol* 1990;139:149–168.
7. Arenella LS, Herndon RM. Mature oligodendrocytes. Division following experimental demyelination in adult animals. *Arch Neurol* 1984;411:1162–1165.
8. Ludwin SK. Proliferation of mature oligodendrocytes after trauma to the central nervous system. *Nature* 1984;308:274–275.
9. Ludwin SK, Bakker DA. Can oligodendrocytes attached to myelin proliferate? *J Neurosci* 1988;8:1239–1244.
10. Wood PM, Bunge RP. The origin of remyelinating cells in the adult central nervous system: the role of the mature oligodendrocyte. *Glia* 1991;4:225–232.
11. Wolswijk G, Noble M. Identification of an adult-specific glial progenitor cell. *Development* 1989;105:387–400.
12. Small RK, Riddle P, Noble M. Evidence for migration of oligodendrocyte-type-2 astrocyte progenitor cells into the developing rat optic nerve. *Nature* 1987;328:155–157.

Advances in Neurology, Vol. 59, edited by
Fredrick J. Seil. Raven Press, Ltd.,
New York © 1993.

10

Source of Remyelinating Oligodendrocytes

Patrick M. Wood and Joseph Mora

The Miami Project to Cure Paralysis, Department of Neurological Surgery, University of Miami School of Medicine, Miami, Florida 33136

During development the first oligodendrocytes appear just prior to the onset of myelination in the central nervous system (CNS). They can only arise through the proliferation and differentiation of primitive progenitor cells. Oligodendrocytes do not normally divide after commencing myelination (1,2). When myelin sheaths or oligodendrocytes in the adult CNS are damaged or destroyed, new myelin and oligodendrocytes can be regenerated in many situations (3). In adult tissue new oligodendrocytes could arise either from a persisting undifferentiated stem cell population or from surviving differentiated oligodendrocytes. In this chapter we review the available evidence that progenitors and differentiated oligodendrocytes can be precursors and evidence from tissue culture studies that mature oligodendrocytes dedifferentiate. Finally, we present some preliminary data comparing the regenerative capacity of "adult progenitors" and differentiated oligodendrocytes and discuss the relevance of these findings in the context of the regeneration of oligodendrocytes and myelin in the adult CNS.

THE ARGUMENT FOR THE ADULT OLIGODENDROCYTE PROGENITOR

There are a number of reasons to suggest that stem cells (progenitors) would be a better source of new oligodendrocytes than differentiated oligodendrocytes. Such stem cells might be expected to be capable of a more immediate response to demyelination, dividing rapidly to expand in number. Because they would be likely to have fewer, less branched processes, they would be more capable of extensive migration to completely populate a demyelinated lesion. In addition, because they begin their response as undifferentiated cells, the progenitors could initiate remyelination by the same sequence of steps as that which occurs during development.

During the last half of the 1980s, data were obtained in several laboratories defining the properties of an oligodendrocyte progenitor in cell cultures prepared from developing rodent CNS (reviewed in refs. 4, 5). These observations provided the basis for a model of oligodendrocyte development that is widely accepted, if still somewhat controversial. A simplified version of this model is illustrated in Fig. 1. In this model the oligodendrocyte progenitor is a motile cell with bipolar morphology that expresses on its surface a glycolipid designated as A2B5. Its division and differentiation are believed to be regulated by the levels of two growth factors, platelet-derived growth factor (PDGF) and basic fibroblast growth factor (bFGF), both of which are produced by astrocytes (6–8). In the presence of high levels of ciliary neuronotrophic factor (CNTF) or serum in the culture medium, the

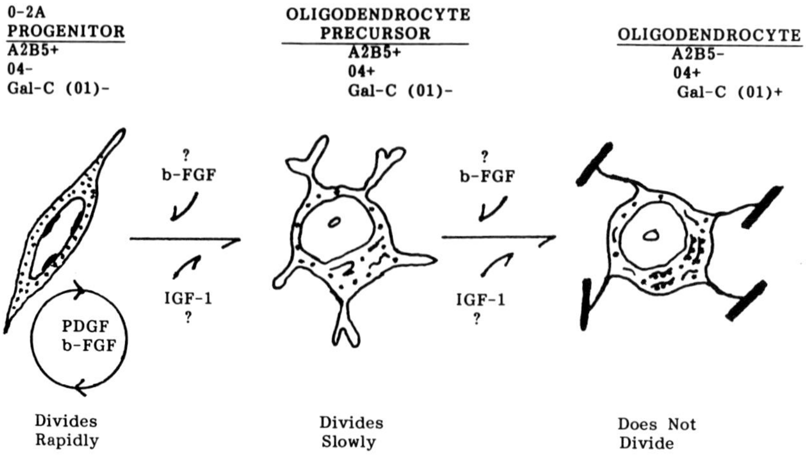

FIG. 1. Pathway of origin of oligodendrocytes during development. This pathway is based on observations from studies of the generation of oligodendrocytes in cultures of cells from developing CNS tissues, primarily of rat optic nerve (for explanation and references see text). Note that the proliferation of the 0-2A progenitor depends on the growth factors PDGF and bFGF, both of which are released by cultured astrocytes. Also note that the acquisition of galC signals the cessation of proliferative activity and the onset of the production of myelin. Whereas IGF-1 may act to promote the maturation of the oligodendrocyte precursors, bFGF may act to retard maturation. Unipolar cells bearing the phenotype of the multipolar precursor ($04^{+}01^{-}$) are found in adult CNS tissue and have been proposed as possible precursors of remyelinating oligodendrocytes. Cells with the phenotype $A2B5^{+}04^{-}$ are rare in adult tissues.

progenitor differentiates into an astrocyte (9); however, the manifestation of this potential *in vivo* is controversial (5,10).

Because the progenitor has demonstrated a potential to differentiate either into an oligodendrocyte or into an astrocyte, it is called the 0-2A progenitor. Depending perhaps on the levels of bFGF and other growth factors in its environment, such as insulin-like growth factor 1 (IGF-1), the progenitor differentiates further into an intermediate oligodendrocyte precursor, retaining A2B5 and acquiring on its surface an undefined differentiation antigen recognized by the monoclonal antibody, 04 (2,11). This intermediate precursor is multipolar and retains some capacity for division and for differentiation into either oligodendrocytes or astrocytes (12). It is tempting to speculate that this intermediate, defined by immunocytochemistry of cells in culture, is identical to the oligodendroblast defined morphologically *in vivo* by Skoff (1,13). Eventually this intermediate precursor differentiates into the myelin-forming oligodendrocyte, thereby losing the expression of A2B5 on its surface, acquiring galactocerebroside (galC), and initiating the first steps in the formation of myelin. It is at this stage that the oligodendrocyte becomes postmitotic.

It should be noted that the experiments on which this model are based were carried out in cultures without neurons, and the ways in which neuron–oligodendrocyte progenitor interactions may influence the course of development are not known. This may explain why there seem to be points of controversy and discrepencies between this model based on tissue culture observations and what has been observed *in vivo*. These points of controversy are the subject of a recent review (5).

The bipolar $A2B5^{+}$ 04^{-} progenitor cell is not thought to persist into adult life. However, a unipolar cell expressing A2B5 and 04 antigens but not galC has been identified in adult tissue and has been designated an "adult 0-2A progenitor" (14,15). There is evidence that cells with this phenotype isolated from adult animals and manipulated in cultures can differentiate into cells that express galC or into cells expressing glial fibrillary acidic protein (GFAP), implying that they, like their neonatal counterparts, are bipotential. Furthermore, they are responsive to the mitogen PDGF (16). However, these adult progenitors do not exhibit response times consistent with a rapid regeneration of oligodendrocytes. They divide (with a cell cycle time of $2\frac{1}{2}$ days) and differentiate (over 7 days) more slowly than does the neonatal progenitor. The question must be raised whether their response to demyelination *in vivo* would be rapid enough to account for observed rates of remyelination. For example, after experimental demyelination caused by lysolecithin injection, extensive remyelination by oligodendrocytes can be observed within 8 days after the injection (17). This short time period would only permit a maximum of three cycles of cell division at the cell cycle time exhibited *in vitro* under the most favorable conditions, and this would not allow time for maturation.

There is some evidence from an *in vivo* study that suggests that adult 0-2A progenitors may be involved in remyelination (18). After demyelination in mice caused by the A59 strain of mouse hepatitis virus, there was a rapid increase in the number of cells of the progenitor phenotype (04^+ only), and these cells could be labeled directly with tritiated thymidine, indicative of cell division, whereas differentiated oligodendrocytes could not. However, as we will demonstrate and discuss in later sections in this chapter, differentiated oligodendrocytes ($galC^+$ as detected by staining with monoclonal 01 antibody) rapidly dedifferentiate into cells expressing the progenitor phenotype (04 only). Thus, in the animal studies there is a strong possibility that some part of the population of proliferating 04-only cells observed after viral infection were derived from the differentiated oligodendrocyte pool.

ARGUMENT FOR THE DIFFERENTIATED OLIGODENDROCYTE

Because oligodendrocytes do not normally divide in adult tissue and seem to be relatively undisturbed by drastic changes in their environment (e.g., in Wallerian degeneration), and because it is difficult to conceive of a mechanism by which a mature oligodendrocyte could disengage itself from the maintenance of one to several myelin sheaths in order to divide, there has been some resistance to the idea that mature myelinating oligodendrocytes might be a major source of new oligodendrocytes to carry out remyelination. However, observations suggestive of mature oligodendrocyte division have been reported repeatedly since the earliest studies of remyelination 30 years ago (19; reviewed in ref. 20). A particularly convincing example of such evidence was presented by Arenella and Herndon (17). They administered a single pulse of tritiated thymidine to adult mice 1 hr prior to perfusion at 2, 5, or 8 days after lysolecithin had been injected into the spinal cord to cause demyelination. Although oligodendrocytes near the injection site were damaged or destroyed by the lysolecithin, they survived, and myelin was retained in the area surrounding the zone of demyelination. In this adjacent zone, thymidine-labeled oligodendrocytes were observed as early as 48 hr following the lysolecithin injection. The labeled oligodendrocytes exhibited a wide range of morphologies, including those classified as light, medium, and dark. It has been proposed that these different morphologies represent different levels of maturation, with the dark class at the most mature end of the spectrum (21). However, as Arenella and Herndon pointed out, and as was discussed further by Wood and Bunge (20), the functional significance of the morphological heterogeneity within the oligodendrocyte family is still not well understood. Nonetheless, it was clear that oligodendrocytes displaying a range of different morphologies were capable

TABLE 1. *Effect of basic FGF on adult rat oligodendrocytes*[a]

Concentration (ng/ml)	Labeling index (01+ cells)	Labeling index (01− cells)	01$^+$ Cells (%)
0	0.4 (0.2, 0.6)	40 (49, 31)	89 (88, 89)
0.1	0.5 (0.6, 0.4)	36 (26, 45)	88 (88, 87)
1.0	10 (8.5, 11.3)	38 (46, 30)	79 (74, 85)
10.0	54 (53, 55)	60 (60, 60)	68 (64, 72)

[a] A cell suspension enriched in adult oligodendrocytes was prepared by plating the crude spinal cord cell suspension overnight on 100-mm culture dishes (Corning) to absorb out microglial cells. The enriched cell suspension was 85% 01$^+$ oligodendrocytes. This suspension was plated at a density of 20,000 cells per 22-mm collagen-coated coverslip. The cells were exposed to recombinant bovine bFGF (Amgen) at indicated concentrations for 6 days, then pulsed with 100 nCi/ml ^{3}H-thymidine for 18 hr, stained with anti-01 antibody and rhodamine conjugated goat anti-mouse IgA + IgG + IgM, fixed and processed for autoradiography. Counts of labeled cells were performed on duplicate coverslips for each condition; at least 500 cells were counted on each coverslip. The values shown are averages with individual values shown in parentheses.

of reactivation to proliferative status. Furthermore, the location of the labeled cells within unaffected myelinated tissue suggests that oligodendrocytes were reactivated to divide at the same time as they were engaged in the maintenance of myelin sheaths.

Because of the extreme thinness and fragility of the processes connecting the oligodendrocyte perikaryon with its myelin segments, the demonstration that oligodendrocytes can be labeled with thymidine while their processes are connected to myelin sheaths is very difficult in adult animals. There is a report of thymidine labeling of myelin-connected oligodendrocytes in areas adjacent to ablation lesions of the cerebral cortex in adult mice (22). However, the clarity of the connection, at least in the published electron micrographs, does not permit an unambiguous conclusion on this point, and the percentage of oligodendrocytes with suggestive connections to myelin profiles that were also thymidine labeled was small.

That some differentiated oligodendrocytes possess the capacity to divide was confirmed by tissue culture observations that galC$^+$ oligodendrocytes derived from adult rat spinal cord could be stimulated to vigorous division by sensory neurons (23). The neurons were mitogenic in either the presence or the absence of serum (P. M. Wood, unpublished observations). Differentiated adult oligodendrocytes can also be stimulated to divide by pituitary-derived or recombinant bFGF (Table 1). In cultures of sensory neurons and oligodendrocytes, the effects of the neuronal mitogen and bFGF may be additive (Table 2). The mechanism by which neurons stimulate oligodendrocyte division is unknown, but it is interesting that neurons also present a potent mitogen to Schwann cells (24,25). It has been demonstrated that the stimulation

TABLE 2. *Effect of sensory neurons and basic FGF on adult rat oligodendrocyte proliferation*[a]

Culture type	Labeling index −FGF	(galC$^+$ cells) +FGF
Oligodendrocytes only	2 (2, 2)	18 (10, 26)
Neurons and oligodendrocytes	23.5 (23, 24)	51 (53, 49)

[a] A cell suspension containing oligodendrocytes (≈50%) was prepared from adult rat spinal cord by centrifugation on a Percoll gradient to remove myelin debris. This suspension was plated at a density of 20,000 cells per culture (22 mm diameter) either onto coverslips coated with collagen or onto coverslips containing a network of purified dorsal root ganglion neurons. Some of each of these types of cultures were exposed to bFGF (prepared from pituitary extract and extensively characterized by Wice; see ref. 27) at bFGF levels giving maximal stimulation of the oligodendrocytes alone (i.e., at a dilution of 1:500). Cultures were exposed to 100 nCi/ml ^{3}H-thymidine in the medium for 18 hr beginning on the sixth day after plating the oligodendrocyte suspension. The cultures were stained with monoclonal anti-galC antibody and rhodamine conjugated goat antimouse IgA + IgG + IgM, fixed and processed for autoradiography. Labeling indices were counted as in Table 1. Average values are shown with individual values in parentheses.

of Schwann cells requires contact between the neuronal and Schwann cell membranes (26), but this requirement has not been demonstrated for the oligodendrocyte. These observations are of interest because they suggest a general mechanism by which oligodendrocyte division could be induced following demyelination. Either bFGF, possibly released by reactive astrocytes in or around lesions, or the axons bared by demyelination could trigger and sustain oligodendrocyte proliferation.

MATURE OLIGODENDROCYTES CAN DEDIFFERENTIATE

The results discussed in the last section constitute strong evidence that differentiated oligodendrocytes can be activated to divide. There are at this time little data to indicate the fate of the cells generated by that division or whether these progeny ultimately are responsible for remyelination. It is reasonable that remyelination occurs by a repetition of the same processes by which myelination is accomplished during development. In that case, highly differentiated, myelin-maintaining oligodendrocytes may not be capable of carrying out the initial steps of new myelin formation, i.e., the recognition and segregation of myelin-receptive axons, the formation of mesaxons, and the elongation of the ensheathing process around and along the axon to produce the first uncompacted spiral of myelin. This raises the question of whether the mature oligodendrocytes must first dedifferentiate to allow a repetition of the orderly sequence of gene expression underlying normal myelin formation.

We have recently reported evidence obtained from tissue culture studies that indicates that differentiated oligodendrocytes can at least partially dedifferentiate (20). Unfractionated cell suspensions from adult rat spinal cord typically contain about 50% 01^+ (differentiated) oligodendrocytes, 2% progenitors (04^+01^-), and 35% to 40% microglia and other unidentified cells. When this crude suspension was added to cultures containing purified sensory neurons, the following events occurred sequentially: (a) 01^+ oligodendrocytes incorporated thymidine and divided (after 1 week); (b) the cultures became extensively populated with newly generated oligodendrocytes (after 2 weeks); and (c) many axons were myelinated by oligodendrocyte processes (after 3 to 4 weeks). To clarify or establish a direct relationship between the dividing 01^+ oligodendrocytes seen at 1 week and the myelinating oligodendrocytes at 4 weeks, we compared oligodendrocyte generation and myelination in cultures to which were added either cells from an 01^+ cell fraction prepared by flow cytometry or cells from the 01^- cell fraction (20). Initially the 01^- cell fraction contained six times more cells with the progenitor phenotype than did the 01^+ cell fraction. However, we observed that cultures receiving cells from the 01^+ cell fraction developed much more myelin than did cultures receiving cells from the 01^- fraction, indicating that cells that were 01^+ at the time of addition were the most likely source of the myelinating oligodendrocytes observed 4 weeks later. We were also surprised to observe, at 1 week after the glial cell addition, many more cells of the progenitor phenotype in cultures receiving cells from the 01^+ cell fraction. This result suggested that 01^+ cells lose their surface galC by dedifferentiating, either independent of or coincident with cell division.

This interpretation was further tested by the following experiment. A suspension of adult spinal cord cells was purified to >97% 01^+ cells by two passages through the flow cytometer. These highly purified 01^+ cells were added at low density to cultures of purified dorsal root ganglion neurons. The number and phenotype of adherent cells were determined at 16 hr after plating. During the following 2 weeks, small discrete colonies of cells were generated by the division of some of the adherent cells. The colonies were counted, and the phenotype of the cells within each colony was determined at 1 week after plating. The results of this experiment

TABLE 3. *Phenotype of cells in colonies developing in cultures of purified sensory neurons after adding 01$^+$ cells*[a]

	1 Week		2 Weeks	
	#1	#2	#1	#2
Total colonies	43	61	46	47
Colonies with both 04$^+$01$^+$ cells and 04$^+$01$^-$ cells	29	33	28	28
Colonies with 04$^+$01$^-$ cells only	11	28	14	15
Colonies with 04$^+$01$^+$ cells only	1	0	0	0
Colonies with 04$^-$01$^-$ cells only	2	0	4	4

[a] Experimental details are given in the text. Average number of cells adhering per culture, 245; percentage 01$^+$ cells of adhering cells, 98.5; average number 04$^+$01$^-$ cells/culture, <1; average number 04$^-$01$^-$ cells/culture, 4.

are summarized in Table 3. Because of the high purity of the starting 01$^+$ cell suspension, the number of contaminating progenitors was vanishingly low. The majority of colonies contained cells expressing the 04$^+$01$^-$ phenotype, and several colonies in each culture contained only 04$^+$01$^-$ cells. Since each culture received fewer than one (on average) progenitor initially, the numbers of 04$^+$01$^-$ colonies observed in each culture rule out the possibility that they derived from contaminating progenitors.

Thus, some 01$^+$ oligodendrocytes clearly possess the capacity for rapid dedifferentiation, as manifest by the loss of surface galC. The loss of galC from the surface of the 01$^+$ oligodendrocyte may denote other fundamental dedifferentiative changes that could facilitate proliferation, migration, and the reinitiation of myelin formation. For example, the morphology of these new 04$^+$01$^-$ cells is different from that of their 01$^+$ parent. The 04$^+$01$^-$ cells have fewer processes and appear more spindle-shaped rather than rounded. It is possible that all the myelin sheaths that are eventually observed in such cultures are produced only by cells that first dedifferentiate, but this remains to be proven.

COMPARISON OF THE MYELINATING POTENTIAL OF 01$^+$ OLIGODENDROCYTES AND 04$^+$01$^-$ PROGENITORS

Although the cells generated by the dedifferentiation of 01$^+$ cells have the same surface phenotype as the adult progenitors with respect to 01 and 04 antigens, these two cell types may have very different properties, including their capacity for generating new myelinating oligodendrocytes. In the experiment described in the preceding section, very little proliferation of 04$^+$01$^-$ cells and little myelination was observed in sensory neuron cultures that had been plated with cells from the 01$^-$ cell fraction, in contrast to vigorous proliferation and extensive myelination in cultures that had been plated with cells from an 01$^+$ cell fraction. Since the 01$^-$ cell fraction initially had 6 times the number of progenitors as the 01$^+$ fraction, this experiment suggested that the progenitors had less capacity for proliferation, and thus the generation of new myelinating cells, than did the differentiated oligodendrocytes.

To test this interpretation, we have isolated the progenitors from adult spinal cord cell suspension at higher purity and have been able to add comparable numbers of either 01$^+$ oligodendrocytes or of 04$^+$01$^-$ progenitors to the neuronal test cultures. The cord cell suspension was sequentially stained with 01 antibody followed by 04 antibody and separated by flow cytometry (see Fig. 2). By this procedure the 01$^+$ cells were double labeled, and the 04$^+$01$^-$ cells were single labeled. Because the frequency of progenitors in the starting suspension was only 2%, the yield of cells with the 04$^+$01$^-$ phenotype was low; however, the purity (85%) was comparable to that of the 01$^+$ cell fraction (97%). The purified neuronal cultures were plated with either 01$^+$ cells or with 04$^+$01$^-$ cells at equal starting

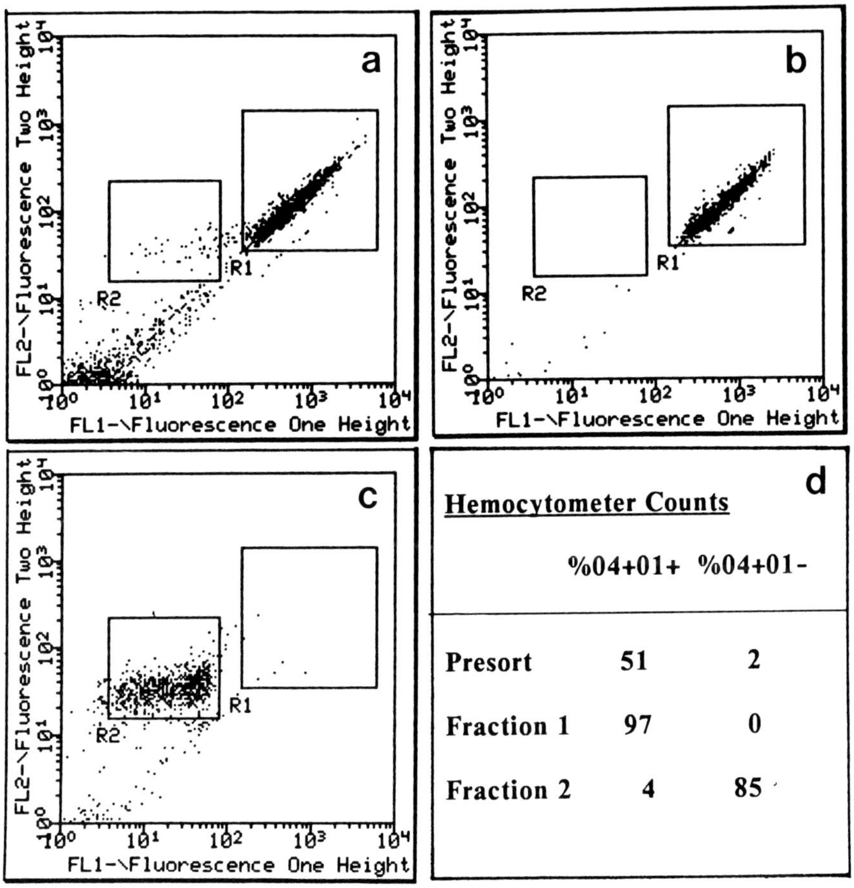

	%04+01+	%04+01-
Presort	51	2
Fraction 1	97	0
Fraction 2	4	85

FIG. 2. Separation of 01^+ and 04^+01^- cell fractions by flow cytometry. A suspension of cells from adult rat spinal cord was sequentially stained with 01 antibody, then with fluorescein-conjugated goat antimouse IgA + IgG + IgM, followed by 04 antibody, and finally with phycoerythrin-conjugated goat antimouse kappa chain. By this procedure oligodendrocytes were double labeled green (01^+) and red (04^+), whereas progenitors were red (04^+) only. (**a**) Plot of green (FL1) and red (FL2) fluorescence of particles in the whole-cell suspension. The population of particles selected as double labeled (01^+) cells is indicated by *rectangle* 1, whereas the 04^+01^- population is indicated by *rectangle 2.* (**b**) Plot of the fluorescence of particles in the 01^+ cell fraction (fraction 1) after resorting. (**c**) Plot of the fluorescence of particles in the 04^+01^- cell fraction. Note the presence of a few contaminating 01^+ cells or particles in this fraction. (**d**) Phenotypes of the cells in the purified cell fractions as determined by cell counts (of 1,000 cells) using a hemocytometer and Hoechst nuclear stain to distinguish cells from myelin debris.

densities per culture. Cultures were maintained in medium containing bFGF and PDGF for 1 week to promote proliferation of both progenitors and differentiated oligodendrocytes, then switched to medium without these added growth factors to permit differentiation. Cultures were fixed at 4 weeks and stained for 01 and 04 antigens and myelin.

The results of this experiment are illustrated in Fig. 3 and Table 4. Figure 3 shows a comparison of the cell density and phenotype of the cells in the two groups of cultures. An increase in the number of 04^+01^- and 01^+ cells was observed in both groups of cultures; however, this increase was much greater in cultures receiving 01^+ cells. Furthermore, cultures receiving 04^+01^- cells initially had little myelin by 4 weeks, in contrast to cul-

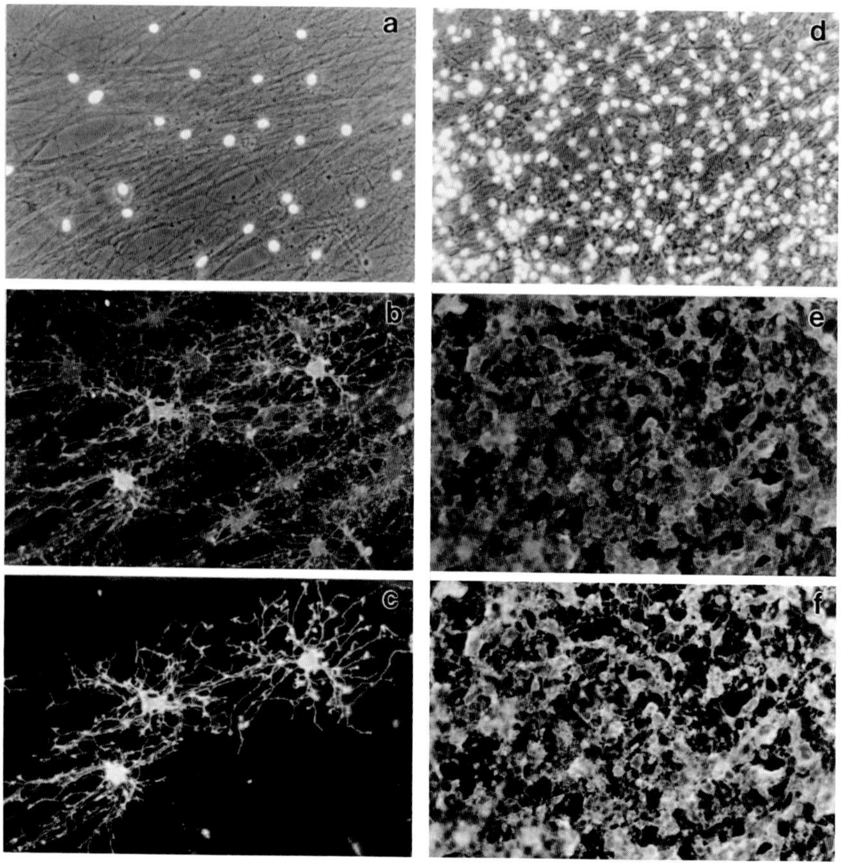

FIG. 3. Comparison of density and phenotypes of cells developing in purified neuronal cultures receiving cells from the 04^+01^- or from the 01^+ cell fraction. (**a**) Phase-contrast micrograph of a representative field in a culture receiving 04^+01^- cells. The culture was stained 4 weeks after the addition of 04^+01^- cells. The position and number of cells are indicated by fluorescence from the Hoechst nuclear stain. (**b**) Fluorescence from 04 staining of the field shown in **a.** Note that most of the cells exhibit multipolar processes and moderate (not bright) 04 staining intensity. (**c**) Fluorescence from 01 staining in the field shown in **a,** showing three 01^+ cells. Most of the cells were 01^-. Note the many long, slender processes that each 01^+ cell has generated. (**d**) Phase-contrast micrograph of a representative field in a culture receiving 01^+ cells demonstrates an increased density of cells when compared to **a.** This culture was also stained 4 weeks after the addition of 01^+ cells. (**e**) Fluorescence from 04 staining in the field shown in **d.** (**f**) Fluorescence from 01 staining in the field shown in **d.** Compare the morphology of cells in **e** and **f** with that of cells in **b** and **c** respectively.

tures receiving 01^+ cells, which were moderately well myelinated by 4 weeks (Table 4).

The results of this experiment suggest that the progenitors actually have less regenerative capacity than do the differentiated 01^+ oligodendrocytes or the 04^+01^- cells derived from the 01^+ oligodendrocytes. The slow proliferation rate of the progenitors coupled with their low frequency in the tissue argues against the progenitors making a major contribution in remyelination. The question must be raised whether the 04^+01^- cells in adult CNS tissue function primarily as stem cells, as has been proposed, or whether they may have some alternative function in the tissue. The 04^+01^- state may be, for them, a

TABLE 4. *Comparison of the amount of myelin formed in neuronal cultures receiving adult 01⁺ or 04⁺01⁻ cells[a]*

Phenotype of added cells	Myelin quantity (arbitrary units)	Percentage of fields with myelin
01^+	188 (266, 55)	36 (20, 52)
04^+01^-	0 (0, 0)	0 (0, 0)

[a] Cultures were fixed at 4 weeks after the addition of glial cells and stained with Sudan black. Myelin quantity was assessed using an eyepiece grid divided into 100 squares. Twenty-five fields selected by stage coordinates were examined in duplicate cultures with each phenotype. The number shown in the average of total number of grid squares crossed by a meylin segment. Values in parentheses are individual values for each of the duplicate cultures. To determine the percentage of fields with myelin, 64 fields in each culture selected by stage coordinates were assessed for the presence of myelin. The magnification used for counting was ×200.

mature state. In this regard, the observations of Gard and Pfeiffer (2) on neonatal progenitor differentiation in culture is of interest. They observed that some 0-2A progenitors never fully differentiated into galC-expressing oligodendrocytes but appeared to be blocked at the 04^+ $galC^-$ stage of differentiation. They whimsically called these cells procrastocytes and offered the suggestion that these could be equivalent to the 04^+ $galC^-$ cells found in adult tissue and might function to slowly replace oligodendrocytes lost to natural causes. We would offer the suggestion, based on the observations we have reviewed here, that a primitive stem cell with robust regeneration potential does not actually reside as such in adult CNS tissue and that re-

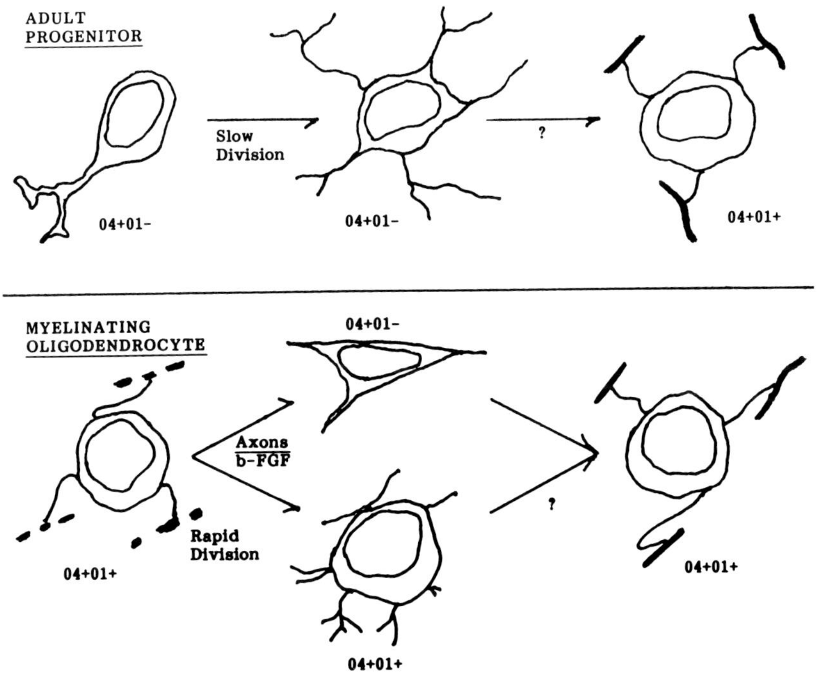

FIG. 4. Possible pathways of origin of remyelinating oligodendrocytes in adult CNS. This diagram represents an interpretation of the data reviewed or presented in this chapter. We propose that cells bearing the progenitor phenotype make a relatively minor contribution in the generation of new oligodendrocytes because of their slow rate of division and differentiation. Thus, the rapid regeneration of oligodendrocytes for remyelination would depend on the activation of differentiated oligodendrocytes, which would first become partially dedifferentiated, rapidly divide to generate the required number of cells and then reinitiate myelination.

myelination ultimately may depend heavily on the reactivation of surviving differentiated oligodendrocytes.

CONCLUSION

We have reviewed the evidence regarding the origin of remyelinating oligodendrocytes in adult animals and presented new evidence obtained from studies with neuron–oligodendrocyte cultures in which both proliferation and myelination occur. We have used this culture system to test the regenerative capacity of the cells that are the most probable candidates (04^+01^- cells and differentiated oligodendrocytes) for the role of oligodendrocyte precursor in the adult. We have consistently observed a much greater potential for proliferation, for the generation of cells with less differentiated phenotype (04^+01^-), and for the generation of myelinating oligodendrocytes among cells that were initially differentiated (01^+). On the basis of these observations, we propose the following model, illustrated in Fig. 4, to account for the generation of oligodendrocytes in adult tissue. According to this model, the 04^+01^- cells that reside in low numbers within the tissue are themselves not normally dividing but are carrying out an unknown function. In response to a change in the status quo (i.e., demyelination), they respond by slow division and may even generate a few oligodendrocytes. We suggest that they will mainly produce other 04^+01^- cells but may make a minor contribution to remyelination. In contrast, differentiated oligodendrocytes that are connected to myelin sheaths, or whose myelin sheaths may break down while cell viability is retained, are activated to divide either by a soluble mitogen such as bFGF or by contact with a mitogen presented on the surface of denuded axons. Some of these reactivated oligodendrocytes dedifferentiate and continue to divide. We suggest that it is this group of dedifferentiated oligodendrocytes (which are transiently 04^+01^-) that ultimately carry out remyelination.

ACKNOWLEDGMENTS

The authors wish to thank Francisco Cruz for excellent technical assistance, Ms. Charlaine Rowlette for unmatched and unruffled skill in preparing the bulk of the manuscript, Ms. Cynthia Jones for assistance in preparing the manuscript, Mr. Art Alamo for cell sorting, and Dr. Melitta Schachner for hybridoma cell lines producing 01 and 04 antibodies.

This work was supported by National Multiple Sclerosis Society grant 2210-A-2 and The Miami Project to Cure Paralysis.

REFERENCES

1. Skoff RP, Price DL, Stocks A. Electron microscopic autoradiographic studies of gliogenesis in rat optic nerve. II. Time of origin. *J Comp Neurol* 1976;169:313–334.
2. Gard AL, Pfeiffer SE. Oligodendrocyte progenitors isolated directly from developing telencephalon at a specific phenotypic stage: myelinogenic potential in a defined environment. *Development* 1989; 106:119–132.
3. Ludwin SK. Regeneration of myelin and oligodendrocytes in the central nervous system. *Prog Brain Res* 1987;71:469–484.
4. Cameron RS, Rakic P. Glial cell lineage in the cerebral cortex: a review and synthesis. *Glia* 1991; 4:124–137.
5. Noble M. Points of controversy in the 0-2A lineage: clocks and type-2 astrocytes. *Glia* 1991;4:157–164.
6. Richardson W, Pringle N, Mosley M, Westermark B, Dubois-Dalcq M. A role for platelet derived growth factor in normal gliogenesis in the central nervous system. *Cell* 1988;53:309–319.
7. Bögler O, Wren D, Barnett SC, Land H, Noble M. Cooperation between two growth factors promotes extended self-renewal and inhibits differentiation of 0-2A progenitor cells. *Proc Natl Acad Sci USA* 1990;87:6368–6372.
8. McKinnon RD, Matsui T, Dubois-Dalcq M, Aaronson SA. FGF modulates the PDGF-driven pathway of oligodendrocyte development. *Neuron* 1990; 5:603–614.
9. Lillien LE, Sendtner M, Rohrer H, Hughes SM, Raff M. Type-2 astrocyte development in rat brain culture is initiated by a CNTF-like protein produced by type-1 astrocytes. *Neuron* 1988;1:485–494.
10. Skoff RP. Gliogenesis in rat optic nerve: astrocytes are generated in a single wave before oligodendrocytes. *Dev Biol* 1990;139:149–168.
11. Dubois-Dalcq M. Characterization of a slowly proliferative cell along the oligodendrocyte differentiation pathway. *EMBO J* 1987;6:2587–2595.
12. Trotter J, Schachner M. Cells positive for the 04 surface antigen isolated by cell sorting are able to differ-

entiate into astrocytes or oligodendrocytes. *Dev Brain Res* 1989;46:115–122.
13. Skoff RP, Knapp PE. Division of astroblasts and oligodendroblasts in postnatal rodent brain: evidence for separate astrocyte and oligodendrocyte lineage. *Glia* 1991;4:165–174.
14. French-Constant C, Raff MC. Proliferating bipotential glial progenitor cells in adult rat optic nerve. *Nature* 1986;319:499–502.
15. Wolswijk G, Noble M. Identification of an adult-specific glial progenitor cell. *Development* 1989; 105:387–400.
16. Wolswijk G, Riddle PN, Noble M. Platelet-derived growth factor is mitogenic for 0-2A adult progenitor cells. *Glia* 1991;4:495–503.
17. Arenella LS, Herndon RM. Mature oligodendrocytes: division following experimental demyelination in adult animals. *Arch Neurol* 1984; 41:1162–1165.
18. Godfraind C, Friedrich V, Holmes K, Dubois-Dalcq M. *In vivo* analysis of glial cell phenotypes during a viral demyelinating disease in mice. *J Cell Biol* 1989;109:2405–2416.
19. Koenig H, Bunge M, Bunge RP. Nucleic acid and protein metabolism in white matter: observations during experimental demyelination and remyelination: a histochemical and autoradiographic study of the spinal cord of the adult cat. *Arch Neurol* 1962;6:177–193.
20. Wood PM, Bunge RP. The origin of remyelinating cells in the adult central nervous system: the role of the mature oligodendrocyte. *Glia* 1991;4:225–232.
21. Mori S, Leblond CP. Electron microscopic identification of three classes of oligodendrocytes and a preliminary study of their proliferative activity in the corpus callosum of young rats. *J Comp Neurol* 1970;39:1–30.
22. Ludwin S, Bakker D. Can oligodendrocytes attached to myelin proliferate? *J Neurosci* 1988;8: 1239–1244.
23. Wood P, Bunge R. Evidence that axons are mitogenic for oligodendrocytes isolated from adult animals. *Nature* 1986;320:756–758.
24. Wood P, Bunge R. Evidence that sensory axons are mitogenic for Schwann cells. *Nature* 1975; 256:662–664.
25. Ratner N, Hong D, Lieberman M, Bunge R, Glaser L. The neuronal cell surface molecule mitogenic for Schwann cells is a heparin-binding protein. *Proc Natl Acad Sci USA* 1988;85:6992–6996.
26. Salzer J, Bunge RP, Glaser L. Studies of Schwann cell proliferation. III. Evidence for the surface localization of the neurite mitogen. *J Cell Biol* 1980;84:767–778.
27. Wice B, Milbrandt J, Glaser L. Control of muscle differentiation in BC3H1 cells by fibroblast growth factor and vanadate. *J Biol Chem* 1987;262: 1810–1817.

Advances in Neurology, Vol. 59, edited by
Fredrick J. Seil. Raven Press, Ltd.,
New York © 1993.

11

The Role of Astrocytes in the Remyelination of Glia-free Areas of Demyelination

R. J. M. Franklin, A. J. Crang, and W. F. Blakemore

Department of Clinical Veterinary Medicine, University of Cambridge, Cambridge CB3 OES, England

When areas of demyelination are created in the white matter tracts of the spinal cord by the injection of gliotoxins such as lysolecithin, 6-aminonicotinamide, or ethidium bromide, astrocytes as well as oligodendrocytes are destroyed to leave demyelinated axons in a glia-free environment (1). An insight into normal repair processes can be obtained by studying the resolution of such lesions. Furthermore, by transplanting different glial cell populations into demyelinating lesions, it is possible to gain a fuller understanding of the cell–cell interactions required to regenerate central nervous system (CNS) glial environments and thereby determine the contributions made by specific cell types (2). This chapter focuses on the role of astrocytes and their interactions with Schwann cells and cells of the O-2A lineage in the reconstruction of the CNS glial environment.

THE ETHIDIUM BROMIDE LESION: A SYSTEM FOR STUDYING GLIAL CELL INTERACTIONS DURING REMYELINATION

The injection of ethidium bromide into the dorsal funiculus of the rat spinal cord results in the local destruction of astrocytes and oligodendrocytes. The axons are thus demyelinated and reside within a glia-free environment. Subsequently, the demyelinated axons are remyelinated by oligodendrocytes and, to a greater extent, by Schwann cells. By 4 weeks after ethidium bromide injection, few axons remain demyelinated (3). The two types of remyelination occur in clearly defined areas of the lesion, with Schwann cell-remyelination dominating the dorsal and central parts of the lesion and oligodendrocyte remyelination being primarily confined to areas adjacent to normal tissue. In terms of astrocyte presence, the two types of repair present a clear contrast. Within areas of oligodendrocyte repair, the remyelinated axons are separated by a fine network of astrocyte processes. Conversely, Schwann cell-repaired regions are largely devoid of astrocytes (Fig. 1). At points where astrocyte processes abut Schwann cells, they are usually covered by a basal lamina (Fig. 2). Thus, observations on the normally repairing ethidium bromide lesion suggest a mutual exclusion between Schwann cells and central glia during the repopulation of glia-deficient environments.

Indeed, in all situations where Schwann cell myelination of CNS axons occurs, both oligodendrocyte and astrocyte intoxication can be illustrated in the early stages of lesion development (3,4). This observation, together with those made on the effect of X-irradiation on the developing (5) or lesioned (6) spinal cord, led to the conclusion that it is the presence of astrocytes that normally pre-

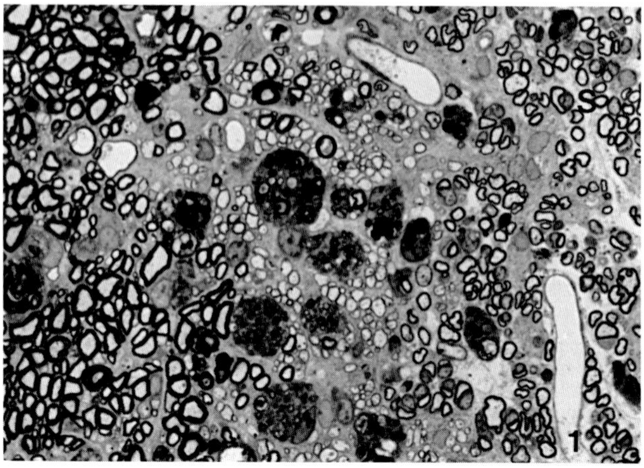

FIG. 1. Following the creation of a glia-free lesion in CNS white matter by the injection of gliotoxic agents such as ethidium bromide, demyelinated axons may be remyelinated by oligodendrocytes (O) or Schwann cells (S). The oligodendrocyte-remyelinated areas also contain a network of astrocyte processes. In contrast, astrocytes are not a feature of areas containing extensive Schwann cell remyelination. Toluidine blue, ×340.

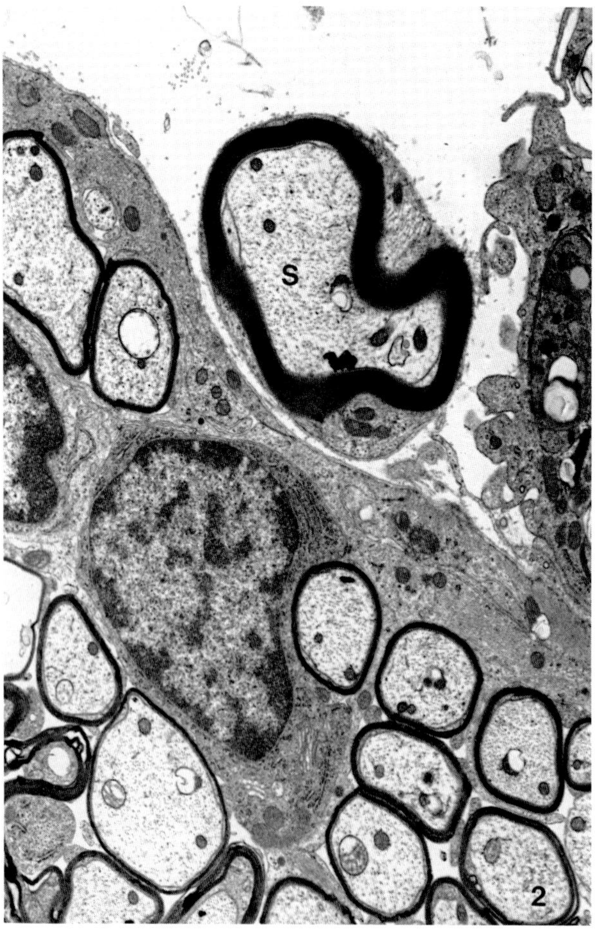

FIG. 2. Oligodendrocyte-remyelinated axons contained within an area bordered by astrocyte processes and covered by a basal lamina. A Schwann-cell-remyelinated axon (S) is excluded from this area. ×9,500.

vents Schwann cells from myelinating or remyelinating CNS axons. Such a role is consistent with the ascribed function of astrocytes in defining the boundary between CNS and peripheral nervous system. Further observations on gliotoxic lesions indicate that astrocytes not only play a role in controlling Schwann cell remyelination of CNS axons but might also influence oligodendrocyte remyelination (7). With the demonstration that it is possible to remyelinate areas of demyelination by transplanting glial cell cultures (8), it has become possible to use the technique of glial cell transplantation to examine in greater detail the effects of astrocytes, in particular the astrocyte phenotype characterized *in vitro* as the type 1 astrocyte (9), on the remyelination of CNS axons.

ASTROCYTES CONTROL THE ENTRY OF SCHWANN CELLS INTO AREAS OF DEMYELINATION

The role of type 1 astrocytes in preventing the entry of Schwann cells into areas of demyelination was demonstrated in experiments that compared the nature of remyelination following the transplantation of mixed CNS glial cell cultures with cultures enriched for cells of the O-2A lineage but depleted of type 1 astrocytes into ethdium bromide lesions made in normal rats (10). When mixed glial cultures were transplanted, the lesions were largely remyelinated by oligodendrocytes, showing that this type of culture could alter the normal repair pattern of the lesion and that supplementation of central glia resulted in more extensive reconstruction of a central glial environment. However, following the injection of the O-2A-enriched, type 1 astrocyte-depleted cultures, the enhancement of oligodendrocyte remyelination was slight, and the majority of axons were remyelinated by Schwann cells in spite of the increased availability of oligodendrocytes and their precursors. The tendency for Schwann cells to predominate over oligodendrocytes in the repair of glia-free lesions is thought to be a reflection of the vigorous mitotic and migratory potential of the Schwann cell compared with its CNS counterpart (11). These results indicate that in the absence of type 1 astrocytes, O-2A lineage cells are not able to secure extensive areas of central-type remyelination when faced with competition from Schwann cells. Moreover, there was evidence that Schwann cell processes were displac-

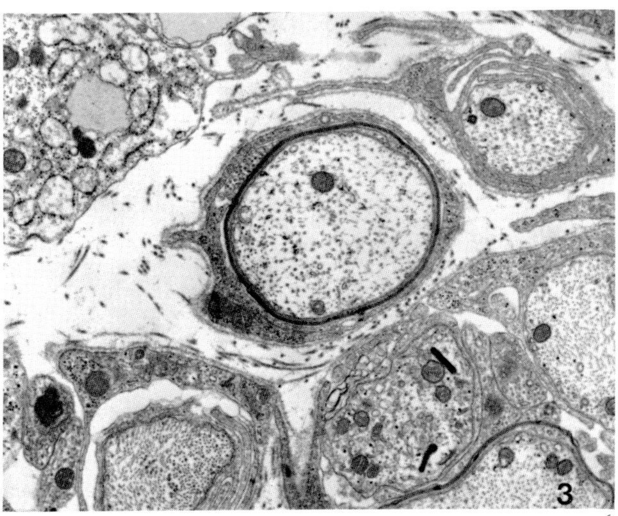

FIG. 3. A Schwann cell, covered with a prominent basal lamina, can be seen wrapping processes around an axon with a thin central myelin sheath. ×12,650.

ing or enveloping oligodendrocyte myelin sheaths (Fig. 3).

ASTROCYTES FAIL TO INHIBIT SCHWANN CELL REMYELINATION OF DEMYELINATED CNS AXONS IN THE ABSENCE OF CELLS OF THE O-2A LINEAGE

Studies on the repair of gliotoxic lesions and the transplantation studies described in the previous paragraph have provided clear evidence for the importance of astrocytes in inhibiting Schwann cell invasion of the CNS following demyelination. In order to further confirm this conclusion, a series of experiments were conducted in which astrocytes alone or together with a controlled number of O-2A lineage cells were co-transplanted with Schwann cells.

The proportion of the different cell types within the transplant suspension can be controlled by various tissue culture manipulations such as separating top-dwelling from bottom-dwelling cells or by immunocytolysis. However, in order to transfer this same control to the *in vivo* environment of the lesion, it was necessary to remove the unquantifiable contribution of host-derived glia. This was achieved using the X-irradiated form of the ethidium bromide lesion in which the host glial response is suppressed. Thus, using the X-irradiated ethidium bromide system, we could be certain that the cellular interactions observed and the repair outcome of the transplanted lesion were reflections of the content of the transplant and were not influenced by the contribution of host glia.

In our experience, CNS glial cultures typically contain a small proportion of Schwann cells (under 5%) (12,13), as revealed by immunostaining with antibodies against L1 and S100 (14). When cultures containing large numbers of cells of the O-2A lineage (top-dwelling cells in mixed glial cell cultures) were injected into irradiated lesions, Schwann cell remyelination was only a minor component of the observed remyelination (8). However, when the same numbers of contaminating Schwann cells were present in cultures that contained mainly type 1 astrocytes and only a low number of oligodendrocytes, only Schwann cell remyelination was observed (11). In a further experiment in which all cells of the O-2A lineage had been removed to produce a culture of almost pure type 1 astrocytes with a small number of Schwann cells, the extent of Schwann cell remyelination was further increased; indeed, the presence of type 1 astrocytes enhanced Schwann cell remyelination (15). Thus, in these studies a high number of type 1 astrocytes within the transplant suspension were unable to control the expansion of the small co-transplanted population of Schwann cells, an observation that appeared *prima facie* to be at variance with the concept developed earlier that Schwann cell remyelination of CNS axons was a consequence of astrocyte destruction in areas of demyelination and that the presence of type 1 astrocytes was required for exclusion of Schwann cells.

An explanation for this apparent paradox lies in a consideration of the arrangements adopted by astrocytes in situations where their presence results in an inhibition of Schwann cell remyelination and where they are unable to exert this inhibition. Where the extent of Schwann cell remyelination is reduced by astrocyte transplantation, extensive areas of central glial reconstruction occur, consisting of numerous oligodendrocyte-remyelinated axons surrounded by a dense and integrated network of astrocyte processes (Fig. 4). These areas are bounded by a surface of astrocyte processes covered by a basal lamina and resemble the normal glial limitans (Fig. 2). Such astrocyte territories are often continuous with normal tissue (Figs. 4 and 5). Conversely, in situations where Schwann cell remyelination is not inhibited and is even enhanced following astrocyte transplantation, the arrangement of astrocytes is quite different. Here, astrocytes form small discrete clumps of cells containing few axons, which usually remain demyelinated (Fig. 6).

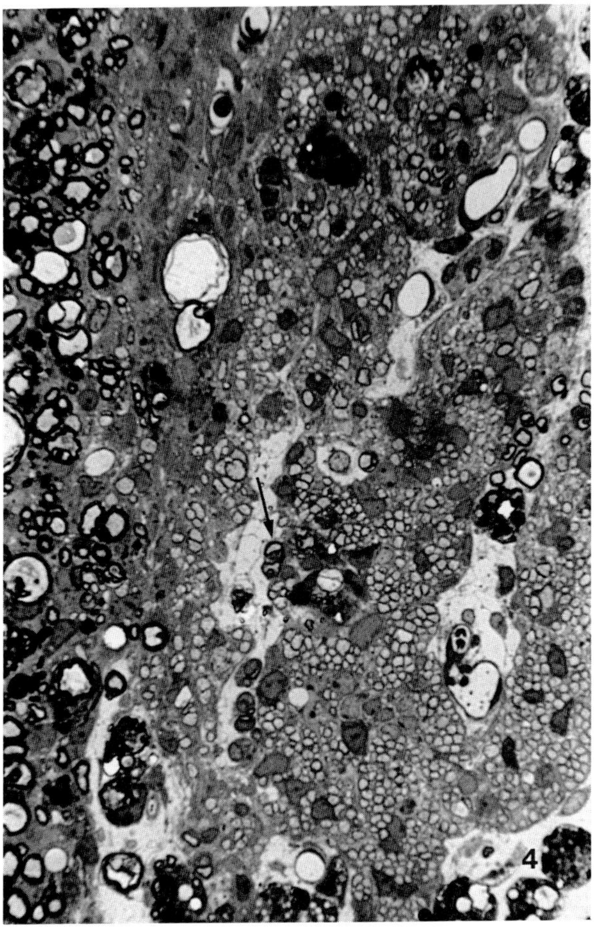

FIG. 4. Areas of extensive central glial reconstruction following transplantation of an O-2A-depleted type 1 astrocyte culture into a non-irradiated ethidium bromide lesion. These areas contain oligodendrocyte-remyelinated axons and numerous astrocytes. Occasional Schwann-cell-remyelinated axons are present on the surface of these central glial terrains (*arrow*). Toluidine blue, ×330.

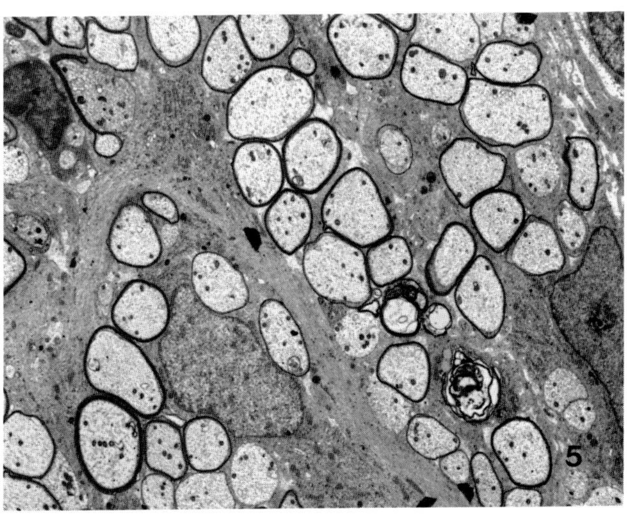

FIG. 5. Electron micrograph showing oligodendrocyte-remyelinated axons in an environment rich in astrocyte processes. Only a few axons have remained demyelinated. ×1,850.

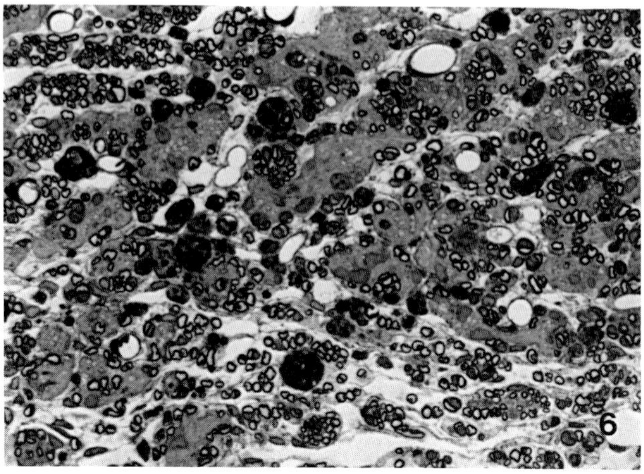

FIG. 6. In areas of the repairing lesion where O-2A lineage cells are absent, astrocytes tend to form clumps of cells rather than contributing to the large areas of reconstruction such as those in Fig. 4. In this arrangement, astrocytes are unable to prevent extensive Schwann cell remyelination. Schwann cell-remyelinated axons can be seen on the surface of the astrocyte clumps, the latter occasionally containing demyelinated axons. Toluidine blue, ×300.

These clumps are bounded by basal laminae and often have Schwann cells closely associated with their surfaces. The key difference between these two arrangements is the presence or absence of O-2A lineage cells. Thus, where astrocytes are able to contribute to extensive reconstruction of glia-deficient areas, one typically finds O-2A lineage cells present. Where these cells are not abundant, astrocytes tend to clump together, forming fragmented islands of cells. There appears, therefore, to be a cooperative interaction between central glial cells in restricting Schwann cell behavior. Although astrocytes are necessary to prevent incursion of Schwann cells into areas of CNS demyelination and thereby allow extensive oligodendrocyte remyelination, the adoption of appropriate arrangements to restrict Schwann cells is dependent on the availability of cells of the O-2A lineage.

ASTROCYTES CAN ENHANCE THE RECRUITMENT OF HOST O-2A LINEAGE CELLS

When cell cultures are introduced into lesions that have a normal repair capacity, it is not possible to identify whether the repair seen following transplantation is carried out by transplanted or host cells without the use of markers that distinguish transplanted cells from host cells. Thus, the extent to which recruited host cells or transplanted cells contribute to the enhanced oligodendrocyte repair observed in the experiments undertaken in non-irradiated tissue is not clear. To resolve this issue, cultures of type 1 astrocytes from which O-2A lineage cells were removed by immunocytolysis and that had no demonstrable ability to generate these cells *in vitro* (Table 1) were transplanted into ethidium bromide lesions. Following transplantation of these cultures into lesions made in normal white matter, a significant increase in oligodendrocyte remyelination was observed, which, since no O-2A lineage cells were transplanted, must have been carried out by host-derived cells (16) (Fig. 6). Support for this interpretation comes from the observation that following transplantation of these same O-2A-depleted, type 1 astrocyte cultures, from which Schwann cells are also absent, into non-repairing X-irradiated lesions, there is no evidence of remyelination after 2 weeks (unpublished observation) (Fig. 7).

TABLE 1. *Composition of type 1 astrocyte cultures*

	GFAP	GalC	O4	A2B5	Fibronectin	L1/S100
Composition before O-2A depletion	>85%	<5%	<5%	<5%	<5%	<5%
Composition at 7, 14, and 28 days after depletion protocol	>90%	0	0	0	<5%	<5%

[a] Cultures of type 1 astrocytes typically contain a small contaminating population of cells of the O-2A lineage (GalC-, O4-, A2B5-positive cells), meningeal cells (intensely fibronectin-positive cells), and Schwann cells (L1/S100-positive cells). O-2A lineage cells can be removed by a combined technique of complement-mediated immunocytolysis and cytosine arabinoside treatment. The cultures are treated with a cocktail of antibodies containing antitetanus-toxin, O4, and A2B5 antibodies (see ref. 16 for details).

There are a number of possible mechanisms by which transplanted astrocytes could potentiate host oligodendrocyte remyelination. (a) Transplanted astrocytes may be a source of diffusible factors that promote the migration of remyelinating cells into the lesion and/or act as mitogens. Platelet-derived growth factor (PDGF) may be one such factor since *in vitro,* PDGF, derived from type 1 astrocytes, is a mitogen (17–19) and chemoattractant for O-2A progenitors (20). Tissue culture studies have also identified a number of other growth factors and cytokines (some shown to be produced by astrocytes) that influence the behavior of O-2A lineage cells, such as fibroblast growth factor (21), transforming growth factor (22), insulin-like growth factor (23), and interleukin 2 (24). (b) The presence of astrocytes may also provide an appropriate matrix on which remyelinating cells can migrate throughout the lesion. In the absence of sufficient astrocyte numbers, and where the cellular environment consists predominantly of demyelinated axons, the migration of oligodendrocyte precursors may be limited. (c) Astrocytes may passively promote oligodendrocyte remyelination by their capacity to control Schwann cells and thus create an environment where oligodendrocytes are freed from competing

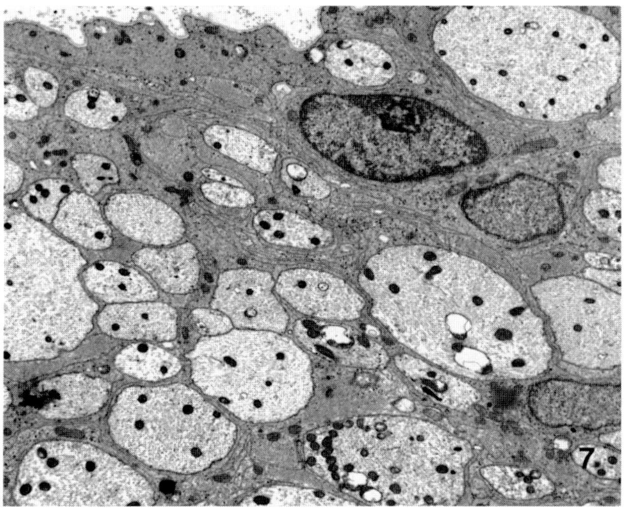

FIG. 7. Following transplantation of O-2A-depleted type 1 astrocyte cultures from which Schwann cells are also absent into X-irradiated ethidium bromide lesions, there is no evidence of either oligodendrocyte or Schwann cell remyelination. The transplanted astrocytes form an integrated astrocytic environment around the demyelinated axons. ×5,200.

with Schwann cells and have unhindered access to demyelinated axons. It is probable that all or a combination of these mechanisms operate in an astrocyte-rich remyelinating environment.

THE RELATIONSHIP BETWEEN ASTROCYTE PRESENCE AND OLIGODENDROCYTE MYELIN SHEATH FORMATION

The ability to manipulate the nature of the repair of a demyelinating CNS lesion by glial cell transplantation has created situations where it is possible to make observations on the integrity of oligodendrocyte myelin sheath formation in areas of different astrocyte density. In areas where there are no astrocytes, myelin sheaths are often not as well formed as in areas where the astrocyte density is similar to that found in normal spinal cord (Fig. 8). Conversely, where the astrocyte density is high, remyelinated sheaths tend to be thicker (Fig. 5). These observations indicate that astrocytes may play some secondary role in relation to myelin sheath formation.

The potentiation of oligodendrocyte remyelination by astrocytes observed in the context of a repairing lesion, both in terms of recruitment and myelin sheath formation, is difficult to resolve with the observation that type 1 astrocytes can inhibit oligodendrocyte myelination in tissue culture (25). These authors suggest that in tissue culture, type 1 astrocytes release soluble factors that inhibit myelin sheath formation and may exert an antiproliferative effect. It seems, therefore, that the behavior of type 1 astrocytes, including the nature of the soluble factors released, may be very different in the *in vitro* and *in vivo* situations. This is an issue that requires further clarification. It is possible that the density of astrocytes within a lesion may exceed an optimal level beyond which the effects on oligodendrocyte remyelination are adverse, perhaps by preventing the remyelinating cell from gaining access to the axon or by masking axonal signals. However, a preliminary series of experiments in which type 1 astrocytes have been transplanted at very high density suggests that this is not the case, since in these experiments oligodendrocyte remyelination is extensive, and myelin sheath formation is normal.

Although much has been gleaned about remyelination and the repopulation of glia-depleted environments from studying the

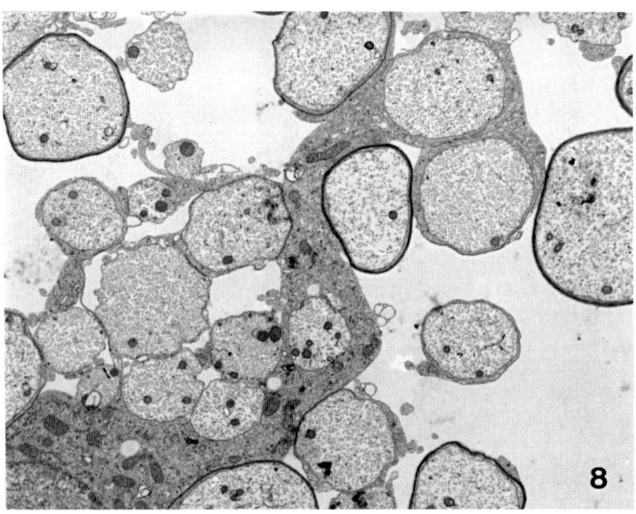

FIG. 8. In areas of repair where astrocytes are absent, oligodendrocyte remyelination is poor. Although oligodendrocyte processes surround many axons, myelin sheath formation has occurred around only a few. ×5,900.

resolution of demyelinating lesions, the technique of transplanting cultured glial cells has provided a means of extending our comprehension of the roles of individual cell types in the repair process. Our studies to date indicate that the astrocytes play a facilitatory role in remyelination and thus challenge the traditional view of neuropathology, based on their association with the non-repairing gliotic plaques of multiple sclerosis, that astrocytes hinder remyelination.

ACKNOWLEDGMENTS

Much of the work described in this chapter was supported by grants from the Multiple Sclerosis Society of Great Britain and the Wellcome Trust. R. J. M. Franklin holds a Wellcome Research Fellowship.

REFERENCES

1. Blakemore WF, Crang AJ, Evans RJ. The effect of chemical injury on oligodendrocytes. In: Mims CA, Cuzner ML, Kelly RE, eds. *Viruses and demyelinating diseases.* London: Academic Press; 1983: 167–90.
2. Blakemore WF, Franklin RJM. Transplantation of glial cells into the CNS. *Trends Neurosci* 1991; 14:323–327.
3. Graça DL, Blakemore WF. Delayed remyelination in rat spinal cord following ethidium bromide injection. *Neuropathol Appl Neurobiol* 1986;12:593–605.
4. Blakemore WF. Remyelination by Schwann cells of axons demyelinated by intraspinal injections of 6-aminonicotinamide. *J Neurocytol* 1975;4:745–757.
5. Sims TJ, Gilmore SA. Interactions between intraspinal Schwann cells and the cellular constituents normally occurring in the spinal cord: an ultrastructural study in the irradiated rat. *Brain Res* 1983;276:17–30.
6. Harrison B. Schwann cell and oligodendrocyte remyelination in lysolecithin-induced lesions in irradiated rat spinal cord. *J Neurol Sci* 1985;76:142–59.
7. Blakemore WF. Observations on remyelination in the rabbit spinal cord following demyelination induced by lysolecithin. *Neuropathol Appl Neurobiol* 1978;4:47–59.
8. Blakemore WF, Crang AJ. Extensive oligodendrocyte remyelination following injection of cultured central nervous system cells into demyelinating lesions in the adult central nervous system. *Dev Neurosci* 1988:10:1–10.
9. Raff MC, Abney ER, Cohen J, Lindsay R, Noble M. Two types of astrocytes in cultures of developing rat white matter: differences in morphology, surface gangliosides and growth characteristics. *J Neurosci* 1983;3:1289–1300.
10. Blakemore WF, Crang AJ. The relationship between type-1 astrocytes, Schwann cells and oligodendrocytes following transplantation of glial cell cultures into demyelinating lesions in the adult rat spinal cord. *J Neurocytol* 1989;18:519–528.
11. Crang AJ, Blakemore WF. The effect of the number of oligodendrocytes transplanted into X-irradiated, glial-free lesions on the extent of oligodendrocyte remyelination. *Neurosci Lett* 1989;193:269–274.
12. Blakemore WF, Crang AJ. The use of cultured autologous Schwann cells to remyelinate areas of persistent demyelination in the central nervous system. *J Neurol Sci* 1985;70:207–223.
13. Blakemore WF, Crang AJ, Evans RJ, Patterson RC. Rat Schwann cell remyelination of demyelinated cat CNS axons: evidence that injection of cell suspensions of CNS tissue results in Schwann cell remyelination. *Neurosci Lett* 1987;77:15–19.
14. Mirsky R, Jessen KR, Schachner M, Goridis C. Distribution of the adhesion molecules N-CAM and L1 on peripheral neurons and glia in adult rats. *J Neurocytol* 1986;15:799–815.
15. Franklin RJM, Crang AJ, Blakemore WF. Type 1 astrocytes fail to inhibit Schwann cell remyelination of CNS axons in the absence of cells of the O-2A lineage. *Dev Neurosci [in press].*
16. Franklin RJM, Crang AJ, Blakemore WF. Transplanted type-1 astrocytes facilitate repair of demyelinating lesions by host oligodendrocytes in adult rat spinal cord. *J Neurocytol* 1991;20:420–430.
17. Noble M, Murray K, Stroobant P, Waterfield MD, Riddle P. Platelet-derived growth factor promotes division and motility and inhibits premature differentiation of the oligodendrocyte/type-2 astrocyte progenitor cell. *Nature* 1988;333:560–565.
18. Richardson WD, Pringle N, Mosley MJ, Westermark B, Dubois-Dalcq M. A role for platelet-derived growth factor in normal gliogenesis in the central nervous system. *Cell* 1988;53:309–319.
19. Wolswijk G, Riddle PN, Noble M. Platelet-derived growth factor is mitogenic for O-2A adult progenitor cells. *Glia* 1991;4:495–503.
20. Armstrong RC, Harvarth L, Dubois-Dalcq ME. Type-1 astrocytes and oligodendrocyte-type-2 astrocyte glial progenitors migrate toward distinct molecules. *J Neurosci Res* 1990;27:400–407.
21. Besnard F, Perraud F, Sensenbrenner M, Labourdette G. Effects of acidic and basic fibroblast growth factors on proliferation and maturation of cultured rat oligodendrocytes. *Int J Dev Neurosci* 1989; 7:401–409.
22. Van Obberghen-Schilling E, Behar T, Sporn MB, Dubois-Dalcq M. Signalling between type-1 astrocytes and glial O-2A progenitors: modulation by transforming growth factor-β (TGF-β). *J Cell Biol* 1987;105:318a.
23. McMorris FA, Dubois-Dalcq M. Insulin-like growth factor I promotes cell proliferation and oligodendroglial commitment in rat glial progenitors developing *in vitro*. *J Neurosci Res* 1988;21:199–209.
24. Benveniste EN, Merrill JE. Stimulation of oligodendroglial proliferation and maturation by interleukin-2. *Nature* 1986;321:610–613.
25. Rosen CL, Bunge RP, Ard MD, Wood PM. Type-1 astrocytes inhibit myelination by adult rat oligodendrocytes *in vitro*. *J Neurosci* 1989;9:3371–3379.

Advances in Neurology, Vol. 59, edited by
Fredrick J. Seil. Raven Press, Ltd.,
New York © 1993.

12

Dynamic Aspects of Sodium Channel Expression in Astrocytes

S. G. Waxman, H. Sontheimer, J. A. Black,
J. E. Minturn, and B. R. Ransom

Department of Neurology, Yale University School of Medicine, New Haven, Connecticut 06510; and PVA/EPVA Neuroscience Research Center, Veterans Administration Medical Center, West Haven, Connecticut 06516

Although astrocytes outnumber neurons in the central nervous system (CNS) by a large margin, the functions of these nonneuronal cells remain enigmatic. Recent studies have demonstrated that the expression of voltage-activated sodium channels is not restricted to neurons but, in addition, occurs in some glial cell types. Sodium currents, for example, have been recorded in cultured Schwann cells (1,2), cultured astrocytes from cortex (3,4) and optic nerve (5,6), and cultured glial precursor cells in cortex (7) and optic nerve (8). In order to better understand astrocytic properties and neuron–astrocyte interactions, we have studied the characteristics of voltage-sensitive sodium channels in astrocytes under a variety of conditions.

Our findings demonstrate that astrocytes express several types of sodium currents. Astrocytes from different CNS regions display different patterns of channel expression. Moreover, our results show that sodium channel expression in these cells is a dynamic process that is subject to modulation by neuronal and glial influences. These findings, together with ultrastructural observations that indicate a close relationship between astrocytic contact and the development of sodium-channel-rich regions along normal and pathological axons, suggest the possibility that alterations in channel expression participate in the response of astrocytes to CNS injury. This chapter briefly outlines our current knowledge with respect to the expression of sodium channels in mammalian astrocytes.

ASTROCYTES *IN VITRO* EXPRESS SODIUM CHANNELS

Both immunocytochemical and electrophysiological methods demonstrate sodium channels in astrocytes *in vitro*. Figure 1 shows indirect immunofluorescence microscopy of astrocytes derived from postnatal day 7 (P7) rat optic nerve examined at 2 days *in vitro* (DIV) with a monoclonal antibody against GFAP (Fig. 1A) and polyclonal antibody 7493 (9), which is directed against rat brain sodium channels (Fig. 1B). At 2 DIV in these cultures, three cell types are present: fibroblast-like $GFAP^+/A2B5^-$ and stellate $GFAP^+/A2B5^+$ astrocytes and $GFAP^-/A2B5^+$ precursors [O-2A progenitor cells according to the terminology of Raff et al., (10)]. As shown in Fig. 1B, at 2 DIV all of these cell types in these cultures exhibit sodium channel immunostaining with antibody 7493 (11).

When studied using patch-clamp methods (6), the two types of astrocytes in optic nerve cultures both express sodium currents at

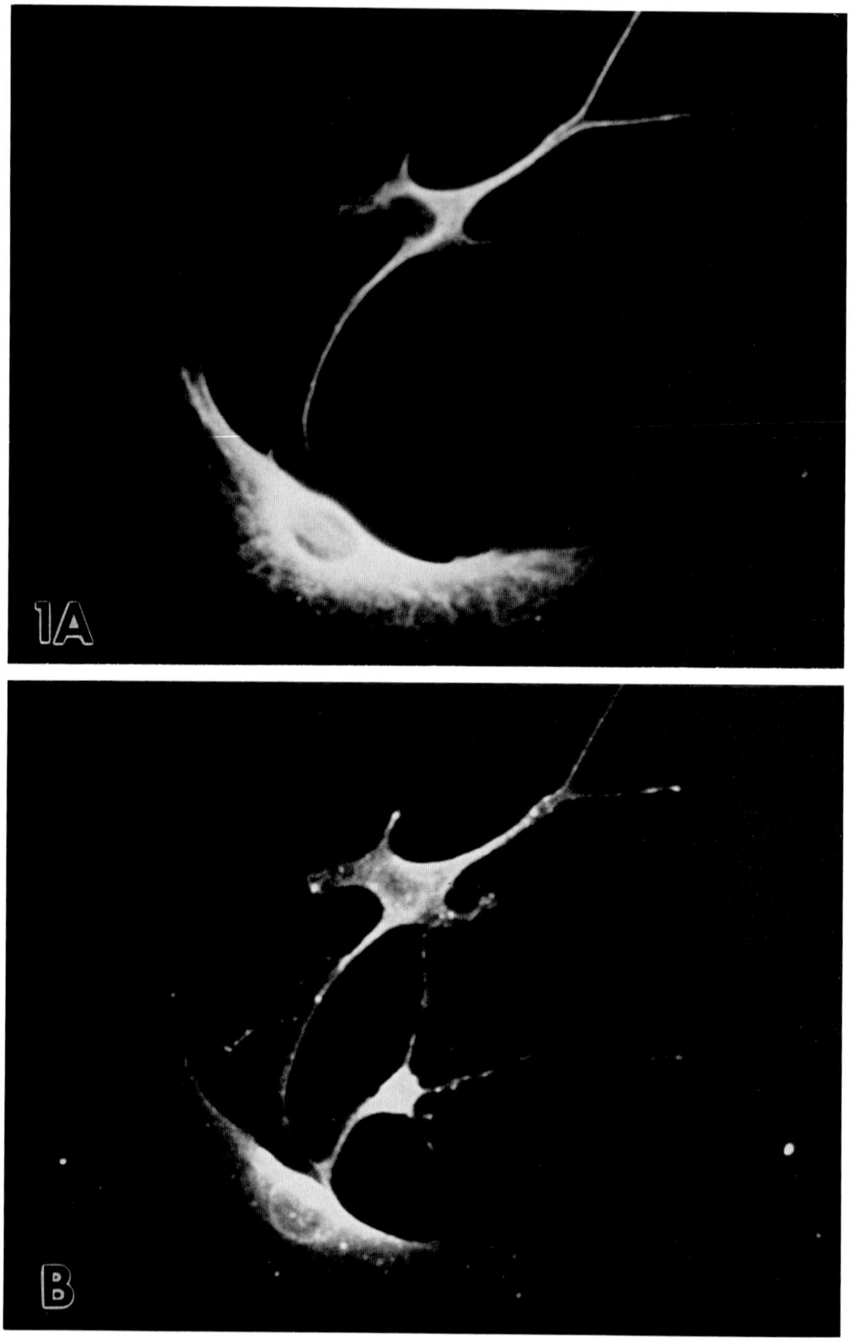

FIG. 1. Sodium channel immunoreactivity in astrocytes from P7 rat optic nerve at 2 DIV. GFAP (**A**) was visualized with rhodamine, and sodium channels (**B**) were detected with antibody 7493 using fluorescein-conjugated secondary antibodies. At 2 DIV, both flat, fibroblast-like and stellate, process-bearing GFAP$^+$ cells exhibit sodium channel immunoreactivity. A tripolar GFAP$^-$ cell, probably an 02-A progenitor, also displays 7493 immunostaining. (Modified from Minturn et al., ref. 11.)

early times *in vitro* (Fig. 2a,c). Inward currents were identified as sodium currents on the basis of sensitivity to tetrodotoxin, insensitivity to $CdCl_2$, and reversal potentials close to E_{Na}. As a measure of sodium channel density, we used the quotient between peak current and whole-cell membrane capacity (see refs. 12, 13 for discussion). During the initial period in culture (<10 DIV), both types of optic nerve astrocyte (A2B5$^+$ and A2B5$^-$) exhibit substantial sodium current densities (9.7 ± 4.6 pA/pF, n = 50, A2B5$^+$; 7.38 ± 6.5 pA/pF, n = 69, A2B5$^-$). Assuming a single-channel conductance of 20 pS and an open-channel probability of 0.25 (5,14), these current densities suggest a density of about 0.25 channels/μm^2 in optic nerve astrocyte membrane (6).

Typical patch-clamp recordings from astrocytes from another region of the CNS, the hippocampus (12,13), are shown in Fig. 3. One day after plating, rat hippocampal astrocytes exhibit a mean whole-cell sodium current density of 34.6 pA/pF, which suggests an estimated density of ~0.9 sodium channels/μm^2 in these cells at early stages in culture (12,13). As described below, sodium channel expression in astrocytes *in vitro* is a

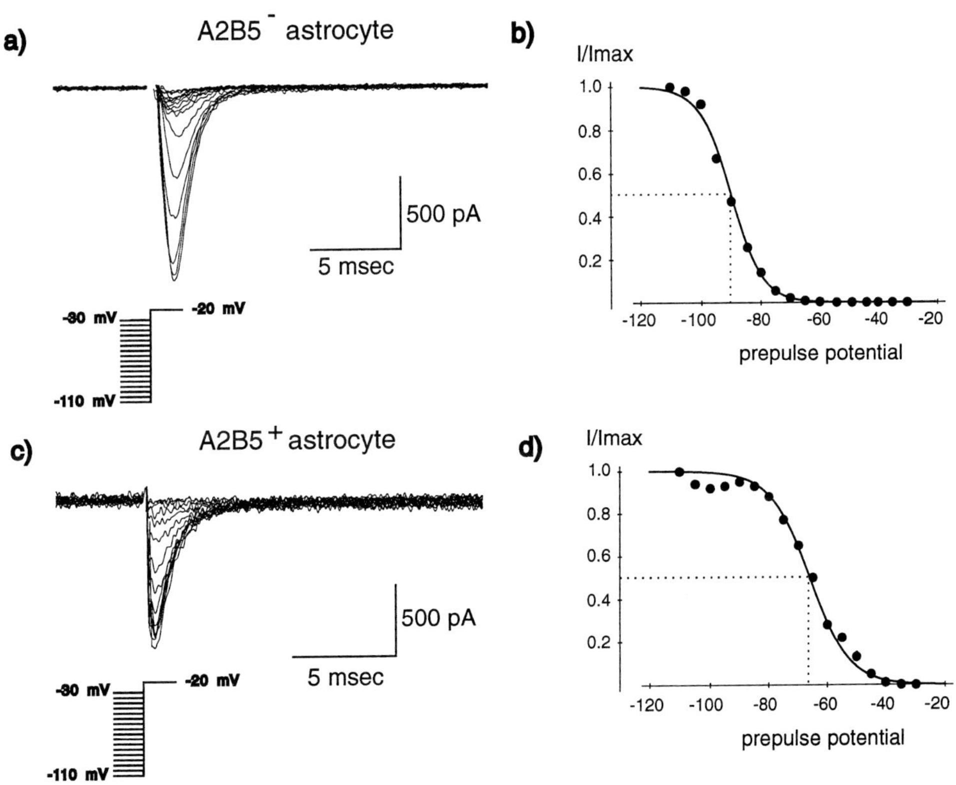

FIG. 2. A2B5$^+$ and A2B5$^-$ optic nerve astrocytes differ in their steady-state inactivation (h_∞) characteristics. The h_∞ curves were obtained by applying a conditioning prepulse protocol: cells were voltage clamped at −70 mV and stepped for 200 msec to the prepulse potential indicated (**inset** to **a,b**). Following this prepulse, currents were activated by stepping the membrane to the potential for maximum current activation (−20 mV). Peak currents were normalized to the largest current (at −110 mV), and the normalized values (I/I_{max}) were plotted as a function of prepulse potential to yield the steady-state inactivation curves shown in **b** and **d.** The data were fitted to a modified Boltzmann equation using an algorithm to minimize the least-squared error (*continuous lines* in **b,d**). The h_∞ curve midpoints were close to −85 mV in A2B5$^-$ astrocytes (**a,b;** *dotted line*) but were close to −65 mV in A2B5$^+$ astrocytes (**c,d**). (Modified from Sontheimer et al., ref. 6.)

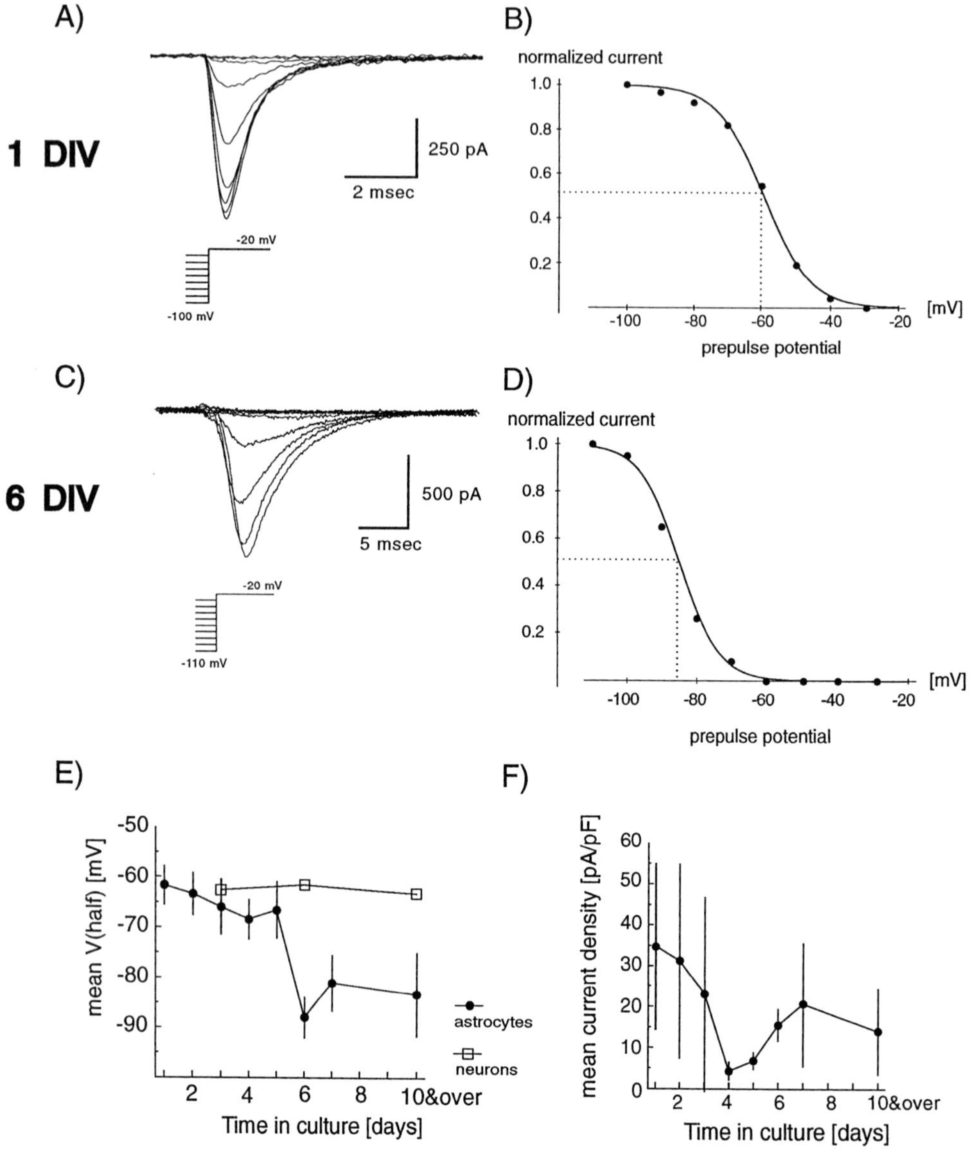

FIG. 3. Na^+ current characteristics in hippocampal astrocytes. Steady-state inactivation (h_∞) curves were obtained as described in the legend to Fig. 2. Current recordings (**A**) and h_∞ curve (**B**) from an astrocyte cultured for 1 day. Prepulse potential was varied from −100 to −30 mV, and currents were activated through a voltage step to −20 mV. Current amplitude was maximal at −100 mV and decreased with more depolarizing voltage steps. The steady-state inactivation curve (**B**) showed its midpoint close to −60 mV and reached base line around −40 mV. **C** and **D:** Same protocol as in **A,** but recordings were obtained from an astrocyte after 6 days in culture. The midpoint of the steady-state inactivation curve was close to −85 mV, and base line was reached at −60 mV. Thus, the entire curve is shifted about 25 mV towards more hyperpolarized potentials when compared to (**A**). Midpoint of the steady-state inactivation curve and Na^+ current density in hippocampal astrocytes are shown as functions of time in culture in **E** and **F,** respectively. **E:** The mean values of the midpoints in the steady-state inactivation curves ($V_{1/2}$) of all cells studied were plotted as a function of time. These values were close to −65 mV during the first 5 days in culture but changed by about 20 mV for

dynamic process, and this channel density is not maintained at a constant value in these cultures.

Astrocytes from still another region of the CNS, the spinal cord, exhibit different properties. We have recently established cultures derived from the spinal cord of the neonatal rat (15). In these cultures, there are several classes of astrocytes including GFAP$^+$ flat fibroblast-like cells with a round outline and GFAP$^+$ stellate, process-bearing astrocytes. The flat astrocytes (which resemble pancakes *en face* and are thus termed "pancake cells") express sodium currents at high densities *in vitro* (whole-cell currents >10,000 pA in most cells after 5 DIV; see Fig. 4A). Sodium current densities in these cells at 7 DIV can exceed 200 pA/pF. In these spinal cord astrocytes *in vitro,* the electrophysiological measurements suggest that there are at least 8 sodium channels/μm^2, a density similar to that seen in some neurons. Notably, sodium currents are expressed in these cells at increasing densities over the first 7 days in culture, at a time when potassium currents are attenuated so that, at 7 DIV, the ratio of peak sodium current to peak potassium current (Fig. 4A) is much greater than in optic nerve or hippocampal astrocytes (or in some neurons). As might be expected from the relatively high sodium channel density and the large ratio of sodium to potassium current (12) in these cells, anode break electrogenesis can be demonstrated in these spinal cord astrocytes *in vitro* (Fig. 4E) (15).

It should be emphasized that this does not imply that, under normal conditions, these astrocytes are excitable. Resting membrane potential in pancake astrocytes is relatively depolarized (about −30 mV, as expected from the low potassium conductance in these cells) so that, at resting potential, sodium channels would be expected to be almost entirely inactivated (15). Regenerative responses have not been recorded from astrocytes *in situ* (see, e.g., ref. 16), either as a result of this inactivation or because of different channel densities and/or distributions *in vitro* and *in situ.* The important conclusion from the *in vitro* patch-clamp studies is that, under at least some conditions, spinal cord astrocytes are capable of synthesizing significant numbers of sodium channels.

The large range of sodium channel densities displayed by astrocytes from different CNS regions (together with differences in the temporal pattern of sodium channel expression described below) illustrates the striking regional heterogeneity that is displayed by these cells (17). Whether different patterns of sodium channel expression reflect intrinsic, preprogrammed differences in these cells or modulation by region-specific influences that are different in various parts of the CNS is not yet known. The distinct patterns of channel expression in these astrocytes, even when studied under similar culture conditions *in vitro* where neuronal influences are minimal, might be interpreted as suggesting that astrocytes from different CNS regions possess inherent, highly differentiated properties. Although regional heterogeneity of glial cells has not been previously emphasized, it is not an unexpected phenomenon, given the strik-

←

astrocytes 6 days and older. In contrast, neurons measured at 3 days, 6 days, or 10 days and older did not show any significant changes in their midpoints and remained close to −60 mV. Note that the step-like change of the mean midpoints plotted corresponds to the occurrence of a second peak in the current density plot shown in **F. F:** Current densities for Na^+ currents were obtained by dividing the peak current measured in a particular cell by its whole-cell capacity. Mean values were plotted as a function of time in culture. The initial Na^+ current density was around 35 pA/pF 1 day after plating. This value dropped to 4 pA/pF within the first 4 days in culture. A second peak in current densities was observed at day 7. The mean value for cells 10 to 20 days in culture was 16 pA/pF. (Modified from Sontheimer et al., ref. 12.)

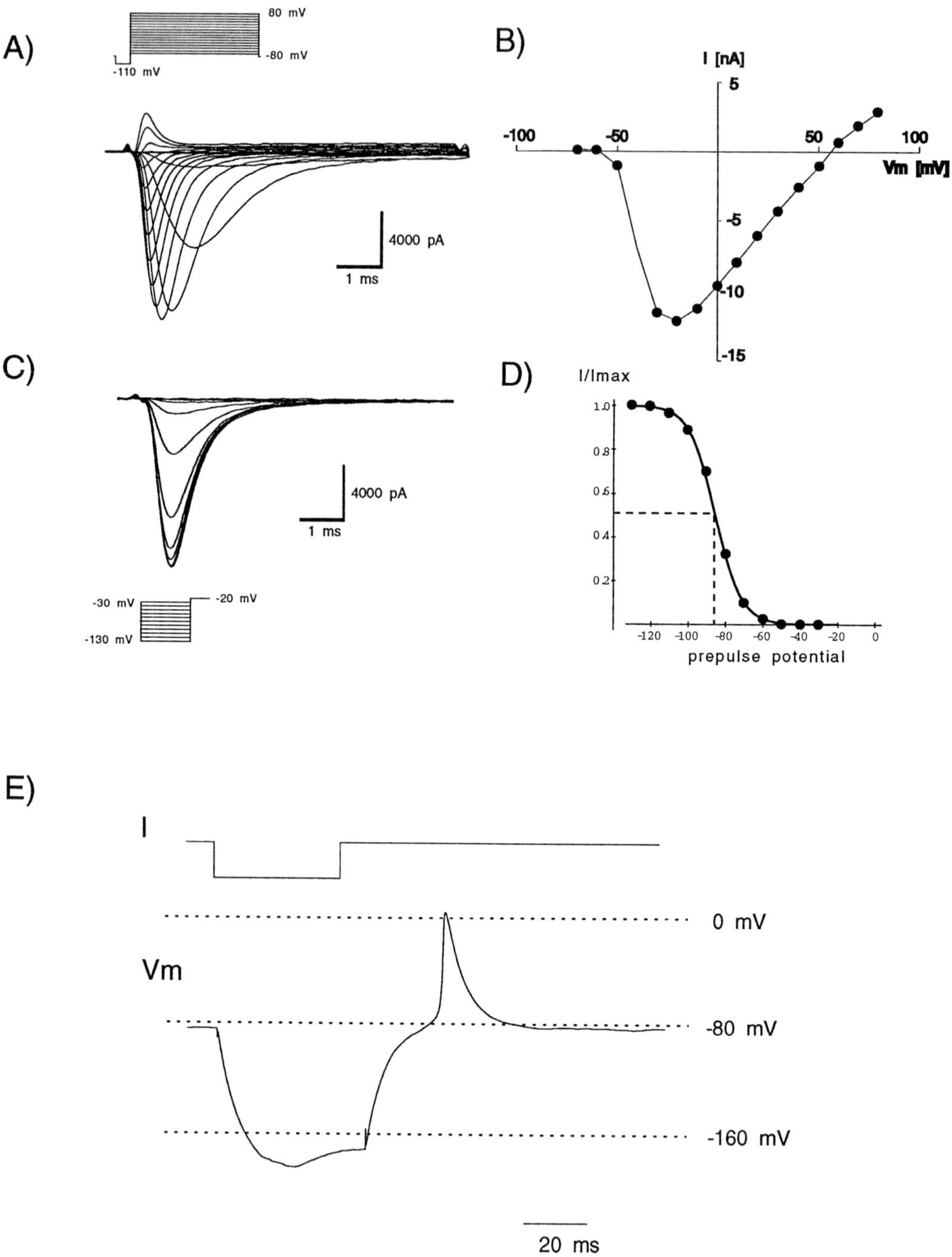

FIG. 4. High levels of sodium channel expression in spinal cord astrocytes. Examples of a recording obtained in a flat (pancake-like) spinal cord astrocyte. Whole-cell currents were recorded at 7 DIV as described in the legend to Fig. 2, but under conditions that allowed both sodium and potassium currents to occur. **A:** Sodium current activation was studied by activating currents from a resting potential of −110 mV to the potentials indicated (**inset**). Potentials more positive than −50 mV activated a transient inward current that inactivated within milliseconds. Currents were largest in response to a voltage step to −20 mV and decreased at more positive test potentials. **B:** Peak currents

ing regional specialization of the other major cell type in the CNS, the neuron, that has been recognized since the earliest neuroanatomic studies.

SOME ASTROCYTES EXPRESS SODIUM CHANNELS WITH PROPERTIES SIMILAR TO THOSE OF NEURONS

Several studies have recently demonstrated that some astrocytes exhibit sodium currents with properties similar to those expressed by neurons. For example, patch-clamp studies by Barres et al. (5) and Sontheimer et al. (6) show that the steady-state inactivation (h_∞) curve for voltage-activated sodium currents from A2B5$^+$ optic nerve astrocytes has a midpoint at about −65 mV (Figs. 2d, 6E), i.e., a midpoint that is shifted about 20 mV in a depolarizing direction compared to other glial-like sodium currents expressed in A2B5$^-$ optic nerve astrocytes. The h_∞ curve for sodium currents in A2B5$^+$ optic nerve astrocytes is similar to that expressed by a variety of neuronal cell types, including retinal ganglion cells (5), hippocampal neurons (12), and dorsal root ganglion neurons (18), and these channels have therefore been termed "neuronal" (5); it should be noted, however, that *I–V* curves for activation and kinetics of these channels differ from those in many types of neurons. Since it is not clear that these astrocytic channels are identical to those expressed by neurons, we prefer the terminology "neuronal-like."

Expression of "neuronal-like" sodium current is not confined to astrocytes derived from white matter. At early times in culture (<6 DIV), astrocytes derived from the CA1 and CA3 regions of neonatal rat hippocampus express sodium currents with similar properties, i.e., with relatively fast kinetics and an h_∞ curve with a midpoint close to −60 mV (Fig. 3B) (12,13). Interestingly, astrocytes in these cultures display a discrete shift in sodium current characteristics with increasing time in culture, initially expressing a "neuronal-like" sodium current but then expressing a "glial-like" sodium current after about 6 days in culture (Fig. 3D,E), as described below.

SODIUM CHANNEL EXPRESSION IN ASTROCYTES CHANGES WITH TIME *IN VITRO*

Figure 5 shows stellate (Fig. 5A,B) and flat, fibroblast-like astrocytes (Fig. 5C,D) derived from P7 rat optic nerve, studied by immunofluorescent microscopy at 20 DIV. All astrocytes in these cultures stain positively with

plotted as a function of membrane potential yield the current activation curve. Sodium current activation curve peaked at close to −20 mV and indicates current reversal at 55 mV, which is close to the sodium equilibrium potential. **C:** Steady-state inactivation of sodium currents was studied using a conditioning prepulse protocol as described in the legend to Fig. 2. Current amplitudes were largest at prepulse potentials more negative than −100 mV and showed steep declines at more positive potentials. **D:** Currents were normalized to the largest current amplitude and were plotted as a function of prepulse potential to yield the steady-state h_∞ curves. The data were fit to the Boltzmann equation. The h_∞ curve showed a midpoint at −85 mV. **E:** Current-clamp recordings in the same cell display the capability to fire anode break spikes under appropriate conditions. The cell for which voltage-clamp recordings were displayed in **A** through **D** was current clamped at a potential of −80 mV, and a hyperpolarizing current pulse of 50-msec duration and 1 nA was applied. Such current injections typically hyperpolarized the cells to potentials more negative than −150 mV. On termination of the voltage step, the cells typically showed an overshooting, action-potential-like response. Note that a large hyperpolarization is required to elicit such a response. Recordings in **A–E** were obtained under conditions where potassium currents were not blocked. As illustrated in this figure, after more than 5 DIV, potassium currents were typically very small in these spinal cord astrocytes and accounted for less than 20% of the cells' peak conductance.

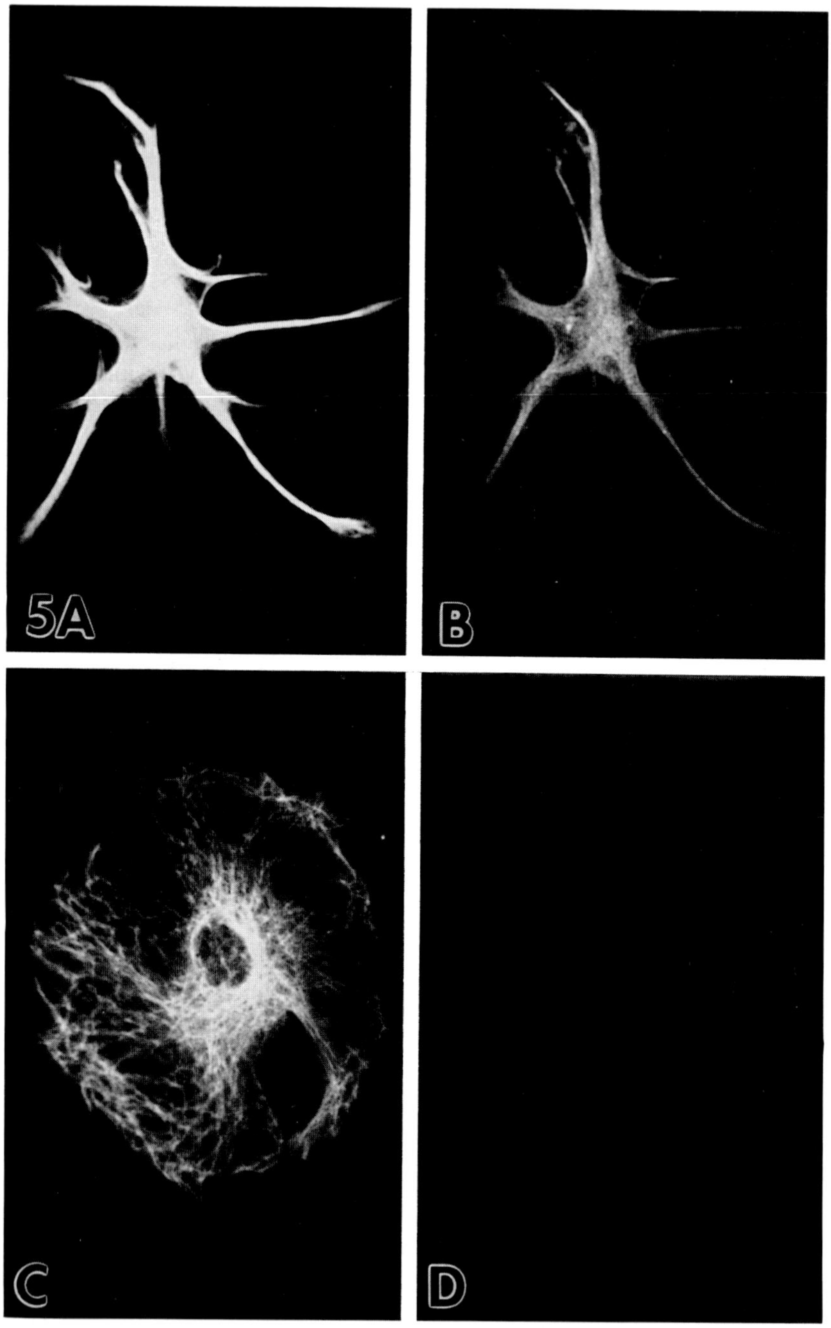

FIG. 5. Different patterns of sodium channel immunoreactivity in stellate and flat astrocytes from P7 optic nerve, examined at 20 DIV. Stellate (**A, B**) and flat (**C, D**) astrocytes exhibit GFAP immunostaining (**A, C**), but only process-bearing astrocytes maintain sodium channel immunoreactivity (**B**). Fibroblast-like astrocytes are not immunostained by 7493 (**D**). (Modified from Minturn et al., ref. 11.)

GFAP (Fig. 5A,C). However, following staining for sodium channels with antibody 7493 in long-term culture, there are different patterns of immunoreactivity in the two types of astrocytes. Stellate optic nerve astrocytes continue to exhibit sodium channel immunoreactivity with antibody 7493 (Fig. 5B) for up to 28 DIV (the longest time point studied), whereas flat astrocytes in these cultures lose sodium channel immunoreactivity after 6 DIV (Fig. 5D) (6). These immunocytochemical results suggest different temporal patterns of sodium channel expression in the two types of optic nerve astrocytes.

As a physiological measure of sodium channel density, we used patch-clamp methods to monitor sodium currents and membrane capacitance in optic nerve astrocytes at various times in culture. In cultures derived from optic nerve, h_∞ curve midpoints in A2B5$^+$ and A2B5$^-$ astrocytes do not change with time *in vitro* (6). Mean values were around −85 mV for sodium currents expressed by A2B5$^-$ astrocytes but were close to −65 mV for A2B5$^+$ astrocytes at all times in culture (Fig. 6E). Since h_∞ curves with intermediate midpoints were not observed, it appears that each type of astrocyte produces a single, distinct type of sodium current.

Mean values for sodium current density in the two types of optic nerve astrocytes are displayed in Fig. 6C,D. A2B5$^-$ astrocytes in these cultures typically showed capacity values between 10 and 200 pF; after an initial rise throughout the first 10 DIV, whole-cell capacity values remained stable at 100 to 150 pF. Capacities measured in A2B5$^+$ astrocytes were considerably smaller and remained below 100 pF for periods up to 16 DIV (the longest period that these cells could be studied in culture). Whole-cell mean peak sodium currents are shown in Fig. 6A,B, and current densities as a function of time in culture are shown in Fig. 6C,D. In these plots, cells that did not exhibit sodium currents were included by calculating mean values with a density of 0 pA/pF. The dotted lines in Fig. 6C,D indicate the average detection limit of 1 pA/pF, corresponding to approximately 0.03 channels/μm^2 in our recording configuration; cells with current densities at or below the 1 pA/pF detection threshold were classified as lacking sodium current expression.

A2B5$^+$ astrocytes displayed sodium current densities ranging from 2.3 pA/pF to 22.5 pA/pF (mean 9.7 pA/pF, S.D. 4.6 pA/pF, n = 50), and sodium current densities did not change substantially with time in culture (Fig. 6D). In contrast, A2B5 astrocytes showed a decrease in current densities with increasing time *in vitro,* and currents were almost completely abolished after 12 DIV. Mean sodium current densities in A2B5$^-$ astrocytes were similar to those in A2B5$^+$ astrocytes up to 6 DIV, but in A2B5$^-$ astrocytes, sodium current densities began to fall at 6 to 8 DIV. The decreasing current densities in A2B5$^-$ astrocytes were caused by both a decrease in the proportion of cells with measurable sodium currents and a decrease in the peak current of the few A2B5$^-$ cells that showed measurable sodium currents (6).

The lag between loss of sodium channel immunoreactivity (at 6 DIV) and loss of physiologically demonstrable sodium currents (which fell to approach the threshold for detection at 14 DIV) may be caused by the fact that antibody 7493 immunostaining can detect sodium channels or channel precursors that are not yet inserted into the plasma membrane (and are thus not yet functional) (19) but can not detect the low sodium channel densities that can be observed in patch-clamp experiments. Assuming that this cytoplasmic pool contains channel precursors that are destined for subsequent insertion into the plasma membrane, its depletion would be expected to lead, after an appropriate lag time, to loss of membrane-associated channels. The estimated half-life of sodium channels incorporated into the plasma membrane of cultured rabbit Schwann cells is 2.2 days (20). The time lag between loss of sodium channel immunoreactivity at 6 DIV and loss of electrophysiological evidence of membrane-associated sodium channels in cultured A2B5$^-$ astrocytes is consistent with depletion of a cytoplasmic pool

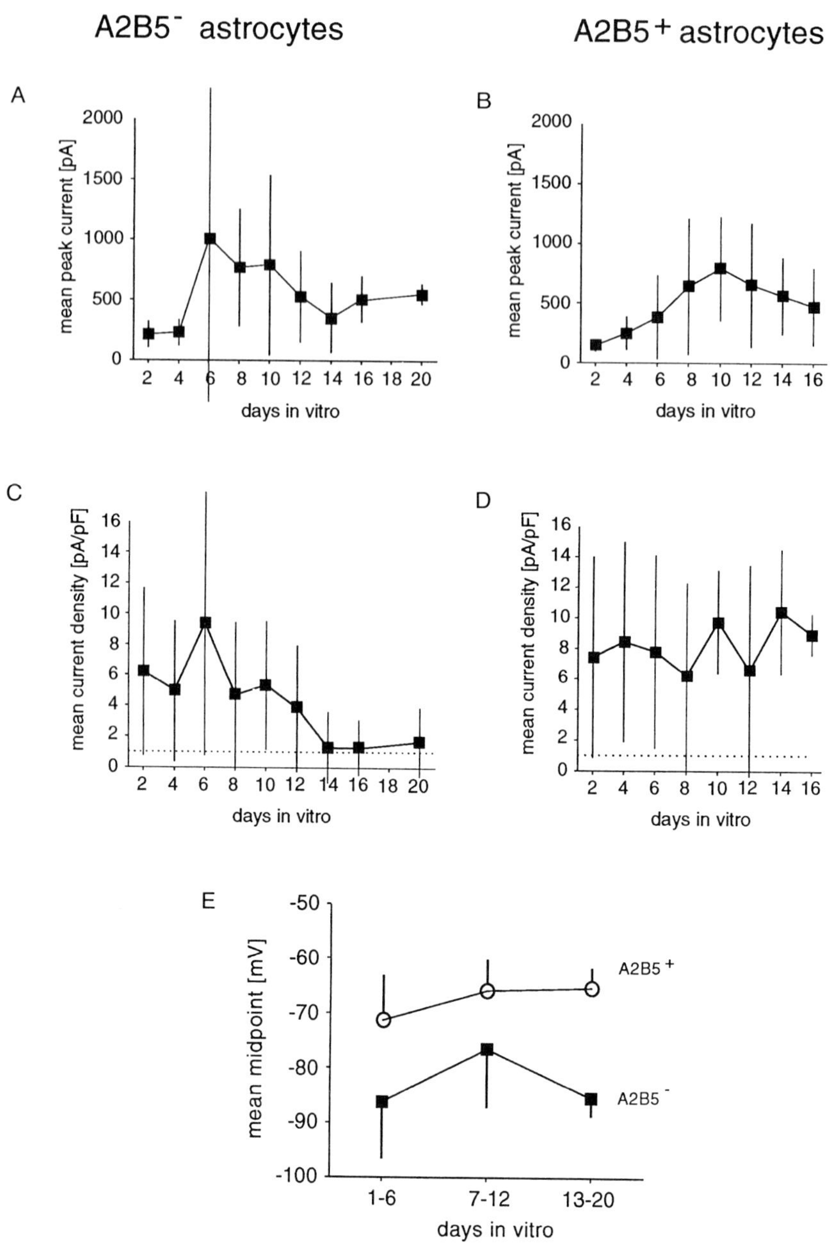

FIG. 6. Time course of Na^+ current expression in rat optic nerve astrocytes. Mean values and S.D. were obtained for the peak Na^+ currents (**A, B**) and Na^+ current densities (i.e., peak current/whole-cell capacity; **C, D**) of optic nerve astrocytes. Mean values for 2-day periods (e.g., days 1 and 2, 3 and 4, etc.) were pooled and plotted as a function of time in culture for A2B5$^-$ astrocytes (**A, C**) and A2B5$^+$ astrocytes (**B, D**). **A,B:** Peak currents in A2B5$^-$ astrocytes were small within the first 4 DIV and after 14 DIV. Values were largest at 6 to 10 DIV. This time course was similar in A2B5$^+$ astrocytes, but variations were less pronounced. **C, D:** Na^+ current densities in A2B5$^-$ astrocytes were between 6 and 10 pA/pF at 1 to 10 DIV. Thereafter current densities dropped to reach values close to the detection level of our recording (1 pA/pF; *dotted lines*). In contrast, mean Na^+ current densities were always close to 9 pA/pF in A2B5$^+$ astrocytes and did not vary significantly with time. **E:** Steady-state inactivation curves (h_∞ curves) were obtained as described in the legend to Fig. 2. The average midpoint values (±S.D.) of the h_∞ curves for all cells were plotted as a function of time in culture. These values were close to −65 mV in A2B5$^+$ astrocytes (*circles*) over the entire time period studied (20 DIV). In contrast, h_∞ midpoints were consistently about 20 mV more negative in A2B5$^-$ astrocytes (*squares*), with mean values close to −85 mV. (Modified from Sontheimer et al., ref. 6.)

of sodium channel precursors *in vitro* at 6 DIV, followed by a loss of membrane-associated sodium channels as these turn over and are not repleted, so that the density of these channels falls to the threshold for physiological detection at 14 DIV.

A different temporal pattern of sodium current expression is seen in rat hippocampal astrocytes *in vitro* (12). In these astrocytes studied at 1 DIV, the midpoint of the h_∞ curve was close to −60 mV (mean −61.7 ± 3.8 S.D. mV) (Fig. 3B,E). In contrast, the midpoint of the h_∞ curves for hippocampal astrocytes studied at 6 DIV (or in astrocytes cultured at P5 at 1 DIV) was almost 25 mV more negative, with a midpoint close to −85 mV (mean −84.5 ± 5.4 mV at 6 and 7 DIV), and remained in this range in astrocytes studied at longer times in culture, up to 20 DIV (the latest time point examined; Fig. 3D,E). This was caused by a discrete shift in sodium current characteristics. Intermediate values of the h_∞ midpoint were not seen, and no overlap in the two types of sodium currents was observed when astrocytes studied before and after 6 DIV were compared. Hippocampal neurons studied in the same cultures exhibited h_∞ midpoints of approximately −60 mV at all times in culture and did not show the shift in steady-state inactivation that was displayed by hippocampal astrocytes (Fig. 3E).

Interestingly, in these hippocampal astrocyte cultures, whole-cell sodium current density, which provided a measure of current expression, exhibited a biphasic time course (Fig. 3F). Sodium current density was highest on the first day after plating (34.6 pA/pF) but dropped by almost an order of magnitude to 4.2 pA/pF after 4 DIV. Sodium current densities then rose again to reach a second peak (20.6 pA/pF) at day 7 and stabilized close to 14 pA/pF from 10 DIV on. The biphasic current density plot appears to reflect an initial loss of sodium channels followed by a second wave of expression beginning at 6 DIV. The development of the second peak of current density, beginning at 5 DIV, is temporally coincident with the occurrence of the shift in h_∞ curves in these cells. Moreover, the first wave of sodium currents in these cells is lost with a time course that is similar to the loss of sodium channel immunoreactivity in A2B5$^-$ optic nerve astrocytes after 6 DIV. These observations in hippocampal astrocytes suggest an early decrease of channel synthesis and attenuation in expression of channels inserted in the plasma membrane at early times in culture, followed by a second wave of channel expression beginning at 5 to 6 DIV.

NEURONS MODULATE ASTROCYTE SODIUM CHANNEL EXPRESSION

The attenuation of sodium channel expression in A2B5$^-$ astrocytes *in vitro* suggests the possibility that channel expression in these cells is subject to neuronal modulation (11). Several laboratories have examined sodium channel expression in optic nerve astrocytes after enucleation (21) or nerve transection (22), maneuvers that result in the development of astrocytes in an axon-deprived environment. These studies indicate that, indeed, neurons appear to play a role in modulating ion channel expression in astrocytes.

Neonatal optic nerve transection results in a profound decrease in the number of oligodendrocytes and A2B5$^+$ astrocytes but has less effect on the number of A2B5$^-$ astrocytes in the optic nerve, demonstrating that axons play a role in the survival of certain glial cell types in the developing optic nerve (23,24). In our studies we used enucleation in the neonatal rat, which produces an optic nerve consisting of a nearly pure glial cell population (24). To test the hypothesis that the *in vitro* environment in optic nerve cultures lacks a neuron-derived factor necessary for the maintenance of sodium channel expression, we studied the expression of sodium channels in astrocytes cultured from enucleated optic nerves (21). In contrast to control cultures derived from normal optic nerves, which exhibited robust sodium channel immunoreactivity, astrocytes from enucleated optic nerves did not display sodium channel immunoreactivity *in vitro*. We also used patch-

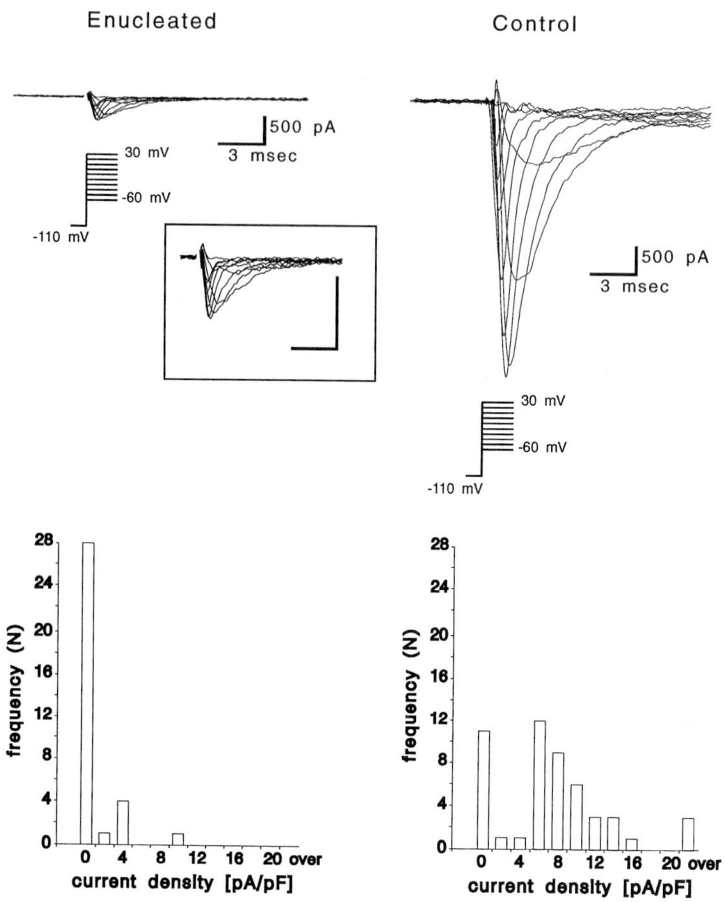

FIG. 7. Na^+ channel expression is down-regulated in axon-deprived optic nerve astrocytes. Na^+ currents recorded in astrocytes from intact and enucleated rat optic nerve. **Top:** Na^+ currents were recorded under whole-cell voltage clamp in response to the series of depolarizing voltage steps indicated. Typical recordings of astrocytes from enucleated rat optic nerve and normal age-matched rat optic nerve that showed measurable Na^+ currents and were of approximately equal size (as judged by whole-cell capacity, which was about 80 pF in both cells) are displayed to scale to demonstrate differences in peak currents. Currents were typically activated at −50 mV and were largest in response to −20 mV voltage steps for both preparations. The majority of astrocytes from intact nerves showed substantial Na^+ currents with amplitudes ranging from 100 to 5,000 pA (mean 500 pA). In contrast, astrocytes from enucleated rat optic nerve typically lacked Na^+ currents, and only six out of 34 cells showed small Na^+ currents, the largest example of which is displayed. **Bottom:** Frequency distribution of Na^+ current densities in astrocytes from intact and enucleated rat optic nerve. Current densities were derived by dividing Na^+ peak currents by whole-cell membrane capacitance for all cells. Current densities were pooled in bins with 2 pA/pF increments and plotted as a function of frequency. The majority of astrocytes cultured from intact nerves showed current densities of 4 to 14 pA/pF. In contrast, the majority of astrocytes cultured from enucleated optic nerves did not show any measurable currents (0 pA/pF). Five cells showed current densities of 2 to 6 pA/pF, and only one cell showed a current density of 9 pA/pF. (Modified from Minturn et al., ref. 21.)

clamp methods to quantitatively determine sodium current densities in cultured astrocytes from enucleated optic nerves and compared them with densities obtained from $A2B5^-$ astrocytes from intact optic nerves (Fig. 7). Control astrocytes exhibited sodium current densities that were scattered around 6 to 16 pA/pF (mean 7.15 ± 1.1 pA/pF). In contrast, sodium currents were not detectable (<1.0 pA/pF) in the majority of astrocytes from enucleated optic nerves, with only six out of 38 astrocytes from enucleated optic nerve exhibiting measurable sodium currents; the mean sodium current density in astrocytes from these axon-deprived optic nerves was 0.66 ± 0.3 pA/pF. Current expression was significantly lower ($p < 0.0001$) in astrocytes derived from enucleated optic nerves compared to astrocytes derived from intact optic nerve (21).

Barres et al. (22), using the "tissue print technique," noted the absence of sodium channels in astrocytes derived from optic nerve following nerve transection. Thus, it has been demonstrated in two laboratories that, following loss of axons in the optic nerve, $A2B5^-$ astrocytes exhibit patterns of sodium channel expression that are different from those seen in astrocytes derived from normal optic nerves. Earlier studies using saxitoxin (STX) binding in the optic nerve following enucleation *in Necturus* (25) or crush injury in the rabbit (26) demonstrated decreased saturable STX uptake compared to normal optic nerves. These observations are consistent with the patch-clamp data in suggesting that sodium channel expression in optic nerve astrocytes is down-regulated following axonal degeneration. The available results provide evidence for neuronal regulation of sodium channel expression in these astrocytes.

SODIUM CHANNEL EXPRESSION IS MODULATED BY ASTROCYTE–ASTROCYTE INTERACTIONS

A variety of influences appear to modulate ion channel expression in astrocytes. There is, for example, evidence suggesting effects of cAMP and neurotransmitters, as well as serum, on channel expression in cultured astrocytes (27,28). There is also evidence for differential effects of nerve growth factor, fibroblast growth factor, epidermal growth factor, and dexamethasone on sodium channel expression in PC12 cells *in vitro* (29).

Because astrocytes are coupled by gap junctions (30–32), which can mediate the diffusion of inorganic and small organic molecules between connected cells (33,34), we examined the relationship between sodium current expression and cell–cell coupling in astrocytes (13). In these studies, we examined astrocytes in primary cultures obtained from the CA1 and CA3 region of the neonatal rat hippocampus. In such cultures dye coupling, demonstrated with the fluorescent dye Lucifer yellow, appears as early as 24 hr after plating, at which time ~20% of all astrocytes that physically contacted neighboring cells showed dye coupling. The percentage of coupled cells in these cultures increases with time and peaks after 10 DIV, when ~50% of astrocytes show coupling (13).

Patch-clamp studies in these cultures reveal that only a subpopulation of astrocytes showed measurable sodium currents. At early times in culture (1 to 2 DIV), ~70% of astrocytes showed detectable sodium currents; at 10 to 20 DIV, however, only 30% of the cells examined showed sodium current expression. In order to determine whether there was a relationship between cell coupling and sodium channel expression, we obtained recordings from 39 astrocytes that exhibited dye coupling to adjacent cells and 87 astrocytes that did not reveal dye coupling. With the exception of two recordings, which were obtained on presumed glial precursor cells at 1 DIV, all coupled astrocytes lacked measurable inward currents. In contrast, 63% of astrocytes that were noncoupled exhibited sodium currents, with amplitudes of up to 5 nA (Fig. 8).

Since the failure to observe sodium currents in coupled astrocytes might, in theory, have been explained by insufficient

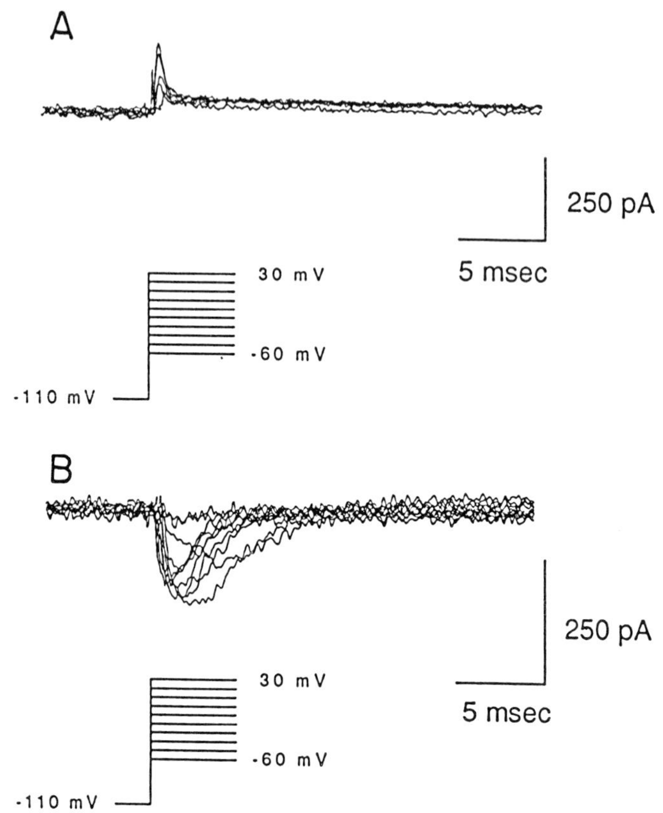

FIG. 8. Na^+ current expression is restricted to hippocampal astrocytes that lack coupling. Examples of Na^+ current recordings in a coupled (**A**) and a noncoupled (**B**) astrocyte were displayed from two cells recorded on the same coverslip after 13 DIV. (**A**) Depolarizing voltage steps were applied to the potentials indicated in **inset.** The cell under observation showed dye coupling to six adjacent cells. No inward currents were observed in response to depolarizing steps of up to 30 mV. Initial outward current transients are uncompensated capacity transients. (**B**) The same protocol of voltage steps as in **A** was applied to an astrocyte on the same coverslip that lacked dye coupling. Voltage steps to potentials more positive than −40 mV activated a transient inward Na^+ current (leakage currents subtracted). (Modified from Sontheimer et al., ref. 13.)

space clamp of the coupled cells, we acutely uncoupled cells by applying 10 μM octanol, which is known to reduce gap junctional permeability (35,36). We substantiated the loss of coupling by observing a significant increase in input resistance and an alteration in the time course of the response to a depolarizing voltage step from a double exponential to a single exponential. Our observation that sodium currents could not be observed in these acutely uncoupled cells supports the idea that sodium channel expression was restricted to noncoupled cells in these hippocampal astrocyte cultures (13).

The strong negative relationship between sodium current expression and coupling in hippocampal astrocytes suggests that there may be a functional relationship between these two events. It has been suggested that sodium channel expression may be modulated by electrical activity (37,38). Coupling of astrocytes would tend to clamp each cell close to the potential of nearby cells and might thus inhibit the expression of sodium channels. Alternatively, it should be recalled that sodium channel expression in cultured neurons, including PC12 cells, is modulated by pathways that involve cAMP-dependent kinase (39) and other second messengers (38). Thus, it is possible that sodium channel expression is suppressed or that channel activity is modulated by a diffusible intracellular signal that enters cells that have become part of the astrocytic syncytium.

ASTROCYTES ARE INTIMATELY ASSOCIATED WITH THE NODE OF RANVIER

Observations on myelinated fibers may provide a clue to the function of astrocytic sodium channels. A variety of lines of evidence, based on morphological, electrophysiological, and immunocytochemical studies, indicate that sodium channels are clustered in high density in the axon membrane at the node of Ranvier (40,41). Hildebrand (42,43) pointed out that astrocyte processes are intimately associated with the node of Ranvier. Observations in a number of mammalian (44–46) and inframammalian (47,48) myelinated tracts indicate that perinodal astrocyte processes will travel for many micrometers to contact the sodium-channel-rich axon membrane at the node of Ranvier. The proximity between these astrocyte processes and the nearby nodal axon membrane has led to the suggestion (3,49) that astrocytes may function as subsidiary sites for the synthesis of sodium channels, which are subsequently transferred to the axon membrane, where they supplement the synthesis of channels in the neuronal cell body. Although this hypothesis remains speculative, it is interesting

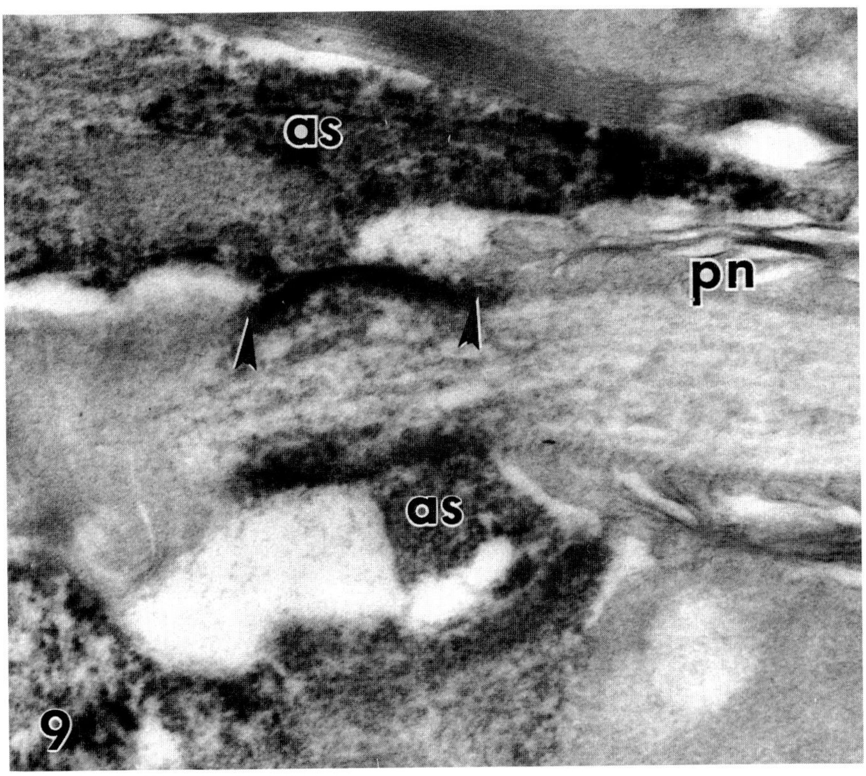

FIG. 9. Sodium channel immunostaining at node of Ranvier with antibody 7493. The axon membrane at the node of Ranvier (between *arrowheads*) exhibits intense sodium channel immunoreactivity, and there is some sodium channel immunoreactivity in the adjacent axoplasm. The axon membrane beneath the paranodal loops (pn) is not immunoreactive. Perinodal astrocyte processes (as) are densely immunostained following exposure to antibody 7493. The cytoplasm of the perinodal astrocyte exhibits sodium channel immunoreactivity. (Modified from Black et al., ref. 50.)

that, as noted below, perinodal astrocytes *in situ* express sodium channels.

Perinodal Astrocytes *in Situ* Express Sodium Channels

Although observations *in vitro* such as those described above demonstrate that sodium channels are present in cultured astrocytes, an important question concerns the degree to which sodium channel expression occurs in similar cells *in vivo*. We have used immunoultrastructural methods to study sodium channel expression in astrocytes *in situ* (50,51). In these studies, we examined astrocytes in rat optic nerve *in situ* after perfusion fixation with 4% paraformaldehyde/0.01% glutaraldehyde. For immunoelectron microscopic localization of sodium channels, tissue was incubated in polyclonal antibody 7493, biotinylated secondary antibody, avidin–horseradish peroxidase complex, and diaminobenzidine hydrogen peroxide.

The immunoultrastructural studies demonstrated that sodium channels are present in astrocytes *in situ* in rat optic nerve. As shown in Fig. 9, sodium channel immunoreactivity is present in the axon membrane at the node of Ranvier, as expected from the high density of sodium channels in this part of the axon membrane. Adjacent paranodal and internodal regions of the axon membrane, which are known to contain a much lower density of sodium channels than the nodal membrane (41), did not display immunoreactivity with antibody 7493. Similarly, sodium channel immunoreactivity was not present in the plasma membrane of oligodendrocytes. Notably, perinodal astrocyte processes *in situ* displayed marked sodium channel immunoreactivity. In most cases sodium channel immunostaining of perinodal astrocytes was distributed through the perinodal astrocyte cytoplasm, and cytoplasmic immunostaining was usually more prominent than staining of the plasma membrane. This may reflect the presence in these cells of a cytoplasmic pool of sodium channels or their precursors, as has been demonstrated in Schwann cells (19).

Astrocytes Contact Sodium Channel-Rich Regions of Demyelinated Axons

Conduction block accounts for much of the clinical deficit in demyelinating diseases such as multiple sclerosis (52) and is largely a result of the exposure of (formerly internodal) regions of the axon membrane with low sodium channel density after injury to the insulating myelin sheath (53). The most common human model of demyelination, multiple sclerosis, is characterized by remissions in which there is functional recovery despite a paucity of remyelination within the brain and spinal cord. Several studies have demonstrated that demyelinated axons can, under some circumstances, recover the capability to conduct action potentials (54,55), and a variety of lines of evidence suggest that demyelinated axon membrane can develop, at least in specialized regions, a sodium channel density that is higher than normal for the internode (56–59).

Figure 10 is an electron micrograph that shows a chronically demyelinated axon in the dorsal columns of rat that had been injected 1 month previously with ethidium bromide, followed by irradiation (56). It shows a demyelinated axon that exhibits a sharply demarcated zone of sodium channel immunoreactivity. The zone of sodium channel immunostaining is coincident with the footprint of a glial process, but there is no sodium channel immunoreactivity at the site where the axon is contacted by a second glial process or where it is not contacted by glial cells. Electrophysiological recordings within the ethidium bromide/irradiation lesion demonstrated that at least some axons were able to conduct action potentials within the lesion, supporting the conclusion that there is a reorganization of sodium channels within the axon membrane of these chronically demyelinated axons (56). Several previous studies have demonstrated "islands" of node-like membrane (presumably with a high sodium channel density) within axons that lack myelin, in specific association with glial processes. Interestingly, at these sites, the axon is

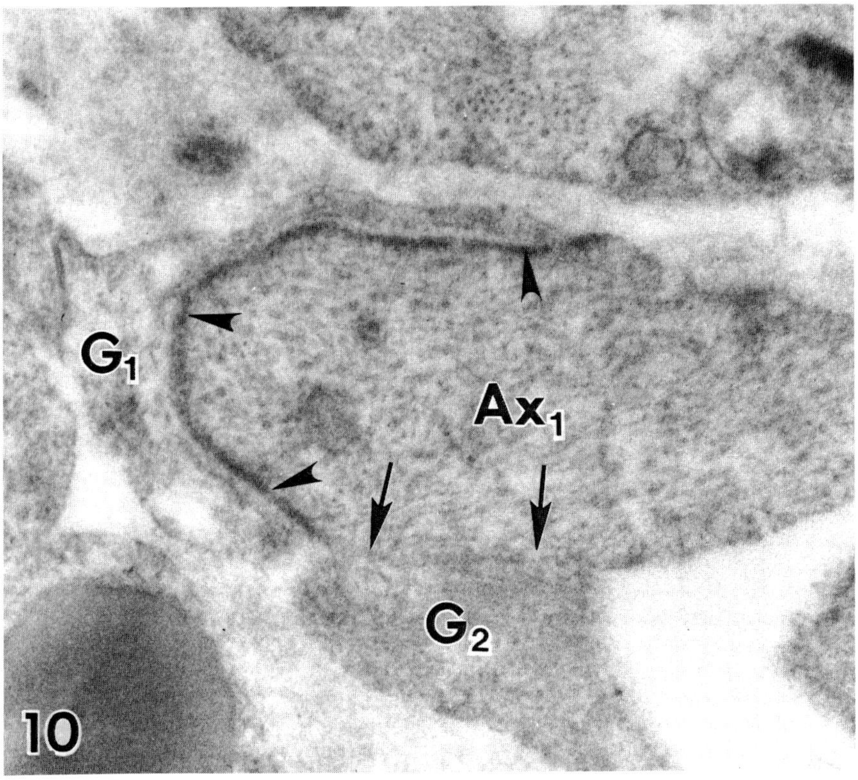

FIG. 10. Sodium channels cluster in chronically demyelinated axons at sites of glial contact. This electron micrograph shows sodium channel immunostaining with antibody 7493 of dorsal column axon 30 days after ethidium bromide/irradiation-induced demyelination. A demyelinated axon (Ax_1) near the periphery of the lesion exhibits a focal zone of sodium channel immunostaining (*arrowheads*) where it is abutted by one glial process (G_1); in contrast, the axolemma (*arrows*) abutted by a second glial process (G_2) and bare axolemma do not display sodium channel immunostaining. (Modified from Black et al., ref. 56.)

contacted by astrocyte processes. For example, some unmyelinated (60,61), dysmyelinated (62–67), and glial-cell-deprived (68) axons exhibit well-delineated regions of node-like axon membrane differentiation at sites of abutment by astrocytes or Schwann cell processes.

Although the role of glial cells in reorganization of the demyelinated axon membrane remains incompletely understood, the differentiation of sodium-channel-rich axon membrane regions at sites of astrocyte contact suggests that glial cells may participate actively in this membrane reorganization. One possibility is that, as suggested by Ritchie and his colleagues (3,49), astrocytes function as sites for the synthesis of sodium channels that are then transferred to the axon. Alternatively, it is possible that astrocytes elaborate extracellular matrix molecules that participate in the targeting or anchoring of sodium channels at specific sites along the axon membrane. A third possibility is that astrocytic contact alters the axon membrane so that sodium channel precursors in the axoplasm are inserted in the axon membrane at sites of astrocyte contact.

COMMENTS AND PERSPECTIVES

Abundant evidence, based on electrophysiological and immunocytochemical studies *in vitro* and on immunocytochemical investigations *in situ*, indicates that astrocytes express voltage-sensitive sodium channels. Notably, some subclasses of astrocytes express sodium channels with properties similar to those of neurons. Channel expression in astrocytes appears to be dynamic in that it changes over time, and it appears to be modulated by both neuronal and glial influences. Given the myriad of soluble factors and cell-surface-associated molecules produced by neurons and glial cells, it would not be surprising to see a complex network of interactions that regulate, in highly specific ways, channel expression in astrocytes. The combinatorial milieu of factors that might influence channel expression, together with differential responsiveness to these factors, could account for the diversity of patterns of sodium channel expression seen in even the limited number of CNS regions (optic nerve, hippocampus, spinal cord) that have been examined in our laboratory thus far.

One theme that is emerging from our studies is that astrocytes constitute a highly heterogeneous cell population. In this regard, it is not unlikely that many subclasses of astrocytes with distinct physiological as well as morphological properties may soon be delineated. In at least some CNS regions such as the optic nerve, the different types of astrocytes display distinct patterns of sodium channel expression and express sodium currents with different gating and kinetic properties. An important question concerns the degree to which these physiological differences in astrocytes represent preprogrammed phenotypic variation or reflect differential regional influences on a single class of progenitor cells.

The demonstration of several types of sodium currents in astrocytes does not answer the question of whether several distinct sodium channel mRNAs, coding for different protein sequences, are present. Alternatively, posttranslational modification of a single type of channel protein molecule could account for the presence of several types of sodium current in astrocytes. It is also possible that physiological properties of channels are modulated by the lipid membrane microenvironment, regulation of channels through their intracellular or extracellular environment, and/or association with other membrane proteins. Molecular biological studies using cDNA or oligonucleotide probes directed against various isoforms of mammalian sodium channels should clarify this issue. The sequential expression of neuronal- and then glial-type sodium currents in hippocampal astrocytes demonstrates that at least some astrocytes are pluripotential in terms of channel expression. In this regard, astrocytes may provide a useful model system in which it is possible to examine the factors that regulate expression of ion currents.

Although the role of sodium channels in cellular function of astrocytes is still incompletely understood, our work and that of others show that channel expression changes in some astrocytes in response to loss of neuronal influences. These findings suggest the possibility that astrocyte channel expression changes in response to injury of nearby neurons or axons *in vivo*. If such changes occur following CNS injury, we are led to speculate that, in addition to hypertrophy and hyperplasia, the *function* of astrocytes may change in response to CNS injury. Moreover, the close association between astrocytes and the sodium-channel-rich membrane at the node of Ranvier, together with the development of sodium-channel-enriched regions along demyelinated axons at sites of astrocyte contact, suggests that the astrocyte may participate in reorganization of the axon membrane following injury in a manner that leads to restoration of action potential conduction. This hypothesis is now under study in several laboratories. It will be interesting, in this regard, to determine whether the altered expression of channels contributes to glial scarring or, alternatively, to a more positive role of astrocytes in neural plasticity and/or functional recovery after injury to the brain and spinal cord.

ACKNOWLEDGMENTS

Work in the authors' laboratories has been supported in part by grants from the National Institutes of Health and the National Multiple Sclerosis Society and by the Medical Research Service, U.S. Department of Veterans Affairs. H. Sontheimer was supported in part by a Spinal Cord Research Fellowship from the Eastern Paralyzed Veterans Association and in part by a grant from the Allen Charitable Trust, and J. A. Black was supported in part by grants from the Daniel Heumann Fund and the Folger Foundation.

REFERENCES

1. Chiu SY, Shrager P, Ritchie JM. Neuronal-type Na^+- and K^+-channels in rabbit cultured Schwann cells. *Nature* 1984;311:156–157.
2. Shrager P, Chiu SY, Ritchie JM. Voltage-dependent sodium and potassium channels in mammalian cultured Schwann cells. *Proc Natl Acad Sci USA* 1985;82:948–952.
3. Bevan S, Chiu SY, Gray PTA, Ritchie JM. The presence of voltage-gated sodium, potassium and chloride channels in rat cultured astrocytes. *Proc R Soc Lond B* 1985;225:229–313.
4. Nowak L, Ascher P, Berwald-Netter Y. Ionic channels in mouse astrocytes in culture. *J Neurosci* 1987;7:101–109.
5. Barres BA, Chun LLY, Corey DP. Glial and neuronal forms of the sodium channel: characteristics and cell-type distribution. *Neuron* 1989;2:1375–1388.
6. Sontheimer H, Minturn JE, Black JA, Ransom BR, Waxman SG. Two types of Na^+-currents in cultured rat optic nerve astrocytes: changes with time in culture and with age of culture derivation. *J Neurosci Res* 1991;30:275–287.
7. Sontheimer H, Trotter J, Schachner M, Kettenmann H. Channel expression correlates with differentiation stage during development of oligodendrocytes from their precursor cells in culture. *Neuron* 1989;2:1135–1145.
8. Barres BA, Koroshetz WJ, Swartz KJ, Chun LLY, Corey DP. Ion channel expression by white matter glia: The O-2A glial progenitor cell. *Neuron* 1990;4:507–524.
9. Elmer LW, Black JA, Waxman SG, Angelides KJ. The voltage-dependent sodium channel in mammalian CNS and PNS: antibody characterization and immunocytochemical localization. *Brain Res* 1990;532:222–231.
10. Raff MC, Abney ER, Cohen J, Lindsay R, Noble M. Two types of astrocytes in cultures of developing rat white matter: differences in morphology, surface gangliosides, and growth characteristics. *J Neurosci* 1983;3:1289–1300.
11. Minturn JE, Black JA, Angelides KJ, Waxman SG. Sodium channel expression detected with antibody 7493 in $A2B5^+$ and $A2B5^-$ astrocytes from rat optic nerve *in vitro*. *Glia* 1990;3:358–368.
12. Sontheimer H, Ransom BR, Cornell-Bell AH, Black JA, Waxman SG. Na^+-current expression in rat hippocampal astrocytes *in vitro*: alterations during development. *J Neurophysiol* 1991;65:3–19.
13. Sontheimer H, Waxman SG, Ransom BR. Relationship between Na^+-current expression and cell–cell coupling in astrocytes cultured from rat hippocampus. *J Neurophysiol* 1991;65:989–1002.
14. Howe JR, Ritchie JM. Sodium currents in Schwann cells from myelinated and nonmyelinated nerves of neonatal and adult rabbits. *J Physiol* 1990; 425:169–210.
15. Sontheimer H, Black JA, Ransom BR, Waxman SG. Ion channels in spinal cord astrocytes *in vitro*: I. Transient expression of high levels of Na^+ and K^+ channels. *J Neurophysiol* (in press).
16. Ransom BR, Goldring S. Ionic determinants of membrane potential of cells presumed to be glia in cerebral cortex of cat. *J Neurophysiol* 1973; 5:855–868.
17. Ransom BR. Vertebrate glial subtypes, lineage and morphology. *Ann NY Acad Sci* 1991;633:19–26.
18. MacDermott AB, Westbrook GL. Early development of voltage-dependent sodium currents in cultured mouse spinal cord neurons. *Dev Biol* 1986;113:317–326.
19. Ritchie JM, Black JA, Waxman SG, Angelides KJ. Sodium channels in the cytoplasm of Schwann cells. *Proc Natl Acad Sci USA* 1990;87:9290–9294.
20. Ritchie JM. Sodium-channel turnover in rabbit cultured Schwann cells. *Proc R Soc Lond [Biol]* 1988;233:423–430.
21. Minturn JE, Sontheimer H, Black JA, Ransom BR, Waxman SG. Sodium channel expression in optic nerve astrocytes chronically deprived of axonal contact. *Glia [in press]*.
22. Barres BA, Koroshetz WJ, Chun LLY, Corey DP. Ion channel expression by white matter glia: The type-1 astrocyte. *Neuron* 1990;5:527–544.
23. David S, Miller RH, Patel R, Raff MC. Effects of neonatal transection on glial cell development in the rat optic nerve: evidence that the oligodendrocyte-type 2 astrocyte cell lineage depends on axons for its survival. *J Neurocytol* 1984;13:961–974.
24. Ransom BR, Yamate CL. The rat optic nerve following enucleation: pure preparation of mammalian glia. *Soc Neurosci Abstr* 1984;10:949.
25. Tang CM, Strichartz GR, Orkand RK. Sodium channels in axons and glial cells of the optic nerve of *Necturus maculosa*. *J Gen Physiol* 1979;74: 629–642.
26. Pellegrino RG, Ritchie JM. Sodium channels in the axolemma of normal and degenerating rabbit optic nerve. *Proc R Soc Lond [Biol]* 1984;222:155–160.
27. Barres BA, Chun LLY, Corey DP. Calcium current in cortical astrocytes: Induction by cAMP and neurotransmitters and permissive effect of serum factors. *J Neurosci* 1989;9:3169–3175.
28. Yarowsky PJ, Krueger BK. Development of saxitoxin-sensitive and insensitive sodium channels in

cultured neonatal rat astrocytes. *J Neurosci* 1989;9:1055–1061.
29. Pollock JD, Krempin M, Rudy B. Differential effects of NGF, FGF, EGFD, cAMP, and dexamethasone on neurite outgrowth and sodium channel expression in PC12 cells. *J Neurosci* 1990;10: 2626–2637.
30. Kettenmann H, Orkand RK, Schachner M. Coupling among identified cells in mammalian nervous system cultures. *J Neurosci* 1983;3:506–516.
31. Kettenmann H, Ransom BR. Electrical coupling between astrocytes and between oligodendrocytes studied in mammalian cell culture. *Glia* 1988;1:64–73.
32. Ransom BR, Kettenmann H. Electrical coupling without dye coupling between mammalian astrocytes and oligodendrocytes in cell culture. *Glia* 1990;3:258–266.
33. Bennett MVL. Physiology of electrotonic junctions. *Ann NY Acad Sci* 1966;137:509–539.
34. Loewenstein WR. Junctional intercellular communication: the cell-to-cell membrane channel. *Physiol Rev* 1981;61:829–913.
35. Somogyi R, Kolb HA. Cell-to-cell channel conductance during loss of gap junctional coupling in pairs of pancreatic acinar and Chinese hamster ovary cells. *Eur J Physiol* 1988;412:54–65.
36. Spray DC, Saez JC, Brosius D, Bennett MV, Hertzberg EL. Isolated liver gap junctions: gating of transjunctional currents is similar to that in intact pairs of rat hepatocytes. *Proc Natl Acad Sci USA* 1986;83:5494–5497.
37. Sherman SJ, Catterall WA. Electrical activity and cytosolic calcium regulate levels of tetrodotoxin-sensitive sodium channels in rat muscle cells. *Proc Natl Acad Sci USA* 1984;81:262–266.
38. Sherman SJ, Chrivia J, Catterall WA. Cyclic adenosine 3′5′-monophosphate and cytosolic calcium exert opposing effects on biosynthesis of tetrodotoxin-sensitive sodium channels in rat muscle cells. *J Neurosci* 1985;5:1570–1578.
39. Kalman D, Wong B, Horvai EA, Cline MJ, O'Lague PH. Nerve growth factor acts through cAMP-dependent kinase to increase the number of sodium channels in PC12 cells. *Neuron* 1990;2:355–366.
40. Black JA, Kocsis JD, Waxman SG. Ion channel organization of the myelinated fiber. *Trends Neurosci* 1990;13:48–54.
41. Waxman SG, Ritchie JM. Organization of ion channels in the myelinated nerve fiber. *Science* 1985;228:1502–1507.
42. Hildebrand C. Ultrastructural and light-microscopic studies of the developing feline spinal cord white matter. I. The nodes of Ranvier. *Acta Physiol Scand* [*Suppl*] 1971;364:81–101.
43. Hildebrand C. Ultrastructural and light-microscopic studies of the nodal region in large myelinated fibres of the adult feline spinal cord white matter. *Acta Physiol Scand* [*Suppl*] 1971;364:43–71.
44. Hildebrand C, Waxman SG. Postnatal differentiation of rat optic nerve fibers: Electron microscopic observations on the development of nodes of Ranvier and axoglial relations. *J Comp Neurol* 1984;224:25–37.
45. Raine CS. On the association between perinodal astrocyte processes and the node of Ranvier in the CNS. *J Neurocytol* 1984;13:21–27.
46. Waxman SG, Black JA. Freeze–fracture ultrastructure of the perinodal astrocyte and associated glial junctions. *Brain Res* 1984;308:77–87.
47. Bodega G, Suarez J, Fernandez B. Fine structured relationships between astrocytes and the node of Ranvier in the amphibian and reptile spinal cord. *Neurosci Lett* 1987;80:7–10.
48. Sims TJ, Gilmore SA, Waxman SG. Radial glia give rise to perinodal processes. *Brain Res* 1991; 549:25–36.
49. Gray PT, Ritchie JM. Ion channels in Schwann and glial cells. *Trends Neurosci* 1985;8:411–415.
50. Black JA, Friedman B, Waxman SG, Elmer LW, Angelides KJ. Immuno-ultrastructural localization of sodium channels at nodes of Ranvier and perinodal astrocytes in rat optic nerve. *Proc R Soc Lond* [*Biol*] 1989;238:38–57.
51. Black JA, Waxman SG, Friedman B, Elmer LW, Angelides KJ. Sodium channels in astrocytes of rat optic nerve in situ: immunoelectron microscopic studies. *Glia* 1989;2:353–369.
52. Waxman SG. Clinicopathological correlations in multiple sclerosis and related diseases. In: Waxman SG, Ritchie JM, eds. *Demyelinating disease: basic and clinical electrophysiology,* New York: Raven Press; 1981:169–182.
53. Waxman SG. Conduction in myelinated, unmyelinated, and demyelinated fibers. *Arch Neurol* 1977;34:585–590.
54. Bostock H, Sears TA. The internodal axon membrane: electrical excitability and continuous conduction in segmental demyelination. *J Physiol* 1978;280:273–301.
55. Waxman SG, Brill MH. Conduction through demyelinated plaques in multiple sclerosis: computer simulations of facilitation by short internodes. *J Neurol Neurosurg Psychiatry* 1978;41:408–417.
56. Black JA, Felts P, Smith KJ, Kocsis JD, Waxman SG. Distribution of sodium channels in chronically demyelinated spinal cord axons: Immuno-ultrastructural localization and electrophysiological observations. *Brain Res* 1991;544:59–70.
57. England JD, Gamboni F, Levinson SR, Finger TE. Changed distribution of sodium channels along demyelinated axons. *Proc Natl Acad Sci USA* 1990;87:6777–6786.
58. Foster RE, Whalen CC, Waxman SG. Reorganization of the axonal membrane of demyelinated nerve fibers: morphological evidence. *Science* 1980; 210:661–663.
59. Smith KJ, Bostock H, Hall SM. Saltatory conduction precedes remyelination in axons demyelinated with lysophosphatidyl choline. *J Neurol Sci* 1982;54:13–31.
60. Black JA, Waxman SG, Hildebrand C. Membrane specialization and axo-glial association in the rat retinal nerve fibre layer: freeze–fracture observations. *J Neurocytol* 1984;13:417–430.
61. Hildebrand C, Waxman SG. Regional node-like membrane specializations in nonmyelinated axons of rat retinal nerve fiber layer. *Brain Res* 1983;258:23–32.

62. Bray GM, Cullen MJ, Aguayo AJ, Rasminsky M. Node-like areas of intramembranous particles in the unensheathed axons of dystrophic mice. *Neurosci Lett* 1979;13:203–208.
63. Ellisman M. Molecular specializations of the axon membrane at the node of Ranvier are not dependent upon myelination. *J Neurocytol* 1979;8:719–735.
64. Rosenbluth J. Aberrant axon–Schwann cell junctions in dystrophic mouse nerves. *J Neurocytol* 1979;8:655–672.
65. Rosenbluth J. Intramembranous particle patches in myelin-deficient rat mutant. *Neurosci Lett* 1985; 62:19–24.
66. Rosenbluth J, Blakemore WF. Structural specializations in cat of chronically demyelinated spinal cord axons as seen in freeze–fracture replicas. *Neurosci Lett* 1984;48:171–177.
67. Waxman SG, Black JA, Duncan ID, Ransom BR. Macromolecular structure of axon membrane and action potential conduction in myelin deficient and myelin deficient heterozygote rat optic nerves. *J Neurocytol* 1990;19:11–27.
68. Black JA, Sims TJ, Waxman SG, Gilmore SA. Membrane ultrastructure of developing axons in glial cell deficient rat spinal cord. *J Neurocytol* 1985;14:79–104.

Advances in Neurology, Vol. 59, edited by Fredrick J. Seil. Raven Press, Ltd., New York © 1993.

13

Spinal Cord Injury

Physiology and Transplantation

W. Z. Rymer

Rehabilitation Institute of Chicago and Departments of Physical Medicine and Rehabilitation, Physiology, and Biomedical Engineering, Northwestern University, and Veterans Administration Medical Center, Lakeside, Chicago, Illinois 60611

Several of the chapters in this volume relating to spinal cord injury explore factors guiding regeneration and/or recovery of function in damaged axons in the mammalian spinal cord. Although this approach is enormously important and represents the ultimate solution to recovery from human spinal cord injury, there are important interim lessons to be gleaned from studies of residual function in subjects with either partial or complete spinal cord injury. This information is applicable to our understanding of the control mechanisms operating in the normal intact cord and of the clinical movement disturbances that arise in incomplete spinal cord injury. These disturbances are manifested as several types of functional impairment, such as weakness of voluntary movement, spasticity, and abnormal muscular coordination.

In this chapter I deal briefly with several aspects of altered motor function in incomplete spinal cord injury that may help to explain the weakness of voluntary movement that is a major symptom in subjects with incomplete spinal cord injury. I address changes in the so-called "intrinsic" properties of spinal motoneurons as well as alterations in the patterns of recruitment and rate modulation in the neurons of the motoneuron pool. In addition, I briefly review abnormalities in segmental reflex responses that arise in clinical spinal cord injury. These various abnormalities also underlie the major clinical disturbances of motor function in spinal cord injury, such as spasticity and disturbed motor coordination, but these are not addressed here. For more detailed review of spasticity issues, see Katz and Rymer (1).

MECHANISMS OF MUSCULAR WEAKNESS IN SPINAL CORD INJURY

There are several potential mechanisms by which lesions of the neuraxis may give rise to weakness of voluntary movement. First, the traditional view, enunciated by Hughlings Jackson (2), is that weakness for voluntary movement develops because there is a loss of descending excitatory input to the spinal cord from major pathways such as the corticospinal and rubrospinal systems. This mechanism of weakness is clearly important, but it may not be the only one, and in some circumstances, it may not even be the most significant (see further below). Furthermore, from a practical standpoint, the loss of a major source of excitatory synaptic drive, such as that originating in descending corticospinal and rubrospinal systems, cannot be readily replaced by other means in the foreseeable future, and there are no methods currently available by which the major descending pathways can be helped to reestablish their spinal synaptic connections. It follows that other types of disturbances in motor output, if present, may be more amenable to therapeutic intervention.

For example, in addition to the aforementioned loss of descending excitatory input, two other types of physiological disturbances may contribute to muscular weakness. First, there is evidence that the activation of the motoneuron pool may be severely disorganized, displaying severe abnormalities of electromyographic (EMG) output, motoneuron rate, and recruitment (3–5). Second, there will often be associated disorganization of spatial and temporal features of muscle activation, producing severe incoordination of voluntary movement (6). If such alternative mechanisms of muscular weakness turn out to be significant, they may in fact be more amenable to therapeutic intervention than those attributable to loss of descending excitatory input.

I begin by providing evidence for disorganization of the output of the motoneuron pool and then address potential mechanisms for the observed phenomena.

ABNORMALITIES OF FORCE–EMG RELATIONS

Animal Models

A number of studies of spinal-lesioned animals have reported severe disruptions in the stretch reflex response coupled with marked alterations in the relationship between EMG activity and the resulting force (3–5). For example, in the typical decerebrated cat preparation, stretch of the soleus muscle will result in a significant increase in reflex muscle force, which increases with increasing amplitude and/or velocity of stretch. This is the well-known tonic stretch reflex. If dorsolateral white matter of the cord is then lesioned surgically, or if the dorsolateral spinal quadrants are cooled, there is a swift transformation from stretch-induced excitation (i.e., the tonic stretch reflex) to stretch-induced inhibition (3,7). This is the so-called "clasp-knife reflex."

We now know that this reflex is not mediated by the classical encapsulated receptors (spindles and tendon organs) but appears to be mediated by the discharge of small-caliber afferents (group III and IV), which arise from free nerve endings in muscle (3,8,9). Many of these free nerve ending mechanoreceptors are excited by stretch (albeit weakly), by muscle contraction (sometimes strongly), and by surface manipulation of the muscle aponeuroses and tendons (very strongly) (9). The role of these small-caliber afferents and their reflex connections are addressed further below. However, it is worth noting that they may also mediate the disruption of motor output in other ways, perhaps by altering the patterns of interneuronal activity in the spinal cord.

For example, the same spinal-lesioned cat preparation that manifests stretch-induced inhibition of muscle (described in the previous paragraph) usually displays a substantial alteration in the relationship between mean rectified EMG levels and the associated force change (3,4). Within 15 to 20 min of a spinal cord dorsal hemisection (placed usually at the midthoracic level), there is a striking increase in the amount of EMG electrical activity produced, unaccompanied by any comparable force increase. In addition, there is often a "gritty" irregular tremor accompanied by a substantial increase in the variance (or total power) of both the EMG and force traces (see below) (4). This change in the force–EMG relationship is visible over a wide range of forces, so that there is typically an increase in the slope of the force–EMG relationship, which may reach values three to four times greater than is seen in the normal (unlesioned) cord. These changes develop so quickly that there is little likelihood of altered neuromuscular transmission or of change in muscle mechanical properties. It appears most likely that the changes in the force–EMG relationship result from severe reductions in minimum firing rate of spinal motoneurons, coupled with alterations in the normal recruitment rank order, and perhaps with increased synchrony of neuronal discharge (5). These abnormalities may arise from changes in the intrinsic properties of motoneurons or from altered patterns of synaptic input, driven by changes in interneuronal responsiveness.

As documented further below, each of these functional disturbances appears to play some role in mediating muscular weakness. However, it would be helpful to establish first whether these animal models are clinically relevant and whether similar abnormalities arise in human subjects after either spinal or supraspinal lesions.

Human Subjects

Although the data are relatively scarce, it appears likely that there are also substantial disturbances in motor output evident in patients with either spinal or supraspinal injury. In spastic hemiplegia induced by stroke, for example, Tang and Rymer (10) reported a substantial change in force–EMG relationships that was consistent with a disorganization of motoneuron pool output. Similarly, in human spinal cord injury, Latash (11,12) reported significant changes in EMG spectra, consistent with abnormalities of motoneuron activation. Comparisons of force and EMG power spectral density plots in human limbs of spinal-cord-injured subjects (11,12) with normal controls also provide evidence for abnormalities of motoneuron activation, but we do not yet know how they develop, and it is unclear whether abnormalities of rate, recruitment, or increased synchrony predominate.

ABNORMALITIES OF MOTONEURON ACTIVATION IN SPINAL CORD INJURY

Under normal conditions, there is a relatively precise rank order for recruitment of spinal motoneurons within a motoneuron pool, as excitatory drive is increased. This order of recruitment is correlated with both the size of the motoneuron and the tetanic force that is produced by the associated muscle unit. There is also an orderly, if somewhat more complex, relationship between the rank order of motoneuron recruitment and the rate of discharge of a motoneuron, so that high-threshold motoneurons characteristically display steeper rate–force relationships than do low-threshold motoneurons.

Many of these features of motoneuron pool behavior appear to be seriously disrupted in incomplete spinal cord injury, especially when dorsolateral quadrant descending spinal pathways are interrupted (3–5). Under these conditions, both motoneuron recruitment rank order and discharge rates are seriously disordered. In animal models of spinal cord injury, motoneuron discharge rate at recruitment is characteristically much lower than in normal muscles, and recruitment is compressed and the order sometimes even reversed, so that normally high-threshold units may be activated at lower stimulus intensities than low-threshold units (5). In addition, because the force generated by each motor unit is ineffectual, the total numbers of motor units activated is greatly increased for any level of force, producing substantial alterations in force–EMG relationships and abnormal force and EMG power spectra (4). Although we do not know whether these changes are present in chronic spinal cord injury in man, preliminary observations (see above and refs. 11,12) suggest that such changes in force–EMG spectra are likely.

FUNCTIONAL AND THERAPEUTIC IMPLICATIONS

If motor unit activation is inefficient, then many more motor units need to be activated in order to reach a given force level. This means that for many voluntary activities, high-threshold and potentially more readily fatigable units are activated prematurely and at much lower forces, increasing the likelihood that the muscle will be unable to sustain the commanded force, because the subject will experience a greater sense of effort and premature fatigue.

Although most of our knowledge on incomplete spinal cord injury is derived from animal models, there is increasing evidence that similar abnormalities of motor unit recruitment and rate modulation appear in supraspinal and spinal disorders in man.

INTRINSIC MOTONEURON PROPERTIES

Our views of the intrinsic properties of motoneurons have changed quite radically in recent years. Until recently, our conceptual model of the spinal motoneuron was relatively simple. The motoneuron was seen as incorporating classic Hodgkin–Huxley sodium and potassium voltage-gated conductances together with transmitter-evoked conductance changes generating classical excitatory and inhibitory postsynaptic potentials. The voltages induced by these synaptic effects were assumed to be summed passively and to give rise to action potential formation originating in the initial segment of the neuron. Many of these conductances were treated in essentially the same way as proposed by Eccles and colleagues working in Canberra in the 1950s and 1960s.

We now know that this view of the motoneuron is incomplete and even incorrect, at least partly because spinal motoneurons have been studied in barbiturate-anesthetized preparations. Under the latter conditions, many descending pathways and interneuronal systems are suppressed, and their transmitter and modulator actions are not manifested. Indeed, there is now substantial evidence that in unanesthetized preparations, motoneurons display a much broader range of conductances, including voltage and calcium activated channels, many of which are sensitive to ambient neuromodulators such as the monoamines (13). In effect, motoneurons are now seen to display many of the conductances that have already been described in other mammalian neurons such as those of cortex, cerebellum, and brainstem.

One neuromodulator that may prove to be particularly important in motor behavior is serotonin, which is released in the cord by fibers descending from nuclei in the raphe system in the brainstem. Hultborn and colleagues (14,15) have shown that in the presence of serotonin, a transient depolarizing current (such as might be induced by glutamate exposure) can give rise to a sustained voltage change or "plateau potential," which may last seconds or minutes and induce sustained and rapid neuronal discharge. This plateau potential can be "reset" either by an inhibitory synaptic input or simply by injecting a hyperpolarizing current. Although the mechanisms generating these plateau potentials have not been fully examined in mammalian preparations, similar response patterns in reptilian spinal motoneurons have been attributed to calcium currents and/or to their effects on calcium-sensitive potassium conductances.

FUNCTIONAL IMPLICATIONS OF MOTONEURON PLATEAU POTENTIALS

If spinal cord injury interrupts descending serotonergic input to spinal segments, then motoneuron plateau potentials will be substantially diminished or even abolished, altering the relationship between excitatory synaptic input and motoneuron discharge, so there is less discharge elicited for a given excitation. This amounts to a form of gain reduction in the input/output properties of the motoneuron and may well contribute to muscular weakness. We do not know, however, whether plateau potentials are expressed in all motoneurons or whether they are reserved for high levels of motor output that associated with strong synaptic drive. Regardless of the operating range of the serotonin effects, it is clear that loss of the serotonergic input may alter motoneuronal input/output relations in an adverse manner.

ABNORMAL REFLEX FUNCTION

There are also profound disturbances in spinal reflex function in both complete and incomplete injury. These disturbances range from flexor spasms of limb musculature to more subtle disturbances of reflex function, such as the Babinski and other cutaneous reflexes. We do not fully understand the origins of such altered flexor reflexes, but presumably they depend at least partly on the actions of spinal segmental interneurons that have been released from descending control by the spinal lesion. These altered interneuronal discharge patterns may also contribute to the abnormal patterns of motoneuron activation.

For example, it is now well known that dorsolateral white matter lesions in the spinal cord of the cat will induce a significant change in reflex patterns in which stretch-induced excitation is converted to stretch-induced inhibition or a "clasp-knife reflex" (see refs. 3, 7, 8). We now know that this stretch-induced inhibition is an outcome of the actions of fine-caliber mechanoreceptor afferents, which begin in free nerve endings in muscle. There does not seem to be any change in the pattern of group III and IV afferent discharge following the spinal lesion, so that it appears likely that the inhibitory effects are mediated by a change in interneuronal responsiveness, especially for interneurons connecting with motoneurons innervating extensor muscles. When such extensor muscles are stretched, the inhibition arises as muscle is stretched to near-maximum length, and it is exacerbated by increasing initial tension. These response patterns conform with the patterns of responsiveness of group III and some group IV mechanoreceptors. In addition, this extensor inhibition is accompanied by strong concurrent excitation of flexors, so that the net effect of stretching an extensor muscle is a powerful flexion response (8). This effect is manifested so readily in the spinal-lesioned preparation that it is tempting to speculate that many of the features of spinal spasticity in man are related to the actions of a similar class of afferents, together with changes in the responses of inhibitory interneurons and their reciprocally activated interneurons.

The actions of many spinal interneurons, especially those in lamina I and laminae V, VI, and VII of spinal cord dorsal gray matter, are very strongly influenced by discharge of free nerve afferents. Many of these stain strongly for substance P in their terminals. Although substance P may not be the primary transmitter released, it may still be possible to influence the frequency and/or severity of flexor spasms, and perhaps of spasticity of flexor muscles, by reducing afferent inflow to the cord from this class of afferents. There are a number of agents, such as capsaicin analogs, that appear capable of depleting terminals of such group III and IV afferents, and they may be well worth pursuing for their therapeutic value.

SUMMARY AND CLINICAL IMPLICATIONS

It is now clear that the spinal cord has extensive computational power, as evidenced by the capacity to adaptively modify short-latency reflexes, to emit patterned goal-directed motor output, and to induce locomotion. These various features may prove to be important in the restoration of function in the spinal-lesioned human subject in the future. In the interim, as the changes in muscle responsiveness after spinal cord injury are increasingly understood, it is evident that changes in segmental reflex patterns are common and may give rise to abnormal performance, which impairs motor activity of the human subject. If these alterations in segmental behavior are mediated by neuromodulators that are released from descending pathways in a continuous or slowly changing manner, then we may be able to improve clinical performance by substituting for these agents by intrathecal or parenteral administration.

ACKNOWLEDGMENTS

Preparation of this chapter was supported by VA merit review and by NIH grants NS 28076 and NS 30295.

REFERENCES

1. Katz R, Rymer WZ. Spastic hypertonia: mechanisms and measurement. *Arch Phys Med Rehab* 1989;70:144–155.
2. Jackson JH. In: Taylor J, ed. *Selected writings of John Hughlings Jackson,* Vol II. London: Hodder and Stoughton, 1932.
3. Rymer WZ, Houk JC, Crago PE. Mechanisms of the clasp-knife reflex studied in an animal model. *Exp Brain Res* 1979;37:93–113.
4. Blaschak MJ, Powers RK, Rymer WZ. Disturbances of motor output in a cat hindlimb muscle following acute dorsal hemisection of the spinal cord. *Exp Brain Res* 1988;71:377–387.
5. Powers RK, Rymer WZ. The effects of acute dorsal spinal hemisection on motoneuron discharge in the medial gastrocnemius of the decerebrate cat. *J Neurophysiol* 1988;59:1540–1556.
6. Bourbonnais D, Vanden Noven S, Carey K, Rymer WZ. Abnormal spatial patterns of elbow muscle activation in hemiparetic human subjects. *Brain* 1989;112:85–102.
7. Burke D, Knowles L, Andrews C, Ashby P. Spasticity, decerebrate rigidity and the clasp-knife phenomenon: an experimental study in the cat. *Brain* 1972;95:31–48.
8. Cleland CL, Rymer WZ. Neural mechanisms underlying the clasp-knife reflex in the cat I. Characteristics of the reflex. *J Neurophysiol* 1990;64: 1303–1318.
9. Cleland CL, Rymer WZ. Neural mechanisms underlying the clasp-knife reflex in the cat II. Stretch sensitive muscular free nerve endings. *J Neurophysiol* 1990;64:1319–1330.
10. Tang A, Rymer W. Abnormal force–emg relations in paretic limbs of hemiparetic human subjects. *J Neurol Neurosurg Psychiatr* 1981;44:690–698.
11. Latash ML. Spectral analysis of the electromyogram (EMG) in spinal trauma patients: I. Different types of EMG and corresponding spectra. *Electromyogr Clin Neurophysiol* 1988;28:319–327.
12. Latash ML. Spectral analysis of the electromyogram (EMG) in spinal trauma patients: II. Motor unit and interference power spectra. *Electromyogr Clin Neurophysiol* 1988;28:319–327.
13. Carp J, Rymer WZ. Serotonin enhances tonic stretch and vibration reflexes. *Exp Brain Res* 1986;62:111–122.
14. Hounsgard J, Hultborn H, Jesperson B, Kiehn O. Intrinsic membrane properties causing a bistable behavior of alpha-motoneurones. *Exp Brain Res* 1984;55:391–394.
15. Hounsgard J, Hultborn H, Jesperson B, Kiehn O. Bistability of alpha motoneurones in the decerebrate cat and in the acute spinal cat after intravenous 5-hydroxy tryptophan. *J Physiol* 1988;405:345–367

Advances in Neurology, Vol. 59, edited by
Fredrick J. Seil. Raven Press, Ltd.,
New York © 1993.

14

Adaptive Plasticity in Spinal Cord

Jonathan R. Wolpaw and Jonathan S. Carp

Wadsworth Laboratories, New York State Department of Health and State University of New York, Albany, New York 12201-0509

The central nervous system (CNS) is distinguished by its ability to adapt to the changing demands of external and internal environments. Although capacity for adaptive change is ascribed to the entire CNS, the conventional view is that this capacity is not distributed uniformly throughout the neuraxis. Adaptive plasticity in response to environmental demands, development, and trauma is thought to be concentrated at higher CNS levels, in the cerebral hemispheres, and particularly in cortex. These levels are associated with the most common and easily recognized forms of adaptation, such as single-trial learning phenomena, and include the structures believed to be most intimately involved in memory.

The spinal cord is traditionally conceded little capacity for adaptation. It is often viewed as a hard-wired structure that responds in unchanging and stereotyped fashion to afferent input from the periphery and to descending commands from supraspinal levels. This perception has a lengthy pedigree. Prior to the 19th century, the role of the spinal cord, beyond its clear function as a conduit to and from the brain, was obscure (1). The elucidation of spinal reflex function that began in the 18th century with Whytt and others and culminated in the description of the "excitory-motor" (or spinal reflex) system by Marshall Hall in the 19th century revealed the complex intrinsic capabilities of the spinal cord (2). In response to this new knowledge, some scientists, most especially Pfluger, argued that the spinal cord, like the brain, possessed a soul (3). This radical position, a vitalist anachronism in the late 19th century, met with minimal and transient success. The mainstream, led particularly prominently by Sherrington and Sechenov, adopted spinal reflex functions into the modern hierarchical conception of CNS organization (4,5). In this formulation, the most sophisticated functions of the CNS, such as the capacity for adaptation, are concentrated at and help define the highest levels of the nervous system.

Although plasticity at the spinal level has received little attention until recently, extensive clinical and laboratory evidence for it has been accumulating throughout this century. In the past decade, the fact that spinal cord plasticity can be adaptive has become clear. This adaptive capacity has significant experimental and clinical implications and is likely to receive increasing attention in the future.

PLASTICITY IN THE SPINAL CORD

Until recently, spinal cord plasticity was evident primarily in the presence of damage to supraspinal or peripheral structures. If such damage distorts or eliminates activity in descending pathways from supraspinal structures or activity in sensory afferents, and if this change in activity continues long enough, intrinsic changes in the spinal cord can occur. For example, spinal cord injury in humans (6–10) or surgical transection in cats (11) causes the gradual development of abnormal spinal reflexes below the lesion. In humans, the long-term consequences of injury commonly include increased resistance to passive muscle stretch, especially in leg extensors and ankle flexors with the associated clasp-knife phenomenon, and increased stretch reflexes manifested by hyperactive deep tendon reflexes and clonus. These findings comprise the syndrome of spasticity. They are accompanied by changes in electrophysiological measures. For example, H-reflexes change gradually after spinal cord injury (12). Furthermore, vibratory inhibition of the H-reflex, which increases immediately after injury (13,14), eventually becomes abnormally low (15,16).

Exposure of spinal circuitry to distorted supraspinal influence for even brief periods of time can alter the spinal cord. Perhaps the most striking evidence comes from experiments first conducted by Anna DiGiorgio in the 1920s and repeated by a number of others since (17–20). In these studies, hemicerebellar lesions created asymmetric hindlimb postures, and, after a delay, transection of the thoracic spinal cord removed the descending influence of the damaged cerebellum. If the delay between the cerebellar lesion and the transection was at least 40 min, the hindlimb asymmetry persisted for weeks. Related studies indicated that the crucial changes are in the spinal cord itself, not in the periphery, and that comparable phenomena occur with a variety of supraspinal lesions.

Clinical evidence indicates that the evolution of spinal reflexes in normal development depends on descending influences, since it may fail to occur in the presence of supraspinal damage (21). The capacity of altered peripheral input to produce intrinsic cord changes is illustrated by evidence that the isolated spinal cord can be classically conditioned (22), by studies of flexor reflex plasticity after thermal injury (23), and by biochemical and physiological evidence for dorsal horn plasticity from peripheral inflammation (24). These data show that, with the correct impetus over sufficient time, the spinal cord has the capacity for intrinsic and persistent change.

Studies at the neuronal and synaptic levels give some insight into the mechanisms underlying spinal cord plasticity. After cord transection, Ia afferent excitatory postsynaptic potentials (EPSPs) in motoneurons undergo substantial changes in size that evolve over months (25). Partial axotomy of Ia afferents by dorsal column hemisection enhances monosynaptic transmission from undamaged Ia afferent branches to motoneurons (26). Chronic depression of Ia input by application of tetrodotoxin to the peripheral nerve markedly increases amplitude of Ia EPSPs (27). Changes in spinal circuitry involved in presynaptic inhibition of Ia fibers contribute to spinal reflex abnormalities in humans with spasticity (28) and in cats with chronic cord lesions (29). Diazepam, which enhances presynaptic inhibition in acutely lesioned animals, does not do so in chronically lesioned animals (29). Motoneuron excitability increases in persons with spinal cord injury (12). In cats, motoneuron membrane properties are different for acute and chronic spinal lesions (30). These data suggest that multiple sites in the spinal cord undergo gradual changes after trauma distorts or removes supraspinal and/or peripheral influences. Furthermore, they direct particular attention to Ia afferents and to α-motoneurons as possible sites of spinal cord plasticity.

PROBABILITY AND SIGNIFICANCE OF ADAPTIVE PLASTICITY IN SPINAL CORD

The evidence that chronic pathological or developmental change in descending activity changes the spinal cord suggests that the spinal cord also changes during the learning of motor skills, if the learning involves significant and persistent changes in descending activity. Motor skills requiring prolonged change would presumably include common behaviors like walking or jumping and more specialized ones such as dancing, skiing, writing, or playing the piano. That spinal cord changes might constitute an important part of the learning of these skills is further suggested by the prolonged practice over lengthy periods required for their mastery. This gradual acquisition is reminiscent of the gradual changes in spinal function that occur during development and after injury. For example, Goode and van Hoeven found that lower leg stretch reflexes and H-reflexes are reduced in ballet dancers and that this reduction correlates with the number of years spent in training (31).

The probability that the spinal cord has significant adaptive capacity has both theoretical and practical importance. First, as noted above, this capacity could play an important role in acquisition of motor skills. Second, because the spinal cord is simpler and more accessible than other CNS structures, spinal cord adaptive plasticity could prove a felicitous model with which to study the processes of learning and the substrates of memory. Third, understanding of the adaptive capacity of the spinal cord may lead to new therapeutic approaches to the abnormal segmental function caused by spinal cord injury, stroke, and other lesions that remove or distort descending activity (32). Although such new therapeutic approaches could have substantial use at present, their true value might well become evident only when methods for producing significant CNS regeneration are developed. For example, after regeneration of a transected spinal cord pathway, normal function will almost certainly not redevelop automatically. Techniques for utilizing the adaptive capacity of the spinal cord to retrain reestablished pathways will be essential.

OPERANT CONDITIONING OF THE SPINAL STRETCH REFLEX

The possibility that spinal cord plasticity might provide a model for defining substrates of memory in a higher vertebrate was the principal impetus for a sequence of experiments that have taken place in our laboratory over the past decade (reviewed in ref. 33). The work began with the hypothesis that if an animal learned a task in which long-term, tonic alteration in descending activity increased reward probability, adaptive changes in the spinal cord would occur as part of the learning process. These changes would be part of the CNS plasticity underlying the adaptive change in behavior and would therefore constitute substrates of memory located in the spinal cord and thus relatively accessible to detailed study.

All animal procedures were in accord with DHEW Publication No. (NIH) 85-223, *Guide for the Care and Use of Laboratory Animals,* and had been reviewed and approved by the Wadsworth Center Animal Welfare Committee.

The initial experiments developed an operant conditioning task that demanded chronic change in supraspinal influence on the spinal cord (34,35). In an effort to maximize the simplicity and accessibility of any adaptive changes that occurred in the spinal cord, this task focused on the behavior mediated by the simplest stimulus–response pathway in the vertebrate CNS, the two-neuron pathway of the spinal stretch reflex (SSR).

The SSR, known clinically as the tendon jerk, is the first response to sudden muscle stretch (36–39). As illustrated in Fig. 1A, it is wholly spinal and largely monosynaptic, a product of the two-neuron pathway consisting of the muscle spindle, the Ia afferent fiber, and the α-motoneuron. The SSR amplitude, measured as electromyographic (EMG) activity, reflects the number of α-motoneurons that fire in response to the sudden stretch. Although the SSR is the product of a two-neuron spinal pathway, the state of this pathway, and therefore the SSR amplitude, is affected by activity in descending pathways that influence the Ia synapse and/or the motoneuron itself. It is this descending activity that the task was designed to operantly condition.

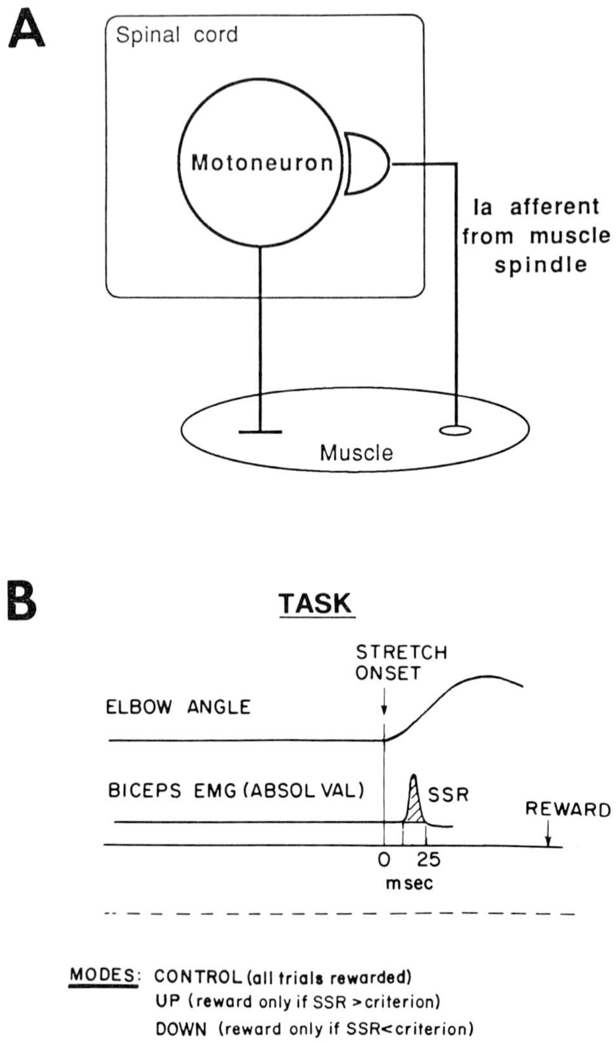

FIG. 1. (A) Two-neuron monosynaptic arc of the spinal stretch reflex (SSR). It is made up of the Ia afferent neuron, its synapse on the α-motoneuron, and the motoneuron itself. Sudden muscle stretch lengthens the muscle spindle and stimulates the Ia afferent. The Ia afferent synapse stimulates the α-motoneuron and causes muscle contraction. **(B)** Original operant conditioning task. Animal keeps elbow angle (i.e., muscle length) and biceps EMG within defined limits against constant background extension torque. At the termination of a randomly varying 1.2 to 1.8-sec period, a short pulse of additional extension torque extends the elbow and evokes the biceps SSR. In the control mode, a liquid reward is always given 0.2 sec after the pulse. In the SSRup or SSRdown mode, a reward is given only if the SSR (measured by EMG) is above or below a criterion value. Animals usually average 3,000 to 4,000 trials per day. (Modified from refs. 33,34.)

The task is shown in Fig. 1B. Monkeys (*Macaca nemestrina*) with chronically implanted fine wire EMG electrodes learned to change biceps SSR amplitude without change in initial muscle length or background α-motoneuron tone as measured by EMG (34,40–47). Since the stretch eliciting the reflex occurred at an unpredictable time, and since the SSR occurred before any other possible CNS response, the task required continual change in supraspinal influence on the spinal arc of the reflex for the 5 to 7 hr/day the animals spent on the task. When they first encountered the requirement to increase (SSRup mode) or decrease (SSRdown mode) the reflex, SSR amplitude changed appropriately by about 8% within 6 hr (44). After this rapid small phase I change, very gradual phase II change of 1% to 2% per day occurred over subsequent weeks as the animal continued to work at the task. Under the SSRup mode, SSR amplitude eventually rose to over 150% of control. Under the SSRdown mode, it eventually fell to about 50% of control. Figure 2 illustrates the prolonged course of change in an SSRup animal and an

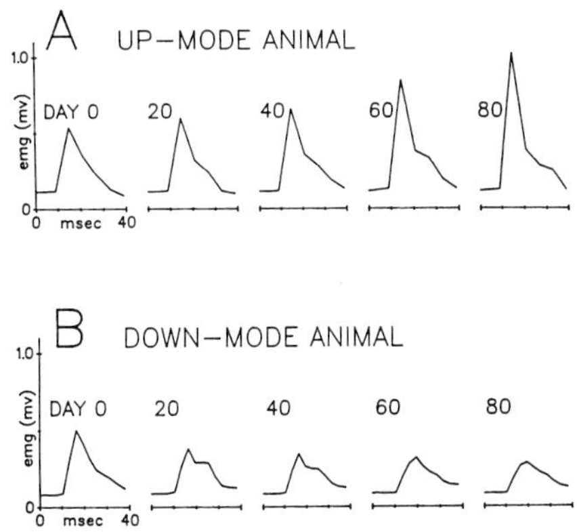

FIG. 2. Chronic effects of SSRup and SSRdown modes on SSR amplitude. (**A**) Representative data from an animal exposed to the SSRup mode for 80 days. The graphs show average daily SSR amplitude for every 20th day beginning with onset of the SSRup mode. The SSR amplitude grows steadily without change in background EMG (represented here by the 12 msec before SSR onset). (**B**) Analogous results from an animal exposed to the SSRdown mode. Steady decrease in SSR amplitude occurs without change in background EMG. (Modified from ref. 44.)

SSRdown animal. When the requirement was reversed, amplitude change reversed in the same two-phase fashion (35,41). Change was greatest in the agonist muscle and lasted for weeks without continued task performance (46,47).

Ongoing studies by Wolf, Segal, and their colleagues are demonstrating that humans have a similar capacity for adaptive change in the SSR (48,49). These studies are exploring the potential therapeutic significance of this capacity in patients with spinal cord injury or other supraspinal lesions. Their hypothesis is that appropriate operantly conditioned change in SSR amplitude will be accompanied by improvement in motor function (32).

In a highly relevant study of monkeys trained to oppose limb perturbations as quickly as possible, Meyer-Lohmann et al. (50) found that the SSR component of the response grew gradually over months and years of training until it was responsible for a major portion of the effective response. This change may be related to the reflex changes found in dancers (31) and to those that normally occur during development of basic motor skills (21).

ADAPTIVE PLASTICITY IN SPINAL CORD

The studies described above indicated that spinal reflex function can undergo adaptive change, but they did not prove that the adaptive plasticity occurs in the spinal cord itself. The most likely interpretation of the results appeared to be that phase I change reflects rapid operantly conditioned change in supraspinal influence on the spinal reflex arc, whereas subsequent phase II change, occurring over weeks and months, reflects slow changes in the spinal cord resulting from chronic exposure to the tonic descending influence responsible for phase I (43,44). However, the SSR change might be produced and maintained solely by tonic descending input from supraspinal areas or might be caused by change in the peripheral sensory organ, the muscle spindle. Only a demonstration that change persisted in the absence of descending control and without the participation of the muscle spindle would constitute strong evidence for adaptive plasticity in the spinal cord itself.

To prepare the way for determining whether intrinsic spinal cord changes did occur, the task was modified to operantly condition the H reflex, the electrical analog of the SSR, in the triceps surae muscle of the leg (51,52). The key difference is that the H-reflex is produced by direct electrical stimulation of the peripheral nerve, so that the muscle spindle is removed from the reflex arc. In addition, in this new protocol, the triceps surae H-reflex was measured in both legs simultaneously while reward was controlled only by the H-reflex in one leg, the conditioned leg. The other leg was an internal control. This modified task produced operant conditioning of the H-reflex in the conditioned leg (35,53). Like the SSR change, the H-reflex change in the conditioned leg progressed steadily over weeks. The H-reflex in the control leg changed very little (54). Figure 3 illustrates the H-reflex asymmetry that results. The H-reflex in the conditioned leg rises under the HRup mode or falls under the HRdown mode, while the H-reflex in the control leg remains close to its initial (i.e., control mode) amplitude.

Besides eliminating the muscle spindle as a possible site for plasticity, H-reflex operant conditioning in the lower limb prepared the way for testing the possibility of wholly supraspinal plasticity. If H-reflex conditioning changes the spinal cord, then change should remain even after all supraspinal control is removed. The arc of the triceps surae H-reflex is located in the lumbosacral spinal cord, which can be freed from supraspinal control by thoracic cord transection.

In the next experiments, animals in which the triceps surae H-reflex in one leg had been increased or decreased by operant conditioning were deeply anesthetized and surgically prepared (55,56). The triceps surae nerve volley responses to direct dorsal root stimulation were measured before and for up to 3 days after thoracic cord transection under continued anesthesia. The still-anesthetized animals were then sacrificed by anesthetic overdose.

In both HRup and HRdown animals, reflex asymmetries consistent with the effects of conditioning persisted after cord transection. Several days after transection removed supraspinal influence, reflexes of HRup animals remained significantly larger in HRup legs than in control legs, and reflexes of HRdown animals remained significantly smaller in HRdown legs than in control legs. Figure 4 shows representative responses to dorsal root stimulation in conditioned and control legs of an HRup and an HRdown monkey 2 to 3 days after thoracic cord transection. Reflex asymmetries consistent with the effects of conditioning are prominent.

These results demonstrate that operant conditioning of the H-reflex changes the spinal cord. Thus, they confirm the initial hypothesis that a task requiring chronic change in descending influence on a spinal pathway would lead to adaptive plasticity in the spinal cord. This plasticity may be viewed as a physi-

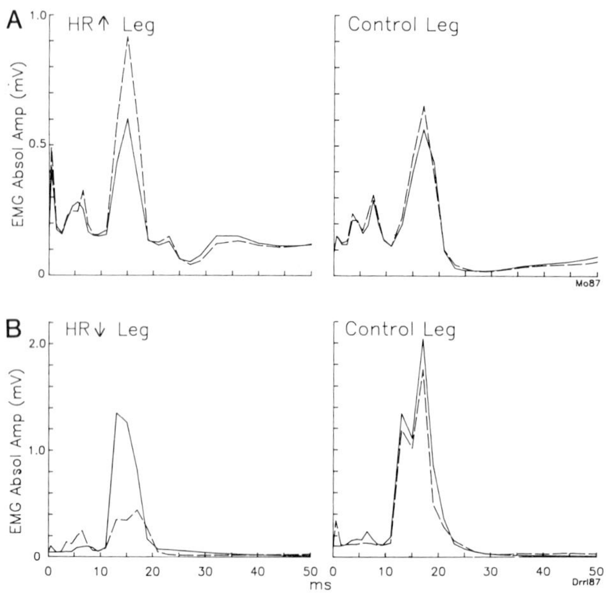

FIG. 3. **(A)** Average triceps surae H-reflexes in HRup leg and control leg of an animal for two different days, one under the control mode (*solid*) and the other after prolonged exposure to the HRup mode (*dashed*). The HRup mode exposure increases the H-reflex in the HRup leg, while the H-reflex in the control leg changes little. Threshold M responses precede the H-reflexes. **(B)** Average triceps surae H-reflexes from another animal on two different days, one under the control mode (*solid*) and the other after prolonged HRdown mode exposure (*dashed*). The HRdown mode exposure decreases the H-reflex in the HRdown leg, while the H-reflex in the control leg changes little. (Modified from ref. 54. See refs. 51 and 64 for full details of method.)

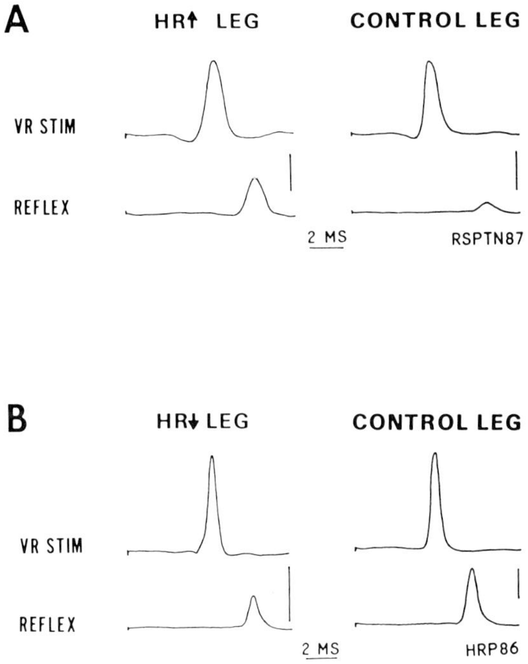

FIG. 4. Evidence for adaptive plasticity in the spinal cord. Responses to ventral root (VR) stimulation and monosynaptic reflex responses to dorsal root stimulation from triceps surae nerve branches in conditioned and control legs of an HRup animal and an HRdown animal, both under deep pentobarbital anesthesia, 2 to 3 days after thoracic spinal cord transection eliminates supraspinal influence. To facilitate interleg comparison in each animal, its responses are scaled so that the responses to VR stimulation (i.e., the maximum possible responses) are equal in height. *Vertical bars* are 100 μV. Mode-appropriate reflex asymmetry is evident in both animals. In the HRup animal **(A)**, the reflex is larger in the conditioned leg than in the control leg, and in the HRdown animal **(B)** it is smaller in the conditioned leg than in the control leg. In addition, the reflex in the control leg of the HRdown animal is much bigger than the reflex in the control leg of the HRup animal. Both of these effects of conditioning were evident throughout the several days of posttransection study under continued anesthesia. (Reprinted from ref. 65. See ref. 66 for full presentation.)

ological analog of the pathological spinal cord plasticity produced in the DiGiorgio experiments (17–20).

EVIDENCE FOR COMPLEX CHANGES IN SPINAL CORD

In the awake behaving animal, the only substantial effect of H-reflex conditioning is appropriate change in the H-reflex of the conditioned leg. The H-reflex in the control leg changes little, so that in the days prior to anesthesia and transection it was close to its original control mode value. However, the studies of the anesthetized transected animal (55,56) indicated that H-reflex conditioning did more than produce plasticity responsible for reflex increase (HRup animals) or decrease (HRdown animals) in the conditioned leg. Although task-appropriate reflex asymmetry was evident in the anesthetized transected animal (e.g., Fig. 4), another wholly unexpected effect of conditioning was also seen. Reflexes in the control legs of HRdown animals were much larger than reflexes in the control legs of HRup animals and remained larger throughout the 3 days of study under continued anesthesia. Like the asymmetry, this effect is illustrated in Fig. 4.

In sum, the removal of descending activity by anesthesia and transection uncovered an effect of H-reflex conditioning that was not apparent in the awake, behaving animal. Table 1 compares the major findings in the awake, behaving animals with those in the same animals after anesthesia and transection (55,56). (The arrows in the right-hand column were obtained by comparing the nerve volley data from conditioned animals with comparable data from naive animals.) The difference between the results in the awake, behaving state, when supraspinal influence was present, and the results in the anesthetized transected state, when supraspinal influence was absent, indicates that the

TABLE 1. *Summary of major effects of H-reflex operant conditioning*

		Test method	
Training mode	Leg	H-reflex in awake behaving animal	Nerve volley in anesthetized transected animal
HR_{up}	Up	↑↑	↑
	Control	Unchanged	↓
HR_{down}	Down	↓	↑
	Control	Unchanged	↑↑

behavior that was conditioned (i.e., appropriate change in H-reflex amplitude in the awake, behaving animal) was produced by a combination of spinal plasticity and continued supraspinal influence.

The respective supraspinal and spinal contributions to the behavior of the awake behaving animal remain to be defined. At this point, the simplest possible interpretation is that spinal cord plasticity is responsible for the change in the control leg reflexes (decrease in HRup animals and increase in HRdown animals), which is the main effect seen in the anesthetized transected state (right data column of Table 1), and that supraspinal influence produces bilateral symmetrical change (increase in HRup animals and decrease in HRdown animals), which combines with the spinal cord plasticity to produce the results seen in the awake, behaving state (left data column of Table 1). However, concurrent intracellular studies of triceps surae motoneurons in conditioned animals suggest that the situation is much more complex (57).

Our current physiological and anatomical studies at the level of the individual triceps surae motoneurons and their Ia synaptic connections seek to define the location(s) of the spinal cord plasticity underlying H-reflex conditioning. Identification of these locations will lead to investigation of the specific supraspinal influences that interact with the spinal plasticity to produce the conditioned behavior and to studies of the processes through which the spinal cord plasticity is produced. The possible sites of spinal cord plasticity fall into three categories: (a) the two-neuron arc itself, composed of the Ia synapse and the motoneuron, (b) other oligosynaptic spinal pathways that could conceivably contribute to the reflex, and (c) spinal interneurons that provide tonic input to the two-neuron arc. These possibilities are discussed in detail elsewhere (58). The intracellular studies intended to differentiate among them are still under way. As indicated above, preliminary analysis of the intracellular data suggests a pattern of spinal and supraspinal plasticity even more complex than that implied by the results summarized in Table 1 (57).

The occurrence of a complex pattern of spinal and supraspinal changes in response to an apparently simple operant conditioning task was unexpected and at first inexplicable. However, when this complexity is considered either in the context of the animal's full repertoire of behaviors or in the context of the individual neuronal or synaptic sites that contribute to the conditioned behavior, the conclusion must be that it not only is explicable but could have been anticipated.

THE CONTEXT OF THE ANIMAL'S ENTIRE BEHAVIORAL REPERTOIRE

Laboratory studies seeking to isolate and describe the substrates of adaptive plasticity or memory typically proceed by exposing an animal to a learning experience and then searching for persistent changes in the CNS. Thus, in our case, we operantly conditioned animals to increase or decrease the monosynaptic reflex in one muscle and set out to isolate the plasticity responsible for the amplitude change. The usual assumption in this approach is that the principal changes that occur are those responsible for the behavioral change that is the intended product and marker of the learning and that the research goal is to locate and describe these changes. One of the inferences suggested by the results summarized in Table 1 is that this common assumption lacks proper appreciation of the complexity of the problem that any learning experience, however simple, presents for the animal.

The new demand on CNS performance presented by a learning experience is not only that the CNS change so that a specific behavior is modified. Certainly, the CNS should change so that the specific behavior is modified. But, in addition, it should change so that the previous behavioral repertoire of the animal is still performed in a satisfactory manner in spite of the presence of the change responsible for the new behavior. Thus, in our example, the H-reflex should change while other behaviors that also involve the motoneuron and Ia synapse continue as before. Since the motoneuron is, in Sherrington's phrase, the final common pathway for motor behavior, and the Ia synapse is closely related to it, change at either site could affect a wide variety of important behaviors. In the case of the triceps surae motoneurons involved here, the asymmetric H-reflex changes created by our task could affect walking, jumping, or climbing. As a result, mastery of the conditioning task probably involves not only plasticity that appropriately changes H-reflex amplitude but plasticity that preserves other behaviors in spite of the plasticity responsible for the H-reflex change. These two classes of plasticity might be called "intended" (i.e., by the experimenter) and "compensatory" (55).

The likelihood of both intended and compensatory plasticity renders the results summarized in Table 1 less surprising. The behavior of the awake, behaving animal reflects the entire pattern of supraspinal and spinal intended and compensatory plasticity and thus is as required: the H-reflex in the conditioned leg is appropriately altered, and other behavior, here represented by the H-reflex in the control leg, is little changed. In contrast, the behavior of the anesthetized and transected animal reflects only the intended and compensatory plasticity that resides in the spinal cord. Thus, it provides a different picture: the task-appropriate reflex asymmetry is present, but, in addition, control leg reflexes are altered. In the present stage of ignorance, we can say little more. A substantive explanation of the specific pattern of spinal changes seen awaits the results of further studies like the physiological and anatomical investigations now under way (57).

THE CONTEXT OF INDIVIDUAL NEURONAL AND SYNAPTIC LOCATIONS

Each synapse or neuron in the CNS is subjected to a specific set of neuronal influences reaching it from elsewhere and has a specific set of reactions to them. These reactions may be acute, such as excitation or inhibition, or chronic, such as gradual sensitization or desensitization. The cause of a particular influence does not affect the reaction to it. Whether the influence is the product of trauma, development, conditioning, or some other event, the reaction of the synapse or neuron is the same. As a result, individual elements of the pattern of CNS plasticity produced by learning may, when viewed in isolation, bear little obvious relation to the behavioral change intended or produced. Furthermore, the probability that some stereotyped local changes will actually impede performance of the conditioned behavior should ensure that most learning will of necessity involve a complex pattern of plasticity.

For example, Webb and Cope (27) have shown that prolonged decrease in Ia synaptic activity produced by chronic application of tetrodotoxin to the peripheral nerve leads over several weeks to a large increase in the amplitude of Ia EPSPs. In this instance, a chronic decrease in synaptic activity produces supersensitization. This effect appears comparable to the supersensitivity that follows denervation at the neuromuscular junction or decreased activity at a variety of CNS synapses (59). Their finding may eventually prove highly relevant to the puzzle presented by Table 1. The Ia synapse is subject to presynaptic inhibition from supraspinal and peripheral sites (60,61). This inhibition plays a role in motor function acutely (62,63) and could help produce the operantly conditioned H-reflex changes of interest here; e.g., increased presynaptic inhibition could contribute to H-reflex decrease under the HRdown mode. The data of Webb and Cope (27) suggest that the decrease in transmitter release caused by the increased inhibition would eventually produce supersensitivity of the synapse. This supersensitivity would not be apparent in the behaving animal because of the continued presence of increased presynaptic inhibition but might become evident after anesthesia and transection had removed presynaptic influences. That is, a reflex that had been smaller than control in the awake, behaving state might be normal or larger than normal in the anesthetized transected state. An opposite picture might appear with HRup conditioning.

This example cannot by itself account for the entire pattern present in Table 1, nor can it completely account for the even more complex pattern emerging from intracellular studies (57). Nevertheless, it indicates that consideration of events on the neuronal and synaptic levels, like consideration of the requirements of the animal's full behavioral repertoire, makes complexity like that apparent in Table 1 more explicable.

SUMMARY

Recent studies indicate that the primate spinal cord has significant adaptive capacity. Monkeys and humans can gradually increase or decrease the amplitude of the spinal stretch reflex in response to an operant conditioning task. Plasticity in the spinal cord itself contributes to this behavioral change. Current evidence indicates that this spinal cord plasticity is complex. In the awake behaving animal, it combines with supraspinal influence to produce the operantly conditioned reflex change.

Adaptive plasticity in spinal cord may play a significant role in acquisition of a wide variety of motor skills. Furthermore, because of the relative simplicity and accessibility of the spinal cord, its adaptive capacity provides a new model for investigation of the neuronal and synaptic bases of adaptive change in behavior. Finally, spinal cord plasticity could furnish the basis for a new therapeutic approach to the abnormal spinal reflex function that accompanies distortion or loss of supraspinal control.

ACKNOWLEDGMENTS

Our studies have been supported in part by NIH grant NS22189, the United Cerebral Palsy Research and Educational Foundation, and the Paralyzed Veterans of America Spinal Cord Research Foundation.

REFERENCES

1. Clarke E, O'Malley CD. *The human brain and spinal cord.* Berkeley: University of California Press; 1968.
2. Liddell EGT. *The discovery of reflexes.* Oxford: Clarendon Press; 1960.
3. Clark E, Jacyna LS. *Nineteenth-century origins of the neuroscientific concepts.* Berkeley: University of California Press; 1987.
4. Sherrington CS. *The integrative action of the nervous system.* London: Constable; 1906.
5. Sechenov IM. *Reflexes of the brain.* Cambridge: The MIT Press; 1965.
6. Riddoch G. The reflex functions of the completely divided spinal cord in man, compared with those associated with less severe lesions. *Brain* 1917;40:264–402.
7. Kuhn RA. Functional capacity of the isolated human spinal cord. *Brain* 1950;73:1–51.
8. Henneman E. Organization of the spinal cord and its reflexes. In: Mountcastle VB, ed. *Medical Physiology,* Vol 1. St. Louis: CV Mosby; 1980;780–785, 793–801.
9. Landau WM. What is it? What is it not? In: Feldman RG, Young RR, Koella WP, eds. *Spasticity: disor-*

dered motor control. Chicago: Year Book; 1980:17–24.
10. Dimitrijevic MR, Faganel J, Lehmkuhl D, Sherwood A. Motor control in man after partial or complete spinal cord injury. In: Desmedt JE, ed. *Advances in neurology,* Vol 39. Motor control mechanisms in health and disease. New York: Raven Press; 1988:915–926.
11. Fujimori B, Kato M, Matsushima S, Mori S, Shimamura M. Studies on the mechanism of spasticity following spinal hemisection in the cat. In: Granit R, ed. *Muscular afferents and motor control.* New York: John Wiley & Sons; 1966;397–413.
12. Little JW, Halar EM. H-reflex changes following spinal cord injury. *Arch Phys Med Rehab* 1985; 66:19–22.
13. Ashby P, Verrier M, Lightfoot E. Segmental reflex pathways in spinal shock and spinal spasticity in man. *J Neurol Neurosurg Psychiatry* 1974;37: 1352–1360.
14. Ashby P, Verrier M. Neurophysiological changes following spinal cord lesions in man. *Can J Neurol Sci* 1975;2:91–100.
15. Burke D, Ashby P. Are spinal "presynaptic" inhibitory mechanisms suppressed in spasticity? *J Neurol Sci* 1972;15:321–326.
16. Delwaide PJ. Human monosynaptic reflexes and presynaptic inhibition. In: Desmedt JE, ed. *New developments in electromyography and clinical neurophysiology,* Vol 3. Basel: Karger; 1973:508–522.
17. DiGiorgio AM. Persistenza nell'animale spinale, di asymmetrie posturali e motorie di origine cerebellare: I, II, III. *Arch Fisiol* 1929;27:518–580.
18. Manni E. Localizzazoni cerebellari corticali nella cavia. Nota 1:II "corpus cerebelli." *Arch Fisiol* 1950;49:213–237.
19. Gerard RW. The fixation of experience. In: Gerard RW, Konorski J, eds. *Brain mechanisms and learning.* Oxford: Blackwell; 1961:21–32.
20. Kandel ER, Spencer WA. Cellular neurophysiological approaches in the study of learning. *Physiol Rev* 1968;48:65–134.
21. Myklebust BM, Gottlieb GL, Agarwal GC. Stretch reflexes of the normal human infant. *Dev Med Child Neurol* 1986;28:440–449.
22. Patterson MM. Mechanisms of classical conditioning of spinal reflexes. In: Thompson RF, Hicks LH, Shvyrkov VB, eds. *Neural mechanisms of goal-directed behavior and learning.* New York: Academic Press; 1980;263–272.
23. Woolf CJ, McMahon SB. Injury-induced plasticity of the flexor reflex in chronic decerebrate rats. *Neuroscience* 1985;16:395–404.
24. Dubner R, Ruda MA. Activity-dependent neuronal plasticity following tissue injury and inflammation. *Trends Neurosci* 1992;15:96–102.
25. Nelson SG, Collatos TC, Niechaj A, Mendell LM. Immediate increases in Ia-motoneuron synaptic transmission caudal to spinal cord transection. *Neurophysiol* 1979;42:655–664.
26. Decima EE, Morales FR. Long-lasting facilitation of monosynaptic pathway as a result of "partial" axotomy of its presynaptic elements. *Exp Neurol* 1983;79:532–551.
27. Webb CB, Cope TC. Modulation of Ia EPSP amplitude: the effects of chronic synaptic inactivity. *J Neurosci* 1992;12:338–344.
28. Desmedt JE. Mechanisms of vibration-induced inhibition or potentiation: tonic vibration reflex and vibration paradox in man. In: Desmedt JE, ed. *Advances in neurology,* Vol 39. Motor control mechanisms in health and disease. New York: Raven Press; 1983;671–683.
29. Schlosser W, Franco S, Bautz G, Horst DW, Naftchi NE. Alterations of various physiological and biochemical parameters during the development of spasticity in the chronic spinal cat. In: Naftchi NE, ed. *Spinal cord injury.* New York: SP Medical and Scientific Books; 1982:115–131.
30. Gustafsson B, Katz R, Malmstem J. Effects of chronic partial deafferentiation on the electrical properties of lumbar alpha-motoneurons in the cat. *Brain Res* 1982;246:23–33.
31. Goode DJ, Van Hoeven J. Loss of patellar and Achilles tendon reflex in classical ballet dancers. *Arch Neurol* 1982;39:323.
32. Wolf SL, Segal RL. Conditioning of the spinal stretch reflex: implications for rehabilitation. *Phys Ther* 1990;70:652–656.
33. Wolpaw JR, Carp JS. Memory traces in spinal cord. *Trends Neurosci* 1990;13:137–142.
34. Wolpaw JR, Braitman DJ, Seegal RF. Adaptive plasticity in the primate spinal stretch reflex: initial development. *Neurophysiol* 1983;50:1296–1311.
35. Wolpaw JR, Herchenroder PA. Operant conditioning of H-reflex in freely moving monkeys. *J Neurosci Meth* 1990;31:145–152.
36. Magladery JW, Porter WE, Park AM, Teasdall RD. Electrophysiological studies of nerve and reflex activity in normal man. IV. The two-neuron reflex and identification of certain action potentials from spinal roots and cord. *Bull Johns Hopkins Hosp* 1951;88:499–519.
37. Matthews PBC. *Mammalian muscle receptors and their central actions.* Baltimore: Williams & Wilkins; 1972.
38. Lee RG, Tatton WG. Motor responses to sudden limb displacements in primates with specific CNS lesions and in human patients with motor system disorders. *Can J Neurol Sci* 1975;2:285–293.
39. Henneman E, Mendell LM. Functional organization of motoneuron pool and inputs. In: Brooks VB, ed. *Handbook of physiology. Sect I. The nervous system. Vol II. Motor control. Part I.* Baltimore: Williams & Wilkins; 1981:423–507.
40. Wolpaw JR. Change in short-latency response to limb displacement in primates. *Fed Proc* 1982;41:2156–2159.
41. Wolpaw JR. Adaptive plasticity in the primate spinal stretch reflex: Reversal and re-development. *Brain Res* 1983;278:299–304.
42. Wolpaw JR. Adaptive plasticity in the spinal stretch reflex: an accessible substrate of memory? *Cell Mol Neurobiol* 1985;5:147–165.
43. Wolpaw JR, Kieffer VA, Seegal RF, Braitman DJ, Sanders MG. Adaptive plasticity in the spinal stretch reflex. *Brain Res* 1983;267:196–200.
44. Wolpaw JR, O'Keefe JA. Adaptive plasticity in the primate spinal stretch reflex: evidence for a two-phase process. *J Neurosci* 1984;4:2718–2724.

45. Wolpaw JR, O'Keefe JA, Kieffer VA, Sanders MG. Reduced day-to-day variation accompanies adaptive plasticity in the primate spinal stretch reflex. *Neurosci Lett* 1985;54:165–171.
46. Wolpaw JR, O'Keefe JA, Noonan PA, Sanders MG. Adaptive plasticity in the primate spinal stretch reflex: Persistence. *J Neurophysiol* 1986;55:272–279.
47. Wolpaw JR, Seegal RF, O'Keefe JA. Adaptive plasticity in the primate spinal stretch reflex: behavior of synergist and antagonist muscles. *J Neurophysiol* 1983;50:1312–1319.
48. Evatt ML, Wolf SL, Segal RL. Modification of human spinal stretch reflexes: preliminary studies. *Neurosci Lett* 1989;105:350–355.
49. Segal RL, Wolf SL. Initial studies on the modification of spinal stretch reflexes in spinal cord injured patients. *Soc Neurosci Abst* 1991;17:198.
50. Meyer-Lohmann J, Christakos CN, Wolf H. Dominance of the short-latency component in perturbation induced electromyographic responses of long-trained monkeys. *Exp Brain Res* 1986;64:393–399.
51. Wolpaw JR. Operant conditioning of primate spinal reflexes: the H-reflex. *Neurophysiol* 1987;57: 443–458.
52. Herchenroder PA, Wolpaw JR. Reflex measurement and modification in unrestrained primates. *Soc Neurosci Abstr* 1988;14:62.
53. Wolpaw JR. Operant conditioning of primate spinal reflexes: the H-reflex. *J Neurophysiol* 1987;57: 443–458.
54. Wolpaw JR, Lee CL, Calaitges JG. Operant conditioning of primate triceps surae H-reflex produces reflex asymmetry. *Exp Brain Res* 1989;75:35–39.
55. Wolpaw JR, Lee CL. Memory traces in primate spinal cord produced by operant conditioning of H-reflex. *J Neurophysiol* 1989;61:563–572.
56. Wolpaw JR, Carp JS, Lee CL. Memory traces in spinal cord produced by H-reflex conditioning: effects of posttetanic potentiation. *Neurosci Lett* 1989;103:113–119.
57. Carp JS, Chen XY, Wolpaw JR. Motoneuron physiology after H-reflex change by operant conditioning. *Soc Neurosci Abstr* 1991;17:645.
58. Carp JS, Wolpaw JR. Possible mechanisms of operantly conditioned plasticity in motoneuron response to Ia afferent input. In: Wernig A, ed. *Restorative neurology,* Vol 5. Plasticity of motoneuronal connections. Amsterdam: Elsevier; 1991:435–442.
59. Thesleff S. Denervation sensitivity. In: Adelman G, ed. *Encyclopedia of neuroscience,* Vol 1. Boston: Birkhauser; 1987:322–323.
60. Baldissera F, Hultborn H, Illert M. Integration in spinal neuronal systems. In: Brooks VB, ed. *Handbook of physiology. Sect I. The nervous system. Vol. II. Motor control. Part I.* Baltimore: Williams & Wilkins; 1981:509–595.
61. Burke RE, Rudomin P. Spinal neurons and synapses. In: Kandel ER, ed. *Handbook of physiology. The nervous system. Cellular biology of neurons.* Baltimore: Williams & Wilkins; 1978:877–944.
62. Capaday C, Stein RB. Amplitude modulation of the soleus H-reflex in the human during walking and standing. *J Neurosci Methods* 1987;21:91–104.
63. Capaday C, Stein RB. Difference in the amplitude of the human soleus H reflex during walking and running. *J Physiol* 1987;392:513–522.
64. Wolpaw JR, Herchenroder PA. Operant conditioning of the H-reflex in freely moving monkeys. *J Neurosci Methods* 1990;31:145–152.
65. Wolpaw JR, Lee CL, Carp JS. Operantly conditioned plasticity in spinal cord. In: Wolpaw JR, Schmidt JT, Vaughan TM, eds. *Activity-driven changes in learning and development.* New York: New York Academy of Science; 1991:338–348.
66. Wolpaw JR, Lee CL. Memory traces in primate spinal cord produced by operant conditioning of H-reflex. *J Neurophysiol* 1989;61:563–572.

Advances in Neurology, Vol. 59, edited by Fredrick J. Seil. Raven Press, Ltd., New York © 1993.

15

Inhibitory Control of Reflex Excitability Following Contusion Injury and Neural Tissue Transplantation

Floyd J. Thompson, Paul J. Reier, Ronald Parmer, and Christopher C. Lucas

Departments of Neuroscience and Neurosurgery, University of Florida Health Science Center, Gainesville, Florida 32610

It is well known that human spinal cord injury often results in the progressive onset of spasticity of motor functions controlled by cord segments caudal to the level of injury (1,2). Since the exaggeration of segmental reflexes occurs in time and in proportion to the presentation of spasticity (3), this condition of hyperreflexia is considered to be largely responsible for the expression of overt behavioral spasticity (4,5). Because hyperreflexia with the associated spasticity continues to be a major problem (6), one aspect of spinal cord injury research has focused on the pathophysiological changes that may contribute to the evolution of this condition (7–10).

Reflex excitability is known to be governed by two mechanisms, excitatory processes that initiate reflexes and regulatory processes that decrease them. A balance between these two is critical for normal reflex excitability. Studies of various experimental models of spinal cord injury have demonstrated that some features of hyperreflexia may be produced in laboratory animals (9,11). It has been shown at the cellular level that there is an immediate increase in the excitatory postsynaptic potentials (EPSPs) from muscle afferents to motoneurons subsequent to spinal cord transection (12,13). Acute dorsal hemisections also produced an increase in the ease of motoneuron recruitment (14) along with a shortening of the after hyperpolarization of slow-conducting motoneurons (15). These increased EPSPs, however, were not exhibited by lumbar motoneurons caudal to chronic thoracic spinal transections (16). Therefore, no compelling evidence exists for postsynaptic excitatory processes that would account for the long-lasting increase in reflex excitability.

Several reports of human hyperreflexia have consistently remarked on the potential alterations in reflex regulatory processes as a critical factor in the altered expression of reflex excitability. Correlations between the progressive onset of hyperreflexia and the loss of reflex depression, normally induced by reflex repetition, have been particularly suggestive of a relationship between exaggerated reflexes and decreased regulatory or inhibitory processes (3,7).

With these issues in mind, we began a series of studies to address two specific questions. (a) Subsequent to spinal cord injury, what quantitative changes in reflex excitability occur that relate to the development of hyperreflexia? (b) Can the magnitude of these physiological changes be regulated by an experimental therapeutic approach involving neural tissue transplantation?

Particular interest was directed at quantification of specific neurophysiological features induced by spinal cord injury that could serve as an index of functional loss. Such measures of reflex excitability could also provide a quantitative index of the therapeutic impact of intraspinal neural tissue transplantation on certain functional deficits precipitated by experimental spinal cord injury (see also refs. 17, 18; Nornes et al., this volume).

We chose the contusion injury model because this reproduces many of the histopathological features of human traumatic spinal cord injury (19). In addition, contusion-induced lesions exhibit a progressive pathology and often show some surviving white matter. The contusion injury model offers an opportunity to examine the ability of fetal central nervous system (CNS) grafts to either spare some functions or otherwise exert an influence via persisting fiber tracts.

Following contusion injury of the adult rat spinal cord, segmental reflex activity exhibits several interesting patterns of alteration that are progressive in onset and permanent once established (20). The most striking change is a significant reduction in rate-sensitive depression of test reflexes. In this chapter, we review some of these findings and describe the use of rate-sensitive depression as a quantitative probe of the efficacy of neural tissue transplantation to promote patterns of lumbar reflex functions closer to those recorded in normal rats.

RATE-SENSITIVE REFLEX DEPRESSION AND PRESYNAPTIC INHIBITION

Since reflex magnitude represents an accurate index of synchronous motoneuron discharge, comparison of monosynaptic reflex (MSR) magnitudes has been a useful means of testing specific influences on reflex excitability. It is known that the MSR varies in proportion to the intensity of afferent stimulation as well as the frequency of reflex repetition (21–23). These observations emphasized (21,24,25) that recent activity in a reflex pathway produced long-lasting changes in the excitability of the components of that pathway, particularly the presynaptic elements (26). Eccles and Rall (21) reported that the amplitude of a compound monosynaptic reflex was reduced if the interval between reflexes was less than 3 sec (i.e., a repetition rate of 0.3 Hz) and was markedly reduced in a graded fashion as the interval was further decreased by increasing the repetition frequency. Since no changes in excitability were detected postsynaptically to account for the low-frequency rate depression, Frank and Fuortes (26) concluded that the long-lasting depression must be presynaptic. Accordingly, they suggested that it be called presynaptic inhibition. Therefore, reflex amplitude appeared to be determined not only by motoneuron excitability or the type and number of afferent fibers activated in a given reflex pathway (22,27) but also by the excitability of the intraspinal network of primary afferent central connections that comprise the presynaptic component of that reflex pathway (22,23,28).

A complex intraspinal reflex network has been revealed that receives input from segmental afferents (29,30) as well as descending fiber systems (31) that, via interneurons that terminate axo-axonally on the primary afferent fibers (32), influence the excitability of the primary afferent terminals. These interneurons include GABAergic cells that terminate on $GABA_B$ receptors on the primary afferent terminals and can produce long-lasting decreases in calcium conductance (33). Because transmitter release is dependent on calcium influx, an afferent volley reaching the primary afferent terminal during a phase of decreased calcium conductance will elicit release of significantly less transmitter (33). In normal reflex pathways, presynaptic inhibition following a single segmental afferent test volley has an onset latency of 10 to 20 msec, a maximal inhibition from 40 through 100 msec, and a progressively decrementing inhibition trailing out to 3,000 msec (21,23,29). Normally, segmental afferent input to presynaptic inhibitory interneurons is continuous, and, in addition, descending fiber systems converge onto these interneurons and contribute both tonic and event-related conditioning of the presynaptic pathways (34). Presynaptic inhibition has thus been ascribed an important role in regulating reflex excitability without directly altering the responsiveness of motoneurons (35,36). Therefore, each segmental afferent volley that enters the spinal cord normally reaches motoneurons through an intraspinal presynaptic network whose terminal excitability is continuously modulated.

Because each reflex event produces a long-lasting change in the excitability of presynaptic components, a strategy for testing the level of influence of this presynaptic regulatory mechanism is to compare reflex amplitudes produced by stimuli at relatively long intervals (e.g., 0.3 Hz) to those elicited at shorter intervals (e.g., 1 to 20 Hz). In the normal spinal cord, a rate-sensitive decrease in the amplitude of the lumbar monosynaptic reflexes is significant by 1 Hz and can be expressed as the percentage of the 0.3-Hz control reflex amplitude at this and higher test frequencies (21,23,25). Clinical tests have routinely included an evaluation of rate-sensitive depression of spinal monosynaptic reflexes because of the correlation between the loss of rate-sensitive reflex depression and the onset, as well as the magnitude, of spasticity (3,7). Accordingly, decreases in presynaptic regulatory processes are thought to contribute, at least in part, to the development of hyperreflexia following CNS injuries (7,10). Therefore, measures of rate-sensitive depression of MSRs were selected for our present studies because of their suggested clinical relevance, correlation with processes that govern reflex expression, and the opportunity they present for quantitative comparisons across animals.

BASIC METHODS

Contusions were produced using a modification of the Allen weight-drop method (37,38) in 4% chloral-hydrate-anesthetized animals (10 ml/kg, i.p.). Each animal also received a preoperative dose of penicillin (Longicil, 100,000 U, i.m.). Following laminectomy at T-8, a 10-g weight was dropped from a height of 2.5 cm onto a Teflon impounder that had been gently placed on the dura. Terminal physiological recording sessions were carried out at either 28 or 60 days subsequent to injury.

Recordings were performed in animals anesthetized by constant infusion of ketamine (i.p.). The axial skeleton was immobilized with spinal clamps, and the lumbar enlargement was exposed by laminectomy. The reflexes were elicited by stimulation of the L-4 and L-5 dorsal roots. The monosynaptic reflexes were recorded from the tibial nerve exposed in the popliteal fossa and prepared for monophasic recordings. Thirty-two consecutive test reflexes were obtained at seven test frequencies of 1, 2, 3, 4, 5, 10, and 20 Hz. The attenuation of the tibial MSR amplitude as a function of stimulus frequency was compared across groups using a one-factor, multilevel ANOVA followed by *post hoc* t-tests; data are expressed ± the standard error. Reflex magnitude responses as a function of repetition rate were obtained using maximal reflexes at a control repetition rate of 0.3 Hz, consistent with criteria standardized in the original studies of rate-sensitive depression (21,24). Reflex magnitudes were measured as the base-line-to-base-line integration of the monosynaptic waveform.

ALTERATIONS IN LUMBAR REFLEX EXCITABILITY SUBSEQUENT TO CONTUSION INJURY OF THE THORACIC SPINAL CORD

As noted earlier, in normal animals, rate-sensitive depression results in a substantial reduction in the activation of reflex pathways by tonic or repetitive stimuli. A typical waveform to illustrate this process is shown in Fig. 1A. In this example, the magnitude of the MSR elicited at 10 Hz was attenuated by

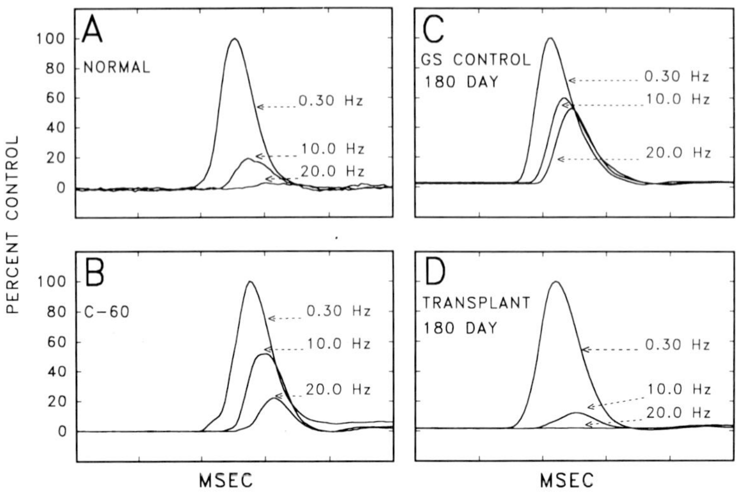

FIG. 1. (A) Tibial monosynaptic reflexes (MSRs) recorded from a normal animal at 0.3 Hz, 1.0 Hz, and 5.0 Hz, respectively. All waveforms shown in this and subsequent figures are the signal average of 32 consecutive waveforms. **(B)** Tibial MSRs recorded from a 60-day postcontusion animal at the same frequencies as in **A**. (Data from Thompson et al., ref. 20.) **(C)** Tibial MSRs recorded from a glucose–saline control animal 180 days post-contusion. **(D)** Tibial MSRs recorded from an E14-transplanted animal, 180 days post-contusion.

more than 80% of the control reflex elicited at 0.3 Hz; at 20 Hz, the reflex was attenuated to approximately 1% of the control. Group mean responses to 1- to 20-Hz stimulation frequencies are graphed in Fig. 2 to further illustrate this point (see also refs. 21,23,26). Based on these data, it would be expected that a loss of rate-sensitive depression should permit higher levels of tonic or repetitive afferent stimuli to influence spinal reflex pathways.

When tested at 28 days after contusion and later, the tibial MSR magnitudes were significantly less attenuated in response to repetition than those observed in normal animals at corresponding frequencies ($p \leq 0.05$, ANOVA). A sample waveform from a 60-day postcontusion animal is shown for comparison in Fig. 1B. The magnitude of the MSR elicited at 10 Hz was only attenuated to 50% of the control, and even at 20 Hz, the magnitude was nearly 20% of the 0.3-Hz con-

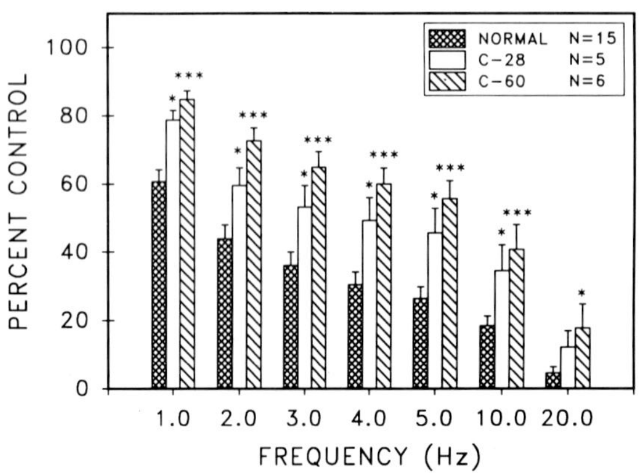

FIG. 2. Group means for rate-sensitive depression in normal, 28-day, and 60-day postcontusion animals, respectively. (Asterisks denote significantly different from normal ANOVA; * $p \leq .05$; *** $p \leq .005$). (Data from Thompson et al., ref. 20.)

trol. The graphed means for data recorded in 28-day and 60-day postcontusion animals (Fig. 2) clearly indicate that a larger proportion of the control reflex magnitude was recorded at all test frequencies in the postcontusion animals than in the normal animals. In the 60-day postcontusion animals, these differences were significant at each test frequency from 1 to 20 Hz.

In summary, these studies revealed an enduring decrease in rate-sensitive depression subsequent to contusion injury of the midthoracic spinal cord. Since tonic and repetitive stimuli are present in many forms of proprioceptive input to the spinal cord, a significant decrease in rate-sensitive depression could be expected to lead to exaggerated levels of reflex expression (i.e., hyperreflexia). Therefore, the changes in spinal reflex excitability that we have observed can provide quantitative differences between normal and spinal contusion-injured animals. In addition, these changes are relevant to altered patterns of reflex excitability observed in human spinal cord injury.

STUDIES OF LOW-FREQUENCY DEPRESSION IN CONTUSED ANIMALS WITH TRANSPLANTS INTRODUCED AT A SUBCHRONIC PERIOD SUBSEQUENT TO INJURY

During the past few years, the successful intraspinal transplantation of fetal spinal neural tissue has been demonstrated in a variety of injury models (reviewed in refs. 39,40). Anatomically, such grafts exhibit a high degree of differentiation and often restore rostral–caudal structural continuity through the lesion, with some anatomic integration occurring at points of host–graft apposition. For example, transplants of fetal spinal cord tissue into the neonate promote the growth of serotonergic fibers across the site of transection (41) and enhance the recovery of locomotor function after spinal injury (42). Recent evidence also indicates that fetal spinal cord grafts into lesions of the adult spinal cord can promote some improvement in certain locomotor tasks (43–45). In addition, fetal grafts have also been shown to prevent axotomy-induced retrograde cell death in supraspinal and segmental neuronal populations of neonatal (46) and adult (47) recipients, respectively. Though specific details are still incomplete, such results suggest that fetal grafts may affect the host nervous system by way of a variety of circuits and nonsynaptically mediated mechanisms.

Having observed quantifiable and reproducible neurophysiological deficits after contusion injury, we initiated studies to determine whether fetal tissue grafts would have a therapeutic benefit specific to this physiological measure. For this first phase of our work, we tested a 1-week delay between injury and transplantation. For these experiments a suspension of dissociated E14 fetal spinal cord cells (approximately 1.6×10^6 viable cells/ml, 40 to 60 μl total volume) was injected into the lesion epicenter. Control animals received only a glucose–saline vehicle used in the preparation of the suspension. The recording experiments were performed at 6 months following the initial contusion injury.

The frequency attenuation patterns in the control animals (C-180G) differed significantly from those obtained in normal animals at all seven test frequencies. A sample waveform is shown in Fig. 1C, and group means are compared in Fig. 3. Collectively, the marked decrease in rate-sensitive depression observed in postcontusion animals at 28, 60, and 180 days indicated the presence of a severe and lasting alteration in reflex excitability.

In contrast, the tibial MSRs recorded from those animals that had received grafts demonstrated significantly more rate-sensitive depression compared to the time-matched controls. Shown in Fig. 1C, the reflex magnitude recorded from a 180-day glucose–saline control animal maintained approximately 50% of the 0.3-Hz magnitude, whereas waveforms recorded from the transplant recipient at 20 Hz (Fig. 1D) resembled the nearly total reflex attenuation observed in the normal wave-

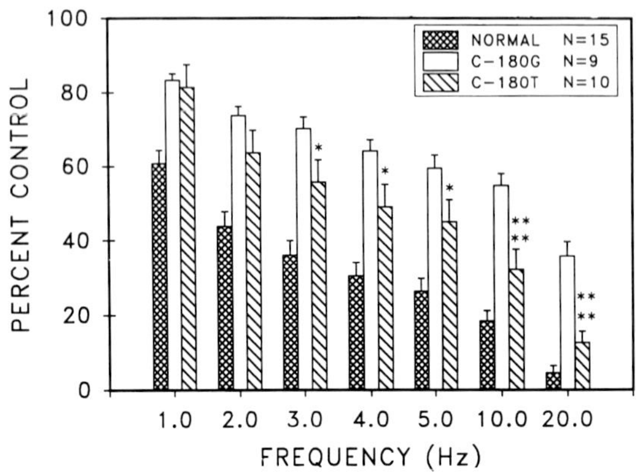

FIG. 3. Group means for rate-sensitive depression in normal, glucose–saline control animals 180 days post-contusion, and E14-transplant animals 180 days post-contusion. (Asterisks denote significantly different from glucose saline controls. ANOVA; * $p \leq .05$; **** $p \leq .001$).

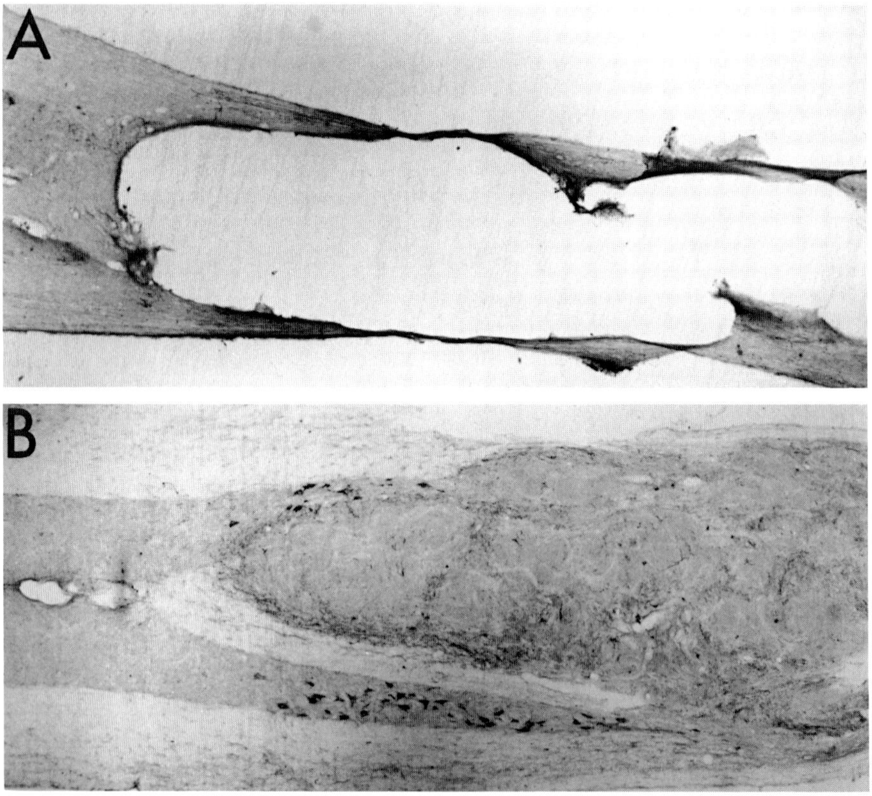

FIG. 4. Histological comparison of longitudinal section through the epicenter of glucose–saline animal 180 days subsequent to contusion injury **(A)**, ×30, compared to E14-transplant animal **(B)**, ×30, also 180 days post-contusion. The section of the spinal cord shown in **B** was stained with antibody to calcitonin gene-related peptide. Motoneuron cell bodies can be seen in the gray matter caudal to the lesion, with some in close proximity to the graft.

form (Fig. 1A). These findings are also reflected in the group means in which the waveforms recorded from the 180-day graft recipients are significantly more attenuated than those recorded from the 180-day controls at five of the seven test frequencies (Fig. 3).

Histological evaluations of cord specimens from fetal transplant recipients in these experiments revealed large grafts that often filled the entire lesion epicenter and formed continuous rostral–caudal appositions with the host spinal cord (Fig. 4). The contusion sites in the glucose–saline controls were characterized by large cystic cavitations that involved all of the gray matter and spared only a thin rim of white matter (Fig. 4A,B).

DISCUSSION

Recent neurophysiological characterization of segmental reflex activity following contusion injury of the adult rat spinal cord revealed several interesting patterns of alteration that were progressive in onset and of enduring duration (20). These findings comprise a model in which specific segmental reflex patterns and the underlying neurophysiology can be tested. In this chapter, we highlighted the use of one aspect of this model as a quantitative probe to determine whether fetal grafts in the injured spinal cord could participate in the normalization of specific features of lumbar segmental reflex patterns altered by midthoracic contusion injury.

Reflexes recorded in animals at 1 month and 2 months post-contusion were observed to express significantly decreased rate-sensitive depression, a regulatory process that greatly attenuates repetitive afferent signals. Spinal reflex responses to repetitive stimuli in postcontusion animals were increased two to three times over those recorded in normal animals at comparable frequencies. Functionally, this means that reflex activations that are normally attenuated in response to repetitive stimuli were being expressed at two to three times the normal magnitude. Input to the spinal cord from a variety of proprioceptors includes a wide range of repetitive afferent signals that, in the normal spinal cord, are subject to considerable attenuation. Decreased rate-sensitive depression would permit a larger proportion of repetitive afferent signals to reach spinal reflex pathways and thereby contribute significantly to exaggerated levels of reflex activation (28). This alteration in a fundamental regulatory process is thus proposed to contribute to post-injury patterns of hyperreflexia. This deficit was also observed 6 months post-injury and is therefore interpreted as a permanent alteration in the reflex excitability of the lumbar spinal cord following thoracic contusion injury. The specific mechanisms for the post-traumatic alterations could involve changes in the reflex pathways utilizing presynaptic inhibition. It can not be excluded, however, that plasticity-related enhancement of primary afferent terminals secondary to central deafferentation may also be involved (48).

These findings underscore the importance of gaining an increased understanding of the neural substrates that regulate reflex excitability in normal animals as well as in animals with spinal cord lesions. In this regard, we were particularly interested in determining if the deficit that we have observed in rate-sensitive depression is unique to the contusion injury or whether it may also be produced by a more controlled unilateral lesion. Preliminary observations have shown that hemisection lesions produced at the T-8 level (the same level as was used for the contusion injuries) are also followed by the progressive onset of a deficit in rate-sensitive depression ipsilateral to the lesion (49). As with the contusion injury, the deficit was observed to be significantly established by 28 days. To identify a specific neuroanatomic substrate, we are currently exploring the possibility that interruption of selected pathways can result in significant loss of rate-sensitive reflex depression.

This issue of the specific neural substrate is of particular interest in light of our findings that therapeutic intervention at 1 week following the contusion injury produced significant normalization of reflex excitability. Animals with fetal spinal cord grafts demonstrated more normal patterns of rate-sensitive depression than those observed in time-matched controls. These observations suggest that transplantation of neural tissue into the injured spinal cord can provide a functional benefit tested against a specific physiological marker. Since a portion of the rate-sensitive depression has been ascribed to presynaptic inhibition, it is possible that a part of the transplant-mediated benefits relate to preserving descending and segmental influences that normally converge on inhibitory interneurons. Whether this preservation relates to specific descending fibers or to a generalized decreased setting for segmental plasticity subsequent to central deafferentation (48) are topics of current studies.

Other studies using a different approach have also examined graft-mediated modulation of segmental reflex excitability. These studies have demonstrated that intraspinal transplants of fetal CNS tissue containing catecholamine cells can strengthen segmental reflexes previously weakened by chemical lesion of central noradrenergic systems (17, 18; see also Nornes et al., this volume). The extent of segmental reflex enhancement correlated with the proportion of catecholamine-containing donor cells in these chemically axotomized spinal cords (18). These results are of considerable interest and further support the potential of cell transplantation for promoting spinal cord functional repair.

Further studies of these transplantation approaches and the quantitative evaluation of their potential to address specific injury-related problems will require an even more extensive repertoire of interdisciplinary strategies. Behavioral improvement or sparing obviously represents the ultimate goal and index of the success of any repair technique, but behavioral measures involve the summation of many neurophysiological processes. It is noteworthy that although hyperreflexia and associated spasticity are a conspicuous hallmark of human spinal cord injury, spasticity *per se* is rarely observed in laboratory models of spinal cord injury (9,11). It appears that although there may be similarities in fundamental organization of spinal reflexes, the complex interactions required to produce overt behavior illustrate, if not amplify, species differences. Therefore, insight into the parallels of physiological changes subsequent to spinal cord injury that occur in both humans and animal models may be revealed at the fundamental reflex level but may not always be obvious at the level of the more complex interactions required for behavior. Therefore, knowing whether some fundamental reflex mechanisms are more responsive to a particular treatment than others is essential if systematic evaluation is to be achieved, since failure to see an immediate behavioral response might undermine estimates of the usefulness of any given strategy.

Whether the transplants served to enhance anatomic sparing, improve function of existing anatomy, or facilitate alternative pathways for descending modulation of reflex excitability are interesting issues around which we are continuing to pose new studies.

ACKNOWLEDGMENTS

The authors gratefully acknowledge the superb technical assistance of Barbara O'Steen and Minnie Ann Smith. These studies were supported in part by NIH-NINCDS (NO1-NS-7-2300 and 5-PO1-NS-27511), the Mark F. Overstreet Chair for Spinal Cord Regeneration Research (University of Florida Foundation), and by the State of Florida Impaired Drivers and Speeders Trust Fund.

REFERENCES

1. Kuhn RA, Macht MB. Some manifestations of reflex activity in spinal man with particular reference to the occurance of extensor spasm. *Bull Johns Hopkins Hosp* 1948;84:43–75.
2. Taylor S, Ashby P, Verrier M. Neurophysiological

changes following spinal cord lesion in man. *J Neurol Neurosurg Psychiatry* 1984;47:1102–1108.
3. Ishikawa K, Ott K, Porter RW, Stuart D. Low frequency depression of the H wave in normal and spinal man. *Exp Neurol* 1966;15:140–156.
4. Guttman L. *Spinal cord injuries, Comprehensive management and research.* London: Blackwell Scientific Publishers; 1976.
5. Lazorthes Y, Sallerin-Caute B, Verdie J, Bastide R, Carillo J. Chronic intrathecal baclofen administration for control of severe spasticity. *J Neurosurg* 1990;72:393–402.
6. Katz RT, Rymer WZ. Spastic hypertonia: mechanisms and measurement. *Arch Phys Med Rehab* 1989;70:144–155.
7. Delwaide PJ. Human monosynaptic reflexes and presynaptic inhibition: an interpretation of spastic hyperreflexia. In: Desmedt JE, ed. *New developments in electromyography and clinical neurophysiology.* Basel: Karger; 1973:508–522.
8. Lance JW. Symposium synopsis. In: Feldman RG, Young RR, Koella WP, eds. *Spasticity: disordered motor control.* Chicago: Year-Book Publishers; 1980:485–494.
9. Hultborn H, Malmsten J. Changes in segmental reflexes following chronic spinal cord hemisection in the cat. I. Increased monosynaptic and polysynaptic ventral root discharges. *Acta Physiol Scand* 1983;119:405–422.
10. Burke D. Spasticity as an adaptation to pyramidal tract injury. In: Waxman SG, ed. Advances in neurology, Vol 47. *Functional recovery in neurological disease.* New York: Raven Press; 1988:401–423.
11. Malmsten J. Time course of segmental reflex changes after chronic spinal cord hemisection in the rat. *Acta Physiol Scand* 1983;119:435–443.
12. Nelson SG, Collatos TC, Niechaj A, Mendell LM. Immediate increase in Ia-motoneuron synaptic transmission caudal to spinal cord transection. *J Neurophysiol* 1979;42:655–664.
13. Cope TC, Hickman KR, Botterman BR. Acute effects of spinal transection on EPSPs produced by single homonymous Ia-fibers in soleus alpha-motoneurons. *J Neurophysiol* 1988;60:1678–1694.
14. Carp JS, Rymer WZ. Enhancement by serotonin of tonic vibration and stretch reflexes in the decerebrate cat. *Exp Brain Res* 1986;62:111–122.
15. Carp JS, Powers RK, Rymer WZ. Alterations in motoneuron properties induced by acute dorsal spinal hemisection in the decerebrate cat. *Exp Brain Res* 1991;83:539–548.
16. Munson JB, Foehring RC, Lofton SA, Zengel JE, Sypert GW. Plasticity of medial gastrocnemius motor units following cordotomy in the cat. *J Neurophysiol* 1986;55:619–634.
17. Buchanan JT, Nornes HO. Transplants of embryonic brainstem containing the locus coeruleus into spinal cord enhance the hindlimb flexion reflex in adult rats. *Brain Res* 1986;381:225–236.
18. Moorman SJ, Whalen LR, Nornes HO. A neurotransmitter specific functional recovery mediated by fetal implants in the lesioned spinal cord of the rat. *Brain Res* 1990;508:194–198.
19. Kakulas BA. Pathology of spinal injuries. *CNS Trauma* 1985;1:117–129.
20. Thompson FJ, Reier PJ, Lucas CC, Parmer R. Lumbar spinal reflex excitability following contusion injury of the mid-thoracic spinal cord. *J Neurophysiol* [*in press*].
21. Eccles JC, Rall W. Effects induced in a monosynaptic reflex by its activation. *J Neurophysiol* 1951;14:353–376.
22. Hunt CC. Monosynaptic reflex response of spinal motoneurons to graded afferent stimulation. *J Gen Physiol* 1955;38:813–852.
23. Lloyd DPC, Wilson VJ. Reflex depression in rhythmically active monosynaptic reflex pathways. *J Gen Physiol* 1957;40:409–426.
24. Jefferson AA, Schlapp W. Some effects of repetitive stimulation of afferents on reflex conduction. In: Malcolm JL, Gray JAB, eds. *The Spinal Cord.* London: Churchill; 1953:99–119.
25. Beswick FB, Evanson JM. Reflex effects of repetitive stimulation of group I muscle afferent fibres. *J Physiol* 1955;128:83P–84P.
26. Frank K, Fuortes MGF. Presynaptic and postsynaptic inhibition of monosynaptic reflexes. *Fed Proc* 1957;16:39–40.
27. Rall W. Experimental monosynaptic input–output relations in the mammalian spinal cord. *J Cell Comp Physiol* 1955;46:413–438.
28. Kernell D, Hultborn H. Synaptic effects on recruitment gain: a mechanism of importance for the input–output of motoneurone pools? *Brain Res* 1990;507:176–179.
29. Eccles JC, Kostyuk PG, Schmidt RF. Central pathways responsible for depolarization of primary afferent pathways. *J Physiol* 1962;161:237–257.
30. Jankowska E, McCrea D, Rudomin P, Sykova E. Observations on neuronal pathways subserving primary afferent depolarization. *J Neurophysiol* 1981;46:506–516.
31. Rudomin P, Engberg I, Jimenez I. Mechanisms involved in presynaptic depolarization of group I and rubrospinal fibers in cat spinal cord. *J Neurophysiol* 1981;46:532–548.
32. Fyffe RE, Light AR. The ultrastructure of group Ia afferent fibre synapses in the lumbosacral spinal cord of the cat. *Brain Res* 1984;300:201–209.
33. Lev-Tov A, Meyers DRE, Burke RE. Activation of $GABA_b$ receptors in the intact mammalian spinal cord mimics the effects of reduced presynaptic calcium influx. *Proc Natl Acad Sci USA* 1988; 85:5330–5334.
34. Rudomin P, Jimenez I, Solodkin M, Duenas S. Sites of action of segmental and descending control of transmission on pathways mediating PAD of Ia and b afferent fibers in cat spinal cord. *J Neurophysiol* 1983;50:743–769.
35. Wall PD. Excitability changes in afferent fiber terminations and their relation to slow potentials. *J Physiol* 1958;142:1–21.
36. Eccles JC, Schmidt RF, Willis WD. The location and mode of action of the presynaptic inhibitory pathways on to group I afferent fibers from muscle. *J Neurophysiol* 1963;26:506–522.
37. Wrathall JR, Pettegrew RK, Harvey F. Spinal cord contusion in the rat: production of graded, reproducible injury groups. *Exp Neurol* 1985;88:108–122.
38. Kerasidis H, Wrathall JR, Gale K. Behavioral as-

sessment of functional deficit in rats with contusive spinal cord injury. *J Neurosci Methods* 1987; 20:167–189.
39. Reier PJ, Stokes BT, Thompson FJ, Anderson DK. Fetal cell grafts into resection and contusion/compression injuries of the adult rat and cat spinal cord. *Exp Neurol* 1992;115:177–188.
40. Reier PJ, Anderson DK, Thompson FJ, Stokes BT. Neural tissue transplantation and CNS trauma: anatomical and functional repair of the injured spinal cord. *J Neurotrauma* 1992;9:S223–S246.
41. Bregman BS. Spinal cord transplants permit the growth of serotonergic axons across the site of neonatal spinal cord transection. *Dev Brain Res* 1987;34:265–279.
42. Kunkel-Bagden E, Bregman BS. Spinal cord transplants enhance the recovery of locomotor function after spinal cord injury at birth. *Exp Brain Res* 1990;81:25–34.
43. Anderson DK, Reier PJ, Wirth ED, Theele DP, Mareci T, Brown SA. Delayed grafting of fetal CNS tissue into chronic compression lesions of the adult cat spinal cord. *Restor Neurol Neurosci* 1991; 2:309–325.
44. Kunkel-Bagden E, Reier PJ, Dai H, Bregman BS. Influence of fetal spinal cord transplants on recovery of motor function after spinal cord injury. *Soc Neurosci Abstr* 1991;17:236.
45. Stokes BT, Reier PJ. Fetal grafts alter chronic behavioral outcome after contusion damage to the adult rat spinal cord. *Exp Neurol* [*in press*].
46. Bregman BS, Reier PJ. Neural tissue transplants rescue axotomized rubrospinal cells from retrograde death. *J Comp Neurol* 1986;244:86–95.
47. Himes BT, Goldberger ME, Tessler A. Grafts of fetal CNS tissue rescue axotomized Clark's nucleus neurons in adult and neonatal operates. *Soc Neurosci Abstr* 1990;16:818.
48. Goldberger ME, Murray M. Patterns of sprouting and implications for recovery of function. In: Waxman SG, ed. *Advances in neurology,* Vol 47. Functional recovery in neurological disease, New York: Raven Press; 1988:361–385.
49. Thompson FJ, Parmer R, Reier PJ. Alterations in lumbar motoneuron excitability following thoracic contusion compared to hemisection spinal cord injury. *Soc Neurosci Abstr* 1991;17:161.

16

Intraspinal Transplants of Catecholamine-Containing Cells and Fetal Spinal Cord and Iris Tissues in the Adult Rat

H. O. Nornes, S. J. Moorman, A. R. Mihajlov, B. E. Pulford, and L. R. Whalen

Department of Anatomy and Neurobiology, Program in Neuronal Growth and Development, Colorado State University, Fort Collins, Colorado 80523

Tello (1) and Ramón y Cajal (2) observed that transplants of peripheral nerve into the spinal cord promote central nervous system (CNS) regeneration. Since these early findings, investigators have used transplants to examine the underlying mechanisms of CNS regeneration and to reconstruct the injured CNS (reviewed in refs. 3–6).

There are two basic rationales for transplanting tissue in the lesioned CNS: (a) to replace lost inputs and (b) to provide tissue with maintenance factors and bridging substrates to prevent retrograde cell death and promote regeneration. It is well documented that transplants of fetal CNS tissue interact with the adult CNS in a specific manner with respect to both target localization (7–11) and function (12–16). In the experiments reviewed in this chapter, we show that catecholamine (CA)-containing cells transplanted into the adult spinal cord restore a CA-specific deficit, and we describe the regeneration of host fibers into intraspinal transplants of fetal spinal cord and adult iris tissues.

The CA-dependent long-latency component (LLC) of the hindlimb withdrawal reflex, first described by Anden and Jankowska (17,18), was used to assess functional recovery following transplantation (19). In the acute spinal rat, the LLC and associated force are elicited only after CA activation with L-dopa. Chemical denervation of the spinal CA system with 6-hydroxydopamine (6-OHDA) results in loss of both the LLC and the associated force. Transplants of fetal CA-containing cells from the locus ceruleus partially restore the LLC and accompanying force 2 and 4 months post-transplantation. This response is blocked with the α-adrenergic receptor antagonist phentolamine, and the average maximum force correlates with the number of surviving CA cells in the transplant. These two results indicate that the response from the transplant is CA specific.

Subsequent to these initial experiments, we determined if similar responses occur using a neurosecretory transplantation model. Cultured neonatal adrenal chromaffin cells, which secrete catecholamines (20), were implanted into the CA-denervated spinal cord. Animals tested 3 months post-transplantation had partially restored LLCs and associated forces. Histological examination revealed the presence of CA-immunoreactive cells at the implantation sites.

The rationale of using transplants as a "bridge" at the site of the lesion has been tested in a variety of systems in the CNS (reviewed in refs. 3–6). The combination of fetal hippocampal tissue and NGF infusions enhances both the survival and regeneration of forebrain cholinergic neurons into the hippocampus (21,22). A variety of tissues, including peripheral nerve (23–25), collagen matrix (26), and cultured Schwann cells (27), have been used as tissue "bridges" in the adult spinal cord, and the results basically mimic the original Tello and Cajal observations—host axons regenerate into the transplant but fail to reenter the host spinal cord from the transplant. In the lesioned neonatal rat spinal cord, implanted fetal spinal cord tissue prevents retrograde cell loss of rubrospinal tract neurons and provides a substrate for regeneration of descending serotonergic fibers across the transection and into the distal cord (28). It remains unclear, however, whether fetal transplants might serve as a functional "bridge" in the adult spinal cord. Fetal spinal cord tissue, when placed into cavities in the adult rat spinal cord, grows, differentiates, and integrates well with the host tissue (29–35). In spite of this tissue continuity, the regeneration of host fibers into these transplants is minimal (32–34,36).

The fetal spinal cord tissue used in the above experiments was from rat embryos at a developmental stage in the latter half of neurogenesis (crown–rump 12 to 15 mm; day 14 and greater of gestation). Neurons of the spinal cord of rat originate on days 11 to 16 of gestation (37). We review in this chapter our observations of descending CA fiber regeneration into fetal spinal cord transplants that are developmentally in the first half of neurogenesis (8 and 11 mm crown–rump; days 12 to 14 of gestation) (38). This regeneration into fetal tissue was also compared with the regeneration of this same spinal fiber system into transplants of adult iris. Catecholamine fibers have been shown to regenerate into adult iris implanted into the brainstem (39).

TRANSPLANTS OF CATECHOLAMINE-CONTAINING CELLS RESTORE A CA-SPECIFIC DEFICIT OF THE HINDLIMB WITHDRAWAL REFLEX

Role of Descending CA Fibers in the Withdrawal Reflex

Flexor reflex afferent fibers (FRAs), which include group II and III muscle afferents, joint afferents, and low- and high-threshold cutaneous afferents, converge on interneurons within the spinal cord. Lundberg (40) postulates that these fibers are capable of evoking the withdrawal reflex by activating neuronal networks that excite flexor α-motoneurons in the ventral horn of the cord. This reflex is modulated by norepinephrine (NE) fibers from the locus ceruleus (brainstem), which synapse bilaterally in the spinal cord dorsal, intermediolateral, and ventral horns (41). Jankowska et al. (18) found that electrical stimulation of the FRAs prior to administration of L-dopa in spinal animals elicits a low-threshold, short-latency-to-onset response from the biceps femoris muscle, and stimulation after injection of L-dopa evokes a large-amplitude discharge in flexor motoneurons having both a longer latency to onset and longer duration of evoked muscle activity. Monoamine oxidase inhibitors such as pargyline produce a tenfold potentiation of the L-dopa effects. Anden (17) has also shown that α-adrenergic receptor blockers such as phenoxybenzamine and phentolamine are capable of blocking the L-dopa effects on the withdrawal reflex.

Restoration of the CA-Activated Long-Latency Component (LLC) with Fetal Transplants

Cells from Fetal Locus Ceruleus Tissue, When Transplanted into the Adult Rat Spinal Cord, Survive and Extend Processes

Intraspinal transplants of fetal monoamine-containing cells survive and extend

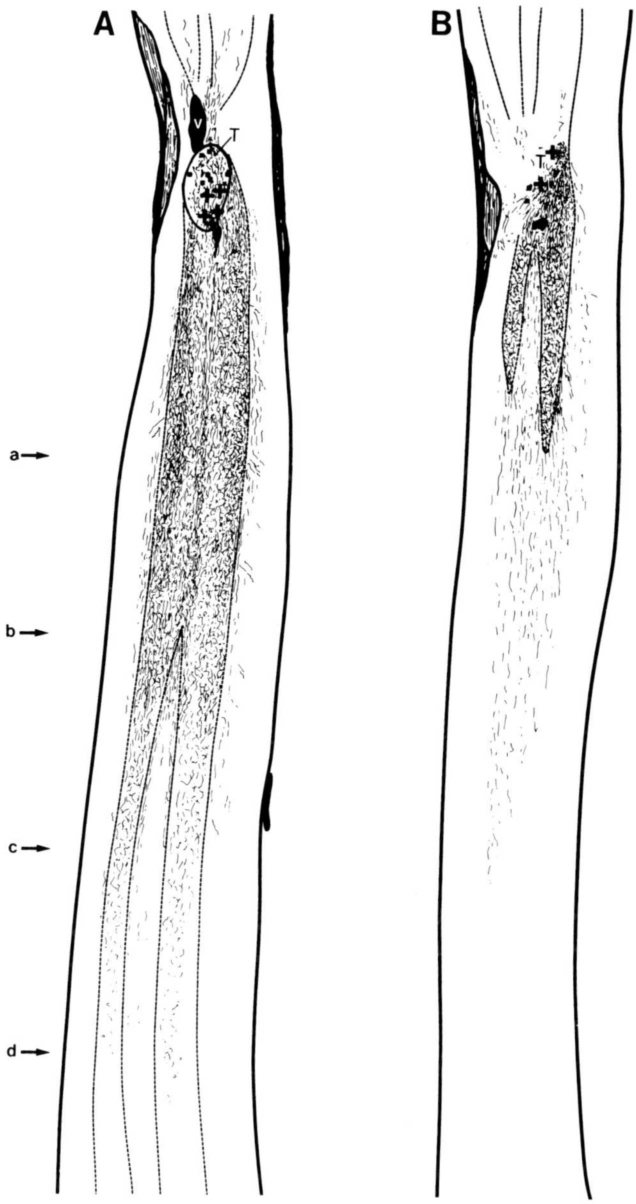

FIG. 1. Camera lucida drawings of the distribution of CA fibers from a locus ceruleus transplant into an adult rat spinal cord (6 months post-transplantation). The tissue was processed histochemically for monoamine histofluorescence (54). The transplant was dissected from a 16-mm fetus and placed into a small subpial cavity in the lower thoracic region. The host spinal cord had been denervated of its CA fibers with the neurotoxin 6-OHDA prior to transplantation. (**A**) Drawing from a horizontal section through the intermediate gray including the transplant (T) and the ventral gray more caudally. Note that the transplant fuses well with the host tissue, and the CA-containing cell bodies (*small squares*) are scattered throughout the transplant. An ependymal-lined cavity (V) is associated with the transplant. Also note that CA fibers have grown from the transplant bilaterally in the intermediate and ventral gray matter, with normal density of CA fibers up to about 3 to 5.5 mm from the transplant (levels a, b). They gradually become more sparse 8.5 mm (level c) and 11 mm (level d) from the graft. (**B**) Drawing of a section ventral to the section in **A.** Note the presence of CA fibers in the ventral gray matter with a few extending into the white matter beyond 5.5 mm. (Reproduced from Nornes et al., ref. 46, with permission.)

processes several millimeters in length (42–45). In our initial experiment, pieces of fetal brainstem containing the anlage of the catecholamine-containing neurons of the locus ceruleus nucleus were transplanted into the lesioned spinal cords of adult rats (46). The descending CA fibers in the host were lesioned with an intrascisternal injection of 250 μg of 6-OHDA 14 days prior to transplantation. Figure 1 illustrates the growth of processes from a solid transplant inserted into a subpial intraspinal cavity (caudal thoracic) of an adult rat 6 months post-transplantation. The CA-fluorescing fibers from the transplant extended primarily into the gray matter of the host. The density of fibers

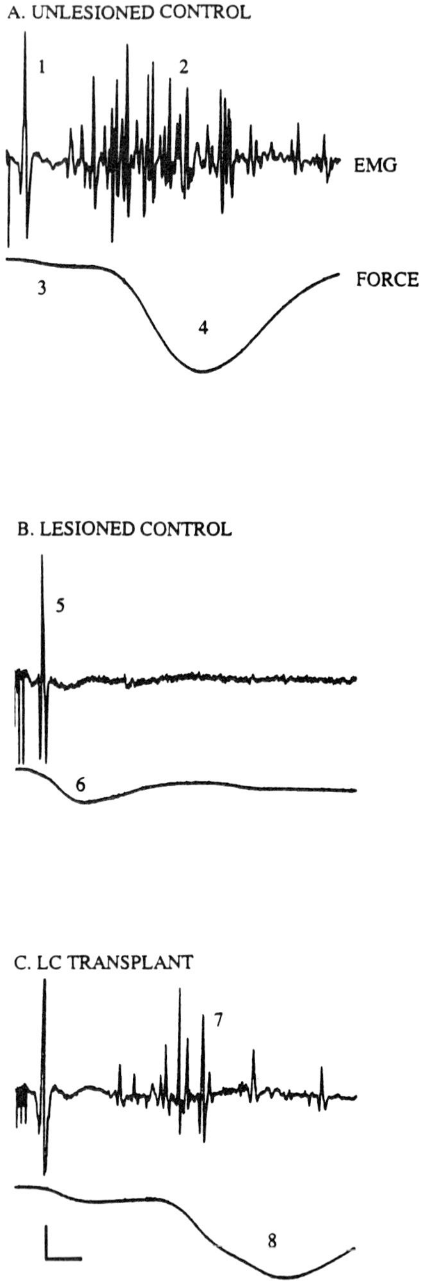

FIG. 2. Recovery of long-latency component and associated force of the withdrawal reflex following intraspinal transplantation of fetal locus ceruleus cells. The top trace in each pair is a recording of the reflex-evoked electrical activity in a muscle (EMG) that produces force during the withdrawal reflex. The bottom trace in each pair is a recording of the force production associated with the reflex (downward deflection, increase in force). (**A**) Unlesioned control animal after administration of L-dopa: (1) the short-latency component of the reflex; (2) the long-latency component of the reflex; (3) the force associated with the short-latency component of the reflex; and (4) the force associated with the long-latency component of the reflex. (Scale bars: horizontal, 15 msec; vertical, 50 μV for EMG, 47 g for force). (**B**) 6-OHDA-lesioned control animal after administration of L-dopa: (5) the short-latency component of the reflex and (6) the force production associated with the short-latency component of the reflex. There is no long-latency component of the reflex or associated force production. (Scale bars: horizontal, 15 msec; vertical, 50 μV for EMG, 19 g for force). (**C**) 6-OHDA-lesioned animal with a transplant of fetal locus ceruleus cells before administration of L-dopa: (7 and 8) the long-latency component of the reflex and its associated force production. (Scale bars: horizontal, 15 msec; vertical, 50 μV for EMG, 19 g for force). (Reproduced from Moorman et al., ref. 19, with permission.)

was greatest within the 5.5 mm of host spinal cord adjacent to the transplant–host boundary and was gradually reduced, with a few fibers fluorescing at a distance of 11 mm from the transplant.

Reflex Activity Can Be Partially Restored with Fetal Locus Ceruleus Implants

A neurochemical lesion with 6-OHDA of the descending CA fiber system results in loss of the LLC of the flexion reflex, and lesioned animals with transplants of fetal CA-containing cells have this specific component restored. The descending spinal CA fibers were lesioned in adult female rats (14 weeks of age) as described in the previous section. Ten to 14 days post-lesion, separate cell suspensions of the anlagen of both the locus ceruleus (LC) and the rhombic lip (RL) were prepared from 13- to 14-mm rat embryos. These suspensions were injected intervertebrally into three sites on the left side of the lumbar spinal cord from L-1 to L-4.

The rats receiving transplants were divided into two equal groups, and their hindlimb withdrawal reflexes were tested at either 2 or 4 months post-transplant. The spinal cord was transected at T-5 in all rats prior to reflex testing. In this type of preparation in an unlesioned control rat, thc LLC component of the flexion reflex is elicited by electrical stimulation only after the administration of L-dopa (Fig. 2A). The lesioned controls, 2 months post-lesion, lack this component after either pargyline or L-dopa administration (Fig. 2B). Lesioned control rats 4 months post-lesion show an inconsistent response to stimulation after administration of pargyline and L-dopa, and the size of the LLC is not linked to stimulus intensity. In lesioned animals with LC transplants 2 months post-transplantation, 40% (4/10) had a LLC prior to the administration of L-dopa. Following L-dopa administration, stimulation elicited a LLC in 80% of the lesioned rats (Fig. 2C). In the 4-month post-transplantation LC group, LLCs were evoked in 75% (6/8) of the rats both before and after L-dopa administration. This response prior to L-dopa administration indicates that the CA cells in the transplant are spontaneously releasing NE. Also, the LLC responses in the animals with LC transplants are highly correlated with stimulus strengths, which suggests that the transplanted cells are contributing to the recovery of the flexor reflex.

The rats transplanted with cell suspensions prepared from the rhombic lip (RL) were intended to be controls, i.e., fetal transplants lacking CA-containing cells. To our surprise, stimulation of the hindpaw of lesioned animals that received RL transplants also elicited LLCs. LLCs were observed before the administration of L-dopa in two of the seven rats tested 2 months post-transplantation and in five of the nine rats tested at 4 months. Histological examination revealed that the rhombic lip transplants also contained CA cell bodies, which explains this seemingly inconsistent result.

Force Production Associated with the Restored LLC

The size of the LLC is correlated to the force produced during the withdrawal reflex.

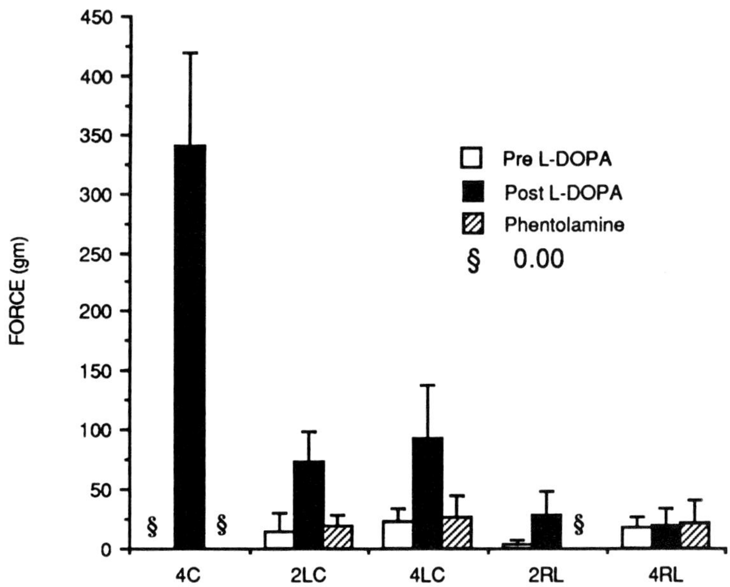

FIG. 3. Average maximum force production per implant group before administration of L-dopa, after L-dopa, and after administration of phentolamine. 4C, 4-month unlesioned control group; 2LC, 2-month locus ceruleus implant group; 4LC, 4-month locus ceruleus implant group; 2RL, 2-month rhombic lip implant group; 4RL, 4-month rhombic lip implant group. Error bars, S.E.M. (Reproduced from Moorman et al., ref. 19, with permission.)

In the unlesioned control animals, the LLC and its associated force are evoked only after the administration of L-dopa (Fig. 3). Similarly, lesioned control animals (16 of 18) lacked a LLC and its associated force before the administration of L-dopa. In contrast to unlesioned control rats, however, 14 of these same lesioned animals still lacked a LLC after drug administration. In LC transplant animals, both 2 and 4 months post-transplantation, stimulation of the hindpaw resulted in a LLC in 10 of 18 rats prior to L-dopa administration. This number increased to 14 of 18 animals after drug administration, and the force of withdrawal increased four- to fivefold (Fig. 3). After

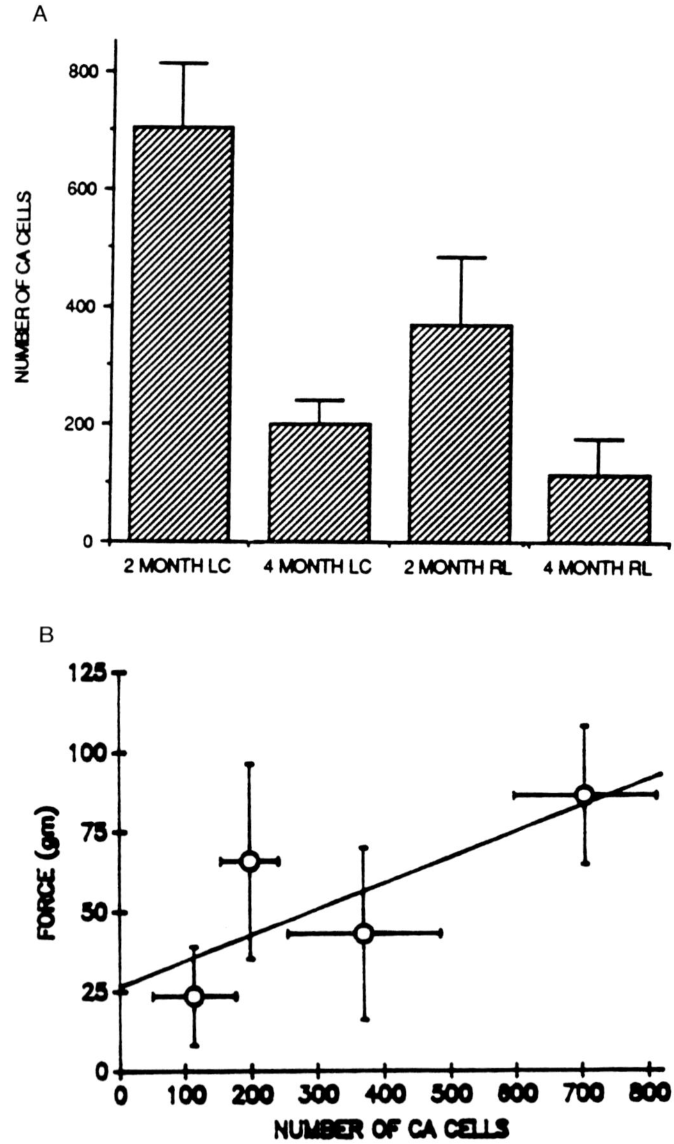

FIG. 4. (**A**) Average number of CA-fluorescent cells per implant group. Error bars, S.E.M. (**B**) Plot of average number of CA-fluorescent cells per implant group versus average maximum force produced in grams per implant group. Linear regression line $r = 0.78$. Error bars, S.E.M. (Reproduced from Moorman et al., ref. 19, with permission.)

administration of phentolamine, an α-adrenergic receptor antagonist (47), the force returned to levels seen before L-dopa administration in both the unlesioned control and LC-transplant animals (Fig. 3). This demonstrates that the increase in force associated with L-dopa administration is mediated by NE.

Catecholamine Cell Counts in Transplants versus Force

A plot of the average number of CA cells in each implant group versus the average maximum force associated with the LLC from each group has a correlation coefficient of 0.78 (Fig. 4B). This positive correlation further supports the hypothesis that the transplants play a role in the evoked CA-specific response in the host animals.

These observations were made on LC-implanted spinal cords processed for catecholamine histofluorescence (48). The number of CA cells found in the sectioned spinal cord tissue of the implanted animals ranged from 36 to 1,036, and CA-fluorescing fibers were found along the entire length of gray matter between implantation sites. No CA cells were found in the spinal cords of either the lesioned or unlesioned control animals. The average number of CA cells in the 4-month post-transplantation groups was found to be less than in the 2-month groups (Fig. 4A). This same trend of declining cell numbers with time was observed in our previous work using the same model system (45). This points out the need for investigating ways to promote implanted cell survival.

Restoration of the Long-Latency Component of the Flexion Reflex with Transplants of Cultured Adrenal Medullary Cells

A fundamental question is whether the transplants evoke their function via a synaptic or neurosecretory mechanism. This question was investigated indirectly by using the same CA-dependent functional test as described above following implantation of cultured adrenal medullary (AM) chromaffin cells. Previous studies have shown that AM chromaffin cells survive implantation into the spinal cord but fail to grow processes into the host tissue (49). We also attempted to induce fiber growth of the implanted AM chromaffin cells by cotransplanting Schwann (SC) cells with the AM cells. In *in vitro* conditions, NGF, which is secreted by SC cells, induces AM chromaffin cells to extend long CA-containing processes (50,51).

Cell suspensions of cultured neonatal AM chromaffin cells, SC cells, or a mixture of the two cell types were implanted into the lumbar region of the rat spinal cord 2 weeks after catecholamine denervation by intracisternal injection of 6-OHDA. Chromaffin cells from 7-day neonates were cultured for 10 days in the presence of NGF (40 ng/ml). The SC cells were prepared from sciatic nerve of the same age rat pups and cultured for 1 to 3 days in the presence of cytosine arabinoside to reduce fibroblast proliferation. Three months after implantation of the cell suspensions, the extent of implant-associated recovery of reflex activity was determined electrophysiologically.

The LLCs and associated force measurements of the hindlimb withdrawal reflex were partially restored in animals that received cell suspensions of cultured neonatal chromaffin cells (Fig. 5). Implanting SC cells conjointly with chromaffin cells did not aid in the recovery of this reflex (Fig. 5). This latter result is in contrast to previous studies in which SC cells enhanced AM cell survival and function (52). Implanting SC cells alone also did not aid in recovery of the reflex, which indicates that nonspecific effects from implanting cells into the spinal cord are not responsible for the observed functional recovery of the AM group. A small percentage (<1%) of the chromaffin cells initially injected at each site survived. The CA-immunoreactive cells were round in shape with short or no processes and were well integrated into the parenchyma of the spinal cord.

In this investigation, we demonstrated that cultured neonatal chromaffin cell implants

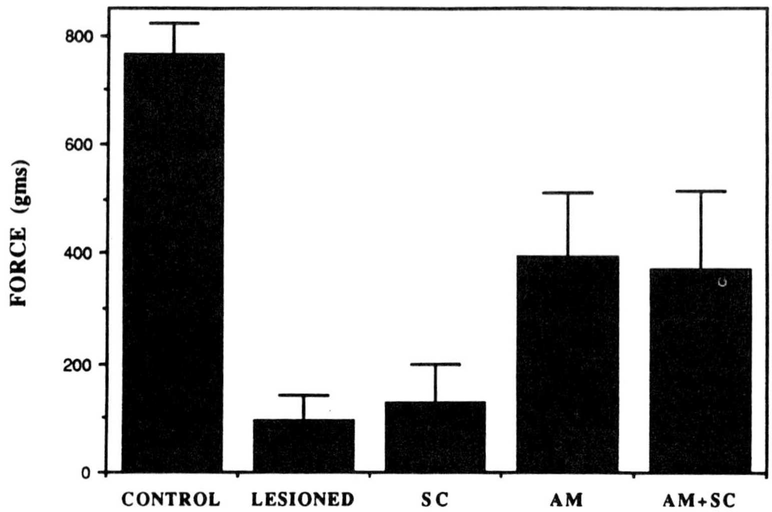

FIG. 5. Average maximum force produced during the long-latency component of the withdrawal reflex after L-dopa administration by each experimental group of host rats 3 months post-transplantation. The adrenal medullary (AM) and AM + Schwann (SC) implant groups produced significantly more force than did the 6-OHDA-lesioned control or SC implantation groups but significantly less force than the unlesioned control animals. There was no statistical difference between the AM and AM + SC groups or between lesioned and SC cell implant rats.

are able to survive for 3 months in the rat spinal cord and are as effective as fetal tissue implants at restoring hindlimb withdrawal reflex function. The question concerning the potential benefits of implanting Schwann cells along with chromaffin cells in order to increase viability and induce morphological changes in the chromaffin cells remains unanswered.

INTRASPINAL TRANSPLANTS OF FETAL SPINAL CORD AND ADULT IRIS

Fetal Spinal Cord Implants

Pieces of fetal spinal cord tissue dissected from 8- and 11-mm rat embryos were transplanted into subpial cavities in the lower thoracic region of adult rats. The extent of the spinal cavities ranged from hemisection to nearly complete transection of the cord. Seventeen animals were analyzed 2.5 to 12 months post-transplantation, and 14 animals had surviving transplants.

The transplanted fetal spinal cord tissue grows and forms tissue continuity with the host cord (Fig. 6A,a,B,b). Silver-stained preparations show that host fibers in the white matter die back from the transplant–host boundary; however, in the gray matter, the fibers extend up to and course along the transplant–host boundary. It appears that the fibers of the gray matter sprout along the boundary; however, few if any cross the transplant–host boundary (Fig. 6C,c,D,d). The results were similar for both the 8- and 11-mm developmental stages.

Catecholamine-histofluorescent preparations of these intraspinal transplants reveal minimal regeneration of host descending CA-fluorescing fibers into the fetal transplants. Figure 7 illustrates a typical CA-histofluorescent preparation where there was intense fluorescence from the descending CA fibers on the cranial side of the host–transplant boundary. In regions with good tissue continuity, a few CA fibers cross the boundary and extend less than 1 mm into the transplant tissue. This lack of regeneration is similar for both developmental stages.

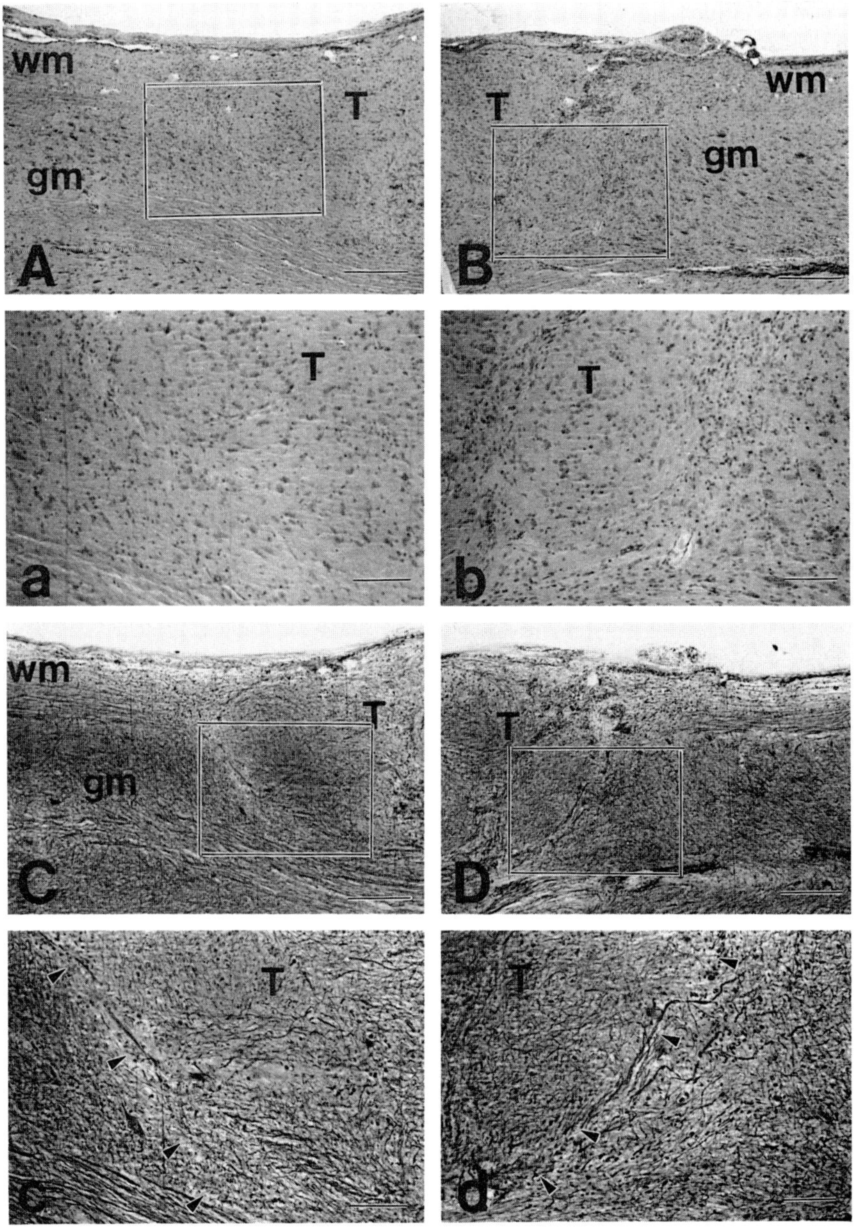

FIG. 6. Horizontal sections of fetal spinal cord transplant (T) in adult spinal cord of rat 8 months post-transplantation. Donor tissue was dissected from an 8-mm rat fetus (day 12) and inserted into a subpial cavity in the lower thoracic region. (**A**) Tissue integration at the rostral boundary of the transplant and host tissues. (**a**) Enlargement of the square in **A.** (**B**) Tissue integration at the caudal boundary of the transplant and host tissues. (**b**) Enlargement of the square in **B.** (**C** and **D**) Alternate section to **A** and **B** above stained with a fiber stain (Bodian). Note the dieback of the fibers in the white matter (wm) and the coursing of fibers up to and along the boundary of the host and transplant in the gray matter (gm). (**c** and **d**) Enlargements of the squares indicated in **C** and **D;** *arrowheads,* host–transplant boundary. Magnification bars in **A, B, C,** and **D,** 300 μm; in **a, b, c,** and **d,** 100 μm.

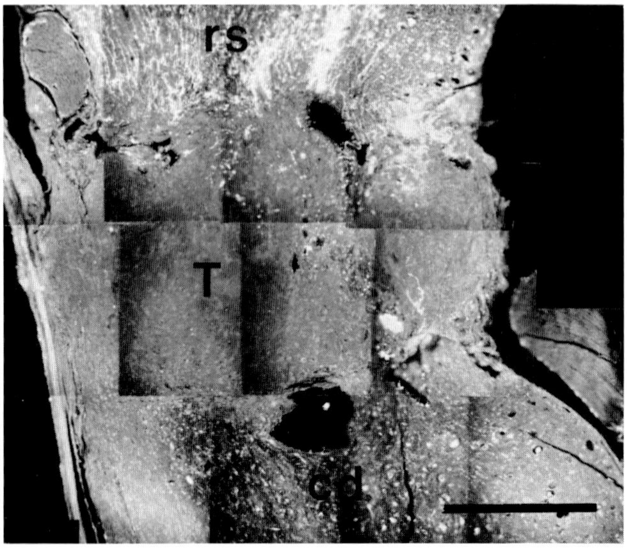

FIG. 7. Horizontal section of intraspinal transplant of fetal spinal cord tissue processed for catecholamine histofluorescent chemistry (54) 5.5 months post-transplantation. The fetal tissue was dissected from an 11-mm rat fetus and inserted into a nearly complete subpial transection, which was prepared by gentle suction in the lower thoracic region of an adult rat. The transplant (T) filled most of the site of transection and established tissue continuity with both the rostral (rs) and caudal (cd) stumps of the host spinal cord. Note the abundance of CA fluorescing in the rostral stump of the host cord and the few CA-fluorescing fibers that had regenerated into the transplant. Magnification bar, 400 μm.

Adult Iris Implants

Iris tissue was dissected from adult rats and implanted into subpial cavities in the lower thoracic region of nearly completely transected spinal cords of adult rats. The transplants were homotypic. Five of the nine animals analyzed had surviving transplants. Descending CA-fluorescing fibers from the rostral stump of the host spinal cord cross the transplant–host boundary and extend into the entire iris transplant (Fig. 8A). When the iris tissue is inserted into the transplant cavity, the tissue folds as it settles into the confines of the cavity. In some specimens, the highest density of CA fibers was around the perimeter of the transplant (Fig. 8B). This strong perimeter fluorescence is typical for the normal rat iris (53) and suggests that the regenerating fibers return to the original CA innervation sites on the transplanted iris.

SUMMARY AND CONCLUSIONS

Intraspinal transplants of CA-containing cells prepared from fetal brainstem or adrenal medulla restore the CA-specific component of the withdrawal reflex, i.e., LLC, and partially restore the associated force levels. This transplant-mediated response is blocked with phentolamine, an α-adrenergic antagonist, which indicates a CA-specific effect from the transplant. Since the transplants of adrenal medullary cells partially restore this CA-specific reflex component in the absence of processes extending into host spinal cord, it is likely that the CA-containing cells in the transplant mediate their function via neurosecretory mechanisms. These two experiments show that the lesioned spinal cord is capable of developing functional interactions with transplanted tissue, in these cases from transplants, and that transplants can be used to

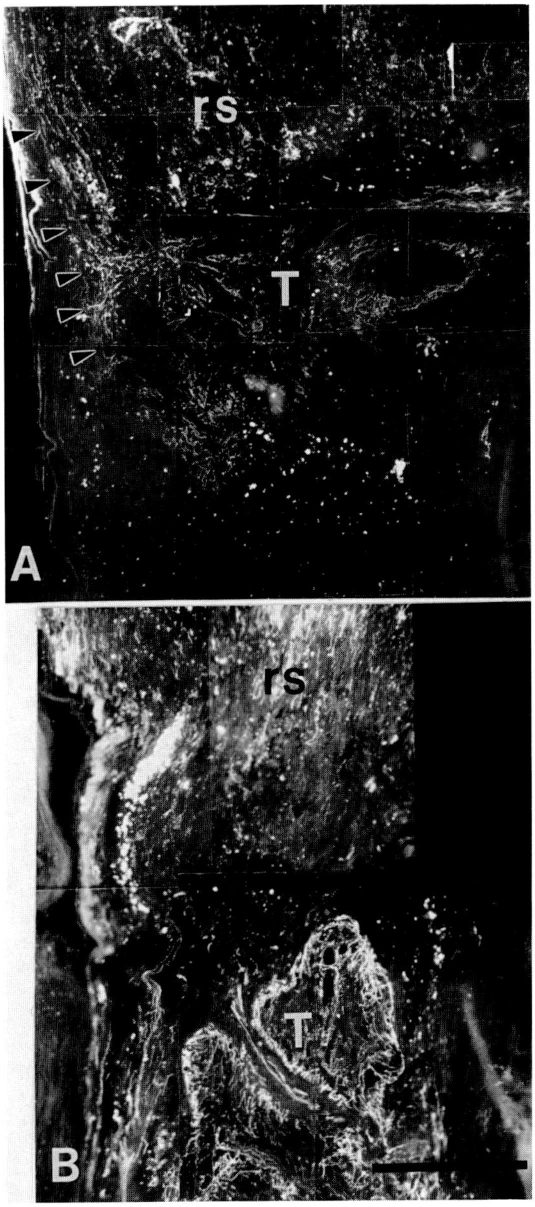

FIG. 8. Horizontal sections of intraspinal transplants (homotypic) of adult iris tissue processed for catecholamine histofluorescent chemistry (54) 5.5 months posttransplantation. The iris tissue was dissected from the host according to Malmfors (53) and inserted into nearly complete subpial transections, which were prepared by gentle suction in the lower thoracic region of adult rats. (**A**) Note the CA-fluorescing descending fibers in the rostral stump (rs) of the spinal cord that cross the host–transplant boundary and extend into the entire iris transplant (T) (*arrowheads*). (**B**) The circular iris tissue has folded into the confines of the subpial cavity. Note the abundance of CA-fluorescing fibers in the rostral stump of the host spinal cord and in the entire iris transplant, particularly along its perimeter. Magnification bar, 400 μm.

deliver molecules to the CNS, in this case a neurotransmitter.

Intraspinal transplants of fetal spinal cord from 8- and 11-mm embryos grow and form tissue continuity with the host spinal cord. Silver-stained preparations and CA histofluorescence reveal few if any neuronal processes crossing the host–transplant boundary. By contrast, there is abundant regeneration of CA fibers into transplants of adult iris. Thus, these particular fibers in the spinal cord have the potential for regeneration if provided with a permissive substrate. Whether the lack of regeneration into the fetal spinal cord transplants was caused by inhibition at the transplant–host boundary or within the fetal tissue itself cannot be determined from these studies. More basic studies examining the molecular and cellular basis of this tissue interaction will be required for further progress.

ACKNOWLEDGMENTS

This research was supported by NIH grant NS21309-05 to H. O. Nornes and a grant from the American Paralysis Association to L. R. Whalen and H. O. Nornes.

REFERENCES

1. Tello F. La influencia del neurotropismo en la regeneracion de los centros nerviosos. *Trab Lab Invest Biol* 1911;9:123–159.
2. Ramón y Cajal S. *Degeneration and regeneration of the nervous system.* London: Oxford University Press; 1928.
3. Björklund A, Stenevi U. Intracerebral neural implants: neuronal replacement and reconstruction of damaged circuitries. *Annu Rev Neurosci* 1984; 7:279–308.
4. Nornes HO, Björklund A, Stenevi U. Transplantation strategies in spinal cord regeneration. In: Sladek JR, Gash DM, eds. *Neural transplants.* New York: Plenum Press; 1984:407–421.
5. Reier PJ, Bregman BS, Wujeck JR, Tessler A. Intraspinal transplantation of fetal spinal cord tissue; an approach toward functional repair of the injured spinal cord. In: Goldberger ME, Gorio A, Murray M, eds. *Development and plasticity of the mammalian spinal cord.* Padova: Liviana Press; 1986:251–269.
6. Das G. Neural transplantation: an historical perspective. *Neurosci Biobehav Rev* 1990;14:389–401.
7. Björklund A, Stenevi U. Reconstruction of brain circuitries by neural transplants. *Trends Neurosci* 1979;2:301–306.
8. Raisman G, Ebner FF. Mossy fibre projection into and out of hippocampal transplants. *Neuroscience* 1983;9:783–901.
9. Zhou CF, Raisman G, Morris RJ. Specific patterns of fibre outgrowth from transplants to host mice hippocampi, shown immunohistochemically by the use of allelic forms of Thy-1. *Neuroscience* 1985; 16:819–833.
10. Zhou CF, Li Y, Raisman G. Embryonic entorhinal transplants project selectively to the deafferented entorhinal zone of adult mouse hippocampi, as demonstrated by the use of Thy-1 allelic immunohistochemistry. Effect of timing of transplantation in relation to deafferentation. *Neuroscience* 1989; 32:349–362.
11. Lewis ER, Mueller JC, Cotman CW. Neonatal septal implants: development of afferent lamination in the rat dentate gyrus. *Brain Res Bull* 1980; 5:217–221.
12. Björklund A, Stenevi U, Dunnett SB, Iversen SD. Functional reactivation of deafferented neostriatum by nigral transplants. *Nature* 1981;289:497–499.
13. Perlow MJ, Freed WJ, Hoffer BJ, Seiger A, Olson L, Wyatt RJ. Brain grafts reduce motor abnormalities produced by destruction of nigrostriatal dopamine system. *Science* 1979;204:643–647.
14. Gash D, Sladek JR, Sladek SD. Functional development of grafted vasopressin neurons. *Science* 1980;210:1367–1369.
15. Krieger DT, Perlow MJ, Gibson MJ, et al. Brain grafts reverse hypogonadism of gonadotropin releasing hormone deficiency. *Nature* 1982;298:468–471.
16. Dunnett SB, Low WC, Iversen SD, Stenevi U, Björklund A. Septal transplants restore maze learning in rats with fornix–fimbria lesions. *Brain Res* 1982;251:335–348.
17. Anden NE, Jukes MGM, Lundberg A, Vyklicky L. The effect of DOPA on the spinal cord. 1. Influence on transmission from primary afferents. *Acta Physiol Scand* 1966;67:373–386.
18. Jankowska E, Jukes MGM, Lund S, Lundberg A. The effect of DOPA on the spinal cord: 6. Half center organization of interneurons transmitting effects from the flexor reflex afferents. *Acta Physiol Scand* 1967;70:389–402.
19. Moorman SJ, Whalen LR, Nornes HO. A neurotransmitter specific functional recovery mediated by fetal implants in the lesioned spinal cord of the rat. *Brain Res* 1990;508:194–198.
20. Livett BG, Dean DM, Whelen LG, Udenfriend SA, Rossier J. Co-release of enkephalin and catecholamine from cultured adrenal chromaffin cells. *Nature* 1981;289:317–319.
21. Kromer LF, Björklund A, Stenevi U. Regeneration of the septohippocampal pathways in adult rats is promoted by utilizing embryonic hippocampal implants as bridges. *Brain Res* 1981;210:173–200.
22. Tuszynski MH, Buzsaki G, Gage FH. Nerve growth factor infusions combined with fetal hippocampal grafts enhance reconstruction of the lesioned septohippocampal projection. *Neuroscience* 1990;36: 33–44.
23. Richardson PM, McGuiness UM, Aguayo AJ. Axons from CNS neurons regenerate into PNS grafts. *Nature* 1980;284:264–265.
24. David S, Aguayo AJ. Axonal elongation into PNS "bridges" after central nervous system injury in adult rats. *Science* 1981;214:931–933.
25. Wrathall J, Rigamonti DD, Braford MR, Kao CC. Reconstruction of the contused cat spinal cord by the delayed nerve graft technique and cultured peripheral non-neuronal cells. *Acta Neuropathol* 1982;57:59–69.
26. Gelderd JB. Evaluation of blood vessel and neurite growth into a collagen matrix placed within a surgically created gap in rat spinal cord. *Brain Res* 1990;511:80–92.
27. Kuhlengel KR, Bunge MB, Bunge RP. Implantation of cultured sensory neurons and Schwann cells into lesioned neonatal rat spinal cord. II. Implant characteristics and examination of corticospinal tract growth. *J Comp Neurol* 1990;293:74–91.
28. Bregman BS. Spinal cord transplants permit the growth of serotonergic axons across the site of neona-

tal spinal cord transection. *Dev Brain Res* 1987;34:265–279.
29. Patel U, Bernstein J. Growth, differentiation and viability of fetal rat cortical and spinal cord implants into adult rat spinal cord. *J Neurosci Res* 1983;9:303–310.
30. Bernstein JJ, Patel U, Kelemen M, Turtil S. Ultrastructure of fetal spinal cord and cortex implants into adult rat spinal cord. *J Neurosci Res* 1984;11:359–372.
31. Das GD. Neural transplantation in the spinal cord of adult rats. *J Neurol Sci* 1983;62:191–210.
32. Pallini R, Fernandez E, Gangitano C, Del Fa A, Olivieri-Sangiacomo C, Sbriccoli A. Studies on embryonic transplants to the transected spinal cord of adult rats. *J Neurosurg* 1989;70:454–462.
33. Reier PJ, Bregman BS, Wujek JR. Intraspinal transplantation of embryonic spinal cord tissue in neonatal and adult rats. *J Comp Neurol* 1986; 247:275–296.
34. Houle JD, Reier PJ. Transplantation of fetal spinal cord tissue into the chronically injured adult rat spinal cord. *J Comp Neurol* 1988;269:535–547.
35. Jakeman LB, Reier PJ, Bregman BS, et al. Differentiation of substantia gelatinosa-like regions in intraspinal and intracerebral transplants of embryonic spinal cord tissue in the rat. *Exp Neurol* 1989;103:17–33.
36. Nothias F, Peschanski M. Homotypic fetal transplants into an experimental model of spinal cord neurodegeneration. *J Comp Neurol* 1990;301: 520–534.
37. Nornes HO, Das GD. Temporal pattern of neurogenesis in spinal cord of rat. I. An autoradiographic study—time and sites of origin and migration and settling patterns of neuroblasts. *Brain Res* 1974; 73:121–138.
38. Olson L, Seiger A. Early prenatal ontogeny of central monoamine neurons in rat: fluorescent histochemical observations. *Z Anat Entwickl Gesch* 1972;137:301–316.
39. Björklund A, Stenevi U. Growth of central catecholamine neurones into smooth muscle grafts in the rat mesencephalon. *Brain Res* 1971;31:1–20.
40. Lundberg A. Multisensory control of spinal reflex pathways. In: Granit R, Pompeiano O, eds. *Progress in brain research, Vol. 50. Reflex control of posture and movement.* Amsterdam: Elsevier/North-Holland Biomedical Press; 1979:11–28.
41. Björklund A, Skagerberg B. Descending monoaminergic projection to the spinal cord. In: Sjolund B, Björklund A, eds. *Brainstem control of spinal mechanisms.* Amsterdam: Elsevier/North-Holland Biomedical Press; 1982:55–87.
42. Nygren LO, Olson L, Seiger A. Monoaminergic reinnervation of the transected spinal cord by homologous brain grafts. *Brain Res* 1977;129:227–235.
43. Commissiong JW. Fetal locus coeruleus transplanted into the transected spinal cord of the adult rat: some observations and implications. *Neuroscience* 1984;12:839–853.
44. Privat A, Mansour H, Rajaofetra N, et al. Intraspinal transplants of serotonergic neurons in the adult rat. *Brain Res Bull* 1989;22:123–129.
45. Buchanan JT, Nornes HO. Transplants of embryonic brainstem containing the locus coeruleus into spinal cord enhance the hindlimb flexion in adult rats. *Brain Res* 1986;381:225–236.
46. Nornes H, Björklund A, Stenevi U. Reinnervation of the denervated adult spinal cord of rats by intraspinal transplants of embryonic brain stem neurons. *Cell Tissue Res* 1983;230:15–35.
47. Biscoe TJ, Curtis DR, Ryall RW. An investigation of catecholamine receptors of spinal interneurons. *Int J Neuropharmacol* 1966;5:429–434.
48. de la Torre JC. Standardization of the SPG histofluorescence method for monoamine transmitters. *Soc Neurosci Abstr* 1981;7:33.
49. Jones CL, Buchanan JT, Nornes HO. Adrenal medulla implants in the adult rat spinal cord. *Soc Neurosci Abstr* 1983;9:696.
50. Unsicker K, Krisch B, Otten U, Thoenen H. Nerve growth factor-induced fiber outgrowth from isolated rat adrenal chromaffin cells. Impairment by glucocorticoids. *Proc Natl Acad Sci USA* 1978; 75:3498–3502.
51. Grothe C, Hofman H-D, Verhofstad AAJ, Unsicker K. Nerve growth factor and dexamethasone specify the catecholaminoergic phenotype of cultured rat chromaffin cells: dependence on developmental stage. *Dev Brain Res* 1985;21:125–132.
52. Kordower JH, Fiandaca MS, Notter MFD, Hansen JT, Gash DM. NGF-like trophic support from peripheral nerve for grafted rhesus adrenal chromaffin cells. *J Neurosurg* 1990;73:418–473.
53. Malmfors T. Studies on adrenergic nerves. *Acta Physiol Scand [Suppl]* 1965;248:1–93.
54. Loren I, Björklund A, Falck B, Lindvall O. The aluminum–formaldehyde (ALFA) histofluorescence method for improved visualization of catecholamines and indoleamines. I. A detailed account of the methodology for central nervous tissue using paraffin, cryostat or Vibratome sections. *J Neurosci Methods* 1980;2:277–300.

Advances in Neurology, Vol. 59, edited by
Fredrick J. Seil. Raven Press, Ltd.,
New York © 1993.

17

Steroid Hormones and Neuronal Regeneration

Alejandro F. De Nicola

Laboratory of Neuroendocrine Biochemistry, Instituto de Biologia y Medicina Experimental, 1428 Buenos Aires, Argentina

Steroid hormones convey molecular information to target cells in the body. In the case of the central nervous system (CNS), steroids secreted from the adrenals, ovary, testis, and placenta or those produced directly by the CNS (neurosteroids) regulate neuronal firing, neurotransmitter metabolism, the activity of genes and enzymes, protein synthesis, cellular development and differentiation, neuroendocrine systems, and behavior. In addition to these well-known actions, steroids have neurotrophic properties and also affect neuronal regeneration.

There are two mechanisms by which steroids interact with nervous system cells. A slow-acting mechanism involves control of genomic expression because of the high-affinity interaction of steroids with intracellular receptors, which, on hormone binding, are transformed into DNA-binding proteins (1). In this context, steroid receptors belong to a superfamily of ligand-activated transcription factors, comprising the glucocorticoid, mineralocorticoid, androgen, estrogen, progesterone, and vitamin D_3 receptors and receptors for nonsteroid members such as thyroid hormone and retinoic acid (1,2). Biochemical, autoradiographic, immunocytochemical, and, more recently, molecular biology techniques have disclosed the discrete localization of steroid receptors and their mRNA in the CNS and the mechanisms for their regulation (3–7; R. B. Simerly, this volume). The second is a fast-driven nongenomic mechanism related to hormone interaction with putative steroid membrane receptors (8,9) or with neurotransmitter receptors such as the GABA–benzodiazepine site (10). Neurosteroids made locally in the CNS most often utilize this system (11), accounting for their anesthetic properties. Binding or recognition of steroids by one of these systems leads to changes in neuronal and glial cell function, which are summarized below when related to neurotropism and regeneration.

ANDROGENS

Most available data come from reports on the sexually dimorphic nuclei (SDN) located in the preoptic area (POA) and the lumbar spinal cord nucleus innervating the bulbocavernosus (SNB), a muscle subserving copulatory functions. Both areas are heavily populated by androgen receptors (12,13). Thus, the area of the SDN-POA is increased by androgens acting in the perinatal period; both neuronal number and dendritic trees of hypothalamic target cells come under androgenic influence (14,15). In the case of the SNB, this nucleus is larger in male than female rodents as a result of postnatal neuronal death in the females from lack of testosterone (16). In humans, a sexual dimorphism has been described in an equivalent area called Onuf's nucleus of the sacral spinal cord (17). In rats, androgen treatment increases neuronal number and prevents their death in females (16). In castrated males, these hormones also increase dendritic membranes, synaptic contacts, neuron–neuron contacts, and double synapses (18). Finally, it has been shown that gap junctions, which are electrical synapses allowing passage of ions and small molecules among cells, are increased in the SNB by testosterone treatment of castrates (19).

Besides the sexually dimorphic nuclei, other neuronal groups are influenced by androgens. In the spinal cord, these hormones increase the dendritic trees of neurons (20) and promote survival of murine fetal lumbosacral neurons in culture (21). There are also reports that testosterone affects the development and functioning of sites in the spinal cord responsive to thyrotropin-releasing hormone (22) that are needed for conduction of electrical impulses. Loss of these sites was linked to the reduction in androgen receptors caused by motoneuron death in patients with amyotrophic lateral sclerosis (23). These effects can be explained in terms of the localization of androgen receptors in motoneurons (24). In birds, there are centers of the brain related to singing in which androgens increase neurogenesis, neuronal migration, dendritic length, and axonal branching (25). On the basis of the time course of action, they most likely represent a genomic effect of androgens.

Finally, androgens increase axonal regeneration after experimental lesion of the hypoglossal and anterior tibialis nerves (26,27). They also enhance the neuron's capacity to repair itself after injury, as shown after crushing the hamster facial motoneuron axon (K. J. Jones, this volume). Altogether, these demonstrations testify that male hormones have profound trophic effects on specialized regions of the CNS, and they may also affect the response to injury.

ESTROGENS

The most pronounced effects of estradiol (E_2) on neuronal process growth and sprouting have been found in regions subserving female reproductive function and behavior. Thus, nuclei within a hypothalamic region rich in E_2 receptors are well-known targets of E_2 action (5,7,28), although some effects have been reported in the limbic system, which contains few E_2 receptors but has a measurable quantity of mRNA for the receptor (29). In the ventromedial nuclei (VMN) of the hypothalamus, an area critical to control of neuroendocrine functions, E_2 provokes morphological changes consisting of increments of stacked rough endoplasmic reticulum (RER) and dense-core vesicles (30). These changes occur to a more limited extent in the arcuate nucleus, POA, or midbrain central gray (31). Typical changes observed in the VMN were nuclear and nucleolar swelling, increases in rRNA and polyadenylated RNA, and increased spine density of neurons (30). A trophic, growth-like effect has been described in the developing hypothalamus under the influence of E_2 (32), and increased length of neuronal processes was observed in the POA area of hypothalamus (33).

Spine density of neurons is also under E_2 control in the VMN and in the pyramidal cells of the hippocampus situated in the CA1 subfield (34,35). Spine density of the CA3 area or dentate gyrus does not change after castration or after E_2 replacement (35), indicating a specialized function of CA1 neurons after hormonal treatment. This finding correlates with changes in hippocampal physiology caused by gonadal steroids (36). Moreover, following removal of the fimbria–fornix afferents to the hippocampus, there is an ingrowth of vascular-associated sympathetic axons originating in the superior cervical ganglion (37). The axonal sprouting is greater in female rats than in males, the change being ascribed to developmental differences in endogenous steroid levels (37).

PROGESTERONE AND RETINOIC ACID

There is a paucity of information regarding these receptor ligands. For progesterone, it has been shown that neuron loss in the hypoglossal and facial motor nuclei after nerve transection could be prevented by progesterone treatment (38).

Retinoic acid enhances regeneration of peripheral neurons located at the dorsal root ganglion cells and neurons of the mouse and human fetal spinal cord. In these cells, retinoic acid, the active metabolite of vitamin A, increases neurite length (with formation of growth cones) but not neurite number, which distinguishes this effect from sprouting (39). Therefore, it has been proposed that retinoic acid is a morphogen because of its ability to induce differentiation (40).

GLUCOCORTICOIDS

Glucocorticoids bind to two receptor types in the CNS. There is a high-affinity receptor (type I) localized preferentially, although not exclusively, in the limbic system and a lower-affinity type II site with widespread distribution in the brain and spinal cord (3–6,41). Additionally, nongenomic effects, which presumably are independent of the classical glucocorticoid receptor, have been described in several regions (9). Whatever the originating mechanism, actions of glucocorticoids can be classified into beneficial or stimulatory for cell function and regeneration and effects inhibitory or deleterious for these parameters.

Inhibitory or deleterious effects have been observed in hippocampus, brain cortex, and pheochromocytoma cells in culture. In hippocampus, corticosterone treatment of male rats decreases axonal sprouting after lesions of the entorhinal cortex (42). Treatment with natural or synthetic glucocorticoids leads to glucocorticoid receptor down-regulation in hippocampus (43) and, if prolonged sufficiently, to dramatic alterations in pyramidal neurons of the CA3 subfield, ranging from low branching to death if high doses are employed chronically (44,45). Other deleterious effects include exacerbation of the toxicity of certain agents (e.g., kainic acid), impaired glucose utilization, increased Ca^{2+} uptake and neuronal necrosis from ischemia, supporting the hypothesis that glucocorticoids are neurotoxic in the hippocampus (45,46). These mechanisms would be involved in the neuronal loss and astrocyte reactivity described in the aged brain, as aging animals show progressively increased levels of circulating glucocorticoids (47). The contribution of the high density of glucocorticoid receptors in hippocampus to these changes is likely, although not yet proven.

Furthermore, glucocorticoid treatment of rats immediately after birth stunts the growth of neurons in the parietal, visual, and cerebellar cortex (48). In PC-12 cells, a clonal cell line derived from a pheochromocytoma tumor, dexamethasone application reduces the low-affinity receptor for nerve growth factor (NGF) (49). The NGF action is needed in these cells to differentiate them fully into sympathetic neurons (50).

Not less numerous are the beneficial or stimulatory roles of adrenal steroids described in the CNS. In the hippocampus, female rats (as opposed to males) respond with sprouting after lesion of the entorhinal cortex (51). Increased homotypic sprouting of serotoninergic fibers has been observed following lesions of the raphe–hippocampal pathway (52). Another example is the granule cells of the dentate gyrus, which are highly dependent on glucocorticoids for survival; after glucocorticoid withdrawal by adrenalectomy, these cells become smaller and less branched, and 3 to 4 months later there is a selective neuronal death in this region. Glucocorticoid treatment restores neuronal size and shape and prevents death (44,53). This contrasts with the effects on the CA3 subfield of hippocampus mentioned above, in which glucocorticoid treatment causes less branching and, if prolonged for 12 weeks, kills large CA3 neurons (45). In addition to the cells of the dentate gyrus, glucocorticoids are beneficial to other neurons, such as those of the fetal rabbit brain in culture, in which case betamethasone addition prolongs survival of neurons *in vitro* (54).

In the spinal cord, numerous reports attest to the beneficial effect of glucocorticoids after trauma. In patients with acute spinal cord injury, treatment with methylprednisolone improves neurological recovery when the medication is given in the first 8 hr, as shown by the Second National Acute Spinal Cord Injury Study (55). This property has been tested experimentally, and the mechanisms proposed for glucocorticoids involve prevention of posttraumatic ischemia and neurofilament protein degradation (56) and reduction of lipid peroxidation with enhancement of the activity of Na^+,K^+-ATPase (57). It has been hypothesized that glucocorticoid effects mediated by receptors lead to neuronal damage, whereas the protective effect is receptor independent and involves inhibition of oxygen free radical lipid peroxidation (58). In support of this, glucocorticoid effects could be duplicated by nonsteroidal lipid antioxidants (see E. D. Hall, this volume).

In spinal-cord-injured rats, treatment with methylprednisolone reduces damage; however, other agents such as tirilazad (a lipid peroxidation inhibitor) and cyclosporin A (an immunosuppressor) are also effective, suggesting that immunosuppression may be a final common pathway in the effect of these drugs (see W. Young, this volume). The antioxidant property of glucocorticoids may also be involved in the retardation of posttraumatic degeneration of peripheral nerves. Thus, surgical transection of the soleus nerve causes anterograde axonal degeneration, an effect delayed by methylprednisolone or triamcinolone, steroids preserving the ability of the soleus to transmit single and repetitive stimuli (59).

GLUCOCORTICOID RECEPTORS AND ACTIONS IN THE SPINAL CORD: IMPLICATIONS FOR TRAUMA AND REGENERATION

Glucocorticoids have many physiological and biochemical effects in the spinal cord (60,61). The type II glucocorticoid receptor seems the more abundant class in this tissue, and segmental distribution suggests a higher concentration of sites binding ^{3}H-dexamethasone in the cervical and lumbar enlargements, i.e., areas rich in motoneurons (62). However, glial cells also contain glucocorticoid receptors (63). Clearly, spinal cord receptors present biochemical, stereospecific, and physicochemical properties similar to those found in other regions of the CNS.

However, the type II glucocorticoid receptor of the spinal cord shows lower affinity than the hippocampal type II site after different protocols are employed to measure binding parameters (64). These differences in equilibrium dissociation constants (K_d) indicate that the milieu of the tissue can influence receptor function, and it could account for a difference in sensitivity of the two systems in the physiological and pharmacological adrenal hormone range. The enrichment of high-affinity type I and type II receptors in the hippocampus correlates with its participation in feedback mechanisms requiring fine sensitivity (3), with a high degree of receptor plasticity in response to hormonal levels (43), with the neuronal loss in aging rats (45,47), and with the reported neurotoxicity in the CA3 subfield (45). In comparison, there are no reports of neuronal loss in the spinal cord after prolonged exposure to adrenal steroids; on the contrary, pharmacological amounts of synthetic glucocorticoids often result in fast recovery from spinal cord injury and in clinical improvement of patients with degenerative diseases (55).

In the spinal cord, enzymes under glucocorticoid control include ornithine decarboxylase (ODC), glycerol phosphate dehydrogenase (GPDH), and Na^+,K^+-ATPase (57,65). The ODC, a rate-limiting enzyme in polyamine synthesis, is present in astrocytes and neurons (66). It increases 4 hr after a single dexamethasone injection; 6 hr afterwards, it further increases, with a return toward normal at 20 hr (65). The induction is found in the ventral horn and lateral funiculus (67). We also found that surgical transection of the spinal cord, while markedly increasing ODC activity *per se*, potentiates the effects of dexamethasone on this enzyme (67). Moreover, spinal cord injury is causally related to generation of free radicals, lipid peroxidation, and membrane damage (58). Glucocorticoids, which reduce recovery time after spinal cord injury, prevent lipid peroxidation (E. D. Hall, this volume). They may do so by stimulating trophic factors, including polyamines involved in glial cell proliferation and in axonal regeneration, since ODC has been mapped immunologically in dendrites, axons, and nerve terminals (66). Therefore, the possibility exists that both neurons and glial cells could synthesize polyamines; notably, it has been reported that the spinal cord is the region of the CNS with the highest content of polyamines (68). Support for a linkage among induction of ODC, prevention of tissue damage, and regeneration is provided by the crush lesion or transection of nerves, in which increases in ODC and polyamines by the neuronal perikaryon are necessary for survival and regeneration of sensory fibers (69,70). In the case of the spinal cord, glucocorticoid-induced ODC could provide a useful marker to determine the repair of axons following transection.

In contrast to ODC, induction of GPDH after a single dose of glucocorticoids is a slow process, with maximal induction at 20 hr still persisting at 46 hr (46). Inasmuch as GPDH is synthesized by myelin-producing oligodendrocytes, activation of these cells by glucocorticoids would enhance axonal remyelination after injury.

The enzyme Na^+,K^+-ATPase is under glucocorticoid and mineralocorticoid control in the CNS (71,72). In the spinal cord, it is inhibited during trauma and recovers following methylprednisolone treatment (57,61), possibly because of hormonal prevention of lipid peroxidation. We have observed that binding of ^{3}H-ouabain to the α subunit of Na^+,K^+-ATPase in membranes obtained from the ventral horn decreases after adrenalectomy and increases after treatment with dexamethasone (unpublished observations). The mRNA for the β subunit of the enzyme, determined by *in situ* hybridization, is also under positive control by glucocorticoids. Inasmuch as Na^+,K^+-ATPase is responsible for the outward Na^+ movement, enzyme activity is needed to repolarize the membrane following depolarization by electrical or chemical stimuli. Enhancement of spinal cord function by glucocorticoids may therefore involve stimulation of the activity and genesis of Na^+,K^+-ATPase subunits, important for reestablishment of neurotransmission.

Recent immunocytochemical studies of the type II glucocorticoid receptor of the spinal cord carried out in our laboratory demonstrated that 2 days after cordotomy, staining is enhanced in motoneurons of lamina IX. These neurons also present a significant increase in immunoreactive satellite cells of the astroglial type (unpublished observations). It is possible that an unknown signal released following transection activates astrocytes and other glial cells and that they then up-regulate their glucocorticoid receptors. These receptors, in addition to other proteins, may be transferred from astrocytes to neurons via the reported glial–neuronal communication system (73,74). In turn, the perineuronal glial cells may provide neurons with trophic factors that activate transcription of the neuronal glucocorticoid receptor, ODC, and Na^+,K^+-ATPase. Therefore, induction of the glucocorticoid receptor would increase the biological activity of endogenous or exogenous glucocorticoids, which is needed for a cell on the verge of regeneration.

Another important topic is the influence of gonadal steroids on biochemical events regulated by glucocorticoids. Not only the progestin receptor but also the glucocorticoid receptor increases in brain after E_2 treatment in rats (75). We recently observed that 4 days of E_2 administration to ovariectomized rats increases ^{3}H-dexamethasone binding exclusively in the dorsal horn of the spinal cord. Since this treatment potentiates the effects of dexamethasone on ODC induction in the ventral horn and lateral funiculus but not the dorsal horn, a transsynaptic effect of the sex steroid hormone was postulated (unpublished material).

In conclusion, it seems that glucocorticoids have neurotrophic properties in the spinal cord. The mechanisms involved are intricate and influenced by the structure of the administered steroid, the intermediacy (or not) of the steroid receptor and the genome, the type of cells involved (neurons and glia), the sex of the animal, and the presence or absence of injury. Therefore, interplay of these factors is of paramount importance when hormonal effects on regeneration are considered.

ACKNOWLEDGMENTS

Research on this topic in the author's laboratory is supported by the National Institutes of Health (RO1 NS20866), the National Research Council of Argentina (PID 3-010200), and the University of Buenos Aires.

REFERENCES

1. Schwabe JWR, Rhodes D. Beyond zinc fingers: steroid hormone receptors have a novel structural motif for DNA recognition. *Trends Biochem Sci* 1991;16:291–296.
2. Carson-Jurica MA, Schrader WT, O'Malley BW. Steroid receptor superfamily: structure and function. *Endocr Rev* 1990;11:201–220.
3. McEwen BS, De Kloet ER, Rostene W. Adrenal steroid receptors and actions in the nervous system. *Physiol Rev* 1986;66:1121–1188.
4. Fuxe K, Wikstrom AC, Okert S, et al. Mapping of glucocorticoid receptor immunoreactive neurons in the rat tel- and diencephalon using a monoclonal antibody against rat liver glucocorticoid receptor. *Endocrinology* 1985;117:1803–1812.
5. Stumpf WE, Sar M. Autoradiographic localization of estrogen, androgen, progestin and glucocorticosteroid in target tissues and non-target tissues. In: Pasqualini JR, ed. *Receptors and mechanism of action of steroid hormones. Modern pharmacology–toxicology,* Vol 8. New York: Marcel Dekker; 1976:41–84.
6. Van Eekelen JAM, Jiang W, De Kloet ER, Bohn MC. Distribution of the mineralocorticoid and the glucocorticoid receptor mRNA in the rat hippocampus. *J Neurosci Res* 1988;21:88–94.
7. Simerly RB, Chang C, Muramatsu M, Swanson LW. Distribution of androgen and estrogen receptor mRNA-containing cells in the rat brain: an *in situ* hybridization study. *J Comp Neurol* 1990;294: 76–95.
8. Orchinik M, Murray TF, Moore FL. A corticosteroid receptor in neuronal membranes. *Science* 1991;252:1848–1851.
9. McEwen BS, Coirini H, Schumacher M. Steroid effects on neuronal activity: when is the genome involved? In: Chadwick D, Widdow K, eds. *Steroids and neuronal activity.* London: John Wiley & Sons; 1990:3–12.
10. Maggi A, Perez J. Estrogen-induced up-regulation of gamma-aminobutyric acid receptors in the CNS of rodents. *J Neurochem* 1986;47:1793–1797.
11. Baulieu E-E, Robel P. Neurosteroids: a new brain function? *J Steroid Biochem Mol Biol* 1990; 37:395–403.
12. Handa RJ, Reid DL, Resko JA. Androgen receptors in brain and pituitary of female rats: cyclic changes and comparisons with the male. *Biol Reprod* 1986;34:293–303.
13. Breedlove SM, Arnold AP. Hormone accumulation in a sexually dimorphic motor nucleus of the rat spinal cord. *Science* 1980;210:564–566.
14. Arnold AP, Gorski RA. Gonadal steroid induction of structural sex differences in the central nervous system. *Annu Rev Neurosci* 1984;7:413–442.
15. Toran-Allerand CD. On the genesis of sexual differences of the central nervous system: morphogenetic consequences of steroidal exposure and possible role of α-fetoprotein. *Prog Brain Res* 1984;61:63–97.
16. Breedlove SM, Arnold AP. Hormonal control of a developing neuromuscular system. II. Sensitive periods for the androgen-induced masculinization of the rat spinal nucleus of the bulbocavernosus. *J Neurosci* 1983;3:424–432.
17. Forger NG, Breedlove SM. Sexual dimorphism in human and canine spinal cord: role of early androgen. *Proc Natl Acad Sci USA* 1986;83:7527–7531.
18. Matsumoto A, Micevych PE, Arnold AP. Androgen regulates synaptic input to motoneurons of the adult rat spinal cord. *J Neurosci* 1988;8:4168–4176.
19. Matsumoto A, Arnold AP, Zampighi GA, Micevych PE. Androgenic regulation of gap junctions between motoneurons in the rat spinal cord. *J Neurosci* 1988;8:4177–4183.
20. Hauser KF, Toran-Allerand CD. Testosterone increases cell number in organotypic cultures of fetal mouse spinal cord. *Soc Neurosci Abstr* 1985;11:898.
21. Hauser KF, Toran-Allerand CD. Androgen increases the number of cells in fetal mouse spinal cord cultures: implications for motoneuronal survival. *Brain Res* 1989;485:157–164.
22. Miller SC, Warnick JE. Protirelin (thyrotropin-releasing hormone) in amyotrophic lateral sclerosis. *Arch Neurol* 1989;46:330–335.
23. Weiner L. Possible role of androgen receptors in amyotrophic lateral sclerosis. *Arch Neurol* 1980;37:129–131.
24. Sar M, Stumpf EW. Androgen concentration in motor neurons of cranial nerves and spinal cord. *Science* 1977;197:77–79.
25. Alvarez-Buylla A, Nottebohm F. Migration of young neurons in adult avian brain. *Nature* 1988;335:353–354.
26. Yu WHA. Effect of testosterone on the regeneration of the hypoglossal nerve in rats. *Exp Neurol* 1982;77:129–141.
27. Vita G, Dattola R, Girlanda P, et al. Effects of steroid hormones on muscle reinnervation after nerve crush in rabbit. *Exp Neurol* 1983;80:279–287.
28. Pfaff DW, Keiner M. Atlas of estradiol-concentrating cells in the central nervous system of the female rat. *J Comp Neurol* 1973;151:121–158.
29. Maggi A, Susanna L, Bettini E, Mantero G, Zucchi I. Hippocampus: a target for estrogen action in mammalian brain. *Mol Endocrinol* 1989;3:1165–1170.

30. Jones KJ. Steroid hormones and neurotrophism: relationship to nerve injury. *Metab Brain Dis* 1988;3:1–18.
31. Meisel RL, Pfaff DW. Brain region specificity in estradiol effects on neuronal ultrastructure in rats. *Mol Cell Endocrinol* 1985;40:159–166.
32. Carrer HF, Aoki A. Ultrastructural changes in the hypothalamic ventromedial nucleus of ovariectomized rats after estrogen treatment. *Brain Res* 1982;240:221–233.
33. Uchibori M, Kawashima S. Stimulation of neuronal process growth by estradiol-17β in dissociated cells from fetal rat hypothalamus–preoptic area. *Zool Sci* 1985;2:381–388.
34. Frankfurt M, Gould E, Wooley CS, McEwen BS. Gonadal steroids modify dendritic spine density in ventromedial hypothalamic neurons: a Golgi study in the adult rat. *Neuroendocrinology* 1990;51: 530–535.
35. Gould E, Wooley CS, Frankfurt M, McEwen BS. Gonadal steroids regulate dendritic spine density in hippocampal pyramidal cells in adulthood. *J Neurosci* 1990;10:1286–1291.
36. Teyler TJ, Vardaris RM, Lewis DL, Rawitch AB. Gonadal steroids: Effects on excitability of hippocampal pyramidal cells. *Science* 1980;209:1017–1019.
37. Milner TA, Loy R. Hormonal regulation of axonal sprouting in the hippocampus. *Brain Res* 1982;491:379–382.
38. Yu WH. Survival of motoneurons following axotomy is enhanced by lactation or by progesterone treatment. *Brain Res* 1989;491:379–382.
39. Quinn SDP, De Boni U. Enhanced neuronal regeneration by retinoic acid of murine dorsal root ganglia and of fetal murine and human spinal cord *in vitro*. *In Vitro Cell Dev Biol* 1991;27A:55–62.
40. Slack JMW. We have a morphogen. *Nature* 1987;327:553–554.
41. Moses DF, Gonzalez S, Orti E, De Nicola AF. Heterogeneity and properties of transformation of corticosteroid receptors in spinal cord and hippocampus. *Brain Res* 1989;481:317–324.
42. Scheff SW, Cotman CW. Chronic glucocorticoid therapy alters axon sprouting in the hippocampal dentate gyrus. *Exp Neurol* 1982;76:644–654.
43. Tornello S, Orti E, De Nicola AF, Rainbow TC, McEwen BS. Regulation of glucocorticoid receptors in brain by corticosterone treatment of adrenalectomized rats. *Neuroendocrinology* 1982;35:411–417.
44. Gould E, Wooley CS, McEwen BS. Short term glucocorticoid manipulation affects neuronal morphology and survival in the adult hippocampal formation. *Neuroscience* 1990;37:367–375.
45. Sapolsky R, Krey L, McEwen BS. The neuroendocrinology of stress and aging: the glucocorticoid cascade hypothesis. *Endocr Rev* 1986;7:284–301.
46. Kerr DS, Campbell LW, Hao S-Y, Lanfield PW. Corticosteroid modulation of hippocampal potentials: increased effect with aging. *Science* 1989;245: 1505–1509.
47. Lanfield P, Waymire J, Lynch G. Hippocampal aging and adrenocorticoids: quantitative correlations. *Science* 1978;202:1098–1102.
48. Schapiro S. Some physiological, biochemical and behavioral consequences of neonatal hormone administration of cortisol and thyroxine. *Gen Comp Endocrinol* 1968;10:214–228.
49. Tocco MD, Contreras ML, Koizumi S, Dickens G, Guroff G. Decreased levels of nerve growth factor receptors on dexamethasone-treated PC12 cells. *J Neurosci Res* 1988;20:411–419.
50. Harper GP, Thoenen H. Target cells, biological effects and mechanism of action of nerve growth factor and its antibodies. *Annu Rev Pharmacol Toxicol* 1981;21:205–209.
51. Scheff SW, Morse JK, Dekosky ST. Hydrocortisone differentially alters lesion-induced axon sprouting in male and female rats. *Exp Neurol* 1988;100: 237–241.
52. Zhou FC, Azmitia EC. The effect of adrenalectomy and corticosterone on homotypic collateral sprouting of serotonergic fibers in hippocampus. *Neurosci Lett* 1985;54:111–116.
53. Sloviter RS, Valiquette G, Abrams GM, et al. Selective loss of hippocampal granule cells in the mature rat brain after adrenalectomy. *Science* 1989;243: 535–538.
54. Kari B, Gilbertson J, Barrada I. Effects of the synthetic glucocorticoid betamethasone on the survival of neurons in fetal rabbit brain cell culture. *Brain Res* 1985;339:1–7.
55. Bracken MB, Shepard MJ, Collins WF, et al. A randomized, controlled trial of methylprednisolone or naloxone in the treatment of acute spinal cord injury. *N Engl J Med* 1990;322:1405–1411.
56. Braughler JM, Hall ED. Effects of multi-dose methylprednisolone sodium succinate administration on injured cat spinal cord neurofilament degradation and energy metabolism. *J Neurosurg* 1984;61: 290–295.
57. Braughler JM, Hall ED. Acute enhancement of spinal cord synaptosomal (Na+K)-ATPase activity in cats following intravenous methylprednisolone. *Brain Res* 1981;219:464–469.
58. Hall ED. Steroids and neuronal destruction or stabilization. In: Chadwick D, Widdows K, eds. *Steroids and neuronal activity.* London: John Wiley & Sons, 1990:206–219.
59. Hall ED, Wolf DL. Methylprednisolone preservation of motor nerve function during early degeneration. *Exp Neurol* 1984;84:715–720.
60. De Nicola AF, Moses DF, Gonzalez S, Orti E. Adrenocorticoid action in the spinal cord: some unique molecular properties of glucocorticoid receptors. *Cell Mol Neurobiol* 1989;9:179–192.
61. Hall ED. Glucocorticoid effects on central nervous excitability and synaptic transmission. *Int Rev Neurobiol* 1982;23:165–195.
62. Orti E, Corini H, De Nicola AF. Properties and distribution of glucocorticoid binding sites in cytosol of the spinal cord. *Neuroendocrinology* 1985;40:225–231.
63. Fuxe K, Harfstrand A, Agnati LF, et al. Immunocytochemical studies on the localization of glucocorticoid receptor immunoreactive nerve cells in the lower brainstem and spinal cord of the male rat using a monoclonal antibody against rat liver glucocorticoid receptor. *Neurosci Lett* 1985;60:1–6.
64. Moses DF, Gonzalez S, McEwen BS, De Nicola AF. Glucocorticoid type II receptors of the spinal cord show lower affinity than hippocampal type II recep-

tors: binding parameters obtained with different experimental protocols. *J Steroid Biochem Mol Biol* 1991;39:5–12.
65. Orti E, Moses DF, Grillo C, De Nicola AF. Glucocorticoid regulation of glycerolphosphate dehydrogenase and ornithine decarboxylase activities in the spinal cord of the rat. *J Neurochem* 1987;48: 425–431.
66. Cintra A, Fuxe K, Agnati LF, et al. Evidence for the existence of ornithine decarboxylase immunoreactive neurons in the rat brain. *Neurosci Lett* 1987;76:269–274.
67. Gonzalez S, Moses DF, De Nicola AF. Glucocorticoid receptors and enzyme induction in the spinal cord of rats: effects of acute transection. *J Neurochem* 1990;54:834–840.
68. Scalabrino G, Monzio-Compagnoni B, Ferioli ME, Lorenzini EC, Chiodini E, Candiani R. Subacute combined degeneration and induction of ornithine decarboxylase in spinal cords of totally gastrectomized rats. *Lab Invest* 1990;62:297–304.
69. Kanje M, Fransson I, Edstrom A, Lowkvist B. Ornithine decarboxylase activity in dorsal root ganglia of regenerating frog sciatic nerve. *Brain Res* 1986;381:24–28.
70. Soifer AI, Moretto A, Spencer PS, Sabri MI. Axotomy-induced ornithine decarboxylase activity in the mouse dorsal root ganglion is inhibited by the vinca alkaloids. *Neurochem Res* 1988;13:1169–1173.
71. Elkouby A, Ledig M, Mandel P. Effect of hydrocortisone and thyroxine on ATPase activities of neuronal and glial cells in culture. *Neurochem Res* 1982;7:387–397.
72. Grillo C, Vallée S, Piroli G, Angulo JA, McEwen BS, De Nicola AF. Effects of deoxycorticosterone treatment on β-subunit mRNA for (Na+K)-ATPase in brain regions determined by *in situ* hybridization. *Cell Mol Neurobiol* 1991;11:347–356.
73. Berkley KJ, Contos N. A glial–neuronal–glial communication system in the mammalian central nervous system. *Brain Res* 1987;414:49–67.
74. Tytell M, Greenberg SG, Lasek RJ. Heat shock-like protein is transferred from glia to axon. *Brain Res* 1986;363:161–164.
75. Ferrini M, De Nicola AF. Estrogens up-regulate type I and type II glucocorticoid receptors in brain regions from ovariectomized rats. *Life Sci* 1991; 48:2593–2601.

Advances in Neurology, Vol. 59, edited by Fredrick J. Seil. Raven Press, Ltd., New York © 1993.

18

Distribution and Regulation of Steroid Hormone Receptor Gene Expression in the Central Nervous System

Richard B. Simerly

Division of Neuroscience, Oregon Regional Primate Research Center, Beaverton, Oregon 97006

Steroid hormones secreted by the gonads and adrenal gland are powerful humoral agents that act on the brain to coordinate diverse aspects of physiology and behavior. These hormones produce their effects by altering neuronal activity and membrane conductance, modifying neuronal ultrastructure and synaptic morphology, as well as by inducing changes in protein synthesis (see refs. 1–7 for reviews). However, steroid hormones do not merely activate preexisting neural pathways in response to specific environmental cues; they also determine the developmental fate of hormone-sensitive neurons and modify the morphology and biochemistry of these cells throughout life. Thus, exposure to critical levels of gonadal steroid hormones such as testosterone and estrogen during development influences cell survival, morphology, and neurotransmitter phenotype (8–11). Similarly, glucocorticoids secreted by the adrenal cortex affect neuronal morphology, activity, and survival (6,12). Together these observations support the notion that steroid hormones are not simply mediators of adult physiology but also act as potent neurotrophic agents capable of affecting neuronal architecture and synaptic efficacy during development and throughout the life of the individual (see refs. 13,14 for reviews). As described in subsequent reviews in this volume, the ability of steroid hormones to influence neuronal plasticity may have profound implications for neural mechanisms involved in cellular responses to injury (15–17).

STEROID HORMONES AND BRAIN DEVELOPMENT

Sex steroid hormones exert their most pronounced effects on neuronal development during a critical perinatal period. Numerous studies have shown that the morphological organization of certain brain regions known to mediate sexually differentiated functions, such as the control of copulatory behavior, gonadotropin release, and certain cognitive functions, is sexually dimorphic (13,18–20). Moreover, a large body of evidence now supports the notion that the brain is essentially bipotential and differentiates in response to circulating sex steroids present in males during the perinatal period (13). Thus, treatment of female neonates with sex steroids has been shown to alter the number of neurons residing in certain nuclei as well as the morphology, synaptology, and neurotransmitter expression of individual neurons (8,10,11,21,22).

Although numerous studies suggest that neonatal exposure to sex steroids induces changes in cell number by promoting the survival of steroid-sensitive cells (9), sexual dimorphisms are not produced by this mechanism alone. For example, the anteroventral periventricular nucleus of the hypothalamus is larger in female rats (23,24) and contains more dopaminergic and opioid-peptide-containing neurons than that in males (25,26). Treatment of neonatal females with testosterone decreases the numbers of both types of cells, suggesting that sex steroid hormones may selectively promote the death of these neurotransmitter-specific neurons (21,22,26, 27). Alternatively, the neonatal hormone environment may regulate the number of putative dopaminergic and opioid-peptide-containing cells that are formed or that successfully migrate to their final location. It is also possible that such neurochemical sexual dimorphisms are caused by the permanent suppression of neurotransmitter expression within hormone-sensitive populations of neurons brought about by exposure to sex steroids during discrete perinatal critical periods. Although progesterone-induced changes in neuronal number and morphology have not been identified, clinical studies report behavioral correlations that suggest a possible involvement of progesterone in the development of certain cognitive functions (28).

Adrenal steroids appear to exert an overall inhibitory influence on brain development (see refs. 6,12 for reviews). Corticosteroid treatment induces changes in synaptic morphology and causes a general suppression of cell proliferation (6). Consistent with this suggestion of an inhibitory role for glucocorticoids on neural development is the observation that adrenalectomy increases cell proliferation (29) with a concomitant enhancement of myelination (30). That glucocorticoids enhance age-related loss of neurons in the hippocampus (31) indicates that the regressive influences of adrenal steroids (32) may not be limited to the perinatal period. In contrast, glucocorticoids appear to promote development of neurotransmitter expression. For example, treatment of neonatal mice with glucocorticoids increases tyrosine hydroxylase activity in the locus ceruleus (33) and phenylethanolamine-N-methyltransferase in the medulla (34). Similarly, adrenalectomy prevents the normal postnatal rise in tryptophan hydroxylase, the rate-limiting enzyme for serotonin synthesis (35).

MECHANISMS OF ACTION

The cellular mechanisms mediating the actions of steroid hormones on the brain appear to be similar to those characterized in peripheral tissues. These hormones diffuse into neurons where they bind to specific, saturable receptor molecules that act at the level of DNA to influence the function and developmental fate of hormone-sensitive cells. Biochemical receptor assays and autoradiographic studies indicate that steroid hormone receptors are detectable in the developing rodent brain, and concentrations of these nuclear proteins remain low during early life but increase during the perinatal period (36,37).

One of the most significant advances in the understanding of the molecular mechanisms underlying the hormonal control of brain function and development has been the cloning and characterization of genes that encode steroid hormone receptors (38–42). Analysis of the structural and functional properties of gonadal and adrenal steroid hormone receptors has led to their inclusion in a superfamily of genes that function as ligand-activated transcription factors and has shown that they share a common domain structure. Each of these molecules contains a centrally located region of highly conserved cysteine residues that are essential for DNA binding as well as for the specificity of target-gene activation (38,43). The "hormone-binding" domain of each receptor, located near the carboxy terminus, is required for ligand binding and regulates transformation of the receptor to an active form (44,45). Because the capacity of ligand-activated hormone receptors to recognize and regulate target genes is determined by their ability to bind specific DNA sequences in the promoter region of hormone-sensitive genes, designated hormone response elements (HREs), the similarity in the DNA-binding domains of related receptors implies that such receptors may activate overlapping sets of genes by acting through common hormone response elements. Thus, the glucocorticoid and progesterone receptors can bind to the same HRE with high affinity *in vitro* (39), and the number and arrangement of these elements determine the impact of hormone treatment on transcription (46). In addition, coexpressed estrogen receptors enhance the ability of glucocorticoid receptors to activate transcription, suggesting that the presence or absence of heterogeneous HREs can dictate the level of transcriptional control by steroid hormones (47).

Deletion mutagenesis experiments have determined that a discrete region of the DNA-binding domain (the P-box) plays a crucial role in determining specificity of transcriptional activation (39). For example, if three amino acids in the P-box of the estrogen receptor are replaced with the corresponding amino acids of the glucocorticoid receptor, the mutant receptor specifically recognizes the glucocorticoid but not the estrogen response element (48). Conversely, both the glucocorticoid and mineralocorticoid receptors can activate transcription through the same HRE (49). Thus, although the DNA-binding sequence of each receptor specifies which HREs are recognized, closely related receptors are nevertheless capable of binding to the same promoter, but often with differential effects on gene expression. Minor differences in the sequences of HREs may therefore contribute to the broad range of cell-specific patterns of hormone responsiveness. Based on the mechanism by which steroid receptors recognize HREs, they can be divided into generalized subfamilies (39, 42,50). The androgen receptor (AR), mineralocorticoid receptor (MR), glucocorticoid receptor (GR), and progesterone receptor (PR) belong to the GR-like subfamily, whereas the estrogen receptor (ER)-like subfamily includes the ER as well as thyroid hormone receptors.

In brain the ER appears to be encoded by a single mRNA (51–53). However, there may be two distinct forms of AR mRNA in rat brain (54,55), although the functional significance of these subtypes is unknown. Two distinct forms of functional PRs also appear to be expressed in brain tissue (56; O. K. Park and K. E. Mayo, personal communication), but as is the case with ARs, it is not known if each receptor subtype has a unique physiological role. Two separate genes expressed in the mammalian brain encode functional corticosteroid receptors (57,58). The first of these binds glucocorticoids with high affinity and is designated the "type I" corticosteroid receptor (49,59), whereas the second, or "type II" receptor, has a lower affinity for glucocorticoids. On the basis of its characteristic ligand binding profile, the type II receptor is identified as the classical GR (60,61). The GR was the first of the steroid hormone receptors to be cloned, and its structure has served as a model for all members of this growing superfamily of proteins. Surprisingly, the type I neuronal corticosteroid receptor appears to be encoded by the same gene that encodes the MR in the kidney (49,62). Together, these two receptors appear to be capable of activating overlapping sets of genes and may therefore provide a complex binary response mechanism for large changes in circulating levels of glucocorticoids (57).

Shared molecular mechanisms of transcriptional activation between steroid hormone receptors indicate that, together with other nuclear proteins, steroid hormone receptors possess considerable combinatorial potential to modulate gene expression. Moreover, support is emerging for the idea that the level of each such factor within an individual cell determines its relative influence on gene expression and thereby influences the cell's functional activity or developmental fate. It should be kept in mind, however, that the physiological activity of many hormone receptors requires covalent modifications such as phosphorylation events. For instance, phosphorylation appears to be required for activation of androgen (63), glucocorticoid (64), and estrogen (65) receptors but not for progesterone (66) receptors. Despite considerable progress on the molecular biology of steroid hormone receptors, we do not yet fully understand their functional role in controlling neural development. This is in part because of the complexity of possible interactions between members of this superfamily of transcription factors but is also complicated by the apparent involvement of other nuclear proteins yet to be identified (67). Thus, a particularly valuable way of evaluating the impact of these receptors on naturally occurring neuronal processes is to study their expression *in situ*.

DISTRIBUTION OF mRNAs ENCODING STEROID HORMONE RECEPTORS

Steroid hormone receptors are not constituitively expressed in all neurons. Therefore, it is the selective expression of these potent transcriptional factors by distinct and possibly functionally related neural systems that makes such pathways responsive to changes in the endocrine environment. Much of what we currently know regarding the distribution of hormone-sensitive neurons in the mammalian brain derives from biochemical studies that utilized receptor-binding techniques to assess levels of receptors in microdissected tissue samples (12,68–72) or from steroid autoradiographic anatomic studies (12,37, 73,74). The cloning of cDNAs for steroid hormone receptors has greatly facilitated our study of hormone-sensitive neural systems because we are now able to use *in situ* hybridization to map the distribution of neurons that express mRNAs encoding the AR, MR, GR, PR, and ER. The results of these studies are largely consistent with those demonstrated previously with autoradiographic (75–81) and immunohistochemical methods (32–86) and indicate that each receptor has a unique distribution that partially overlaps with those of the other receptors. However, in contrast to steroid autoradiography, the ability to perform *in situ* hybridization is not dependent on the endocrine state of the experimental subjects. Thus, the regulation of hormone receptor gene expression can be assessed in pharmacologically manipulated animals. Because the relative levels of steroid hormone receptors expressed within individual neurons may determine the relative impact of acute changes in circulating hormones on gene expression, a clear understanding of the detailed distribution and hormonal regulation of these ligand-activated transcription factors is a prerequisite for meaningful insight into their role in modulating functional neural systems.

Androgen Receptor

Although antibodies have been generated to AR fusion protein (87), the detailed distribution of AR-immunoreactive neurons in the brain has not been reported. Neurons containing AR mRNA are widely distributed throughout the rat brain (88) with at least moderate densities of AR mRNA-containing neurons present in each major subdivision of the central nervous system, in agreement with earlier steroid autoradiographic studies (37). Consistent with their acknowledged role in modulating reproductive function, many of the cell groups displaying the greatest abundance of AR mRNA are found in the hypothalamus (see Fig. 2 of ref. 88). Thus, the medial preoptic nucleus and ventromedial nucleus of the hypothalamus, which have been implicated in the control of copulatory behavior, contain high densities of heavily labeled AR mRNA-containing neurons. Similarly, the arcuate and ventral premammillary nuclei of the hypothalamus are thought to modulate hormone secretion from the anterior pituitary and to contain a substantial number of AR mRNA-containing neurons. In telencephalic regions the greatest densities of labeled cells are found in areas that supply strong afferents to the hypothalamus, such as the medial nucleus of the amygdala, lateral septal nuclcus, and bed nuclei of the stria terminalis.

Several cortical regions contain AR mRNA-containing neurons, but the most extensive labeling is found in the hippocampal formation. The pyramidal layer of each subdivision of Ammon's horn (CA1 to CA3) and both dorsal and ventral parts of the subiculum express at least moderate levels of AR mRNA, but the dentate gyrus is consistently unlabeled in hybridization histochemical material. The AR mRNA-containing neurons are largely restricted to layers II and III of the isocortex, but a few labeled neurons are reliably found in the deeper layers. One of the most striking aspects of the distribution of AR mRNA-containing neurons in the telencephalon is the relatively abundant expression in olfactory regions such as mitral cells of the main olfactory bulb, the anterior olfactory nucleus, layer II of the piriform cortex, and the endopiriform nucleus.

In general, only low to moderate levels of AR mRNA can be detected histochemically in the thalamus, but several lightly labeled neurons in the region of the A13 dopaminergic neurons of the zona incerta are reliably detected. Moderate densities of AR mRNA-containing neurons in brainstem regions such as the vestibular and cochlear nuclei suggest that androgen may modulate these sensory modalities. In addition, more intense hybridization signals for AR mRNA are found over areas that relay visceral sensory information, such as the nucleus of the solitary tract, the area postrema, and the lateral division of the parabrachial nucleus. Regions involved in somatosensory processes contain only scattered, lightly labeled cells, but the mesencephalic nucleus of the trigeminal nerve contains a moderate density of AR mRNA-containing neurons, as do the substantia gelatinosa and nucleus proprius of the spinal cord.

Several regions that contain somatic motor neurons also contain clearly labeled AR mRNA-containing neurons, including the branchiomotor nuclei of the fifth, seventh, and 12th cranial nerves as well as the nucleus ambiguus and ventral motoneurons of the spinal cord. In addition, strong hybridization signals are found over Purkinje neurons of the cerebellum as well as over cell groups that provide strong inputs to the cerebellum, such as the pontine gray and inferior olive.

Corticosteroid Receptors

The diverse and potent actions of glucocorticoids on the mammalian brain appear to be mediated by two distinct receptors. The distributions of both the MR (type I corticosteroid receptor) and GR (type II corticosteroid receptor) have been mapped in great detail with autoradiographic (12,75,76,80), immunohistochemical (82,83), and *in situ* hybridization histochemical (49,89–93) methods. The results of these studies are generally consistent, and the following description is based on observations of *in situ* hybridization histochemical material (see Fig. 4 of ref. 49 and Fig. 1). Compared with AR mRNA-containing neurons, cells that express detectable levels of MR and GR mRNA are somewhat more widely distributed throughout the central nervous system. This difference is most pronounced in the telencephalon, but like AR mRNA-containing neurons, regions associated with olfaction contain moderate to high densities of MR and GR mRNA-containing cells. These regions include the piriform cortex, the olfactory tubercle, and the endopiriform nucleus. Both MR and GR mRNA are abundant in each major division of isocortex, with the greatest density of MR mRNA-containing neurons in layers II, III, and V. The GR mRNA-containing neurons are also abundant in the same cortical layers, but in addition, layer VI contains moderately labeled cells, especially at caudal levels through the cortex.

The hippocampal formation contains the greatest overall density of MR and GR mRNA-containing neurons of any brain region, but each receptor has a unique distribution in the hippocampus. Whereas MR

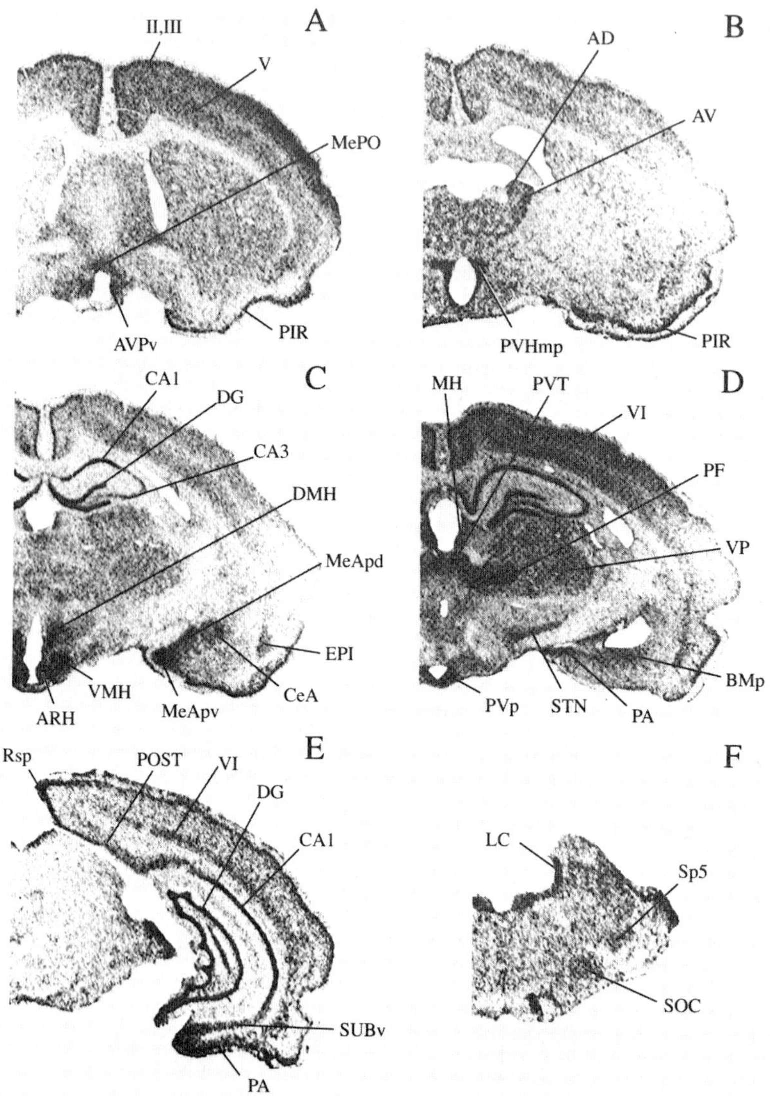

FIG. 1. The GR mRNA in rat brain. A series of autoradiographic images (8-day exposure) derived from coronal sections (analyzed from rostral to caudal, A–F) through the rat brain to show the distribution of GR mRNA expression. *In situ* hybridization was carried out as described (88). Abbreviations: n, nucleus; AD, anterior n (thalamus); ARH, arcuate n (hypothalamus); AV, anteroventral n (thalamus); AVPv, anteroventral periventricular n (hypothalamus); BMp, basomedial n (amygdala) posterior part; CA1-CA3, fields of Ammon's horn; CeA, central n (amygdala); DG, dentate gyrus; DMH, dorsomedial n (hypothalamus); EPi, endopiriform n; LC, locus ceruleus; MeApd, medial n (amygdala) posterodorsal part; MeApv, medial n (amygdala) posteroventral part; MePO, median preoptic n; MH, medial habenula; MM, medial mammillary n; PA, posterior n (amygdala; a.k.a. amygdalo-hippocampal transition area); PF, parafasicular n; PIR, piriform cortex; POST, postsubiculum; PVp, periventricular n (hypothalamus) posterior part; PVHmp, paraventricular n (hypothalamus) medial parvocellular part; PVT, paraventricular n (thalamus); Rsp, retrosplenial area; SOC, superior olivary complex; Sp5, spinal n of trigeminal nerve; STN, subthalamic n; SUBv, subiculum (ventral part); VB, ventral basal complex (thalamus); VMH, ventromedial n (hypothalamus); VP, ventral posterior complex (thalamus); II, III, V and VI, layers of isocortex.

mRNA appears to be most abundant in CA3, only low levels of GR mRNA are expressed in this field of Ammon's horn, with the highest abundance of GR mRNA found in field CA1 (49,89–91). That nearly all neurons of each field express MR and GR mRNAs suggests that the MR and GR are coexpressed in the majority of pyramidal cells of the hippocampal region. However, the differential abundance of the MR and GR in discrete fields of Ammon's horn indicates that certain elements of the hippocampal trisynaptic circuit (see ref. 82) may be differentially sensitive to hormonal influences mediated by circulating glucocorticoids. Both MR and GR mRNAs are extremely abundant in neurons of the ventral subiculum, which has strong projections to the lateral septum and hypothalamus (94,95).

The MR and GR mRNAs are somewhat less abundant in the amygdala than in the hippocampal formation, but distinct differences in the distribution of the two receptors are clearly apparent. High densities of moderately labeled MR mRNA-containing neurons are found in the cortical and basomedial nuclei, and only low levels of labeling are apparent over the medial, central, and lateral nuclei. In contrast, relatively low levels of GR mRNA are found in the cortical nuclei, but the intensity of labeling is considerably higher over the medial and central nuclei. The highest density of MR mRNA-containing neurons is found in the posterior nucleus of the amygdala (the amygdalohippocampal transition area), which, like the medial nucleus, provides strong projections to the hypothalamus (96). Most of the cells in the posterior nucleus express low to moderate levels of GR mRNA. The massive projections of the posterior nucleus of the amygdala to the periventricular zone of the hypothalamus and to the ventral premammillary nucleus, which provides strong inputs to the anteroventral periventricular, arcuate, and paraventricular hypothalamic nuclei (97), suggest that the posterior nucleus of the amygdala may play an important but largely unappreciated role in mediating glucocorticoid feedback on neuroendocrine physiology.

In marked contrast to the distribution of AR mRNA, very few cell groups in the hypothalamus express detectable levels of MR mRNA. However, the hypothalamic distribution of GR mRNA-containing neurons is quite extensive, with the highest densities of labeled cells found in the periventricular zone. Thus, the pariventricular and arcuate nuclei of the hypothalamus, which harbor neurons that secrete neuroendocrine releasing factors (98), as well as the anteroventral periventricular nucleus of the preoptic region, which supplies strong inputs to these nuclei, all contain significant numbers of GR mRNA-containing neurons. In the medial zone of the hypothalamus, regions with the highest densities of GR mRNA-containing neurons have strong connections with the periventricular zone, including the medial part of the medial preoptic nucleus (99) and ventral premammilary nucleus, both of which contain a moderate density of lightly labeled neurons. The functional significance of the relatively high levels of GR mRNA expressed in the dorsomedial and ventromedial nuclei of the hypothalamus remains unclear. MR mRNA is not abundant in the thalamus, but a notable exception is the reticular nucleus of the thalamus. In contrast, GR mRNA is widely distributed throughout most thalamic complexes, but the reticular nucleus appears to lack GR mRNA-containing neurons, and only a few regions such as the medial habenula and parafasicular nucleus contain heavily labeled cells.

On a cellular level, MR mRNA is much more abundant in the brainstem and spinal cord than is GR mRNA. As is the case for nuclei that contain AR mRNA-containing neurons, regions that express MR and GR mRNA can be divided into two major functional categories: those relaying sensory information and those containing somatic motoneurons. At least moderate labeling is found over the vestibular and cochlear nuclei as well as over layers III and V of the superior colliculus, suggesting that the MR may be involved in modulating the processing of vestibular, auditory, and visual information. Furthermore, the presence of moderate to strongly labeled MR mRNA-containing neurons in nuclei that relay somatosensory information from the dorsal root and trigeminal ganglia indicates that sensory modalities transmitted along these pathways may be influenced by hormonal cues mediated by the MR. The GR may also play a role in modulating somatosensory information, since clearly labeled neurons are present in the inferior colliculus, ventral cochlear nuclei, and substantia gelatinosa of the spinal cord. Glucocorticoids may affect visceral sensory information through either the MR or GR, although perhaps by activating somewhat different pathways. The medial part of the nucleus of the solitary tract and lateral part of the parabrachial nucleus, which project to autonomic regions of the hypothalamus, contain heavily labeled MR and GR mRNA-containing neurons, respectively. Intensely labeled GR mRNA-containing neurons are present in the locus ceruleus, which in addition to projecting to the hypothalamus provides widespread noradrenergic inputs to the cerebral cortex (100–104).

Among the most heavily labeled MR mRNA-containing neurons in the brainstem are the motoneurons in the oculomotor, trochlear, trigeminal, abducens, facial, and hypoglossal cranial nerve nuclei as well as neurons in the nucleus ambiguus. The distribution of GR mRNA-containing neurons is much more restricted, with clearly labeled cells found only in the facial and hypoglossal cranial nerve nuclei and in the nucleus ambiguus. Both MR and GR mRNAs are expressed in motoneurons of the spinal cord, but on a cellular basis, MR mRNA is somewhat more abundant than GR mRNA. Other regions involved in the control of motor systems also contain neurons that express MR and GR mRNA. In the cerebellum GR mRNA is abundant in the granular layer, but cellular labeling for MR mRNA is rather light. In addition to AR mRNA, most Purkinje cells express at least low to moderate amounts of MR and GR mRNA. Whether individual Purkinje cells coexpress these receptors remains to be rigorously tested. Regions that supply strong inputs to the cerebellum, such as the pontine gray, inferior olivary nucleus, and lateral reticular nucleus, contain neurons that express MR mRNA as well as scattered lightly labeled GR mRNA-containing neurons. Similarly, the deep cerebellar nuclei contain numerous MR mRNA-containing neurons but only scattered lightly labeled GR mRNA-containing cells.

Progesterone Receptor

Previous autoradiographic (81) and biochemical (70,71) studies indicate that the progesterone receptor has the most restricted central distribution of any of the steroid hormone receptors. Our preliminary examination of the distribution of neurons that express PR mRNA confirms these findings (Fig. 2). The highest densities of PR mRNA-containing neurons are found in the hypothalamus, particularly in regions that modulate neuroendocrine function such as the medial part of the medial preoptic nucleus, anteroventral periventricular, and arcuate nuclei (see ref. 98 and references therein), although PR mRNA labeling is notably light over the paraventricular nucleus of the hypothalamus. That the ventrolateral part of the ventromedial nucleus of the hypothalamus contains a high density of PR mRNA-containing neurons is consistent with numerous reports describing the action of progesterone on this nucleus in activating female copulatory behavior (see refs. 5,105,106 for reviews). In sharp contrast to other members of the GR subfamily of receptors, the PR does not have an extensive telencephalic distribution. Moderate labeling is found over hippocampal pyramidal cells in region CA3, but labeling for PR mRNA over other regions of the hippocampal formation is either very light or absent. Similarly, very few PR mRNA-containing neurons are found in the amyg-

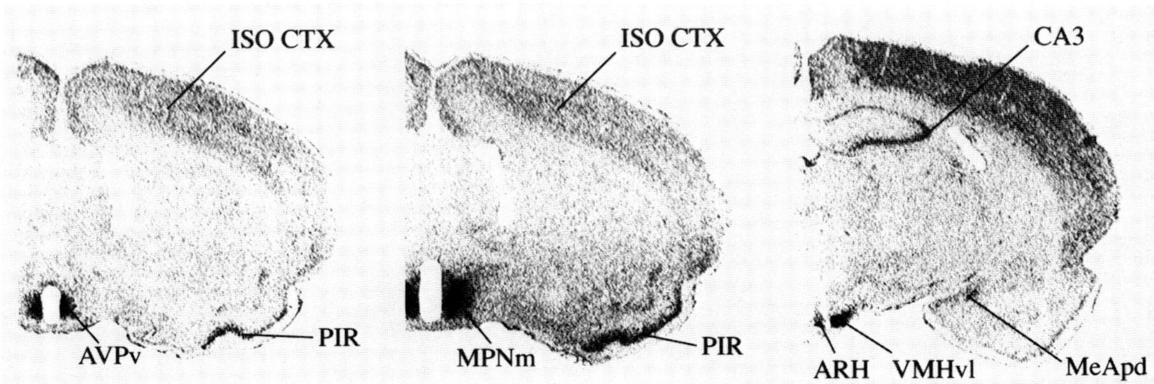

FIG. 2. Progesterone receptor mRNA in rat brain. Three autoradiographic images (4-day cronex film exposure) showing the distribution of PR mRNA expression in the forebrain of the rat. Abbreviations: n, nucleus; AVPv, anteroventral periventricular n (hypothalamus); ARH, arcuate n (hypothalamus); CA3, field of Ammon's Horn; ISO CTX, isocortex; MeApd, medial n (amygdala) posterodorsal part; MPNm, medial preoptic n, medial part; PIR, piriform cortex; VMHvl, ventromedial n (hypothalamus) ventrolateral part.

dala, but moderate labeling over the medial nucleus is a consistent finding. Within the isocortex, low to moderate levels of PR mRNA are detected in layers II and III, and a few lightly labeled neurons are scattered in the deeper layers as well. The PR does not appear to be abundant in the brainstem and spinal cord, but this has not been studied in great detail.

Estrogen Receptor

The distribution of estradiol-concentrating neurons has been mapped in great detail (77,79), and immunohistochemistry has been used to directly localize cells that express the ER (83–85). The distribution of ER mRNA-containing neurons closely matches these accounts (88,107). The greatest densities of ER mRNA-containing neurons are found in the hypothalamus, and there is considerable overlap with the distribution of neurons that express AR mRNA (see Fig. 3 of ref. 88). Moreover, in regions that express both receptors, ER mRNA is generally more abundant (see Table 1 of ref. 88), and many of these regions also contain high densities of PR mRNA-containing neurons (Fig. 2). Neurons that express ER mRNA are particularly abundant in the periventricular zone of the hypothalamus and cell groups in the medial zone that provide strong inputs to the periventricular zone. Thus, intensely labeled neurons are found in the arcuate and anteroventral periventricular nuclei and in all three parts of the periventricular nucleus of the hypothalamus. Medial zone cell groups that contain high densities of ER mRNA-containing neurons include the medial part of the medial preoptic nucleus and the ventrolateral part of the ventromedial nucleus, both of which have been implicated in the control of reproductive function (106,108).

Telencephalic regions that supply strong inputs to the hypothalamus contain the highest densities of ER mRNA-containing neurons, and these regions appear to be a subset of those expressing AR mRNA. The majority of ER mRNA-containing neurons in the amygdala are localized to either the posterodorsal part of the medial nucleus, the anterior and posterior cortical nuclei, or the posterior nucleus of the amygdala (the amygdalohippocampal transition area). In the septal region, the greatest number of heavily labeled cells are localized to the ventral part of the lateral septal nucleus and the encapsulated (principal) nucleus of the bed nuclei of the stria terminalis (109), both of which supply strong inputs to the medial and periventricular zones of the hypothalamus (21,95). The distribution of ER mRNA-containing neurons in cortical regions is quite different from that of the AR or other members of the GR-like subfamily of receptors. In the hippocampal formation ER mRNA is relatively scarce in the pyramidal layer of Ammon's horn, and only low to moderate levels of labeling are seen over the ventral subiculum and presubiculum. Similarly, unlike the GR-like subfamily of receptors, the isocortex is largely free of hybridization signal for ER mRNA, although a few moderately labeled ER mRNA-containing neurons are reliably found in olfactory regions of the cerebral cortex, including the olfactory tubercle, the piriform cortex, and the endopiriform nucleus.

The thalamus is largely free of ER mRNA-containing neurons, but a discrete group of heavily labeled cells is localized to the medial aspect of the lateral habenula and in the paraventricular nucleus. Each part of the zona incerta that has AR mRNA-containing neurons also has at least a few cells that express ER mRNA, including the region of the A13 dopaminergic neurons.

Only a few regions of the brainstem and spinal cord contain significant densities of ER mRNA-containing neurons. The AR, GR, MR, and ER mRNA-containing neurons appear to overlap in the substantia gelatinosa of the spinal cord, but sensory pathways in the rest of the brainstem are largely free of ER mRNA. The medial part of the nucleus of the solitary tract and lateral division of the parabrachial nucleus contain large numbers of ER mRNA-containing neurons, and both regions relay visceral sensory information to the hypothalamus. None of the somatomotor neurons that contain AR, MR, or GR mRNA appear to express ER mRNA, nor is the ER expressed to any great extent in neural systems associated with the cerebellum. One curious exception is the parvicellular division of the dentate nucleus, which contains several intensely labeled ER mRNA-containing neurons. The relative abundance of ER mRNA in the periaqueductal gray is consistent with the suggestion that the behavioral responses mediated by this complex structure may be sensitive to the modulatory effects of circulating estradiol (106). Finally, noradrenergic pathways that may be influenced by circulating estrogen are those arising in the locus ceruleus and A1 cell groups, which contain moderately labeled ER mRNA-containing neurons.

Other members of the ER-like subfamily such as thyroid hormone receptors (110) are generally more widely distributed, but complete mapping studies have not been published.

AUTOLOGOUS REGULATION OF STEROID HORMONE RECEPTORS

Steroid hormone receptors are not normally maintained at constant levels in neurons but rather are subject to regulatory influences of circulating hormones, neurotransmission, and developmental events. Thus, both neural and endocrine factors appear to be capable of modulating the impact of steroid hormones on hormone-sensitive neural systems. The most thoroughly studied regulatory pattern is that mediated by the cognate hormones for each receptor. This autologous regulation is generally negative; increased levels of hormone lead to a suppression of hormone receptor gene expression that is usually brought about by decreasing the rate of transcription and the stability of receptor mRNA (111–113). However, autoregulation of steroid hormone receptor gene expression shows considerable cell and tissue specificity with regard to direction, sensitivity, and temporal organization of the regulatory pattern.

Corticosteroid Receptors

Expression of both the MR and GR in brain appears to be negatively regulated by circulating glucocorticoids (114). Most work on the regulation of MR and GR gene expression has focused on the hippocampus. Analysis of total RNA extracts from whole hippocampus by solution hybridization indicates that both MR and GR mRNAs increase within 24 hr following adrenalectomy but return to control levels by the 16th day (115). However, treatment of adrenalectomized rats with dexamethasone has differential effects on the two mRNAs. Dexamethasone increases MR mRNAs in hippocampus after 2 days of treatment, but these increases are not maintained. Treatment of adrenalectomized rats with dexamethasone appears to maintain GR mRNA at levels similar to those found in intact animals.

A detailed *in situ* hybridization analysis of each subfield of Ammon's horn added greater spatial resolution to these findings, and the results indicate that hormonal regulation of MR and GR gene expression is limited to defined regions of the hippocampus (91). The up-regulation of MR mRNA that follows adrenalectomy appears to be limited to fields CA1 and CA2 and is reversed by treatment with dexamethasone. Adrenalectomy also reversibly increases levels of GR mRNA in fields CA1 and CA2 as well as in the dentate gyrus. In contrast, a different regulatory pattern is observed in the paraventricular nucleus of the hypothalamus (116). Treatment of adrenalectomized rats with corticosterone produces small but significant increases in both MR and GR mRNA in discrete regions of this neuroendocrine nucleus. Whether the observed patterns of regulation are caused by the different hormonal treatments employed or by cell-specific response mechanisms remains to be determined. Nev-

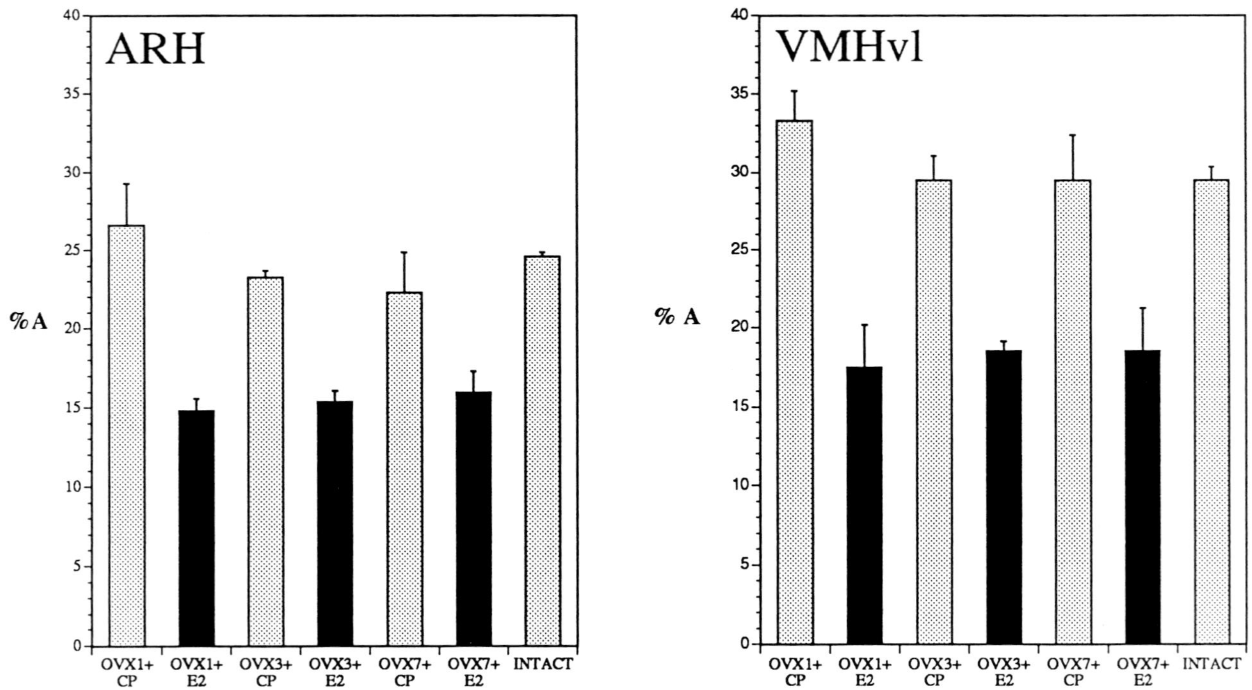

FIG. 3. Autoregulation of ER mRNA. Comparison of hybridization signals for ER mRNA in the arcuate (ARH) and ventromedial (VMHvl) hypothalamic nuclei of female rats. Females were intact (estrous) or were ovariectomized and treated with pellets of estradiol (E_2; 0.5 mg/pellet) or control pellets (CP) for 1, 3, or 7 days before death. *Bars* represent mean percentage absorbance values (±S.E.M.) for each experimental group. *Solid bars* indicate animals with relatively high, and *shaded bars* indicate animals with very low or undetectable levels of circulating estradiol. n = 4 for each experimental group. (Data from ref. 132.)

ertheless, these findings underscore the potential for tissue specificity in hormonal regulation of MR and GR gene expression.

Androgen Receptor

Androgen receptor mRNA also appears to be differentially regulated in various tissues. AR mRNA levels increase within 4 days after orchidectomy in kidney, epididymis, and prostate; treatment of 4-day castrates with androgen for 24 hr reverses these increases (117–120). In whole brain, extracts of total RNA show a similar androgen-reversible increase in AR mRNA after orchidectomy (119). However, we have observed the opposite effect of androgen on AR mRNA in the posterodorsal subdivision of the medial amygdala (MeAp; Fig. 3). The results of this *in situ* hybridization study demonstrate a more than twofold reduction in AR mRNA hybridization in the MeAp of male rats 24 hr after castration, relative to intact animals. This decrease was maintained for at least 3 days, but AR mRNA levels return to those characteristic of intact males by the seventh day. Orchidectomized rats treated with testosterone have AR mRNA hybridization signals that are indistinguishable from those of intact males. Similar results are obtained in female animals: ovariectomy decreases and estradiol treatment increases levels of AR mRNA in the MeAp (Fig. 3). Thus, hormonal regulation of AR mRNA may display cell type specificity, especially in complex heterogeneous tissues such as the brain.

Progesterone Receptor

In the T47D human breast cancer cell line, progesterone suppresses PR gene expression by decreasing transcription and increasing the rate of PR mRNA degradation (111,121, 122). Similarly, progesterone appears to down-regulate the expression of its cognate receptor in tissues of the female reproductive tract (123,124). The autoregulation of PR gene expression in brain has not been addressed with biochemical methods, but a recent report that progesterone increases PR immunoreactivity in estrogen-primed guinea pigs to a greater degree than that found following treatment with estrogen alone (125) suggests that progesterone may induce expression of the PR gene in a tissue-specific manner.

Estrogen Receptor

As is the case for members of the GR-like subfamily of receptors, the hormonal regulation of ER mRNA displays considerable cell and tissue specificity. Circulating estradiol down-regulates levels of both ER mRNA and protein in MCF-7 cancer cells (126–129) as well as in rat uterus (130). However, estrogen treatment appears to cause a significant increase in ER mRNA in rat liver and pituitary (130), as it does in T47D cells (127). In brain, estrogen down-regulates expression of ER mRNA in the ventromedial (131,132) and arcuate nuclei of the hypothalamus (132; Fig. 4) and in the medial nucleus of the amygdala (R. Simerly, unpublished results). These *in situ* hybridization studies are in agreement with immunohistochemical findings, which also indicate an inhibitory effect of estrogen on ER expression (133–136).

Heterologous Regulation

In addition to the autologous regulation described above, at least some steroid hormones exert regulatory influences on the expression of heterologous receptors. For instance, estrogen down-regulates AR (137) and GR (138) gene expression but induces expression of the PR in some but not all regions of the hypothalamus (139,140). Similarly, androgen treatment down-regulates expression of the ER in the hypothalamus (132) but appears to have no effect on PR gene expression (139). Less is known about the influence of progesterone on the expression of other receptors, but it has been shown to suppress expression of the ER in the female re-

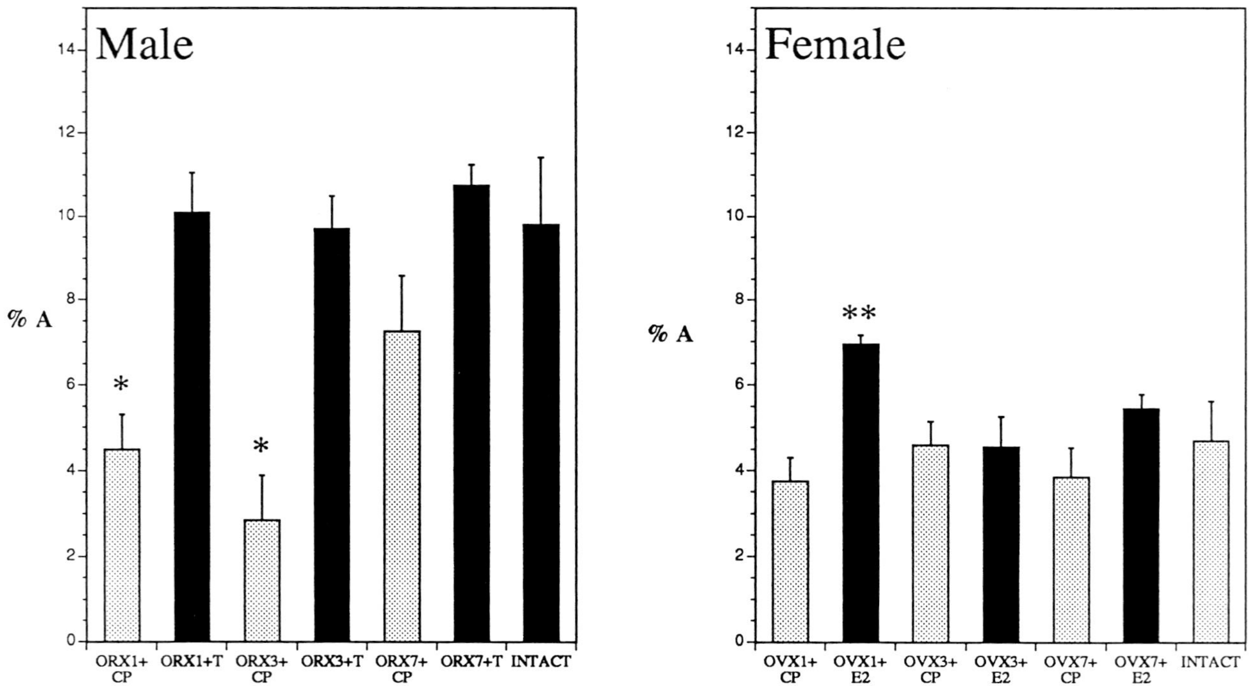

FIG. 4. Autoregulation of AR mRNA. Comparison of hybridization signals for AR mRNA in the MeApd of male and female rats. Intact male rats were compared with animals that were orchidectomized (ORX) and treated with pellets of testosterone (T; 25 mg/pellet) or control pellets (CP) for 1, 3, or 7 days before death. Females were intact (estrous) or were ovariectomized and treated with pellets of estradiol (E_2; 0.5 mg/pellet) or control pellets (CP) for 1, 3, or 7 days before death. Bars represent mean percentage absorbance values (+S.E.M.) for each experimental group (see ref. 132). Solid bars indicate animals with relatively high, and shaded bars indicate animals with very low or undetectable levels of circulating sex steroid hormones; $n = 4$ for each experimental group.

productive tract (141,142). In addition to heterologous hormonal regulation, steroid hormone receptors may be regulated by neural influences mediated by synaptic transmission. For example, removal of the olfactory inputs to the amygdala increases estrogen binding in the medial nucleus of the amygdala (143), and estrogen binding in the hypothalamus is altered following deafferentation (144,145). Changes in estrogen receptor binding have also been observed following pharmacological manipulation of both noradrenergic and dopaminergic neurotransmitter systems (146–148). These changes in hormone binding may relate to activation of steroid receptors by second messenger systems or by other as yet uncharacterized molecular mechanisms (149).

CONCLUSIONS

In the central nervous system, the functional importance of receptor-mediated regulatory events is directly related to the neural pathways in which they occur. Thus, the apparent coexpression of mRNAs encoding the AR, PR, MR, and GR within discrete neurons of the hippocampus suggests that these receptors may activate overlapping sets of genes in pyramidal elements of the trisynaptic circuit (57,150). Cellular factors that lead to the differential expression of these receptors within specific pathways will therefore control the relative impact of each receptor on hippocampal physiology. Similarly, the extensive but only partially overlapping connections between forebrain regions that contain the highest densities of sex steroid hormone receptors provide a possible substrate for the additive influences of the AR and ER on the activity of these complex circuits. Thus, in addition to activating partially overlapping sets of genes within individual neurons, as may be the case in the hippocampus, steroid hormone receptors may regulate gene expression within partially overlapping neural circuitry, whereby an epigenetic level of transsynaptic regulation may be superimposed on the direct genomic effects of the hormone receptors (88). Furthermore, because steroid hormone receptors are themselves subject to the regulatory influences of circulating steroid hormones, the responsiveness of such complex neural systems to hormonal activation can be autoregulated by the hormones themselves.

The unanticipated complexity and diversity of molecular interactions between steroid hormone receptors and their widespread but overlapping distributions in the central nervous system have both illuminated and confounded our understanding of the functional role these powerful factors play in development and in mature physiology. Before we can fully appreciate the role of steroid hormones in modulating neuronal plasticity in general, and neuronal regeneration in particular, it will be necessary to define the expression pattern and complete regulatory profile of steroid hormone receptors within specific neural pathways. Moreover, we will need to determine the combined influence of the different endocrine systems on gene expression and characterize the cellular responses to these hormonally directed molecular events. This information will certainly enhance our understanding of the profound trophic influences on neuronal plasticity mediated by steroid hormones and may ultimately provide new insights into possible strategies for facilitating naturally occurring restorative processes following neuronal injury.

ACKNOWLEDGMENTS

I wish to thank Drs. L. W. Swanson and J. Arriza for their contributions to the work reviewed above and for numerous enlightening discussions. I am also grateful for generous gifts of plasmids from Drs. J. Arriza, C. Chang, M. Muramatsu, O. -K. Park, and K. Mayo. Research in the author's laboratory is supported by PHS grants NS 26723, RR 00163, and the Medical Research Foundation of Oregon. (ORPRC publication # 1854).

REFERENCES

1. Harrison NL, Majewska MD, Meyers DER, Barker JL. Rapid actions of steroids on CNS neurons. In: Lakoski JM, Perez-Polo JR, Rassin DK, eds. *Neural control on reproductive function.* New York: Alan R. Liss; 1989:137–166.
2. Kelly MJ. Electrical effects of steroids in neurons. In: McKerns KW, Pantic V, eds. *Hormonally active brain peptides.* New York: Plenum Press; 1982:253–277.
3. McEwen BS, Davis PG, Parsons B, Pfaff DW. The brain as a target for steroid hormone action. *Annu Rev Neurosci* 1979;2:65–112.
4. McEwen BS, Biegon A, Davis PG, et al. Steroid hormones: humoral signals which alter brain cell properties and functions. *Recent Prog Horm Res* 1982;38:41–92.
5. McEwen BS, Jones KJ, Pfaff DW. Hormonal control of sexual behavior in the female rat: molecular, cellular and neurochemical studies. *Biol Reprod* 1987;36:37–45.
6. Meyer JS. Biochemical effects of corticosteroids on neural tissues. *Physiol Rev* 1985;65:946–1020.
7. Naftolin F, Garcia SLM, Keefe D, Leranth C, MacLusky NJ, Brawer JR. Estrogen effects on the synaptology and neural membranes of the rat hypothalamic arcuate nucleus. *Biol Reprod* 1990;42:21–28.
8. Arai Y, Matsumoto A, Nishizuka M. Synaptogenesis and neuronal plasticity to gonadal steroids: implications for the development of sexual dimorphism in the neuroendocrine brain. *Curr Top Neuroendocrinol* 1986;7:291–307.
9. Arnold AP, Gorski RA. Gonadal steroid induction of structural sex differences in the central nervous system. *Annu Rev Neurosci* 1984;7:413–442.
10. Arnold AP, Jordan CL. Hormonal organization of neural circuits. In: Martini L, Ganong WF, eds. *Frontiers in neuroendocrinology.* New York: Raven Press; 1988:185–214.
11. De Vries GJ. Sex differences in neurotransmitter systems. *J Neuroendocrinol* 1990;2:1–13.
12. McEwen BS, de Kloet ER, Rostene W. Adrenal steroid receptors and actions in the nervous system. *Physiol Rev* 1986;66:1121–1188.
13. Gorski RA. Gonadal hormones as putative neurotrophic substances. In: Cotman C, ed. *Synaptic plasticity,* New York: Guilford Press; 1985:287–310.
14. McEwen BS, Coirini H, Westlind-Danielsson A, et al. Steroid hormones as mediators of neural plasticity. *J Steroid Biochem* 1991;39:223–232.
15. Hall ED. Steroids and neuronal destruction or stabilization. In: Chadwick D, ed. *Steroids and neuronal activity.* Chichester: John Wiley & Sons; 1990:206–219.
16. Hirata F. Glucocorticoids and head injury. *Neurochem Pathol* 1986;7:33–43.
17. Jones KJ. Steroid hormones and neurotrophism: relationship to nerve injury. *Metab Brain Dis* 1988;3:1–18.
18. Goy RW, McEwen BS. *Sexual differentiation of the brain,* Cambridge, MA: MIT Press; 1980.
19. Juraska JM. Sex differences in developmental plasticity in the visual cortex and hippocampal dentate gyrus. *Prog Brain Res* 1984;61:205.
20. Hines M. Prenatal gonadal hormones and sex differences in human behavior. *Psychol Bull* 1982;92:56–80.
21. Simerly RB. Hormonal control of neuropeptide gene expression in sexually dimorphic olfactory pathways. *Trends Neurosci* 1990;13:104–110.
22. Simerly RB. Prodynorphin and proenkephalin gene expression in the anteroventral periventricular nucleus of the rat: sexual differentiation and hormonal regulation. *Mol Cell Neurosci* 1991; 2:473–484.
23. Bleier RW, Byne W, Siggelkow I. Cytoarchitectonic sexual dimorphisms of the medial preoptic and anterior hypothalamic areas in guinea pig, rat, hamster, and mouse. *J Comp Neurol* 1982; 212:118–130.
24. Bloch GJ, Gorski RA. Cytoarchitectonic analysis of the SDN-POA of the intact and gonadectomized rat. *J Comp Neurol* 1988;275:604–612.
25. Simerly RB, Swanson LW, Gorski RA. The distribution of monoaminergic cells and fibers in a periventricular preoptic nucleus involved in the control of gonadotropin release: immunohistochemical evidence for a dopaminergic sexual dimorphism. *Brain Res* 1985;330:55–64.
26. Simerly RB, McCall LD, Watson SJ. Distribution of opioid peptides in the preoptic region: immunohistochemical evidence for a steroid-sensitive enkephalin sexual dimorphism. *J Comp Neurol* 1988;276:442–459.
27. Simerly RB, Swanson LW, Handa RJ, Gorski RA. Influence of perinatal androgen on the sexually dimorphic distribution of tyrosine hydroxylase-immunoreactive cells and fibers in the anteroventral periventricular nucleus of the rat. *Neuroendocrinology* 1985;40:501–510.
28. Sanders SA, Reinisch JM. Behavioral effects on humans of progesterone-related compounds during development and in the adult. In: Ganten D, Pfaff D, eds. *Current topics in neuroendocrinology: actions of progesterone on the brain.* Berlin: Springer-Verlag; 1985:175–206.
29. Meyer JS. Early adrenalectomy stimulates subsequent growth and development of the rat brain. *Exp Neurol* 1983;82:432–446.
30. Meyer JS, Fairman KR. Early adrenalectomy increases myelin content of the rat brain. *Dev Brain Res* 1985;17:1–9.
31. Sapolsky RM, Krey LC, McEwen BS. The neuroendocrinology of stress and aging: the glucocorticoid cascade hypothesis. *Endocr Rev* 1986;7:284–301.
32. Sloviter RS, Valiquette G, Abrams GM, et al. Selective loss of hippocampal granule cells in the mature rat brain after adrenalectomy. *Science* 1989;243:535–538.
33. Markey KA, Towle AC, Sze PY. Glucocorticoid influence on tyrosine hydroxylase activity in mouse locus coeruleus during postnatal development. *Endocrinology* 1982;111:1519–1523.
34. Bohn MC, Black IB. Development of the adrenergic phenotype in rat brain: characterization of a glucocorticoid responsive period. *Soc Neurosci Abstr* 1983;9:306.
35. Sze PY. Developmental-regulatory aspects of brain tryptophan hydroxylase. In: Haber B, Gabay S, eds. *Serotonin. Current aspects of neurochemistry*

and function. New York: Plenum Press; 1981: 507–523.
36. MacLusky NJ, Brown TJ. Control of gonadal steroid receptor levels in the developing brain. In: Lakoski JM, Perez-Polo JR, Rassin DK, eds. *Neural control of reproductive function*. New York: Alan R. Liss; 1989:45–59.
37. Sheridan PJ. Autoradiographic localization of steroid receptors in the brain. *Clin Neuropharmacol* 1984;7:281–295.
38. Evans RM. The steroid and thyroid hormone receptor superfamily. *Science* 1988;240:889–895.
39. Forman BM, Samuels HH. Dimerization among nuclear hormone receptors. *New Biologist* 1990;2:587–594.
40. O'Malley B. The steroid receptor superfamily: more excitement predicted for the future. *Mol Endocrinol* 1990:4:363–369.
41. Tsai SY, Tsai M-J, O'Malley BW. The steroid receptor superfamily: transactivators of gene expression. In: Parker MG, ed. *Nuclear hormone receptors*. London: Academic Press; 1991:103–124.
42. Walhi W, Martinez E. Superfamily of steroid nuclear receptors: positive and negative regulators of gene expression. *FASEBJ* 1991;5:2243–2249.
43. Yamamoto KR. Steroid receptor regulated transcription of specific genes and gene networks. *Annu Rev Genet* 1985·19:209–252.
44. Giguere V, Hollenberg SM, Rosenfeld MG, Evans RM. Functional domains of the human glucocorticoid receptor. *Cell* 1986:46:645–652.
45. Kumar V, Green S, Stack G, Berry M, Jin J-R, Chambon P. Functional domains of the human estrogen receptor. *Cell* 1987;51:941–951.
46. Muller M, Baniahmad C, Kaltschmidt C, Schule R, Renkawitz R. Co-operative transactivation of steroid receptors. In: Parker MG, ed. *Nuclear hormone receptors*. London: Academic Press; 1990:155–174.
47. Ankenbauer W, Strahle U, Schutz G. Synergistic action of glucocorticoid and estradiol responsive elements. *Proc Natl Acad Sci USA* 1988;85: 7526–7530.
48. Mader S, Kumar V, de Verneuil H, Chambon P. Three amino acids of the oestrogen receptor are essential to its ability to distinguish an oestrogen from a glucocorticoid-responsive element. *Nature* 1989;338:271–274.
49. Arriza JL, Simerly RB, Swanson LW, Evans RM. The neuronal mineralocorticoid receptor as a mediator of glucocorticoid response. *Neuron* 1988; 1:887–900.
50. Umesono K, Evans RM. Determinants of target gene specificity for steroid/thyroid hormone receptors. *Cell* 1989;57:1139–1146.
51. Greene GL, Gilna P, Waterfield M, Baker A, Hort Y, Shine J. Sequence and expression of human estrogen receptor complementary DNA. *Science* 1986;231:1150–1154
52. Koike S, Sakai M, Muramatsu M. Molecular cloning and characterization of rat estrogen receptor cDNA. *Nucleic Acids Res* 1987;15:2499–2513.
53. Walter P, Green S, Greene G, et al. Cloning of the human estrogen receptor cDNA. *Proc Natl Acad Sci USA* 1985;82:7889–7893.
54. Bicknell JN, Refsdal CD, Miller MA, Dorsa DM. Androgen and estrogen receptor mRNA expression in the preoptic area of male and female rat brains. *Soc Neurosci Abstr* 1990;16:660.
55. Chang C, Kokontis J, Shutsung L. Structural analysis of complementary DNA and amino acid sequences of human and rat androgen receptors. *Proc Natl Acad Sci USA* 1988;85:7211–7215.
56. Kastner P, Krust A, Turcotte B, et al. Two distinct estrogen-regulated promoters generate transcripts encoding the two functionally different human progesterone receptor forms A and B. *EMBO J* 1990;9:1603–1614.
57. Evans RM, Arriza JL. A molecular framework for the actions of glucocorticoid hormones in the nervous system. *Neuron* 1989;2:1105–1112.
58. Reul JMHM, de Kloet ER. Two receptor systems for corticosterone in rat brain: microdistribution and differential occupation. *Endocrinology* 1985; 117:2505–2511.
59. Arriza JL, Weinberger C, Cerelli G, et al. Cloning of human mineralocorticoid receptor complementary DNA: structural and functional kinship with the glucocorticoid receptor. *Science* 1987;237: 268–275.
60. Hollenberg SM, Weinberger C, Ong ES, et al. Primary structure and expression of a functional human glucocorticoid receptor cDNA. *Nature* 1985;318:635–641.
61. Funder JW, Sheppard K. Adrenocorticosteroids and the brain. *Annu Rev Physiol* 1987;49:397–411.
62. Patel PD, Sherman TG, Goldman DJ, Watson SJ. Molecular cloning of a mineralocorticoid (type I) receptor complementary DNA from rat hippocampus. *Mol Endocrinol* 1989;3:1877–1885.
63. Liao S, Rossini GP, Hiipakka RA, Chen C. Factors that can control the interaction of the androgen–receptor complex with the genomic structure in the rat prostate. In: Bresciani F, ed. *Perspectives in steroid receptor research*. New York: Raven Press; 1980:99–112.
64. Grandics P, Miller A, Schmidt TJ, Litwack G. Phosphorylation *in vivo* of rat hepatic glucocorticoid receptors. *Biochem Biophys Res Commun* 1984;120:59–65.
65. Auricchio R, Migliaccio A, Castoria G, Rotondi A, Lastoria S. Direct evidence of *in vivo* phosphorylation–dephosphorylation of the estradiol-17β receptor. Role of Ca^{2+}–calmodulin in the activation of hormone binding sites. *J Steroid Biochem* 1984;20:31–35.
66. Sheridan PL, Krett NL, Gordon JA, Horwitz KB. Human progesterone receptor transformation and nuclear down-regulation are independent of phosphorylation. *Mol Endocrinol* 1988;2:1329–1342.
67. Murray MB, Towle HC. Identification of nuclear factors that enhance binding of the thyroid hormone receptor to a thyroid hormone response element. *Mol Endocrinol* 1989;3:1434–1442.
68. Handa RJ, Roselli CE, Horton L, Resko JA. The quantitative distribution of cytosolic androgen receptors in microdissected areas of the male rat brain: effects of estrogen treatment. *Endocrinology* 1987;121:233–240.
69. McEwen BS. Steroid receptors in neuroendocrine

tissues: topography, subcellular distribution, and functional implications. In: Naftolin F, Ryan KJ, Davis J, eds. *Subcellular mechanisms in reproductive neuroendocrinology.* Amsterdam: Elsevier; 1976:277–304.

70. McEwen BS, Davis P, Gerlach J, et al. Progestin receptors in the brain and pituitary gland. In: Bardin C, Mauvais-Jarvis P, Milgrom F, eds. *Progesterone and progestin.* New York: Raven Press; 1983:59–76.
71. Parsons B, Rainbow TC, MacLusky NJ, McEwen BS. Progestin receptor levels in rat hypothalamic and limbic nuclei. *J Neurosci* 1982;2:1446–1452.
72. Rainbow TC, Parsons B, MacLusky NJ, McEwen BS. Estradiol receptor levels in rat hypothalamic and limbic nuclei. *J Neurosci* 1982;2:1439–1445.
73. Morrell J, Pfaff DW. A neuroendocrine approach to brain function: localization of sex steroid concentrating cells in vertebrate brains. *Am Zool* 1978;18:447–460.
74. Warembourg M. Steroid receptors in the brain: topography and some functional implications. *Neurochem Int* 1985;7:941–952.
75. Birmingham MK, Stumpf WE, Sar M. Localization of aldosterone and corticosterone in the central nervous system assessed by quantitative autoradiography. *Neurochem Res* 1984;9:333–350.
76. McEwen BS, Weiss JM, Swartz LS. Uptake of corticosterone by rat brain and its concentration by certain limbic structures. *Brain Res* 1969;16:227–241.
77. Pfaff D, Keiner M. Atlas of estradiol-concentrating cells in the central nervous system of the female rat. *J Comp Neurol* 1973;151:121–158.
78. Sar M, Stumpf WE. Distribution of androgen-concentrating neurons in rat brain. In: Stumpf WE, Grant LD, eds. *Anatomical neuroendocrinology.* Basel: Karger; 1975;120–133.
79. Stumpf WE, Sar M, Keefer DA. Atlas of estrogen target cells in rat brain. In: Stumpf WE, Grant LD, eds. *Anatomical neuroendocrinology, International Conference on Neurobiology of CNS–Hormone Interactions, Chapel Hill 1974.* Basel: Karger; 1974:104–119.
80. Stumpf WE, Sar M. Glucocorticoid and mineralocorticoid hormone target sites in the brain: autoradiographic studies with corticosterone, aldosterone, and dexamethasone. In: Jones MT, Dallman MF, Gillham B, Chattopadhyay S, eds. *Interactions within the brain–pituitary–adrenocortical system.* New York: Academic Press; 1979:137–147.
81. Warembourg M. Uptake of ^{3}H labeled synthetic progestin by rat brain and pituitary. A radioautography study. *Neurosci Lett* 1978;9:329–332.
82. Ahima RS, Harlan RE. Charting of type II glucocorticoid receptor-like immunoreactivity in the rat central nervous system. *Neuroscience* 1990;39: 579–604.
83. Fuxe K, Cintra A, Agnati LF, et al. Studies on the cellular localization and distribution of glucocorticoid receptor and estrogen receptor immunoreactivity in the central nervous system of the rat and their relationship to the monoaminergic and peptidergic neurons of the brain. *J Steroid Biochem* 1987;27:159–170.
84. Press MF, Greene GL. Immunocytochemical localization of estrogen and progesterone receptors. In: DeLellis RA, ed. *Advances in immunohistochemistry.* New York: Raven Press; 1988:341–361.
85. Sar M, Parikh I. Immunohistochemical localization of estrogen receptor in rat brain, pituitary and uterus with monoclonal antibodies. *J Steroid Biochem* 1986;24:497–503.
86. Warembourg M, Logeat F, Milgrom E. Immunocytochemical localization of progesterone receptor in the guinea pig central nervous system. *Brain Res* 1986;384:121–131.
87. Takeda H, Chodak G, Mutchnik S, Nakamoto T, Chang C. Immunohistochemical localization of androgen receptors with mono- and polyclonal antibodies to androgen receptor. *J Endocrinol* 1990;126:17–25.
88. Simerly RB, Chang C, Muramatsu M, Swanson LW. Distribution of androgen and estrogen receptor mRNA-containing cells in the rat brain: an *in situ* hybridization study. *J Comp Neurol* 1990;294:76–95.
89. Aronsson M, Fuxe K, Dong Y, Agnati LF, Okret S, Gustafsson J-A. Localization of glucocorticoid receptor mRNA in the male rat brain by *in situ* hybridization. *Neurobiology* 1988;85:9331–9335.
90. Van Eekelen JAM, Jiang W, de Kloet ER, Bohn MC. Distribution of the mineralocorticoid and the glucocorticoid receptor mRNAs in the rat hippocampus. *J Neurosci Res* 1988;21:88–94.
91. Herman JP, Patel PD, Akil H, Watson SJ. Localization and regulation of glucocorticoid and mineralocorticoid receptor messenger RNAs in the hippocampal formation of the rat. *Mol Endocrinol* 1989;3:1886–1894.
92. Sousa RJ, Tannery NH, Lafer EM. *In situ* hybridization mapping of glucocorticoid receptor messenger ribonucleic acid in rat brain. *Mol Endocrinol* 1989;3:481–494.
93. Yang G, Matocha MF, Rapoport SI. Localization of glucocorticoid receptor messenger ribonucleic acid in hippocampus of rat brain using *in situ* hybridization. *Mol Endocrinol* 1988;2:682–685.
94. Canteras NS, Swanson LW. Projections of the ventral subiculum to the amygdala, septum and hypothalamus: a Phal anterograde tract-tracing study in the rat. *J Comp Neurol* [*in press*].
95. Swanson LW, Cowan WM. An autoradiographic study of the organization of the efferent connections of the hippocampal formation in the rat. *J Comp Neurol* 1977;172:49–84.
96. Canteras NS, Simerly RB, Swanson LW. The connections of the posterior nucleus of the amygdala. *J Comp Neurol* [*in press*].
97. Canteras NS, Simerly RB, Swanson LW. The projections of the ventral premammillary nucleus. *J Comp Neurol* [*in press*].
98. Swanson LW. The hypothalamus. In: Björklund A, Hokfelt T, Swanson LW, eds. *Handbook of chemical neuroanatomy.* Amsterdam: Elsevier; 1987: 1–124.
99. Simerly RB, Swanson LW. Projections of the medial preoptic nucleus: a *Phaseolus vulgaris* leucoagglutinin anterograde tract-tracing study in the rat. *J Comp Neurol* 1988;270:209–242.
100. Holets VR, Hokfelt T, Rokaeus A, Terenius L,

Goldstein M. Locus coeruleus neurons in the rat containing neuropeptide Y, tyrosine hydroxylase or galanin and their efferent projections to the spinal cord, cerebral cortex and hypothalamus. *Neuroscience* 1988;24:893–906.
101. Loughlin SE, Foote SL, Grzanna R. Efferent projections of nucleus locus coeruleus: morphologic subpopulations have different efferent targets. *Neuroscience* 1986;18:307–319.
102. McBride RL, Sutin J. Projections of the locus coeruleus and adjacent pontine tegmentum in the cat. *J Comp Neurol* 1976;165:265–284.
103. Sawchenko PE, Swanson LW. The organization of forebrain afferents to the paraventricular and supraoptic nuclei of the rat. *J Comp Neurol* 1983;218:121–144.
104. Simerly RB, Swanson LW. The organization of neural inputs to the medial preoptic nucleus of the rat. *J Comp Neurol* 1986;246:312–342.
105. Etgen AM. Progestin receptors and the activation of female reproductive behavior: a critical review. *Horm Behav* 1984;18:411–430.
106. Pfaff DW, Schwartz-Giblin S. Cellular mechanisms of female reproductive behaviors. In: Knobil E, Neill J, eds. *The physiology of reproduction.* New York: Raven Press; 1988:1487–1551.
107. Pelletier G, Liao N, Follea N, Govindan MV. Mapping of estrogen receptor-producing cells in the rat brain by *in situ* hybridization. *Neurosci Lett* 1988;94:23–28.
108. Sachs BD, Meisel RL. The physiology of male sexual behavior. In: Knobil E, Neill J, eds. *The physiology of reproduction.* New York: Raven Press; 1988:1393–1465.
109. Ju G, Swanson LW, Simerly RB. Studies on the cellular architecture of the bed nuclei of the stria terminalis in the rat: II. Chemoarchitecture. *J Comp Neurol* 1989;280:603–621.
110. Bradley DJ, Young SW III, Weinberger C. Differential expression of α and β thyroid hormone receptor genes in rat brain and pituitary. *Proc Natl Acad Sci USA* 1989;86:7250–7254.
111. Alexander IE, Clarke CL, Shine J, Sutherland RL. Progestin inhibition of progesterone receptor gene expression in human breast cancer cells. *Mol Endocrinol* 1989;3:1377–1386.
112. Dong Y, Poellinger L, Gustafsson J-A, Okret S. Regulation of glucocorticoid receptor expression: evidence for transcriptional and posttranslational mechanisms. *Mol Endocrinol* 1988;2:1256–1264.
113. Shapiro DJ, Barton MC, McKearin DM, et al. Estrogen regulation of gene transcription and mRNA stability. *Recent Prog Horm Res* 1989;45:29–64.
114. Kalinyak JE, Dorin RI, Hoffman AR, Perlman AJ. Tissue-specific regulation of glucocorticoid receptor mRNA by dexamethasone. *J Biol Chem* 1987;262:10441–10444.
115. Reul JMHM, Pearce PT, Funder JW, Krozowski ZS. Type I and type II corticosteroid receptor gene expression in the rat: effect of adrenalectomy and dexamethasone administration. *Mol Endocrinol* 1989;3:1674–1680.
116. Swanson LW, Simmons DM. Differential steroid hormone and neural influences on peptide mRNA levels in CRH cells of the paraventricular nucleus: a hybridization histochemical study in the rat. *J Comp Neurol* 1989;285:413–435.
117. Chang C, Kokontis J, Liao S. Structural analysis of complementary DNA and amino acid sequences of human and rat androgen receptors. *Proc Natl Acad Sci USA* 1988;85:7211–7215.
118. Lubahn DB, Joseph DR, Sar M, et al. The human androgen receptor: complementary deoxyribonucleic acid cloning, sequence analysis and gene expression in prostate. *Mol Endocrinol* 1988; 2:1265–1275.
119. Quarmby VE, Yarbrough WG, Lubahn DB, French FS, Wilson EM. Autologous down-regulation of androgen receptor messenger ribonucleic acid. *Mol Endocrinol* 1990;4:22–28.
120. Tan J-A, Joseph DR, Quarmby VE, et al. The rat androgen receptor: primary structure, autoregulation of its messenger ribonucleic acid, and immunocytochemical localization of the receptor protein. *Mol Endocrinol* 1988;2:1276–1285.
121. Nardulli AM, Katzenellenbogen BS. Progesterone receptor regulation in T-47D human breast cancer cells: analysis by density labeling of progesterone receptor synthesis and degradation and their modulation by progestin. *Endocrinology* 1988;122: 1532–1540.
122. Read LD, Snider CE, Miller JS, Greene GL, Katzenellenbogen BS. Ligand-modulated regulation of progesterone receptor messenger ribonucleic acid and protein in human breast cancer cell lines. *Mol Endocrinol* 1988;2:263–271.
123. Brenner RM, West NB, McClellan MC, Hild-Petito SA, Stouffer RL. Cellular localization of estrogen and progestin receptors in the macaque reproductive system. In: Carlstedt-Duke J, Eriksson H, Gustafsson J-A, eds. *The steroid/thyroid hormone receptor family and gene regulation.* Basel: Birkhauser Verlag; 1989:281–300.
124. Park O-K, Mayo KE. Transient expression of progesterone receptor messenger RNA in ovarian granulosa cells after the preovulatory luteinizing hormone surge. *Mol Endocrinol* 1991;5:967–978.
125. DonCarlos LL, Greene GL, Morrell JI. Estrogen plus progesterone increases progestin receptor immunoreactivity in the brain of ovariectomized guinea pigs. *Neuroendocrinology* 1989;50:613–623.
126. Berkenstam A, Glaumann H, Martin M, Gustafsson J-A, Norstedt G. Hormonal regulation of estrogen receptor messenger ribonucleic acid in $T47D_{co}$ and MCF-7 breast cancer cells. *Mol Endocrinol* 1989;3:22–28.
127. Read LD, Greene GL, Katzenellenbogen BS. Regulation of estrogen receptor messenger ribonucleic acid and protein levels in human breast cancer cell lines by sex steroid hormones, their antagonists, and growth factors. *Mol Endocrinol* 1989;3: 295–304.
128. Ree AH, Landmark BF, Eskild W, et al. Autologous down-regulation of messenger ribonucleic acid and protein levels for estrogen receptors in MCF-7 cells: an inverse correlation to progesterone receptor levels. *Endocrinology* 1989;124:2577–2583.
129. Saceda M, Lippman ME, Chambon P, et al. Regulation of the estrogen receptor in MCF-7 cells by estradiol. *Mol Endocrinol* 1988;2:1157–1162.

130. Shupnik MA, Gordon MS, Chin WW. Tissue-specific regulation of rat estrogen receptor mRNAs. *Mol Endocrinol* 1989;3:660–665.
131. Lauber AH, Romano GJ, Mobbs CV, Pfaff DW. Estradiol regulation of estrogen receptor mRNA in rat mediobasal hypothalamus: an *in situ* hybridization study. *J Neuroendocrinol* 1990;2:605–611.
132. Simerly RB, Young BJ. Regulation of estrogen receptor messenger ribonucleic acid in rat hypothalamus by sex steroid hormones. *Mol Endocrinol* 1991;5:424–432.
133. Blaustein JD, Turcotte JC. Estrogen receptor-immunostaining of neuronal cytoplasmic processes as well as cell nuclei in guinea pig brain. *Brain Res* 1989;495:75–82.
134. Cintra A, Fuxe K, Harfstrand A, et al. On the cellular localization and distribution of estrogen receptors in the rat tel- and diencephalon using monoclonal antibodies to human estrogen receptor. *Neurochem Int* 1986;8:587–595.
135. DonCarlos LL, Monroy E, Malik K, Morrell JI. Estrogen receptor-immunoreactivity in the forebrain of the female guinea pig: distribution and effect of steroid hormone treatment. *Soc Neurosci Abstr* 1989:15:627.
136. Warembourg M, Jolivet A, Milgrom E. Immunohistochemical evidence of the presence of estrogen and progesterone receptors in the same neurons of the guinea pig hypothalamus and preoptic area. *Brain Res* 1989;480:1–15.
137. Stover EP, Krishnan AV, Feldman D. Estrogen down-regulation of androgen receptors in cultured human mammary cancer cells (MCF-7). *Endocrinology* 1987;120:2597–2603.
138. Peiffer A, Barden N. Estrogen-induced decrease of glucocorticoid receptor messenger ribonucleic acid concentration in rat anterior pituitary gland. *Mol Endocrinol* 1987;1:435–440.
139. Lauber AH, Romano GJ, Pfaff DW. Sex difference in estradiol regulation of progestin receptor mRNA in rat mediobasal hypothalamus as demonstrated by *in situ* hybridization. *Neuroendocrinology* 1991;53:608–613.
140. Romano GJ, Krust A, Pfaff DW. Expression and estrogen regulation of progesterone receptor mRNA in neurons of the mediobasal hypothalamus: an *in situ* hybridization study. *Mol Endocrinol* 1989;3:1295–1300.
141. Okulicz WC, Evans RW, Leavitt WW. Progesterone regulation of estrogen receptor in the rat uterus: a primary inhibitory influence on the nuclear fraction. *Steroids* 1981;37:463–470.
142. Okulicz WC, Evans RW, Leavitt WW. Progesterone regulation of the occupied form of nuclear estrogen receptors. *Science* 1981;213:1503–1505.
143. McGinnis MY, Lumia AR, McEwen BS. Increased estrogen receptor binding in amygdala correlates with facilitation of feminine sexual behavior induced by olfactory bulbectomy. *Brain Res* 1985;334:19–25.
144. Carrillo AJ, Sheridan PJ. Estrogen receptors in the medial basal hypothalamus of the rat following complete hypothalamic deafferentation. *Brain Res* 1980;186:157–164.
145. McGinnis MY, Phelps CP, Nance DM, McEwen BS. Changes in estrogen and progestin receptor binding resulting from retrochiasmatic knife cuts. *Physiol Behav* 1982;29:225–229.
146. Blaustein JD, Brown TJ, Swearengen ES. Dopamine-β-hydroxylase inhibitors modulate the concentration of functional estrogen receptors in female rat hypothalamus and pituitary gland. *Neuroendocrinology* 1986;43:150–158.
147. Blaustein JD, Letcher B. Noradrenergic regulation of cytosol estrogen receptors in female rat hypothalamus: possible role of α_2-noradrenergic receptors. *Brain Res* 1987;404:51–57.
148. Woolley DE, Hope WG, Gietzen DW, Thompson MT, Conway SB. Bromocriptine increases ^{3}H-estradiol uptake in brain and pituitary of female, but not of male, gonadectomized adrenalectomized rats. *Proc West Pharmacol Soc* 1982; 25:437–441.
149. Power RF, Mani SK, Codina J, Conneely OM, O'Malley BW. Dopaminergic and ligand-independent activation of steroid hormone receptors. *Science* 1991;254:1636–1639.
150. Swanson LW, Kohler C, Björklund A. The limbic region. I: The septohippocampal system. In: Björklund A, Hokfelt T, Swanson LW, eds. *Handbook of chemical neuroanatomy*. Amsterdam: Elsevier; 1987:125–277.

Advances in Neurology, Vol. 59, edited by
Fredrick J. Seil. Raven Press, Ltd.,
New York © 1993.

19

Gonadal Steroids and Neuronal Regeneration

A Therapeutic Role

Kathryn J. Jones

Departments of Physical Therapy, and Anatomy and Cell Biology, The University of Illinois at Chicago, Chicago IL 60612

Within the brain and spinal cord, extensive receptor systems for all classes of steroid hormones exist (1–4). Through rapidly accumulating evidence in the field of eukaryotic gene expression, steroid hormone receptors have been determined to be transcriptive factors that act to alter gene transcription in a cell- and tissue-specific manner (5). Much recent research on steroidal activation of both neuronal and nonneuronal target tissue has identified many of the cellular and molecular events that occur in response to steroid hormone exposure (5–12). The accumulated evidence indicates that gonadal steroids have profound trophic effects on many aspects of neuronal functioning, including cell survival (13), growth and metabolism (14), elaboration of processes (15), synaptogenesis (16,17), and neurotransmission (18). We initiated a series of experiments designed to exploit the trophic capabilities of steroids as therapeutic agents in neuronal injury and repair (19–21). Two steroid-sensitive model systems are being used for these studies: the hamster facial motoneuron and the rat sciatic motoneuron. In this chapter, summaries of our current understanding of the intracellular receptor-mediated actions of steroids on gene expression in target tissue as well as evidence establishing gonadal steroids as neurotrophic agents are presented initially and are followed by a discussion of our recent data identifying gonadal steroids as therapeutic agents in enhancing the reparative response of motor neurons to injury.

MECHANISM OF STEROID ACTION ON TARGET TISSUE

The generally accepted pathway of the genomic effects of steroids on target tissue involves the interaction of the hormone first with an intracellular receptor and then, as an activated complex, with specific DNA sequences upstream from a steroid-regulated gene (8,22,23). The discovery of hormone-binding molecules in mammalian tissue was originally accomplished through studies of the uptake and binding of radioactively labeled steroidal estrogens (22). Reproductive organs were shown to contain an estrogen-binding protein called estrophilin, i.e., the estrogen receptor, with the uptake and binding of estrogen inhibited by estrogen antagonists. In *in vivo* experiments, it was also shown that most mammalian tissues contain certain amounts of estrophilin, with the unique characteristics of the hormone-responsive tissues being dependent on the magnitude of their estrophilin content.

The use of tritiated steroids in the types of experiments described above paved the way for the mapping of the various classes of steroid hormone receptors in the brain. Originally, biochemical approaches were utilized in mapping steroid binding activity in the brain (24). Cell nuclei were isolated from relatively large regions of the brain, and levels of tritiated steroid binding were assayed. Comparison between the properties of the intracellular steroid-binding macromolecules of the brain and of other organs indicates many similarities, including (a) high-affinity binding, (b) thermolability and the presence of sulfhydryl groups, (c) size, and (d) stereoselectivity toward the appropriate hormone, analogs, and antagonists (24). In the mid-1960s, the steroid hormone autoradiographic technique was pioneered by a number of investigators (2,25). The importance of this approach over the biochemical one is that it allows spatial resolution at the level of the single cell. With this technique, distributions of the various classes of steroid hormones were mapped out for the entire brain (1,26,27). In general, both the biochemical and autoradiographic data agree in terms of location of the different types of receptors. More recently, Simerly et al. (3) used *in situ* hybridization and cDNAs to the various classes of steroid receptors to map the distribution of steroid receptor mRNA-containing neurons within the brain and spinal cord. Their results validated the conclusions from the previous approaches, but from a different point in gene expression. In general, the conclusions from these studies indicate that all vertebrate brains examined to date concentrate steroids in a phylogenetically stable manner (25). Interestingly, both males and females contain similar distribution patterns for both the androgens and estrogens (3).

Until recently, it was thought that the steroid receptor protein resides in its inactivated state within the cytoplasm (28). On binding of the hormone to the receptor, an "activation" process occurs, which results in the translocation of the hormone–receptor complex to the cell nucleus. The activated complex then binds selectively to DNA sites termed hormone response elements (HREs), and alters gene expression in a cell/tissue-specific manner (8). Several studies, both biochemical and immunocytochemical, contradict the translocation process in that the data argue for a nuclear location of the receptor, regardless of whether it is bound to the hormone (29,30). Currently, it appears that the gonadal steroid receptors are predominantly nuclear in location, whereas the glucocorticoid receptor is present in both cytoplasm and nucleus (31–33). The realization that steroid receptors are for the most part nuclear in location, as well as advances in our understanding of eukaryotic gene control, have led to the current expansion in the definition of a steroid receptor. It is now known that the receptor belongs to a superfamily of nuclear proteins that act as ligand-inducible transcription factors (5).

Thus, hormonal regulation of transcription occurs through the interaction of *trans*-acting factors (i.e., specific steroid receptors) with *cis*-acting elements (HREs) present in or around steroid target genes. These *cis*-acting enhancer elements are consensus sequences that consist of inverted repeats separated by several base pairs (23). Considerable progress has been made recently in determining the functional domains of hormone receptors (6,7,12). Currently, six domains (regions A–F) within the receptor molecule have been identified. Comparison of the different amino acid sequences of regions C and E between various classes of steroid receptors as well as across species established a high degree of sequence conservation, which suggested that these two regions have important functions. Using site-directed mutagenesis, Kumar et al. (7) constructed various estrogen receptor deletion mutants and determined that region C corresponds to the DNA binding domain, whereas region E corresponds to the steroid-binding domain. Deletion of region F and the substantial alteration of region D do not alter receptor function appreciably. Subsequent work has demonstrated that region D also encodes a nuclear localization signal (34) and that regions A/B may contain other *trans*-activational functions (7). Within region C are zinc fingers formed by the interaction of four conserved cysteine residues and a zinc molecule (11). Umesono and Evans (11) used *in vitro* mutagenesis of chimeric glucocorticoid, estrogen, and thyroid hormone receptors to examine the molecular basis for target gene specificity for those receptors. They determined that minimal alterations in the amino acid content of the zinc fingers could, for example, convert the target gene specificity of the glucocorticoid receptor into that of the estrogen receptor.

In the estrogen deletion mutant receptor experiments of Kumar et al. (7), it was shown that the steroid hormone must be bound to region E in order for region C to bind to DNA. An estrogen receptor mutant without the hormone-binding domain was still able to bind to its response element. These investigators concluded that an unoccupied hormone-binding domain (region E) masks region C and prevents DNA binding. Hormone binding to region E therefore is thought to "unmask" region C, which is then free to associate with DNA. How this masking effect of region E is actually accomplished is not yet clear. It was also concluded from this study that hormone binding was not the only function of region E, in that estrogen receptor mutants lacking this region were only able to activate transcription poorly. In analyzing the functional activities of region E, Fawell et al. (6) have demonstrated that receptor dimerization, as well as steroid binding, occurs within this domain of the estrogen receptor. In turn, receptor dimerization appears to be important in full transcriptional activation.

GONADAL STEROIDS AS NEUROTROPHIC AGENTS

Gonadal steroids exert major influences on the brain and spinal cord, as evidenced by numerous studies ranging from the structural to the molecular level (6,13,15,35–39). Diverse populations of neurons within the brain and spinal cord, including most cranial and spinal motor neurons, contain gonadal steroid receptors. Both permanent (organizational) and reversible (activational) effects of steroids on neural tissue have been described (40).

Several receptor-concentrating systems have been extensively characterized with regard to the activational effects of steroids, including the actions of estradiol on the ventrolateral portion of the ventromedial nucleus (VL-VMN) of the hypothalamus and of androgens on a sexually dimorphic cluster of spinal motoneurons (SNB or spinal nucleus of the bulbocavernosus) innervating perineal muscles in the male rodent (41–44). Physiological doses of either class of hormone are sufficient to produce major structural changes in their respective target cells (14,45). Short-term exposure of 2 hr to systemic estradiol resulted in a growth-like effect on VL-VMN neurons in the ovariectomized rat (Fig. 1; 14). Nucleolar, nuclear, and somal hypertrophy occurred, as did alterations in nuclear shape from ellipsoid to spherical. The character of the nucleoplasm changed, with a progressive loss of condensed clumps of heterochromatin, and the configuration of the rough endoplasmic reticulum (RER) nuclear envelope was also affected. These cellular changes suggested an early, rapid gene activation geared toward growth and an increased metabolism.

Steroidal regulation of synaptic connections and neurite outgrowth has been demonstrated in a number of systems (45–49). Systemic administration of androgens to castrated male rats maintained the percentage of somatic and proximal dendritic membranes covered with synaptic contacts and also affected the size and number of synaptic contacts in the SNB (16). In addition, androgens have been shown to reduce drastically the normal motoneuron loss that occurs in the SNB during development (13). Numerous *in vitro* studies have shown that the gonadal steroids promote neurite extension in cell and tissue cultures taken from different

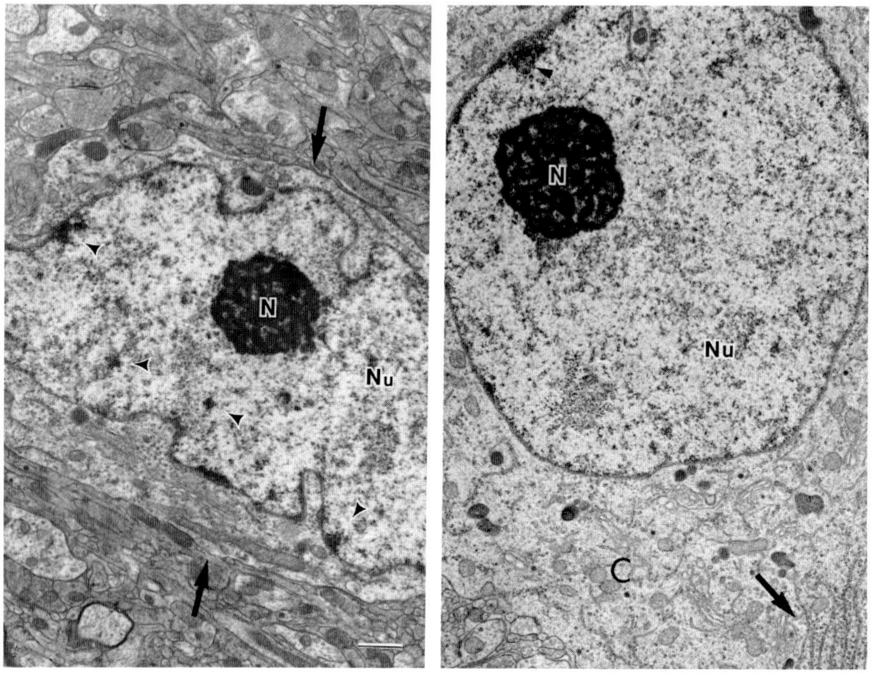

FIG. 1. Changes in ventromedial (VMN) neurons following 2 hr of E_2 treatment. **Left panel:** Control VMN neuron from a sham-operated, ovariectomized (OVX) rat. The nucleus (Nu) is typically small and nonspherical with extensive invaginations of the nuclear envelope. Small clumps of heterochromatin (examples indicated by *arrowheads*) are scattered within the nucleoplasm and along the nuclear envelope. A thin rim of cytoplasm (*arrows*) surrounds the nucleus. Scale bar, 1 μm. **Right panel:** VMN neuron after 2 hr of E_2 administered to OVX rats. Transformation in the shape of the nucleus (Nu) toward spherical and pronounced nuclear and nucleolar (N) swelling have occurred. Fewer clumps of heterochromatin are scattered throughout the nucleoplasm. A single large heterochromatin clump (*arrowhead*) is commonly observed in both the E_2-treated and control neurons. Stacked rough endoplasmic reticulum (RER) (*arrow*) cisternae within the enlarged cytoplasm (C) were frequently found. (Reprinted with permission from Jones et al., ref. 14.)

brain regions (46–48). In a recent study, Ferreira and Caceres (49) demonstrated that estrogen enhances neurite outgrowth through a selective induction of microtubule-stabilizing factors such as the tau proteins.

In target tissues containing steroid receptors, steroid hormones are generally thought to accomplish their actions through mechanisms that involve regulation of gene expression (22). From a molecular perspective, steroidal regulation of a number of gene products within various hormone-responsive neurons in the brain has been documented. In most nonneural target tissue described to date, altered expression of the ribosomal gene has been shown to rapidly occur with exposure to steroids (50). In the brain, rapid activation of the polymerase I system by estrogen has been shown from a structure–function perspective in VL-VMN neurons (see summary, Fig. 2). Initial progress in this area was made by Cohen and Pfaff (35) in ultrastructural studies of the RER in VL-VMN neurons following long-term estrogen treatment. These investigators found significant alterations in the amount of stacked RER following 15 days of estrogen treatment. Other ultrastructural studies of VL-VMN neurons after very short (2 hr) or intermediate (3 days) estrogen treatment also demonstrated significant changes in rRNA-containing components of the cell (14,51). Using *in situ*

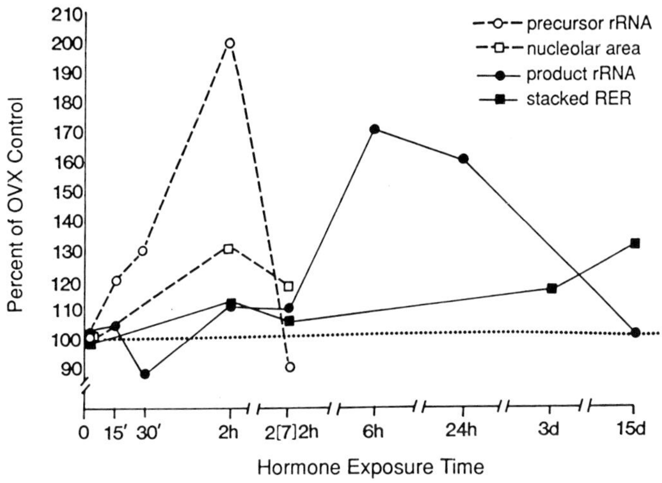

FIG. 2. Summary of the effects of estradiol on the ribosomal system in neurons from the ventrolateral portion of the ventromedial hypothalamus (VL-VMN). The data presented are a compilation of evidence from a number of studies (35,37,38,52). Early after exposure to the hormone in OVX animals, levels of precursor rRNA begin to increase, with a peak at 2 hr. This change in precursor levels is mirrored by an increase and peak in nucleolar hypertrophy, which, in many systems, has been correlated with an heightened level of transcriptional activity of the ribosomal genes. Subsequent to the increased nucleolar activity is a rise in cytoplasmic levels of ribosomes, with a peak in levels of 28 S rRNA occurring at 6 hr and remaining elevated at 24 hr. Despite prolonged exposure to the hormone (15 days), levels of rRNA decline to control values. However, configurational changes in rRNA, as measured by the percentage of neurons containing stacked RER organelles in the cytoplasm, progressively increase throughout exposure to estradiol such that, by 15 days, the number of neurons from hormone-treated animals represents a 30% increase above control levels. This number approximates the number of neurons within the VL-VMN that contain hormone receptors.

hybridization with ribosomal DNA probes (37,38), we correlated the ultrastructural changes with changes in the levels of hybridizable precursor and product rRNA. In these studies, levels of precursor ribosomal RNA were significantly increased in VL-VMN neurons as early as 30 min after systemic exposure to estradiol in ovariectomized rats, whereas levels of product ribosomal RNA were not changed until after at least 6 hr of continuous estrogen (Fig. 2). These data suggest that one of the primary and prolonged genomic effects of steroids on the brain involves activation of the polymerase I system.

In subsequent molecular studies, Romano et al. (52,53) have identified an additional rapid effect of estrogen on gene expression in VL-VMN neurons of ovariectomized rats. They have shown, using proenkephalin (PE) cDNA probes, that estrogen rapidly elevates the levels of PE mRNA in the VL-VMN. Further, they have found that PE gene expression is differentially regulated in male and female rats. Androgens also have been shown to regulate neuropeptide gene expression in the male rat and primate (54,55). *In situ* hybridization was used in conjunction with proopiomelanocortin (POMC) probes to determine that levels of mRNA were significantly increased in the arcuate nucleus of both castrated rats and primates given physiological levels of testosterone.

As evidenced from the discussion above, the actions of steroids on target neurons have now been broadly documented using a variety of techniques and approaches, and their neurotrophic effects have been substantiated from a structure–function perspective. If one can extrapolate from the various studies utilizing the different gonadal steroids, the data argue toward classifying androgens as motor neuron trophic factors.

GONADAL STEROIDS AS THERAPEUTIC AGENTS IN NERVE REGENERATION

Different types of hormones, including gonadal steroids (19–21,56,57), glucocorticoids (58), and thyroid hormones (59–61), have been employed clinically and/or experimentally in the injured or diseased nervous system. With regard to the gonadal steroids, the results of several clinical and experimental studies indicate a potential therapeutic role for these agents in neuropathological processes (62). In clinical trial studies using estrogen to treat postmenopausal women suffering from Alzheimer disease, Fillit et al. (56) determined that estrogen had a positive effect on the performance of these women on a battery of psychometric tests. It has been postulated that a contributing factor in amyotrophic lateral sclerosis, a progressive motoneuron disease, may be androgen receptor deficiencies (63). Yu and collaborators have suggested that injured hypoglossal neurons respond positively to androgen exposure (64–67). They determined that systemic administration of testosterone propionate (TP) immediately after hypoglossal nerve injury increased the number of HRP-labeled neurons within the hypoglossal nucleus. In contrast, Yeagle et al. (68) found no effects of castration or testosterone treatment on the contractile properties of the extensor digitorum longus. Vita et al. (57) examined the effects of a mixture of steroid derivatives with weak androgenic activity on muscle reinnervation after sciatic nerve crush in male rabbits. They found a slight increase in nerve outgrowth distance as well as a larger mean diameter of type 2c fibers within the extensor digitorum longus and soleus muscles.

In view of both the potential therapeutic usefulness of gonadal steroids in neuronal reparative processes and the lack of conclusive mechanistic data to date, we initiated a series of studies designed to examine comprehensively the role of gonadal steroids in nerve regeneration. The model system utilized is that of the hamster facial motoneuron, a well-documented system in which to study nerve regeneration (69). In the adult hamster, facial motoneurons undergo a robust response to crush or cut axotomy of the facial nerve at the level of the stylomastoid foramen. The pattern of the axon reaction in these neurons appears to occur independently of the target muscle, such that the neurons will undergo a defined reactive sequence and return to a "normal" state whether or not reconnection to the facial muscles is allowed to occur. Following injury, the animal displays a characteristic unilateral facial paralysis associated with drooping of one corner of the mouth, flattened and paralyzed vibrissae, and loss of the eyeblink reflex. Return of movement can be readily observed during a 2- to 3-week postoperative period. Finally, it is well established that facial neurons contain androgen receptors (4). Thus, the facial motoneuron represents an ideal system in which to study the effects of androgens on the reparative response after nerve injury.

Effects of Testosterone on Recovery from Facial Paralysis

Our initial studies of gonadal steroid action on injured neurons centered on determining whether subcutaneous administration of TP at the time of facial nerve crush could positively affect functional recovery from the subsequent facial paralysis (21). In the work by Yu and collaborators on the effects of TP on regeneration of crushed hypoglossal axons (64–67), demonstration of HRP-labeled hypoglossal neurons was the criterion used to establish acceleration of reconnection to the target muscles. From this work they hypothesized that TP increases the rate of axonal regeneration. In one of their studies (64), they discussed the possibility that the presence of more HRP-labeled neurons in the TP-treated animals could be caused by a TP-induced increase in the uptake and transport of HRP from the terminals, as opposed to an actual acceleration of the regeneration process. We therefore chose to circumvent this potential problem in data interpretation

TABLE 1. *Timetable of recovery from facial nerve crush following testosterone propionate (TP) injections administered on alternate days*

Experimental groups (total no. of animals)	Days postoperative						
	7	8	9	10	11	12	13
TP injection (4)							
Quivering vibrissae	2	3	4				
Full vibrissae movement							4
Controls (4)							
Quivering vibrissae				4			
Full vibrissae movement							4

Reprinted with permission from Kujawa et al., ref. 21.

by using functional return of movement as our criterion for accelerated recovery. For these experiments, adult male hamsters received right facial nerve crush axotomies and simultaneous silastic implants of TP.

In our preliminary experiment, the amount, frequency, and mode of administration of TP employed by Yu and Srinivasan (66) were utilized, and vibrissae function was monitored, following crush axotomy. Although the initial stages of return of vibrissae function, involving involuntary quivering movements, were accelerated near the end of the first week and beginning of the second week following crush axotomy of the facial nerve, return of full voluntary vibrissae movement was about the same in the TP-treated and control animals (Table 1; data from Kujawa et al., ref. 21).

In the next experiment, the amount and frequency of TP administered to the animals were doubled in order to maximize the accelerative tendency of TP observed in the preliminary experiment. In addition, functional recovery from facial paralysis was further subdivided into return of eye blink, full vibrissae movement, and complete recovery. Complete recovery included full vibrissae movement and return of the vibrissae from a posterior, flattened orientation to the normal anterior orientation observed on the unoperated left side of the animal. The greatest accelerative effect of TP on functional recovery was observed in the second week, with a 4-day difference in demonstration of the full blink reflex present between the hormone-injected and the control animals (Table 2; data from Kujawa et al., ref. 21). A less dramatic but still evident accelerative effect of TP was also noted in return of full vibrissae movement and complete recovery.

Because a greater hormonal effect on recov-

TABLE 2. *Timetable of recovery from facial nerve crush following testosterone propionate (TP) injections administered daily*

Experimental groups (total no. of animals)	Days postoperative														
	4	5	6	7	8	9	10	11	12	13	14	15	16	17	18
TP injection (7)															
Semiblink	4	7													
Blink reflex			2		3	5	7								
Full vibrissae movement									2		7				
Complete recovery											1			2	3
Controls (7)															
Semiblink	2	4	5	7											
Blink reflex					1	4		5	6		7				
Full vibrissae movement										3	5	6			
Complete recovery															1

Reprinted with permission from Kujawa et al., ref. 21.

ery from facial nerve paralysis was noted with the increased dosage of TP, the third experiment of this study involved an alteration in the mode of administration of the hormone from daily injections to subcutaneous implantation of silastic capsules containing 100% crystalline TP. In addition, the surgical procedures were done on castrated male hamsters in order to remove the endogenous source of the hormone. This dual approach allowed separation of endogenous from exogenous hormone effects and the action of a continuous supply of exogenous hormone to be determined within the same experimental paradigm. A pronounced acceleration of recovery of the blink reflex, full vibrissae movement, and normal orientation of the vibrissae were observed in the TP implant group as compared to the castrated control group (Table 3; data from Kujawa et al., ref. 21). As in the previous experiments, the accelerative effect of TP on recovery from facial paralysis was most obvious during the second week following crush axotomy of the facial nerve. Finally, no differences in the regenerative response of castrated control versus noncastrated control animals were found to occur. Instead, addition of a significant amount of exogenous TP to the system may be necessary to observe any functional benefits of the hormone.

In summary, the results of this study (a) suggested that TP accelerates motor neuron axonal regeneration, (b) established that continuous exposure to high levels of exogenous hormone has the greatest effect on functional recovery from facial paralysis, (c) indicated that endogenous hormones contribute little in the way of functional benefits following nerve injury, and (d) suggested that the effects of TP on functional recovery from facial paralysis are exerted at the level of the neuron.

To test the hypothesis that TP acts at the level of the injured neuron rather than the muscle, the temporal requirements of TP exposure necessary for acceleration of recovery from facial paralysis to occur following facial nerve crush were examined in our next study (20). For each of two series of experiments, adult castrated male hamsters were subjected to crush axotomies of the facial nerve at its

TABLE 3. *Timetable of recovery from facial nerve crush axotomy in castrated hamsters following testosterone propionate (TP) replacement via implant and daily injection*

Experimental groups (total no. of animals)	Days postoperative															
	3	4	5	6	7	8	9	10	11	12	13	14	15	16	17	18
TP implant (4)																
Semiblink		1		2	3	4										
Blink reflex								4								
Full vibrissae movement									4							
Complete recovery											4					
TP daily injection (3)																
Semiblink	1	2			3											
Blink reflex								2	3							
Full vibrissae movement											3					
Complete recovery														1		2
Castrated controls (3)																
Semiblink			1	3												
Blink reflex									2	3						
Full vibrissae movement											2	3				
Complete recovery													1			
Controls (3)																
Semiblink				2		3										
Blink reflex										1	3					
Full vibrissae movement											3					
Complete recovery																1

Reprinted with permission from Kujawa et al., ref. 21.

TABLE 4. *Average day of return of facial movements following facial nerve crush*

	Experiment 1 (TP[a] capsule inserted on day 6)		Experiment 2 (TP capsule removed on day 7)	
Average day of return	Hormone treated	Castrated controls	Hormone treated	Castrated controls
Semiblink	5.8	5.8	6.4	7.4
Blink	12.5	12.6	12.8	13.0
Full vibrissae movement	16.0	17.0	15.0	≥16.6
Complete recovery	≥24.8	≥22.2	≥21.0	≥23.0

Reprinted with permission from Kujawa and Jones, ref. 20.
[a] Testosterone propionate.

exit from the stylomastoid foramen. In the first experimental paradigm, one-half of the animals with facial nerve crush axotomies received subcutaneous TP capsules beginning on postoperative (PO) day 6 and continuing throughout the regeneration period, with the remainder of the animals sham implanted. The results indicated that, without the early exposure to TP, the accelerative effects of the hormone on facial nerve regeneration were abolished (Table 4; data from Kujawa and Jones, ref. 20). In the second experimental paradigm, one-half of the animals with facial nerve crush axotomies received subcutaneous TP implants immediately after crush and until PO day 7, with the remainder of the animals sham implanted. The results indicated that an early, discontinuous dose of TP immediately after crush was sufficient to produce a full accelerative effect on the return of the semiblink and complete recovery and a partial accelerative effect on the blink reflex and full vibrissae movement (Table 4; data from Kujawa and Jones, ref. 20).

Effects of Testosterone on the Regenerative Properties of Injured Motoneurons

Collectively, the results from our behavioral studies, as well as data from other systems (57,64,65,68), argue for a priming effect of the hormone exerted predominantly at the neuronal level that may parallel the conditioning lesion effect reported by others (70–72). We therefore hypothesized from these studies that the mechanism of TP action on injured neurons involves alterations in axonal regeneration properties, i.e., the rate of regeneration and/or the delay of sprouting.

This hypothesis was tested using fast axonal transport of radioactively labeled proteins (72). As in the previously described behavioral studies, adult castrated and intact males and intact females were subjected to right facial nerve crush axotomy at the stylomastoid foramen. One-half of the axotomized animals in each group received subcutaneous implants of testosterone, with the remainder of the animals sham implanted. Systemic administration of testosterone resulted in a 26% to 30% increase in the rate of regeneration of the fastest growing population of axons in the male experimental groups, whether the animal was castrated or not (Table 5; data from Kujawa et al., ref. 19) and a 10% increase in the rate of regeneration in the female experimental groups (Table 6; data from Kujawa et al., ref 19). This effect of testosterone on axonal outgrowth rates paralleled that found in conditioning lesion studies utilizing the rat sciatic nerve as a model system (70–73). Oblinger and Lasek (72) found a 25% increase in axonal regeneration rates of sensory neurons when a conditioning lesion preceded the testing lesion. Previous work by McQuarrie (70) identified a 24% increase in the rate of regeneration of motor axons in the sciatic nerve. The conditioning paradigm involves two lesions, an initial "priming" lesion followed later by a "testing" lesion to elicit accelerated outgrowth. It has been suggested that the conditioning phenomenon can be applied to human nerve injuries where the initial insult is considered

TABLE 5. *Summary of the effects of testosterone propionate (TP) on axonal regeneration following facial nerve crush injury in male hamsters*

	Castrated	Intact	Castrated + 1 TP capsule	Castrated + 2 TP capsules	Intact + 2 TP capsules
Rate of regeneration (mm/day)	3.5 (n = 20, r = 0.81)	3.7 (n = 18, r = 0.95)	4.4 (n = 20, r = 0.86)	4.5 (n = 16, r = 0.95)	4.8 (n = 15, r = 0.97)
Delay of sprout formation (days)	1.9	1.7	1.9	2.1	2.5

Reprinted with permission from Kujawa et al., ref. 19.

the conditioning lesion and later removal of the proximal stump neuroma becomes the testing lesion (70). Under this treatment regimen, accelerated return of motor and sensory function might be expected to occur. Our results suggest that systemic administration of testosterone following immediate repair of the severed epineural coverings would eliminate the need for additional surgery involving a testing lesion while capitalizing on the accelerated nerve outgrowth.

It is interesting to note that testosterone increased the rate of regeneration to a greater extent than functional recovery of facial movements (25% to 30% versus 10% to 15%; 19–21). Although the reasons for this are not known, there are a number of possible explanations. First, it may simply be that the behavioral testing is a less sensitive measure than the radioisotopic method for determination of axonal regeneration rates. Second, since the procedures used in this study provide information about only the fastest growing population of axons, there may be differential effects of the steroid on the bulk of more slowly growing fibers. Thus, steroids may affect initial events associated with regrowth of the faster fibers but may not have as pronounced an effect on events associated with subsequent regrowth of the slower fibers. Future electron microscopic studies examining the composition of the regenerating nerve at various distances from the crush site might provide insight into this question

Administration of testosterone to intact females elicited an increase in the rate of axonal regeneration, albeit to a lesser extent than in intact males. In the ovary, aromatase enzymes, under normal physiological conditions, convert testosterone to estradiol (74). These enzymes are present in brain tissue as well as many other peripheral organs and may play an important role in the neuronal processing of testosterone (75). Thus, the reduced effect of TP on axonal regeneration in intact females could have resulted in part from its conversion to estradiol and subsequent inability to bind to androgen receptors within facial neurons (76,77). However, no improvement was noted when the nonaromatizable form of testosterone, dihydrotestosterone (DHT), which has similar biologi-

TABLE 6. *Summary of the effects of testosterone propionate (TP) or dihydrotestosterone (DHT) on axonal regeneration following facial nerve crush injury in female hamsters*

	Intact	Intact + 1 TP capsule	Intact + 1 DHT capsule
Rate of regeneration (mm/day)	4.6 (n = 11, r = 0.94)	5.0 (n = 12, r = 0.91)	5.2 (n = 18, r = 0.92)
Delay of sprout formation (days)	2.5	2.4	2.9

Reprinted with permission from Kujawa et al., ref. 19.

cal effects as TP (78), was utilized in subsequent experiments. Why the female is less responsive, in terms of percentage increase in rate, than the male is unknown but may be related to the inherent differences in the regeneration rates between genders. Since the rate of facial nerve regeneration in intact females not given testosterone is within the same range as that in males administered testosterone, it may be that the system is only capable of achieving a preset maximal level. If so, this implies that intact females with an inherently faster regeneration rate would reach the maximal level with a smaller hormone-induced increase. Examination of the literature supports this idea, in that maximal regeneration rates are, with few exceptions, within ranges similar to those found in hormone-treated females in this study (70,72, 79,80).

A surprising finding of this study was that no significant shortening of the delay of sprout formation by testosterone was observed across the various experimental groups and that, instead, the groups with the highest hormone replacement paradigms (castrated males plus 2 TP, intact males plus 2 TP, and females plus DHT) displayed a lengthening of the delay time (Tables 5 and 6). Examination of the literature indicates that there is considerable variability in the initial time before axonal outgrowth begins, with ranges from 0.4 to 5.2 days (70–73, 79–82). Furthermore, the conditioning lesion may or may not have an effect on the initial delay of sprouting. However, since shortening in the delay of sprout formation did not occur with TP exposure, the significant hormone-induced increases in outgrowth distances could only result from increases in regeneration rate.

These data suggest that the mechanism by which gonadal steroids act in the injured nervous system is partly through the differential regulation of the regenerative properties of the injured cell, presumably via hormone receptor-mediated action at the level of the neuronal genome. If so, what genes would be predicted to be affected by TP following axon injury? As described in the first section of this chapter, gonadal steroids have been shown to affect neurite outgrowth, partly through regulation of cytoskeletal-associated proteins. In the conditioning lesion paradigm, alterations in the synthesis and transport of major cytoskeletal proteins such as tubulin appear to be involved in the mechanism of accelerated growth (83). We have, therefore, initiated a series of experiments designed to examine the effects of gonadal steroids on cytoskeletal gene expression after facial nerve injury. Our preliminary results suggest that TP does differentially regulate the expression of the tubulin gene family after injury. βII-Tubulin mRNA levels were found to be significantly elevated 2 days after axotomy plus TP but not after axotomy alone. By 7 days after axotomy, βII-tubulin levels were elevated in both groups, but to a greater extent in the group supplemented with TP. In contrast, no steroidal effects on βIII-tubulin or α-tubulin were observed.

Effects of Testosterone on the Nerve Cell Body Response to Injury

The evidence we have obtained thus far from the behavioral, regeneration, and tubulin studies suggests that testosterone primes the neuronal cell body in such a way as to accelerate the "switch" from a normal to a reparative state. One way to test this hypothesis is to examine the effects of gonadal steroids on the polymerase I system in an injury paradigm. As stated before, one of the earliest events that occurs in a target cell following exposure to the hormone is activation of the polymerase I system, and the result is a rapid and dramatic increase in ribosomal RNA. Following axotomy, nucleolar changes consistent with increases in rRNA levels also comprise the initial events preceding successful regeneration (84,85). We therefore used *in situ* hybridization and rDNA probes to determine the effects of TP on rRNA levels following axotomy (Fig. 3; 86). The preliminary data indicate that, following axotomy, rRNA levels begin to increase within the first 24 hr after injury, peak at 2 days after axotomy, and then decline. When TP is adminis-

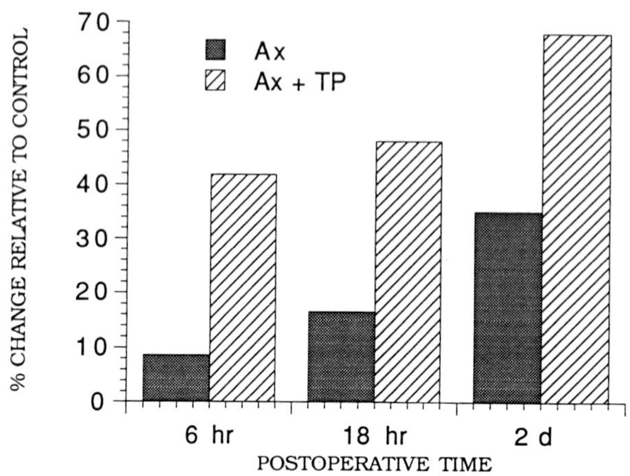

FIG. 3. Effects of axotomy alone and axotomy plus testosterone on levels of hybridizable rRNA in injured hamster facial motor neurons. The data are expressed as ratios of averages of numbers of grains per neuron from axotomized and control facial nuclear groups and compared between animals exposed or not exposed to testosterone after injury. (Reprinted with permission from Kinderman and Jones, ref. 86.)

tered in conjunction with facial nerve cut, the levels of rRNA begin to increase immediately, so that by 6 hr post-injury they already reach the maximum achieved at 2 days with injury alone. In addition, the peak increase in rRNA is approximately double that with injury alone. Thus, it appears that TP activates molecular events associated with the injury response in accordance with the acceleration in functional recovery and regeneration rate.

CONCLUSION

In conclusion, the available evidence to date suggests that many of the aspects of neuronal functioning affected by gonadal steroids under steady-state conditions are also significantly affected by steroids under stress conditions such as axon disconnection. This argues toward a therapeutic usefulness of gonadal steroids in activating and/or accelerating the reparative response of neurons to injury, a concept that will be exciting to test in future clinical studies.

REFERENCES

1. Pfaff DW, Keiner M. Atlas of estradiol-concentrating cells in the central nervous system of the female rat. *J Comp Neurol* 1973;151:121–158.
2. Sar M, Stumpf WE. Androgen concentration in motor neurons of cranial nerves and spinal cord. *Science* 1977;197:77–80.
3. Simerly RB, Chang C, Muramatsu M, Swanson LW. Distribution of androgen and estrogen receptor mRNA-containing cells in the rat brain: An *in situ* hybridization study. *J Comp Neurol* 1990;294:76–95.
4. Yu W-HA, McGinnis MY. Androgen receptor levels in cranial nerve nuclei and tongue muscles in rats. *J Neurosci* 1986;6:1302–1307.
5. Evans RM. The steroid and thyroid hormone receptor superfamily. *Science* 1988;240:889–895.
6. Fawell SE, Lees JA, White R, Parker MG. Characterization and colocalization of steroid binding and dimerization activities in the mouse estrogen receptor. *Cell* 1990;60:953–962.
7. Kumar V, Green S, Stack G, Berry M, Jin JR, Chambon P. Functional domains of the human estrogen receptor. *Cell* 1987;51:941–951.
8. Spelsberg TC, Littlefield BA, Seelke R, et al. Role of specific chromosomal proteins and DNA sequences in the nuclear binding sites for steroid receptors. *Recent Prog Horm Res* 1983;39:463–517.
9. Tsai SY, Carlstedt-Duke J, Weigel NL, et al. Molecular interactions of steroid hormone receptor with its enhancer element: evidence for receptor dimer formation. *Cell* 1988;55:361–369.
10. Tsai SY, Tsai MJ, O'Malley BW. Cooperative binding of steroid hormone receptors contributes to transcriptional synergism at target enhancer elements. *Cell* 1989;57:443–448.
11. Umesono K, Evans RM. Determinants of target gene specificity for steroid/thyroid hormone receptors. *Cell* 1989;57:1139–1146.
12. Webster NJG, Green S, Jin JR, Chambon P. The hormone-binding domains of the estrogen and glucocorticoid receptors contain an inducible transcription activation function. *Cell* 1988;54:199–207.
13. Nordeen EJ, Nordeen KW, Sengelaub DR, Arnold AP. Androgens prevent normally occurring cell death in a sexually dimorphic spinal nucleus. *Science* 1985;229:671–673.
14. Jones KJ, Pfaff DW, McEwen BS. Early estrogen-induced nuclear changes in rat hypothalamic ventromedial neurons: an ultrastructural and morphometric analysis. *J Comp Neurol* 1985;239:255–267.
15. Gould E, Woolley CS, Frankfurt M, McEwen BS. Gonadal steroids regulate dendritic spine density in hippocampal pyramidal cells in adulthood. *J Neurosci* 1990;10:1286–1291.
16. Matsumoto A, Micevych PE, Arnold AP. Androgen

regulates synaptic input to motoneurons of the adult rat spinal cord. *J Neurosci* 1988;8:4168–4176.
17. Matsumoto A, Arnold AP, Zampighi GA, Micevych PE. Androgenic regulation of gap junctions between motoneurons in the rat spinal cord. *J Neurosci* 1988;8:4177–4183.
18. Luine VN. Estradiol increases choline acetyltransferase activity in specific basal forebrain and nuclei and projection areas of female rats. *Exp Neurol* 1985;89:484–490.
19. Kujawa KA, Emeric E, Jones KJ. Testosterone differentially regulates the regenerative properties of injured hamster facial motoneurons. *J Neurosci* 1991;11:3898–3906.
20. Kujawa KA, Jones KJ. Testosterone-induced acceleration of recovery from facial paralysis in male hamsters: temporal requirements of hormone exposure. *Physiol Behav* 1990;48:765–768.
21. Kujawa KA, Kinderman NB, Jones KJ. Testosterone-induced acceleration of recovery from facial paralysis following crush axotomy of the facial nerve in male hamsters. *Exp Neurol* 1989;105:80–85.
22. Jensen EV, Greene GL, Closs LE, DeSombre ER, Nadjii M. Receptors reconsidered: a 20-year perspective. *Recent Prog Horm Res* 1982;38:1–40.
23. Yamamoto KR. Steroid receptor regulated transcription of specific genes and gene networks. *Annu Rev Genet* 1985;19:209–252.
24. McEwen BS, Davis PG, Parsons B, Pfaff DW. The brain as a target for steroid hormone action. *Annu Rev Neurosci* 1979;2:65–112.
25. Pfaff DW. *Estrogen and brain function.* New York: Springer; 1980.
26. Morrell JI, Pfaff DW. Autoradiographic technique for steroid hormone localization. In: Adler NT, ed. *Neuroendocrinology of reproduction.* New York: Plenum Press; 1981:519–531.
27. Morrell J, Pfaff DW. A neuroendocrine approach to brain function: localization of sex steroid concentrating cells in vertebrate brains. *Am Zool* 1978;18:447–460.
28. Gorski J, Toft D, Shyamala G, Smith D, Notides A. Hormone receptors: studies on the interaction of estrogen with the uterus. *Recent Prog Horm Res* 1968;24:45–80.
29. Press MF, Nousek-Goebl NA, Greene GL. Immunoelectron microscopic localization of estrogen receptor with monoclonal estrophilin antibodies. *J Histochem Cytochem* 1985;33:915–924.
30. Welshons WV, Lieberman ME, Gorski J. Nuclear localization of unoccupied estrogen receptors. *Nature* 1984;307:747–749.
31. Fuxe F, Wikstrom AC, Okret S, et al. Mapping of glucocorticoid receptor immunoreactive neurons in the rat tel- and diencephalon using a monoclonal antibody against rat liver glucocorticoid receptor. *Endocrinol* 1985;117:1803–1812.
32. Picard D, Yamamoto KR. Two signals mediate hormone dependent nuclear localization of the glucocorticoid receptor. *EMBO J* 1987;6:3333–3340.
33. Wikstrom AC, Bakke O, Okret S, Bronnegard M, Gustafsson JA. Intracellular localization of the glucocorticoid receptor: evidence for cytoplasmic and nuclear localization. *Endocrinology* 1987;120:1232–1242.
34. Guiochon-Mantel A, Loosfelt H, Lescop P, et al. Mechanisms of nuclear localization of the progesterone receptor: evidence for interaction between monomers. *Cell* 1989;57:1147–1154.
35. Cohen RS, Pfaff DW. Ultrastructure of neurons in the ventromedial nucleus of the hypothalamus in ovariectomized rats with or without estrogen treatment. *Cell Tissue Res* 1981;217:451–470.
36. Goldstein LA, Kurz EM, Sengelaub DR. Androgen regulation of dendritic growth and retraction in the development of a sexually dimorphic spinal nucleus. *J Neurosci* 1990;10:935–946.
37. Jones KJ, Chikaraishi DM, Harrington CA, McEwen BS, Pfaff DW. *In situ* hybridization detection of estradiol-induced changes in ribosomal RNA levels in rat brain. *Mol Brain Res* 1986;1:145–152.
38. Jones KJ, Harrington CA, Chikaraishi DM, Pfaff DW. Estradiol regulation of ribosomal RNA processing in rat ventromedial hypothalamic neurons: early detection by quantitative *in situ* hybridization. *J Neurosci* 1990;10:1515–1521.
39. McEwen BS, Biegon A, Davis PT, et al. Steroid hormones: humoral signals which alter brain cell properties and functions. *Recent Prog Horm Res* 1982;38:41–92.
40. Arnold AP, Gorski RA. Gonadal steroid induction of structural sex differences in the central nervous system. *Annu Rev Neurosci* 1984;7:413–442.
41. Breedlove SM. Cellular analysis of hormone influence on motoneuronal development and function. *J Neurobiol* 1986;3:157–176.
42. Breedlove SM, Arnold AP. Hormonal control of a developing neuromuscular system: I. Complete demasculinization of the male rat spinal nucleus of the bulbocavernosus using the antiandrogen flutamide. *J Neurosci* 1983;3:417–423.
43. Breedlove SM, Arnold AP. Hormonal control of a developing neuromuscular system: II. Sensitive periods for the androgen-induced masculinization of the rat spinal nucleus of the bulbocavernosus. *J Neurosci* 1983;3:424–432.
44. McEwen BS, Jones KJ, Pfaff DW. Hormonal control of sexual behavior in the female rat: molecular, cellular and neurochemical studies. *Biol Reprod* 1987;36:37–45.
45. Kurz EM, Sengelaub DR, Arnold AP. Androgens regulate the dendritic length of mammalian motoneurons in adulthood. *Science* 1986;232:395–398.
46. Faivre-Baumann A, Rosembaum E, Puymirat J, Grouselle D, Tixier-Vidal A. Differentiation of fetal mouse hypothalamic cells in serum-free medium. *Dev Neurosci* 1981;4:118–119.
47. Leedy MG, Beattie MS, Bresnahan JC. Testosterone induced plasticity of synaptic inputs to adult mammalian motoneurons. *Brain Res* 1987;424:386–390.
48. Toran-Allerand D, Leland E, Pfenninger KH. Estrogen and insulin synergism in neurite growth enhancement *in vitro:* mediation of steroids effects by interaction with growth factors. *Dev Brain Res* 1988;41:87–100.
49. Ferreira A, Caceres A. Estrogen-enhanced neurite outgrowth: Evidence for a selective induction of tau and stable microtubules. *J Neurosci* 1991;11:392–400.
50. Whelly SM. Regulation of uterine nucleolar RNA synthesis by estrogens. *Biol Reprod* 1985;33:1–10.
51. Meisel RL, Pfaff DW. Brain region specificity in es-

tradiol effects on neuronal ultrastructure in rats. *Mol Cell Endocrinol* 1985;40:159–166.
52. Romano GJ, Mobbs CV, Howells RD, Pfaff DW. Estrogen regulation of proenkephalin gene expression in the ventromedial hypothalamus of the rat: temporal qualities and synergism with progesterone. *Mol Brain Res* 1988;5:51–58.
53. Romano GJ, Mobbs CV, Lauber A, Howells RD, Pfaff DW. Differential regulation of proenkephalin gene expression by estrogen in the ventromedial hypothalamus of male and female rats: implications for the molecular basis of a sexually differentiated behavior. *Brain Res* 1990;536:63–68.
54. Adams LA, Vician L, Clifton DK, Steiner RA. Testosterone regulates pro-opiomelanocortin gene expression in the primate brain. *Endocrinology* 1991;128:1881–1886.
55. Chowen-Breed JA, Clifton DK, Steiner RA. Regional specificity of testosterone regulation of proopiomelanocortin gene expression in the arcuate nucleus of the male rat brain. *Endocrinol* 1989;124: 2875–2881.
56. Fillit H, Weinreb H, Cholst I, et al. Observations in a preliminary open trial of estradiol therapy for senile dementia–Alzeheimer's type. *Psychoneuroendocrinology* 1986;11:337–345.
57. Vita G, Dattola R, Girlanda P, Oteri G, Lo Presti F, Messina C. Effects of steroid hormones on muscle reinnervation after nerve crush in rabbit. *Exp Neurol* 1983;80:279–287.
58. Bracken MB, Shepard MJ, Collins WF, et al. A randomized, controlled trial of methylprednisolone or naloxone in the treatment of acute spinal-cord injury. *N Engl J Med* 1990;322:1405–1411.
59. Cook RA, Kiernan JA. Effects of triiodothyronine on protein synthesis in regenerating peripheral neurons. *Exp Neurol* 1976;52:515–524.
60. Harvey JE, Srebnik HH. Locomotor activity and axon regeneration following spinal cord compression in rats treated with L-thyroxine. *J Neuropathol Exp Neurol* 1967;26:661–668.
61. Heinicke E. Influence of exogenous triiodothyronne on axonal regeneration and wound healing in the brain of the rat. *J Neurosci* 1977;31:293–305.
62. Jones KJ. Steroid hormones and neurotrophism: relationship to nerve injury. *Metab Brain Dis* 1988;3:1–14.
63. Weiner LP. Possible role of androgen receptors in amyotrophic lateral sclerosis. *Arch Neurol* 1980;37: 129–131.
64. Yu W-HA. Effect of testosterone on the regeneration of the hypoglossal nerve in rats. *Exp Neurol* 1982;77:129–141.
65. Yu W-HA. Sex difference in the regeneration of the hypoglossal nerve in rats. *Brain Res* 1982;238: 404–406.
66. Yu W-HA, Srinivasan R. Effect of testosterone and 5-dihydrotestosterone on regeneration of the hypoglossal nerve in rats. *Exp Neurol* 1981;71:431–435.
67. Yu W-HA, Yu MC. Acceleration of the regeneration of the crushed hypoglossal nerve by testosterone. *Exp Neurol* 1983;80:349–360.
68. Yeagle SP, Mayer RF, Max SR. Contractile properties of rat fast-twitch skeletal muscle during reinnervation: effects of testosterone and castration. *Exp Neurol* 1983;82:344–357.
69. LaVelle A, LaVelle FW. Neuronal reaction to injury during development. In: Almki CR, Finger S, eds. *Developmental neurobiology*. New York: Academic Press; 1984:3–16.
70. McQuarrie IG. Acceleration of axonal regeneration in rat somatic motoneurons by using a conditioning lesion. In: Gorio A, ed. *Posttraumatic peripheral nerve regeneration; experimental basis and clinical implications*. New York: Raven Press; 1981:49–58.
71. McQuarrie IG. The effect of a conditioning lesion on the regeneration of motor axons. *Brain Res* 1978;152:597–602.
72. Oblinger MM, Lasek RJ. A conditioning lesion of the peripheral axons of dorsal root ganglion cells accelerates regeneration of only their peripheral axons. *J Neurosci* 1984;4:1736–1744.
73. Forman DS, McQuarrie IG, Labore FW, et al. Time course of the conditioning lesion effect on axonal regeneration. *Brain Res* 1980;182:180–185.
74. Hadley MC. *Endocrinology*, 2nd ed. Engelwood Cliffs, NJ: Prentice-Hall; 1990.
75. Krey LC, MacLusky NJ, Davis PG, Lieberburg I, Roy EJ. Different intracellular mechanisms underlie testosterone's suppression of basal and stimulation of cyclic luteinizing hormone release in male and female rats. *Endocrinology* 1982;110:2159–2167.
76. Naftolin F, Ryan K, Davies I, et al. The formation of estrogens by central neuroendocrine tissues. *Recent Prog Horm Res* 1975;31:295–319.
77. Naftolin F, Ryan KT. The metabolism of androgens in central neuroendocrine tissues. *J Steroid Biochem* 1975;6:993.
78. Whalen RE, DeBold JF. Comparative effectiveness of testosterone, androstenedione and dihydrotestosterone in maintaining mating behavior in the castrated male hamster. *Endocrinology* 1974;95:1674–1679.
79. Bisby MA. Enhancement of the conditioning lesion effect in rat sciatic motor axons after superimposition of conditioning and test lesions. *Exp Neurol* 1985;90:385–394.
80. Forman DS, Berenberg RA. Regeneration of motor axons in the rat sciatic nerve by labeling with axonally transported radioactive proteins. *Brain Res* 1978;156:213–225.
81. Griffin JW, Drachman DB, Price DL. Fast axonal transport in motor nerve regeneration. *J Neurobiol* 1976;7:355–370.
82. Gutmann E, Guttmann L, Medawar PB, Young JZ. The rate of regeneration of nerve. *J Exp Biol* 1942;19:14–44.
83. McQuarrie IG. Role of the axonal cytoskeleton in the regenerating nervous system. In: Seil FJ, ed. *Nerve, organ and tissue regeneration: research perspectives*. New York: Academic Press; 1983:1–88.
84. Jones KJ, LaVelle A. Differential effects of axotomy on immature and mature hamster facial neurons: a time course study of initial nucleolar and nuclear changes. *J Neurocytol* 1986;15:197–206.
85. Lieberman AR. The axon reaction: a review of the principal features of the perikaryal response to axon injury. *Int Rev Neurobiol* 1971;14:49–125.
86. Kinderman NB, Jones KJ. Testosterone effects on ribosomal RNA levels in injured peripheral motor neurons: a preliminary report. *Metab Brain Dis* 1991;6:157–164.

Advances in Neurology, Vol. 59, edited by Fredrick J. Seil. Raven Press, Ltd., New York © 1993.

20

The Effects of Glucocorticoid and Nonglucocorticoid Steroids on Acute Neuronal Degeneration

Edward D. Hall

Central Nervous System Diseases Research, The Upjohn Company, Kalamazoo, Michigan 49001

Injury to the spinal cord, which commonly results in complete paralysis below the level of the injury site, constitutes one of the most devastating circumstances that can befall a human being. The short- and long-term medical, financial, and social consequences of impaired bodily function and mobility are staggering to the victim's quality of life and to that of his or her family. It is estimated that each year in the United States there are at least 10,000 new injuries. The majority of these are males between the ages of 18 and 35, and the leading causes are automobile and sports-related accidents. As a result of advances in medical and nursing management of these patients, which began to develop during World War II, most of the individuals can look forward to a lengthy life, but one involving severe neurological impairment. The more fortunate cases have an injury low enough in the spinal cord so that normal arm strength remains, allowing them to live independently. However, the largest group have cervical lesions that result in varying degrees of arm as well as leg paralysis. These cases require fairly intensive and sometimes continuous nursing care.

A reason for the persistent belief by neuroscientists that it may be possible to enhance the chances for recovery after spinal cord injury is the long-known fact that most cord injuries do not involve actual transection of the spinal cord. In contrast, the spinal cord is generally contused or compressed by broken or dislocated vertebrae. Indeed, early surgical exposure of the injured spinal cord, when indicated, often reveals little gross damage to the spinal tissue. It appears that a major portion of posttraumatic neuronal necrosis following spinal cord (or brain) injury does not result from diffuse primary injury but rather occurs as a secondary process. A multitude of experimental studies of blunt spinal injury have shown that although a variable degree of immediate mechanical damage to blood vessels, nerve cells, and axons occurs in direct relation to the magnitude of the injury force, much of the posttraumatic destruction is from a progressive secondary pathophysiological process. The initial blunt injury sets in motion a series of molecular and physiological events that lead to gradual tissue (e.g., vascular and neuronal) degeneration, thus destroying the anatomic substrate necessary for neurological recovery to be feasible. Nevertheless, the initial structural integrity of the spinal cord at the injury site suggests that functional recovery could be facilitated if an effective therapy were targeted to interrupt the molecular processes involved in the secondary degeneration phenomenon.

ROLE OF OXYGEN RADICALS IN POSTTRAUMATIC SPINAL CORD DEGENERATION

Extensive evidence from several laboratories using a variety of biochemical indices has shown that free radical generation and cell membrane lipid peroxidation (LP) occur as early events in injured spinal cord tissue (1,2). For instance, there is a rapid loss of tissue vitamin E (3,4) and membrane cholesterol and an increase in the levels of 25-hydroxycholesterol, an autooxidation product of cholesterol (3,5). Demopoulos et al. (5) proposed that the decrease in membrane cholesterol was the result of lipid peroxidation initiated by the trauma to the spinal cord. Other evidence of early posttraumatic LP includes an increase in spinal cord cGMP, reflective of the activation of guanylate cyclase by either oxygen radicals or lipid hydroperoxides (6,7) and a loss of the activity of the phospholipid-dependent enzyme Na^+, K^+-ATPase (8).

The peroxidation of membrane lipids is initiated by free radicals generated by the dislocation or decompartmentalization of endogenous iron and/or hemoglobin, hematin, iron, or other free-radical-producing substances that extravasate into injured spinal cord tissue with blood (1,2). Mechanical trauma, free radicals, or Ca^{2+} released from intracellular stores or leaking into the cell from the extracellular space could all be involved in the stimulation of membrane lipases, resulting in the deacylation of fatty acids. Elevations in free fatty acids together with the loss of cholesterol and lipids by peroxidation can damage cells and affect physiological processes by altering membrane structure, fluidity, permeability, and function. These membrane lipid perturbations can account for the rapid inactivation of the phospholipid-dependent membrane-bound enzyme Na^+, K^+-ATPase and loss of ionic homeostasis causing K^+ to efflux from cells and Ca^{2+} to flood the intracellular compartment from the extracellular space. The membrane potential cannot be maintained, and impulse transmission is lost if Na^+ and K^+ conductances across the membrane are abnormal. High levels of intracellular Ca^{2+} can cause continued or additional activation of membrane phospholipases, mitochondrial dysfunction with compromise of cellular energy metabolism, and activation of Ca^{2+}-dependent protease(s), resulting in degradation of neurofilament proteins. Free arachidonic acid, liberated by calcium-activated phospholipases and lipid peroxidation, is metabolized by cyclooxygenase to prostaglandins and thromboxane and by 5-lipoxygenase to leukotrienes, which may have deleterious actions on the injured spinal cord (3). In addition, it is known that free radicals are produced during the enzymatic conversion of arachidonic acid to the eicosanoids and by activated polymorphonuclear neutrophils. Consequently, both the eicosanoid production and inflammation with later influx of neutrophils that occurs in injured spinal cord can add to the free radical load on this tissue (9).

Thus, it has been reasoned that oxygen free-radical induced LP may play a significant role in the pathochemistry of acute CNS injury. Accordingly, the early administration of compounds with significant lipid antioxidant efficacy and potency may constitute an effective means of interrupting posttraumatic degeneration and thus preserving the anatomic substrate for neurological recovery.

EFFECTS OF THE GLUCOCORTICOID METHYLPREDNISOLONE IN EXPERIMENTAL AND CLINICAL SPINAL CORD INJURY

Over the past several years, the efficacy of the glucocorticoid steroid methylprednisolone (MP) in experimental cerebral nervous system (CNS) trauma has been extensively evaluated. In these studies, a strong correlation between the ability to inhibit CNS tissue LP and positive effects on other pathophysiological processes and neurological recovery is apparent. Moreover, a separation of the glucocorticoid activity from the anti-LP (i.e., antioxidant) and cerebroprotective effects of the steroid has been achieved in the recent discovery of nonglucocorticoid steroids that duplicate or surpass the antioxidant effects of MP.

A major effort has been made to define the neuroprotective pharmacology of MP in experimental spinal cord injury. It has been found that a 30 mg/kg i.v. dose of MP given to cats soon after blunt spinal cord injury can attenuate posttraumatic LP as measured by various biochemical indices (3,5,6,10). In addition, it has been shown that the same dose of MP has other beneficial effects on the injured spinal cord, many of which may be secondary to LP inhibition. These include the support of energy metabolism (11–13), prevention of progressive posttraumatic ischemia (14,15), inhibition of neurofilament degradation (13), reversal of intracellular calcium accumulation (14), and inhibition of vasoactive prostaglandin $F_{2\alpha}$ and thromboxane A_2 formation (3). It is also possible that a 30 mg/kg dose of MP may enhance the acute recovery of somatosensory evoked potentials; an increase in spinal neuronal excitability, another methylprednisolone effect (16), may also be involved in neurophysiological recovery [also see reviews by Hall and Braughler (17) and Hall (18)].

Four observations describe this pharmacological action of MP in spinal cord injury. First is the necessity for large intravenous doses, as described above. Second is the complex, biphasic dose–response curve seen for many beneficial effects of MP; although an intravenous 30 mg/kg dose is required to inhibit LP, doubling the dose causes a loss of that action (6,10,12). The most logical explanation for such a pattern is that the high-dose pharmacology of MP is mediated by a direct membrane action. The third observation is that treatment must be initiated early to achieve a therapeutic effect. The uptake of MP by spinal tissue decreases rapidly with time after injury (19), probably because of secondary posttraumatic tissue loss and a progressive decrease in blood flow to the injury site. More importantly, however, LP-mediated tissue degeneration evolves rapidly after injury and is largely irreversible. A fourth finding is that the time course of MP's protective effects parallels the tissue uptake and elimination of the steroid. Since the half-life of MP in cat spinal tissue is only 2 to 6 hr, frequent doses are necessary to maintain blood flow, improve tissue preservation, and maximize the potential for recovery (12,13).

To demonstrate this, we designed and tested an intravenous dosing regimen in cats with moderately severe spinal injury (3,20). An initial 30 mg/kg bolus was given 30 min after injury, followed with 15 mg/kg doses 2 and 6 hr later, and then a continuous infusion of 2.5 mg/kg per hr for the remainder of the first 48 hr after injury. Cats were blindly evaluated over 4 weeks for their ability to walk, run, and climb stairs, after which they were sacrificed. A histological analysis of the injury site was then conducted. In comparison with vehicle-treated animals, the MP-treated cats showed significantly higher recovery scores beginning at 2 weeks after injury. In addition, a dramatic reduction in posttraumatic spinal tissue loss was observed, the degree of which was inversely correlated with the neurological recovery score (r = 0.88). These studies clearly demonstrate that a dosing regimen centered on an inhibition of posttraumatic LP is associated with both enhanced tissue preservation and functional recovery. Other studies have similarly confirmed that high "antioxidant" doses of MP can enhance the chronic recovery of spinal-cord-injured cats (21,22).

METHYLPREDNISOLONE EFFICACY IN NASCIS 2

The recent publication of the results of the Second National Acute Spinal Cord Injury Study (NASCIS 2) constitutes a major milestone in the search for therapeutic interventions that will interfere significantly with secondary posttraumatic spinal cord degeneration and thereby ameliorate the devastating neurological consequences of spinal cord injury (23). In that study, MP was demonstrated to improve the 6-month recovery of spinal cord injury patients, compared to placebo-treated patients, when administered in an intensive 24-hr intravenous regimen beginning within 8 hr after injury. NASCIS 2 is the first randomized, double-blind, placebo-controlled trial that has unequivocally demonstrated that a pharmacological agent can beneficially modify the course of events after severe CNS injury. The trial was based on extensive studies of MP in experimental models of spinal cord injury. Moreover, the dose level and dosing regimen were derived from careful pharmacological investigations that focused on inhibition of posttraumatic lipid peroxidation as the therapeutic target. The fact that these studies accurately predicted the efficacy of MP has given greater impetus to the pursuit of agents with greater antioxidant activity for acute pharmacotherapy of CNS injury in general.

21-AMINOSTEROIDS

The definition of this high-dose nonglucocorticoid antioxidant action of MP led to the pursuit of nonglucocorticoid steroid analogs of methylprednisolone that also weakly inhibited lipid peroxidation in high concentrations and at high doses were active in models of experimental CNS trauma (24). However, synthetic efforts continued, aimed at preparation of compounds that were even more potent and effective inhibitors of lipid peroxidation, with greater activity in experimental models of CNS trauma and ischemia. This resulted in the discovery of the 21-aminosteroids (e.g., U-74006F, U-74500A) (25,26).

Tirilazad mesylate (U-74006F) has been selected for clinical development for the acute treatment of brain and spinal injury, subarachnoid hemorrhage, and stroke. Phase II clinical trials are currently ongoing for each of those indications. Another 21-aminosteroid, U-74500A, is actually a more potent inhibitor of iron-catalyzed lipid peroxidation than U-74006F, but it has not been chosen for development because of pharmaceutical instability and rapid elimination *in vivo.*

Free Radical Scavenging and Membrane Antioxidant Properties

The 21-aminosteroids have been shown to be potent inhibitors of lipid peroxidation *in vitro.* In an initial study using rat brain homogenates or purified rat brain synaptosomes as the lipid source, U-74006F and U-74500A potently inhibited iron-dependent lipid peroxidation with an efficacy greatly surpassing that of the glucocorticoid steroid MP or the earlier nonglucocorticoids (25,27). These 21-aminosteroids have further been found to decrease iron-induced damage to cultured cortical neurons (28,29).

Although the 21-aminosteroids are potent inhibitors of iron-dependent lipid peroxidation in intact phospholipid environments, they also inhibit lipid peroxidation in systems that do not contain membranes and are free of iron. By using the free radical generator 2,2′-azobis(2,4-dimethyl valeronitrile) to initiate lipid peroxidation in a homogeneous methanol solution of linoleic acid, the 21-aminosteroids have been found to inhibit lipid peroxidation by scavenging lipid peroxyl radicals (LOO·) and thus block lipid radical chain reactions in a manner similar to vitamin E. The LOO· scavenging action of the 21-aminosteroids resides in the amine portion of the molecule and yields an as yet uncharacterized product. During the inhibition of lipid peroxidation, the 21-aminosteroids compete for the same reaction as vitamin E and slow its degradation (30). *In vivo* studies have demonstrated that U-74006F indeed acts to preserve tissue vitamin E levels in injured cat spinal cord, indicative of an inhibition of posttraumatic lipid peroxidation (4).

In addition to scavenging of lipid peroxyl radicals, U-74006F also reacts with hydroxyl radicals generated during *in vitro* Fenton reactions (i.e., $Fe^{2+} + H_2O_2 \rightarrow Fe^{3+} + OH^- + \cdot OH$). Recently, data have been obtained from a mouse head injury model suggesting that the compound may also reduce hydroxyl radical concentration *in vivo*. Administration of salicylate, a hydroxyl radical trap, leads to the posttraumatic formation of dihydroxybenzoic acid (DHBA) in brain tissue when it reacts with hydroxyl radical. U-74006F dosing has been found to decrease DHBA formation in the injured brain, implying either decreased formation or scavenging of hydroxyl radicals (31).

The 21-aminosteroids U-74006F and U-74500A also have stabilizing effects on cell membranes. The release of free arachidonic acid from injured cell membranes is blocked by compounds in this series (32). This effect is not caused by glucocorticoid activity of the compounds (i.e., phospholipase A_2 inhibition) but may be related to their antioxidant actions. In other studies using cultured bovine brain microvascular endothelial cells, U-74006F and U-74500A have been shown to localize within the hydrophobic core of cell membranes and cause an increase in lipid ordering (i.e., decreased fluidity) of the phospholipid bilayer (33). This action may help to inhibit the propagation of lipid peroxidation by restricting the movement of lipid peroxyl and alkoxyl radicals within the membrane so that they are unable to attack the neighboring polyunsaturated fatty acids.

Effects of Tirilazad Mesylate (U-74006F) in Experimental Spinal Cord Injury

U-74006F has been investigated for its ability to promote neurological recovery of cats following a moderately severe compression injury to the lumbar spinal cord (34). Beginning at 30 min after injury, the animals received a 48-hr intravenous regimen of vehicle (sterile water) or U-74006F in a random and blinded protocol similar to that employed in earlier studies with MP (3,20). Initial U-74006F doses ranged from 0.01 to 30 mg/kg. At 4 weeks after injury, vehicle-treated animals consistently remained paraplegic. In contrast, cats that received 48-hr doses of U-74006F ranging from 1.6 to 160.0 mg/kg showed significantly better recovery, regaining approximately 75% of normal neurological function. Histological examination of the injured spinal cord segment showed a modest but statistically significant correlation ($r = 0.57$, $p < 0.001$) between cross-sectional tissue preservation and neurological recovery score, indicating an effect of U-74006F to retard posttraumatic tissue degeneration.

In order to pursue a mechanism by which U-74006F may be acting to promote chronic recovery after blunt spinal cord injury, the acute effects of U-74006F have also been viewed in relation to a possible action to attenuate progressive posttraumatic spinal cord ischemia following spinal cord compression injury (4). In vehicle-treated cats, there was a progressive decline in spinal cord blood flow (SCBF) over the course of the experiment from normal levels immediately after injury. By 4 hr post-injury, SCBF had decreased by 42%. In contrast, the 4-hr SCBF in cats that were treated with any of the three highest dose levels of U-74006F were significantly improved in comparison to the vehicle-treated cats. The molecular mechanism of action of U-74006F in antagonizing posttraumatic ischemia development is believed to involve an inhibition of oxygen radical-mediated microvascular lipid peroxidation. This conclusion is based on the known involvement of lipid peroxidation in posttraumatic ischemia development (35) and the concomitant action of U-74006F to attenuate an injury-induced decline in spinal tissue vitamin E at the same doses that reduce posttraumatic ischemia (4). U-74006F has also been shown to retard posttraumatic ischemia development secondary to a more severe spinal cord contusion injury (36).

Recent studies suggest that U-74006F retains its efficacy in promoting posttraumatic recovery after experimental spinal cord injury even when initiation of treatment is delayed to 4 hr (37). Thus, this novel nonglucocorticoid 21-aminosteroid antioxidant shows considerable promise as a safer and possibly more effective acute treatment of spinal cord injury than MP.

Effects of Methylprednisolone and Tirilazad Mesylate on Anterograde Degeneration of Motor Nerve

In addition to playing a role in posttraumatic microvascular damage and secondary ischemia development in the spinal cord, oxygen radical-induced LP also appears to play a direct role in the degeneration of spinal axons after injury. This has been studied within the context of the anterograde degeneration of surgically sectioned cat soleus motor axons. Specifically, the surgical transection of soleus motor axons at the level of the greater sciatic foramen, followed 48 hr later by an assessment of neuromuscular function in the *in vivo* soleus nerve–muscle preparation, provides a reproducible model for studying the early phases of neuronal anterograde degeneration (38). The 48-hr degenerating motor nerve terminals display subtle but significant defects in neuromuscular transmission that can be quantified by a number of functional parameters.

In this model of cat motor axonal degeneration, it was observed that intensive treatment with glucocorticoids, including triamcinolone (39,40) and MP (41), prior to nerve section could significantly retard the functional degeneration of cat soleus motor nerve terminals. Drakontides (42) has shown that intensive glucocorticoid dosing also exerts an ultrastructural preservation of degenerating rat phrenic motor nerve terminals. Subsequent to the demonstration of the antioxidant properties of glucocorticoids such as MP, it was reasoned that previously demonstrated slowing of motor nerve degeneration may be based on an antioxidant effect. Thus, the effects of pretreatment of cats with high doses of the prototype lipid antioxidant, vitamin E, were studied (43). Five days of vitamin E administration (200 I.U./day orally for 5 days) resulted in an even greater preservation of neuromuscular function in the degenerating soleus nerve–muscle preparations than shown earlier with the glucocorticoid steroids. This suggested that the ability of the steroids to retard anterograde degeneration is indeed a manifestation of their intrinsic antioxidant properties. Moreover, the role of lipid peroxidation in the anterograde degeneration process was implied.

The efficacy of U-74006F has also been viewed in relation to the compound's ability to retard the anterograde degeneration of the cat soleus motor axons (44). Cats were dosed with 7.7, 13.0, or 30.0 mg/kg doses of U-74006F twice daily for 5 days followed by unilateral sciatic nerve section on day 5. At 48 hr after nerve section in untreated animals, the ratio of nerve-evoked (0.4 Hz) contractile tension in the degenerating nerve–muscle preparation was only 52% compared to the contralateral normal preparation. In contrast, the U-74006F-treated (13.0 mg/kg) cats showed a ratio of 86% ($p < 0.01$ versus untreated). U-74006F also significantly improved the ability of the degenerating preparation to maintain high-frequency repetitive transmission. Based on these results, it has been concluded that lipid peroxidation may indeed be a fundamental mechanism of anterograde neuronal degeneration secondary to acute neuronal injury.

SUMMARY

The glucocorticoid steroid methylprednisolone (MP) has been shown to enhance chronic recovery after human spinal cord injury when administered in a 24-hr high-dose regimen beginning within 8 hr. The doses of MP that effect this improved recovery have been demonstrated to inhibit spinal tissue LP, which has been postulated to be a key event in the secondary posttraumatic degenerative cascade. The molecular mechanism of action of the steroid appears to involve intercalation into the cell membrane and blockade of the propagation of LP reactions. At a physiological level, the inhibition of injury-induced LP has been found to result in an attenuation of progressive posttraumatic ischemia and energy failure together with an augmented reversal of intracellular calcium accumulation. However, MP also acts directly to retard secondary neuronal degeneration, as observed in studies showing the steroid's ability to slow the anterograde degeneration of experimentally injured cat soleus motor nerves. The duplication of this effect by the nonsteroidal lipid antioxidant α-tocopherol supports the notion that it is indeed a manifestation of the inhibition of posttraumatic LP. Moreover, the efficacy of MP in limiting lipid peroxidation and secondary spinal cord or motor nerve degeneration has also been duplicated by a nonglucocorticoid 21-aminosteroid, tirilazad mesylate (U-74006F), which suggests the independence of the antioxidant and glucocorticoid effects of MP.

REFERENCES

1. Braughler JM, Hall ED. Central nervous system trauma and stroke: I. Biochemical considerations for oxygen radical formation and lipid peroxidation. *Free Radicals Biol Med* 1989;6:289–301.
2. Hall ED, Braughler JM. Central nervous system trauma and stroke: II. Physiological and pharmacological evidence for the involvement of oxygen radicals and lipid peroxidation. *Free Radicals Biol Med* 1989;6:303–313.
3. Anderson DK, Saunders RD, Demediuk P, et al. Lipid hydrolysis and peroxidation in injured spinal cord: partial protection with methylprednisolone or vitamin E and selenium. *CNS Trauma* 1985;2: 257–267.
4. Hall ED, Yonkers PA, Horan KL, et al. Correlation between attenuation of posttraumatic spinal cord ischemia and preservation of vitamin E by the 21-aminosteroid U-74006F: evidence for an *in vivo* antioxidant action. *J Neurotrauma* 1989;6:169–176.
5. Demopoulos HB, Flamm ES, Seligman ML, Pietronigro DD, Tomasula J, DeCrescito V. Further studies on free radical pathology in the major central nervous system disorders: effects of very high doses of methylprednisolone on the functional outcome, morphology, and chemistry of experimental spinal cord impact injury. *Can J Physiol Pharmacol* 1982;60:1415–1424.
6. Hall ED, Braughler JM. Effects of intravenous methylprednisolone on spinal cord lipid peroxidation and (Na^+, K^+)-ATPase activity. Dose–response analysis during 1st hour after contusion injury in the cat. *J Neurosurg* 1982;49:563–568.
7. Kurihara M. Role of monoamines in experimental spinal cord injury in cats. Relationship between Na^+, K^+-ATPase and lipid peroxidation. *J Neurosurg* 1985;62:743–749.
8. Clendenon NR, Allen N, Gordon WH, Bingham WG. Inhibition of Na^+, K^+-ATPase activity following experimental spinal cord trauma. *J Neurosurg* 1978;49:563–568.
9. Means ED, Anderson DK. The pathophysiology of acute spinal cord injury. In: Davidoff RA, ed. *Handbook of the spinal cord.* New York: Marcel Dekker; 1987:19–61.
10. Hall ED, Braughler JM. Acute effects of intravenous glucocorticoid pretreatment on the *in vitro* peroxidation of cat spinal cord tissue. *Exp Neurol* 1981;73:321–324.
11. Anderson DK, Means ED. Microvascular perfusion and metabolism in injured spinal cord after methylprednisolone treatment. *J Neurosurg* 1982;56: 106–113.
12. Braughler JM, Hall ED. Lactate and pyruvate metabolism in injured cat spinal cord before and after a single large intravenous dose of methylprednisolone. *J Neurosurg* 1983;59:256–261.
13. Braughler JM, Hall ED. Effects of multidose methylprednisolone sodium succinate administration on injured cat spinal cord neurofilament degradation and energy metabolism. *J Neurosurg* 1984;61: 290–295.
14. Young W, Flamm ES. Effects of high dose corticosteroid therapy on blood flow, evoked potentials, and extracellular calcium in experimental spinal injury. *J Neurosurg* 1982;57:667–673.
15. Hall ED, Wolf DL, Braughler JM. Effects of single large dose of methylprednisolone sodium succinate on experimental posttraumatic spinal cord ischemia. *J Neurosurg* 1984;61:124–130.
16. Hall ED. Glucocorticoid effects on central nervous excitability and synaptic transmission. *Int Rev Neurobiol* 1982;23:165–195.
17. Hall ED, Braughler JM. Glucocorticoid mechanisms in spinal cord injury: A review and therapeutic rationale. *Surg Neurol* 1982;18:320–327.
18. Hall ED. The neuroprotective pharmacology of methylprednisolone. *J Neurosurg* 1992;76:13–22.
19. Braughler JM, Hall ED: Uptake and elimination of methylprednisolone from contused spinal cord following intravenous injection of the sodium succinate ester. *J Neurosurg* 1983;58:538–542.
20. Braughler JM, Hall ED, Means ED, et al. Evaluation of an intensive methylprednisolone sodium succinate dosing regimen in experimental spinal cord injury. *J Neurosurg* 1987;67:102–105.
21. Hoerlein BF, Redding RW, Hoff EJ, et al. Evaluation of naloxone, crocetin, thyrotropin releasing hormone, methylprednisolone, partial myelotomy, and hemilaminectomy in the treatment of acute spinal cord trauma. *J Am Anim Hosp Assoc* 1984;21:67–77.
22. Young W, DeCrescito V, Flamm ES, et al. Pharmacological therapy of acute spinal cord injury: studies with high dose methylprednisolone and naloxone. *Clin Neurosurg* 1988;34:675–697.
23. Bracken MB, Shepard MJ, Collins WF, et al. A randomized controlled trial of methylprednisolone or naloxone in the treatment of acute spinal cord injury. *N Engl J Med* 1990;322:1405–1411.
24. Hall ED, McCall JM, Yonkers PA, et al. A nonglucocorticoid analog of methylprednisolone dupli-

cates its high dose pharmacology in models of CNS trauma and neuronal membrane damage. *J Pharmacol Exp Ther* 1987;242:137–142.
25. Hall ED, McCall JM, Braughler JM. New pharmacological treatments for spinal cord trauma. *J Neurotrauma* 1988;5:81–89.
26. Braughler JM, Hall ED, Jacobsen EJ, et al. The 21-aminosteroids: potent inhibitors of lipid peroxidation for the treatment of central nervous system trauma and ischemia. *Drugs Future* 1989;14: 143–152.
27. Braughler JM, Pregenzer JF, Chase RL, et al. Novel 21-aminosteroids as potent inhibitors of iron-dependent lipid peroxidation. *J Biol Chem* 1987; 262:10438–10440.
28. Monyer H, Hartley DM, Choi, DW. 21-Aminosteroids attenuate excitotoxic neuronal injury in cortical cell cultures. *Neuron* 1990;5:121–126.
29. Hall ED, Yonkers PA, Braughler JM, et al. U78517F: a potent inhibitor of lipid peroxidation with activity in experimental brain injury and ischemia. *J Pharmacol Exp Ther* 1991;258:688–694.
30. Braughler JM, Pregenzer JF. The 21-aminosteroid inhibitors of lipid peroxidation: reactions with lipid peroxyl and phenoxyl radicals. *Free Radicals Biol Med* 1989;7:125–130.
31. Althaus JS, Williams CM, Andrus PK, et al. *In vitro* and *in vivo* analysis of tirilazad mesylate (U74006F) as a hydroxyl radical scavenger. *Soc Neurosci Abst* 1991;17:164.
32. Braughler JM, Chase RL, Neff GL, et al. A new 21-aminosteroid antioxidant lacking glucocorticoid activity stimulates ACTH secretion and blocks arachidonic acid release from mouse pituitary tumor (AtT-20) cells. *J Pharmacol Exp Ther* 1988;244: 423–427.
33. Audus KL, Guillot FL, Braughler JM. Evidence for 21-aminosteroid association with the hydrophobic domains of brain microvessel endothelial cells. *Free Rad Biol Med* 1991;11:361–371.
34. Anderson DK, Braughler JM, Hall ED, et al. Effects of treatment with U-74006F on neurological recovery following experimental spinal cord injury. *J Neurosurg* 1988;69:562–567.
35. Hall ED, Wolf DL. A pharmacological analysis of the pathophysiological mechanisms of posttraumatic spinal cord ischemia. *J Neurosurg* 1986; 64:951–961.
36. Hall ED. Effects of the 21-aminosteroid U-74006F on posttraumatic spinal cord ischemia. *J Neurosurg* 1988;68:462–465.
37. Anderson DK, Hall ED, Braughler JM, et al. Effect of delayed administration of U74006F (tirilazad mesylate) on recovery of locomotor function following experimental spinal cord injury. *J Neurotrauma* 1991;8:187–192.
38. Okamoto M, Riker WF. Motor nerve terminals as the initial site of functional changes after denervation. *J Gen Physiol* 1969;53:70–80.
39. Hall ED, Baker T, Riker WF. Glucocorticoid preservation of motor nerve function during early degeneration. *Ann Neurol* 1977;1:263–270.
40. Hall ED, Riker WF, Baker T. Beneficial action of glucocorticoid treatment on neuromuscular transmission during early motor nerve degeneration. *Exp Neurol* 1983;79:488–496.
41. Hall ED, Wolf DL. Methylprednisolone preservation of motor nerve function during early degeneration. *Exp Neurol* 1984;84:715–720.
42. Drakontides AB. The effect of glucocorticoid treatment on denervated rat hemidiaphragm. *Brain Res* 1978;239:175–189.
43. Hall ED. Intensive antioxidant pretreatment retards motor nerve degeneration. *Brain Res* 1987;413: 175–178.
44. Hall ED, Yonkers PA. Preservation of motor nerve function during early degeneration by the 21-aminosteroid antioxidant U-74006F. *Brain Res* 1990;513: 244–247.

Advances in Neurology, Vol. 59, edited by Fredrick J. Seil. Raven Press, Ltd., New York © 1993.

21

Strategies for the Development of New and Better Pharmacological Treatments for Acute Spinal Cord Injury

Wise Young

Department of Neurosurgery, New York University Medical Center, New York, New York 10016

The Second National Acute Spinal Cord Injury Study, NASCIS 2 (1–3), capped nearly a decade of intense animal studies (4) reporting that various drugs can ameliorate tissue damage in injured spinal cords. NASCIS 2 showed for the first time that a treatment delivered after spinal cord injury can improve neurological recovery in humans. High doses (30 mg/kg bolus followed by 5.4 mg/kg per hr for 23 hr) of methylprednisolone, a synthetic corticosteroid, significantly improved motor and sensory recovery compared to placebo or naloxone (5.4 mg/kg bolus followed by 3.0 mg/kg per hr for 23 hr).

An earlier trial, the first National Acute Spinal Cord Injury Study (NASCIS 1), showed no significant difference between a "high" (1,000 mg bolus followed by 1,000 mg/day) and a "low" (100 mg bolus followed by 100 mg/day) dose of methylprednisolone (5). In retrospect, NASCIS 1 failed because of inadequate preclinical data and wishful thinking. Subsequent laboratory studies showed that a 30 mg/kg bolus, or more than twice the dose used in NASCIS 1, was the optimal dose (6–14). Based on the conjecture that secondary injury processes continued for several days, patients were randomized as late as 48 hr after injury. Thus, too little methylprednisolone was given too late in NASCIS 1.

NASCIS 2 was designed to test two hypotheses: (1) that early treatment would be superior to late treatment and (2) that treatment would be ineffective in severely injured patients admitted to hospital with no neurological function below the lesion. The results showed not only that early treatment was better but that late treatment beyond 8 hr after injury was ineffective. The results, however, also disproved the hypothesis that "complete" spinal-injured patients would not benefit from treatment. Although methylprednisolone-treated complete spinal patients did not recover as much as "incomplete" patients with residual sensory or motor function below the lesion level, they did recover approximately 20% of lost motor and sensory function compared to only 8% in placebo-treated patients. Methylprednisolone-treated incomplete patients recovered approximately 79% of lost motor function compared to 59% in placebo-treated patients.

The findings that methylprednisolone must be given within 8 hr to have a beneficial effect and that the drug improves neurological function even in severe spinal cord injury has had and will have far-reaching impacts on spinal cord injury care and research. I first briefly review the impact of NASCIS 2 on clinical care and future clinical studies. I then critically examine the rationale for different variables that must be tested in preclinical studies: dose, treatment initiation time, treatment duration, injury severity, and combining treatments with methylprednisolone. I end with a brief assessment of the challenge that now faces researchers in the field of acute spinal cord injury.

THE IMPACT OF NASCIS 2 ON SPINAL CORD INJURY CARE AND RESEARCH

NASCIS 2 has had and will have a lasting impact on spinal cord injury care, not because it was the first randomized clinical trial to show a treatment effect in human spinal cord injury but because it showed that treatment must be given shortly after injury and that treatment can improve neurological recovery in patients with severe spinal cord injury. Before NASCIS 2, since no treatment was believed to improve neurological recovery, spinal cord injury was often treated in a leisurely fashion. Patients were transported to the nearest emergency room, where they often waited hours for X-rays and consultation. Surgery was often delayed for days or avoided altogether, especially in "complete" patients. NASCIS 2 results suggest a need to reconsider this attitude.

Perhaps the most important legacy of NASCIS 2 is hope. If early treatment with a drug such as methylprednisolone can improve neurological recovery even in "complete" spinal injury, perhaps other interventions, such as surgery, may be helpful. The lessons of NASCIS 2 are that if such treatment is to be applied, it should be as soon as possible, and that spinal injury victims admitted to hospital with no residual motor or sensory function below the lesion level may benefit from the therapy. NASCIS 2 has provided motivation for more aggressive medical and surgical therapy of complete and incomplete spinal injury victims. Thus, spinal cord injury is now on its way to joining the ranks of other urgent medical emergencies such as myocardial infarcts, amputated limbs, and head injury.

The demonstration that methylprednisolone is effective for human spinal cord injury has essentially ruled out further placebo-controlled trials in acute spinal cord injury. New treatments must be compared with the methylprednisolone protocol used in NASCIS 2. Differences between two effective treatments will be smaller and will require more subjects. Comparison of an untested drug with methylprednisolone may be difficult to justify. Given the choice between a proven drug and a drug of unknown efficacy, some patients may refuse to enter the trial. One alternative has been to combine a new treatment with methylprednisolone to see if the combination has an additive effect. Differences between a treatment combined with methylprednisolone and methylprednisolone alone will be even smaller and more difficult to detect.

NASCIS 2 has placed an onerous burden on preclinical studies. To be seriously considered for clinical trial, new drugs must now be shown to be equal or superior to methylprednisolone. Superiority is a subtle quality that can be argued from many vantage points. It is, of course, superior if it causes greater improvements of neurological recovery. However, a drug would also be superior if it were effective over a wider dose–response range, could be given at a later time than methylprednisolone, had fewer side effects, or was effective over a wide range of injury severity. Preclinical trials must now examine at least five additional variables: (a) dose, (b) treatment initiation time, (c) treatment duration, (d) injury severity, and (e) the combination with methylprednisolone.

DOSE–RESPONSE ANALYSES OF NEUROPROTECTIVE THERAPIES

The use of therapy after acute injury presumes the presence of "secondary injury mechanisms." The concept of secondary injury mechanisms represents a singular paradox in biology (15). Neurons are, by definition, the longest-lived cells of our bodies. Unable to regenerate, the neurons that we die with are the same ones that we were born with. Complex cascades of pathological events involving calcium, free radicals, excitatory amino acids, metabolic derangements, blood flow changes, and other destructive changes occur in central nervous tissues shortly after injury. Paradoxically, these important and longest-lived cells of our bodies possess potent autodestructive mechanisms that are initiated by injury and can be ameliorated by treatment. Two general characteristics of the treatments reported to be neuroprotective provide some insights: the requirement for very high doses and the presence of an inverted-U-shaped dose–response curve.

In general, very high doses of drugs are required for neuroprotective effects. For example, effective doses of naloxone and methylprednisolone greatly exceed standard doses of the two drugs as opiate receptor blocker and corticosteroid hormone (16). The dose of methylprednisolone used in NASCIS 2 transcends the definition of "megadose": 30 mg/kg followed by 5.4 mg/kg per hr adds up to nearly 10 g of this potent corticosteroid given intravenously to an average-size person over 24 hr compared to standard doses of 25 to 125 mg. Likewise the 5.4 mg/kg bolus and 3.0 mg/kg per hr dosing protocol for naloxone in NASCIS 2 adds up to nearly 5 g of naloxone, compared to 0.5 mg given to reverse opiate overdoses. At doses that are 10 to 1,000 times the level needed to saturate receptors, these drugs clearly may not be acting through normal mechanisms.

Although very high doses are required, too much is not good. For example, Hall and Braughler (6,8,9,17–19) found that methylprednisolone begins to inhibit lipid peroxidation at 15 mg/kg and peaks at 30 mg/kg for cat spinal cord. However, increasing the dose to 60 mg/kg can actually worsen the tissue damage. Thus, the dose–response curve progresses from threshold to peak and to deleterious effects in a four-fold range. Similar inverted-U-shaped dose–response curves have been reported for naloxone and other opiate antagonists (20,21).

These examples clearly illustrate the importance of doing dose–response analyses in preclinical studies. Neuroprotective drugs have an extremely narrow effective dose range, and overdose can paradoxically lead to deleterious effects. Such dose–response relationships suggest that neuroprotective drugs can be double-edged swords. The studies of Hall and Braughler defining the dose–response curves of steroids not only provide a strong argument that the methylprednisolone is not acting as a hormone (9,22) but are probably the single most important factor underlying the success of NASCIS 2. Detailed dose–response studies are essential.

THE IMPORTANCE OF TREATMENT INITIATION TIME

NASCIS 2 hypothesized that earlier treatment would be better than late treatment. A vast majority of the patients received treatment within 12 hr after injury. Approximately half of the patients received treatment within 8 hr. Patients treated between 8 and 12 hr not only showed no significant benefit from treatment but may have worse motor recovery ($p = 0.08$) than placebo controls at the 1-year follow-up interval (2). It should be emphasized that the 8-hr period was based on the median treatment time rather than any theoretical consideration. The therapeutic time window may be shorter than 8 hr.

The finding that treatment must be delivered early to be effective appears obvious in retrospect. However, before NASCIS 2, most researchers in the field did not realize the importance of treatment timing. Thus, very few researchers (20,21) examined the effects of delayed treatment of spinal cord injury. Delayed treatment with methylprednisolone was simply never examined in animal models. NASCIS 1, in fact, had randomized patients as late as 48 hr after injury on the premise that spinal cord edema and secondary damage to the spinal cord may continue for several days. In light of the NASCIS 2 finding, it becomes clear that spinal cord injury must be treated as a true medical emergency. The study showed not only that treatment can improve recovery but that the treatment must be delivered as rapidly as possible.

Treatment initiation time is a critical factor that must be examined in future preclinical studies. In many ways, we were fortunate that the time limit for randomization turned out to be close to the therapeutic time window for methylprednisolone. If 24 hr had been chosen, the outcome of the study may have been very different, and methylprednisolone may have been dismissed as an ineffective drug for acute spinal cord injury. In the upcoming NASCIS 3 trial, patients will be randomized within 8 hr after injury because there is no longer any rationale and possibly even some contraindication to giving methylprednisolone late. Comparing early and late treatment within the 8-hr period would further narrow down the therapeutic time window.

Examination of the therapeutic time window is also of interest because it may provide some insights into the mechanisms of drug action. For example, tirilazad mesylate is a 21-aminosteroid that is a more potent lipid peroxidation inhibitor than methylprednisolone but has no corticosteroid receptor activity (23–27). Naloxone apparently has a longer therapeutic time window in animal models (20). In a recent study, delaying tirilazad treatment by as long as 4 hr still yielded significant functional improvements in spinal-injured cats, but the drug given at 8 hr was ineffective (28). In contrast, monosialic gangliosides (GM_1) given 48 to 72 hr after spinal cord injury improved functional recovery in humans (29), suggesting a very different mechanism of action.

THE QUESTION OF TREATMENT DURATION

Treatment duration is a question that has seldom been addressed in preclinical studies. Because of the inconvenience of keeping an intravenous line in animals after spinal cord injury, most of the early studies gave drug for only 3 to 6 hr after the injury. The choice of the 24-hr dosing period in NASCIS 2 was made more on the basis of theoretical and safety considerations than on preclinical data. Hall and Braughler (6,8,12,18) had shown that repeated doses were superior to a single dose. Pharmacologically speaking, a continuous infusion should provide more consistent plasma levels. NASCIS 1 had shown a trend for increased infections in patients given 10 days of 1 g/day methylprednisolone. Thus, the NASCIS 2 protocol specified a 24-hr treatment.

A direct comparison of the relative efficacies of methylprednisolone treatments of different durations has not yet been carried out in animals. Thus, although the NASCIS 2 results indicate that a 24-hr treatment course of methylprednisolone is effective and safe, this conclusion cannot be extrapolated to longer or shorter duration treatments. Because spinal cord edema (30) and demyelination (31,32) do not peak until several days after injury, there is good reason to suspect that secondary injury processes can take place over several days. For this reason, the NASCIS 3 study will be comparing 24 hr and 48 hr of methylprednisolone treatment as well as an initial bolus of methylprednisolone followed by 24 hr of tirilazad mesylate.

Investigating treatment duration is really a study of the back end of the therapeutic time window and can provide many insights into treatment mechanisms. Injury initiates a cascade of tissue responses, some of which may start and end early, whereas others may start late and extend for long periods of time. Not all the responses may be deleterious. In fact, the recent finding in NASCIS 2 that patients started on methylprednisolone more than 8 hr after injury may have worse neurological recovery than placebo controls is worrisome because it suggests that very high doses of methylprednisolone at this stage may be inhibiting some beneficial response of the tissue or organism to the injury. For example, although methylprednisolone has well-known antiinflammatory effects on tissues, some of the inflammatory response may play an important role in resolving the injury.

Most of the early studies that showed impressive neurological improvements in animal spinal cord injury in fact employed only early and short-term methylprednisolone treatment. For example, as many as 60% of cats will recover locomotor function when treated with only two bolus doses of 15 mg/kg of methylprednisolone at 45 min and 3 hr after injury (16). Prolonged methylprednisolone treatment may well have deleterious effects, just as 60 mg/kg doses are harmful. In any case, this issue has not yet been resolved in animal studies.

THE INFLUENCE OF INJURY SEVERITY

Injury severity is clearly an important factor. NASCIS 2 showed, to the surprise of many, that methylprednisolone significantly improved neurological recovery in patients admitted to hospital with no motor or sensory function below the lesion level. This finding raises serious questions concerning the current clinical dogma that "complete" spinal-injured patients will not benefit neurologically from treatment and therefore should be conservatively managed. Although some people may argue that the term "complete" spinal cord injury really implies a time period as well as absence of function, few will dispute that patients admitted with no function have been severely injured. An analysis of placebo-treated patients with no motor or sensory function below the injury level on admission shows that these patients recovered an average of less than 6% of lost motor and sensory scores, compared to 59% recovery in those admitted with even the slightest residual motor or sensory function.

It is easy to create an animal model of spinal cord injury in which no treatment, short of regeneration, would be effective. Likewise, it is easy to create a spinal injury model from which most animals will recover without treatment. By carefully titrating trauma dose, researchers can produce spinal cord injury models that are perched on the threshold of recovery and therefore would be sensitive to a variety of treatments that would push it over that threshold. A criticism of this approach to animal modeling is that it may bias the results and would not be predictive of the clinical condition. However, NASCIS 2 findings strongly suggest that many humans may also be on the threshold between "complete" and "incomplete" injuries and that drugs like methylprednisolone can push them over that threshold.

Preclinical studies must include injury severity as one of the variables. A treatment being ineffective in severe injuries does not necessarily mean that it is likewise ineffective in mild or moderate injuries. The opposite can occur; i.e., a drug may work only in severe injuries. It can even happen that a given treatment dose is beneficial for mild injury but deleterious for severe injuries, or vice versa. Robustness of a beneficial drug effect over a wide range of injury severities is a strong argument for the superiority of one drug over another. Finally, investigation of a treatment on a single injury model has a high probability of a false negative.

Dose responses should be studied over a range of injury severities. Laboratory studies have revealed major differences in the spinal cord response to different injuries. For example, white matter blood flow falls in severely (33–35) but not in mildly contused cords (36). The degree of blood–brain barrier breakdown correlates highly with the severity of injuries (37). These factors influence drug delivery and penetration into the injury site. In addition, tissue reaction to injury is more intense in severely injured spinal cords. Thus, the optimal dose may differ depending on injury severity. The assumption that there is one optimal dose and treatment duration for all injury severities should be questioned regularly.

THE PROMISE AND PITFALLS OF COMBINATION TREATMENTS

Human nature impels many of us to hope that if two drugs work, combining the two may yield additive or perhaps even synergistic benefit. After all, injury causes a multivariate cascade of secondary destructive events. There are too many routes to autodestruction, and a single treatment has no hope of stopping all or even a majority of them. Many investigators and drug companies have visions of administering a cocktail of blockers for central nervous system injuries.

Several treatment combinations have been tested in spinal cord injury models. Methylprednisolone was a common component of such therapies. Based on work showing that cooling of the spinal cord is protective (38,39), several investigators examined cooling and steroid therapy (40,41). An antifibrinolytic drug was used with methylprednisolone (42) with positive results. Some combined therapies, however, may be deleterious. Since naloxone improved neurological recovery and blood flow (43–45) in spinal-injured animals, we tested the two drugs together, i.e., 10 mg/kg of naloxone and 15 mg/kg of methylprednisolone given as boluses at 45 min and 3 hr after injury. The two drugs together did not improve neurological function as much as either alone and appeared to be toxic (16). In preparation for NASCIS 3 (unpublished), we gave methylprednisolone (30 mg/kg at 30 min) followed by tirilazad mesylate (6 mg/kg every 6 hr) and found the beneficial effect to be roughly similar to methylprednisolone (30 mg/kg at 30 min and every 6 hr).

Because of the tendency of many drugs to have a narrow inverted-U-shaped dose–response curve, combination therapy is fraught with pitfalls. Careful titration and examination of a wide range of combined doses is necessary to avoid false negatives and the possibility of pushing the dose response into the far side of the U-shaped curve. Unfortunately, combination studies require resources that most laboratories do not have. For example, examining one pair of drugs and varying the dose of each drug over a minimum of three dose levels requires at least seven separate experimental groups examining the combination, six of the two drugs individually, and two vehicle controls. Combined with assessing the 15 treatment mixtures over three injury severities, three treatment initiation times, and two treatment durations yields 270 experimental groups.

Practical considerations, however, are forcing more investigators to examine combination therapy. Because methylprednisolone has been shown to be effective, many clinicians are unwilling to replace it completely with another new and yet unproven drug in a clinical trial. For this reason, many of the newer treatments of spinal cord injury may have to be superimposed on the high-dose methylprednisolone protocol used in NASCIS 2. Unfortunately, little is known about the effects of combining methylprednisolone with other drugs, and each combination must be directly addressed in laboratory and clinical studies.

CONCLUSIONS

The past decade of research has yielded the first effective treatment for acute spinal cord injury. Although methylprednisolone's effect on neurological recovery was highly significant, the effect was modest, and the drug has three drawbacks. First, the drug has a remarkably narrow effective dose. The beneficial effects begin at 15 mg/kg, peaking at 30 mg/kg, and the effects become deleterious at 60 mg/kg. Because actual drug concentrations in the spinal cord cannot be controlled so accurately, drug may be reaching the toxic range in some patients and may be insufficient in others. Second, although NASCIS 2 showed that the short-term high-dose treatment has no significant deleterious effects on the population of spinal-injured patients, it is a potent corticosteroid that is known to cause immunosuppression and other problems when given over a longer period. Third, the finding that delaying treatment with methylprednisolone may result in less neurological recovery than with placebo is disturbing.

NASCIS has vastly complicated both clinical and preclinical investigation of new drugs. Since methylprednisolone was shown to be effective, placebo-controlled clinical trials are no longer feasible. Comparisons must be made with methylprednisolone. The differences between two effective drugs will be smaller, and more subjects will be required to detect treatment effects. A decade ago, preclinical studies simply had to show efficacy to establish a drug as a candidate for clinical trial. Now, preclinical studies must compare a treatment with and in combination with methylprednisolone. Different treatment doses, initiation times, and durations must be examined over a range of injury.

The enormous volume of experiments required to evaluate these variables poses a serious obstacle for developing new and better treatments of acute spinal cord injury. No single laboratory can carry out the *tour de force* alone. Assessing dose response over a range of injury severities while varying treatment dose, time, duration, and combinations may require several thousand experiments. Future preclinical trials may have to be carried out collaboratively between centers, in much the same manner as multicenter clinical trials are being done now. The need for more reproducible injury models and outcome measures has never been greater. Our understanding of drug mechanisms must be improved so that therapeutic protocols are designed rationally.

In summary, NASCIS 2 has not only provided us with the first effective treatment for acute spinal cord injury, it poses a challenge of significant proportions to scientists in the field. The problem of identifying and testing new and better therapies for acute spinal cord injury will not again be as easy as it was preceding NASCIS 2. The issues that have been raised by NASCIS 2 are not unique to spinal cord injury. As the first treatments for stroke and traumatic brain injury are found, these other fields will face the same challenge.

ACKNOWLEDGMENTS

Work in the author's laboratory was supported in part by NIH NINDS grants PO1 NS10164 and NS15590.

REFERENCES

1. Bracken MB, Shepard MJ, Collins WF, et al. A randomized controlled trial of methylprednisolone or naloxone in the treatment of acute spinal-cord injury: results of the Second National Acute Spinal Cord Injury Study. *N Engl J Med* 1990;322: 1405–1411.
2. Bracken MB, Shepard MJ, Collins WF, et al. Methylprednisolone or naloxone in the treatment of acute spinal cord injury: one year follow-up results of the second National Acute Spinal Cord Injury Study. *J Neurosurg* [*in press*].
3. Young W, Bracken MB. The Second National Acute Spinal Cord Injury Study. In: Jane J, Torner J, Anderson D, Young W, eds. *NIH central nervous system status report*. New York: Mary Ann Liebert; 1991:5429–5451.
4. Young W. Clinical trials and experimental therapies of acute spinal cord injury. In: Vincken DJ, ed. *Handbook of neurology*. Amsterdam: Elsevier [*in press*].
5. Bracken MB, Shepard MJ, Hellenbrand KG, et al. Methylprednisolone and neurological function 1 year after spinal cord injury. *J Neurosurg* 1985;63:704–713.
6. Braughler JM, Hall ED. Correlation of methylprednisolone pharmacokinetics in cat spinal cord with its effect on (Na^+–K^+)-ATPase, lipid peroxidation and motor neuron function. *J Neurosurg* 1981;56: 838–844.
7. Hall ED, Braughler JM. Acute effects of intravenous glucocorticoid pretreatment on the *in vitro* peroxidation of cat spinal cord tissue. *Exp Neurol* 1981;73:321–324.
8. Hall ED, Braughler JM. Effects of methylprednisolone on spinal cord lipid peroxidation and (Na^+–K^+)-ATPase activity: dose response analysis during the first hour after contusion injury in the cat. *J Neurosurg* 1982;57:247–253.
9. Hall ED, Braughler JM. Glucocorticoid mechanisms in acute spinal cord injury: a review and therapeutic rationale. *Surg Neurol* 1982;18:320–327.
10. Hall ED, Wolf DL, Braughler JM. Dose response and time action analysis of the effects of a single large dose of methylprednisolone sodium succinate on posttraumatic spinal cord ischemia. *J Neurosurg* 1983;58:1–22.
11. Braughler JM, Hall ED. Lactate and pyruvate metabolism in injured cat spinal cord before and after a single large intravenous dose of methylprednisolone. *J Neurosurg* 1983;59:256–261.
12. Braughler JM, Hall ED. Uptake and elimination of methylprednisolone from contused cat spinal cord following intravenous injection of the sodium succinate ester. *J Neurosurg* 1983;58:538–542.
13. Braughler JM, Hall ED. Effects of multi-dose methylprednisolone sodium succinate administration on injured cat spinal cord neurofilament degradation and energy metabolism. *J Neurosurg* 1984;61: 290–295.
14. Hall ED, Wolf DL, Braughler JM. Effects of a single large dose of methylprednisolone sodium succinate on experimental posttraumatic spinal cord ischemia. Dose–response and time–action analysis. *J Neurosurg* 1984;61:124–130.

15. Young W. The post-injury responses in trauma and ischemia: secondary injury or protective mechanisms. *Cent Nerv Syst Trauma* 1987;4:27–52.
16. Young W, DeCrescito V, Flamm ES, Blight AR, Gruner JA. Pharmacological therapy of acute spinal cord injury: studies of high dose methylprednisolone and naloxone. *Clin Neurosurg* 1988;34:675–697.
17. Braughler JM, Hall ED. Acute enhancement of spinal cord synaptosomal (Na^+–K^+)-ATPase activity in cats following intravenous methylprednisolone. *Brain Res* 1981;219:464–469.
18. Braughler JM, Hall ED. Pharmacokinetics of methylprednisolone in cat plasma and spinal cord following a single intravenous dose of the sodium succinate ester. *Drug Metab Dispos* 1982;10:551–552.
19. Braughler JM, Hall ED, Means ED, Waters TR, Anderson DK. Evaluation of an intensive methylprednisolone sodium succinate dosing regimen in experimental spinal cord injury. *J Neurosurg* 1987; 67:102–105.
20. Faden AI, Jacobs TP, Holaday JW. Comparison of early and late naloxone treatment in experimental spinal injury. *Neurology* 1982;32:677–681.
21. Faden AI, Jacobs TP, Smith MT. Thyrotropin-releasing hormone in experimental spinal injury: dose response and late treatment. *Neurology* 1984;34:1280–1284.
22. Hall ED, Wolf DL. A pharmacological analysis of the pathophysiological mechanisms of posttraumatic spinal cord ischemia. *J Neurosurg* 1986;64: 951–961.
23. Braughler JM, Pregenzer JF, Chase RL, Duncan LA, Jacobsen EJ, McCall JM. Novel 21-amino steroids as potent inhibitors of iron-dependent lipid peroxidation. *J Biol Chem* 1987;262:10438–10440.
24. Hall ED. Beneficial effects of the 21-aminosteroid U74006F in acute CNS trauma and hypovolemic shock. *Acta Anaesth Belg* 1987;38:421–425.
25. Hall ED. Effects of the 21-aminosteroid U74006F on posttraumatic spinal cord ischemia in cats. *J Neurosurg* 1988;68:462–465.
26. Anderson DK, Braughler JM, Hall ED, Waters TR, McCall JM, Means ED. Effects of treatment with U74006F on neurological outcome following experimental spinal cord injury. *J Neurosurg* 1988; 69:562–567.
27. Hall ED, Yonkers PA, Horan KL, Braughler JM. Correlation between attenuation of posttraumatic spinal cord ischemia and preservation of tissue vitamin E by the 21-aminosteroid U74006F: evidence for an *in vivo* antioxidant mechanism. *J Neurotrauma* 1989;6:169–176.
28. Anderson DK, Hall ED, Braughler JM, McCall JM, Means ED. Effect of delayed administration of U74006F (tirilazad mesylate) on recovery of locomotor function after experimental spinal cord injury. *J Neurotrauma* 1991;8:187–192.
29. Geisler FH, Dorsey FC, Coleman WP. Recovery of motor function after spinal-cord injury—a randomized, placebo-controlled trial with GM-1 ganglioside. *N Engl J Med* 1991;324:1829–1838.
30. Lewin MG, Hansebout RR, Pappius HM. Chemical characteristics of traumatic spinal cord edema in cats. Effects of steroids on potassium depletion. *J Neurosurg* 1974;56:106–113.
31. Blight AR. Delayed demyelination and macrophage invasion: a candidate for secondary cell damage in spinal cord injury. *Cent Nerv Syst Trauma* 1985;2:299–315.
32. Blight AR, DeCrescito V. Morphometric analysis of experimental spinal cord injury in the cat: the relation of injury intensity to survival of myelinated axons. *Neuroscience* 1986;19:321–341.
33. Senter HJ, Venes JL. Altered blood flow and secondary injury in experimental spinal cord trauma. *J Neurosurg* 1978;49:569–578.
34. Senter HJ, Venes JL. Loss of autoregulation and posttraumatic ischemia following experimental spinal cord trauma. *J Neurosurg* 1979;50:198–206.
35. Cawthon DF, Senter HJ, Stewart WB. Comparison of hydrogen clearance and ^{14}C-antipyrine autoradiography in the measurement of spinal cord blood flow after severe impact injury. *J Neurosurg* 1980;37:591–596.
36. Lohse DC, Senter HJ, Kauer JS. Spinal cord blood flow in experimental transient paraplegia. *J Neurosurg* 1980;52:335–345.
37. Qu Z-X, Xu J, Perot PL, Hogan EL. A sensitive flurometric method for measurement of vascular permeability in spinal cord injury. *J Neurotrauma* 1991;8:149–156.
38. Albin MS, White RJ, Acosta RG, Yashon D. Study of functional recovery produced by delayed localized cooling after spinal cord injury in primates. *J Neurosurg* 1968;29:113–120.
39. Albin MS, White RJ, Yashon D, Harris LS. Effects of localized cooling on spinal cord trauma. *J Trauma* 1969;9:1000–1008.
40. Black P, Markowitz RS. Experimental spinal cord injury in monkeys: comparison of steroids and local hypothermia. *Surg Forum* 1971;22:409–411.
41. Kuchner EF, Hansebout RR. Combined steroid and hypothermia treatment of experimental spinal cord injury. *Surg Neurol* 1976;6:371–376.
42. Campbell JB, DeCrescito V, Tomasula JJ, Demopoulos HB, Flamm ES, Ortega BD. Effects of antifibrinolytic and steroid therapy on the contused spinal cord of cats. *J Neurosurg* 1974;40:726–733.
43. Faden AI, Jacobs TP, Holaday JW. Opiate antagonist improves neurologic recovery after spinal injury. *Science* 1980;211:493–494.
44. Young W, Flamm ES, Demopoulos HB, DeCrescito V, Tomasula JJ. Effect of naloxone on posttraumatic ischemia in experimental spinal contusion. *J Neurosurg* 1981;55:209–219.
45. Flamm ES, Young W, Demopoulos HB, DeCrescito V, Tomasula JJ. Experimental spinal cord injury: treatment with naloxone. *Neurosurgery* 1982;10: 227–231.

Advances in Neurology, Vol. 59, edited by
Fredrick J. Seil. Raven Press, Ltd.,
New York © 1993.

22

Regulatory Genes in Regeneration and Plasticity

Frank R. Sharp

Department of Neurology, University of California at San Francisco and Veterans Administration Medical Center, San Francisco, California 94121

The induction of immediate early genes and heat shock genes related to brain injury and stimulation is briefly reviewed in this chapter.

IMMEDIATE EARLY GENES

Induction of *c-fos* and other immediate early genes is likely to be very important following brain injury and during subsequent regeneration because these genes are induced by a variety of trophic substances and regulate the transcription of specific target genes (1). Transmitters, peptides, growth factors, and other agents induce *c-fos* and *c-jun* (and other proto-oncogenes). The protein products of these genes, Fos and Jun, form a heterodimer that binds to the AP1 site in the promoter of target genes to regulate their transcription (1). Possible target genes of Fos and Jun include preproenkephalin, dynorphin, vasoactive intestinal polypeptide (VIP), and others. Therefore, extracellular growth factors may exert their effects on cells by inducing one or several protooncogenes which then regulate the expression of target genes that mediate the growth and differentiation of the cells.

A variety of stimuli have been shown to induce the *c-fos* protooncogene in the mammalian brain. Morgan and Curran (2) were the first to show that depolarization of PC-12 cells induced *c-fos* via a calcium-mediated mechanism and that generalized seizures produced by pentylenetetrazol induced *c-fos* throughout the mouse brain (3). The finding that seizures induced *c-fos* was confirmed by Dragunow and Robertson (4). Hunt et al. (5) showed that peripheral cutaneous injury and pain induced *c-fos* in the spinal cord. Sagar et al. (6) first suggested that induction of *c-fos* could be used to map activated neurons in the central nervous system at the cellular level following seizures, cortical stimulation, and dehydration and that *c-fos* and other immediate early gene products might be generally useful for mapping injured and activated cells.

Light has since been shown to induce the *c-fos* gene in the retina (7), suprachiasmatic nucleus (8), and intrageniculate leaflet (8). Dehydration induces *c-fos* in the lamina terminalis, subfornical organ, supraoptic nucleus, and paraventricular nucleus (6,9). Various types of seizures (3,4), stress (9), and adrenalectomy (10) induce *c-fos*. Cortical injury induces Fos protein in neurons throughout the ipsilateral neocortex. This induction, which is likely explained by injury-induced spreading depression, is prevented by NMDA antagonists (11–13).

In order to study the mechanisms of *c-fos* gene induction directly, cultured cortical astrocytes and neurons have been used. We and others (14–18) have shown that agents that promote mitosis and differentiation, including cAMP, epidermal growth factor (EGF), VIP, and fibroblast growth factor (FGF), induce *c-fos* in astrocytic glial cells. Depolarization of astrocytes with potassium slightly induces the *c-fos* gene in some studies (14), but it markedly induces *c-fos* in others (see de Felipe et al., this volume). The reason for these differences is not clear, but it could relate to age, differentiation, or presence of certain receptors on the astrocytes.

Studies of cultured cortical neurons show that *c-fos* mRNA and Fos protein are induced by glutamate, potassium, phorbol ester, basic FGF, zinc, and VIP (19). Glutamate and cAMP induction of *c-fos* mRNA and Fos protein are blocked by N-methyl-D-aspartate (NMDA) antagonists, which also partially block potassium-, zinc-, VIP-, and FGF-induced *c-fos* mRNA expression. However, NMDA antagonists blocked Fos protein expression by all of these agents without affecting total protein synthesis (19). Although there are several possible explanations for these data, the simplest interpretation is that NMDA antagonists block Fos translation without affecting *c-fos* transcription. This suggests that NMDA receptor activation is required for translation of *c-fos* mRNA in cortical neurons following stimulation of multiple intracellular signaling pathways. It is possible that NMDA antagonists prevent cortical plasticity and decrease brain injury from ischemia by blocking induction of the Fos protein and other immediate early gene products that would normally be induced by neurotrophic factors, transmitters, and other substances.

Future studies will address a number of still unanswered questions: the relative role of different proto-oncogenes in different cells; why some stimuli induce *c-fos* in some cells and not in others; the relative role of excitation and inhibition on proto-oncogene induction; the target genes of various proto-oncogenes; and possible roles of proto-oncogenes in differentiation, growth, plasticity, and memory.

HEAT SHOCK GENES

Several laboratories, including ours (20–22) and those of Nowak (23,24), Brown (25), and Nishimura and Dwyer (26,27), have begun to examine the factors responsible for induction of another large class of genes in the nervous system: the heat shock or stress genes. We have found that although normal brain activity does not appear to induce the *hsp72* heat shock gene, stimuli that injure neurons and glia do induce the *hsp72* gene in brain (20,28,29).

Heat shock genes were originally discovered by heating cells (30–33). Once they were cloned and sequenced, it was clear that a large family of stress genes existed that were induced by a variety of stresses including heat, low oxygen, low glucose, heavy metals, peroxidation, etc. These genes can be divided into roughly three classes of proteins of 20 to 30 kD, 70 kD, and 90 to 100 kD (34). Of the stress genes, some exist in normal cells (constituitive) and are induced following stress; others do not exist in normal cells and are then induced following stress. Most studies of brain, to date, have primarily examined the 70-kD genes. There are several members of the 70-kD family in mammalian tissue: *hsp72, hsc73, grp78, hsp60,* and others (34). Of these, *hsc73* has been identified as the clathrin-uncoating ATPase that mediates receptor-activated endocytosis (35). Two different *hsp60* and *hsp70* gene products have been shown to transport, following ATP hydrolysis, fully formed proteins across mitochondrial and across ribosomal membranes (31,36–38). It has been proposed that one of the constituitive *hsp70* proteins binds to normal proteins on ribosomes during their synthesis in order to prevent abnormal folding of the proteins (39). Last, it has been suggested that the inducible *hsp72* gene may bind to partially denatured proteins and prevent them from becoming irreversibly denatured during periods of heat or other stress (34). Almost all of the heat shock proteins appear to bind to other proteins and regulate their activity, availability, or transport or perform some other chaperone function.

Early studies of ischemic brain demonstrated that, although total protein synthesis was decreased, synthesis of heat shock proteins was markedly enhanced (23,40–42). Nowak first showed, using immunocytochemical techniques, that global ischemia in the gerbil induced HSP72 protein primarily in neurons in hippocampus and neocortex and that the pattern of HSP72 induction changed over time (43). Our laboratory first suggested that *hsp72* induction might be a general marker of neuronal injury because focal ischemia, focal status epilepticus, and generalized status epilepticus all induced HSP72 protein in rat brain (20). Gonzalez et al. showed that focal ischemia induced HSP72 protein in neurons within the infarction and in glial cells at the margins of the infarction (20). Dwyer et al. (26) and Ferriero et al. (22) showed that neonatal ischemia in the rat also induced HSP72, primarily in neurons. Status epilepticus produced by kainic acid (20,44) or by gaseous anesthetics (29) induced HSP72 in neurons in regions of brain known to be injured during these seizures. Others have shown that heating whole animals and head trauma also induce the heat shock genes.

Culture studies have shown that heat injury induces HSP72 in astrocytes and neurons (45,46) and that low pH induces HSP72 in astrocytes (27). Moreover, levels of zinc that are likely to be achieved in ischemic brain also induce HSP72 in astrocytes (47).

The significance of HSP72 induction in ischemic and epileptic neurons is uncertain. Vass et al. speculated that HSP72 was induced primarily in ischemic, injured neurons destined to survive (43,44). In our laboratory we tested this hypothesis by administering MK801, ketamine, and phencyclidine (PCP) to animals. These drugs have been shown to induce vacuoles in injured cingulate gyrus neurons that are destined to survive (48). We have shown that these drugs induce HSP72 in vacuolated neurons in the cingulate gyrus (49). Thus, HSP72 appears to be induced primarily in neurons destined to survive the injury, and HSP72 can serve to mark injured neurons in the central nervous system (20). It is still unclear, however, whether HSP72 protein can be induced in neurons destined to die. Nowak (NIH) has recently suggested that *hsp72* mRNA but not HSP72 protein is induced in neurons destined to die (personal communication).

Besides serving as a potential marker of injured cells, heat shock genes appear to be protective in virtually every cell type tested (30,32,33). In mammalian cells, for example, competitive inhibition of *hsp70* gene expression causes thermosensitivity (50). In the mammalian central nervous system, preheating rabbits to induce heat shock genes protects against light damage in the retina (51). Moreover, transient hyperthermia protects against subsequent forebrain ischemic damage (52). These and other data show that heat shock proteins protect cells from injury. Future studies will determine the clinical utility of heat shock proteins.

REFERENCES

1. Morgan JI, Curran T. Stimulus–transcription coupling in the nervous system: Involvement of the inducible proto-oncogenes *fos* and *jun*. *Annu Rev Neurosci* 1991;14:421–451.
2. Morgan JI, Curran T. Role of ion flux in the control of *c-fos* expression. *Nature* 1986;322:552–555.
3. Morgan JI, Cohen DR, Hempstead JL, Curran T. Mapping patterns of *c-fos* expression in the central nervous system after seizures. *Science* 1987; 237:192–196.
4. Dragunow M, Robertson HA. Kindling stimulation induces *c-fos* protein(s) in granule cells of the rat dentate gyrus. *Nature* 1987;329:441–442.
5. Hunt SP, Pini A, Evan G. Induction of *c-fos* like protein in spinal cord neurons following sensory stimulation. *Nature* 1987;328:632–634.
6. Sagar SM, Sharp FR, Curran T. Expression of *c-fos* protein in brain: metabolic mapping at the cellular level. *Science* 1988;240:1328–1331.
7. Sagar SM, Sharp FR. Light induces a Fos-like nuclear antigen in retinal neurons. *Mol Brain Res* 1990;7:17–21.
8. Aronin NA, Sagar SM, Sharp FR, Schwartz WJ. Light regulates expression of a Fos-related protein in rat suprachiasmatic nuclei. *Proc Natl Acad Sci USA* 1990;87:5959–5962.

9. Sharp FR, Sagar SM, Hicks K, Lowenstein D, Hisanaga K. *c-fos* mRNA, Fos, and Fos-related antigen induction by hypertonic saline and stress. *J Neurosci* 1991;11:2321–2331.
10. Jacobson L, Sharp FR, Dallman MF. Induction of Fos-like immunoreactivity in hypothalamic neurons after adrenalectomy in the rat. *Endocrinology* 1990;126:1709–1719.
11. Dragunow M, Robertson HA. Brain injury induces *c-fos* proteins in nerve and glial-like cells in adult mammalian brain. *Brain Res* 1988;455:295–299.
12. Sharp JW, Sagar SM, Hisanaga K, Jasper P, Sharp FR. The NMDA receptor mediates cortical induction of Fos and Fos-related antigens following cortical injury. *Exp Neurol* 1990;109:323–332.
13. Sharp FR, Gonzalez MF, Hisanaga K, Mobley WC, Sagar SM. Induction of Fos-like immunoreactivity in rat forebrain following cortical lesions and NGF injections. *Neurosci Lett* 1989;100:117–122.
14. Hisanaga K, Sagar SM, Hicks KJ, Swanson RA, Sharp FR. *c-fos* protooncogene expression in astrocytes associated with differentiation or proliferation but not depolarization. *Mol Brain Res* 1990; 8:69–75.
15. Arenander AT, Lim RW, Varnum BC, Cole R, de Vellis J, Herschman HR. TIS gene expression in cultured rat astrocytes: induction by mitogens and stellation agents. *J Neurosci Res* 1989;23:247–256.
16. Condorelli DG, Kaczmarek L, Nicoletti F, et al. Induction of protooncogene *fos* by extracellular signals in primary glial cell cultures. *J Neurosci Res* 1989;23:234–239.
17. Szekely AM, Barbaccia ML, Costa E. Activation of specific glutamate receptor subtypes increases *c-fos* proto-oncogene expression in primary cultures of cerebellar granule cells. *Neuropharmacol* 1987; 26:1779–1782.
18. Szekely AM, Barbaccia ML, Alho H, Costa E. In primary cultures of cerebellar granule cells the activation of N-methyl-*d*-aspartate-sensitive glutamate receptors induces *c-fos* mRNA expression. *Mol Pharmacol* 1989;35:401–408.
19. Hisanaga K, Sagar SM, Sharp FR. N-Methyl-*d*-aspartate antagonists block Fos-like protein expression induced via multiple signalling pathways in cultured neurons. *J Neurochem* [*in press*].
20. Gonzalez MF, Shiraishi K, Hisanaga K, Sagar SM, Mandabach M, Sharp FR. Heat shock proteins as markers of neural injury. *Mol Brain Res* 1989;6:93–100.
21. Sharp FR, Lowenstein D, Simon R, Hisanga K. Heat shock protein *hsp72* induction in cortical and striatal astrocytes and neurons following infarction. *J Cereb Blood Flow Metab* 1991;11:621–627.
22. Ferriero DM, Soberano HQ, Simon RP, Sharp FR. Hypoxia–ischemia induces heat shock protein-like immunoreactivity in neonatal rat brain. *Dev Brain Res* 1990;53:145–150.
23. Nowak TS Jr. Synthesis of a stress protein following transient ischemia in the gerbil. *J Neurochem* 1985;45:1635–1641.
24. Nowak TS Jr, Bond U, Schlesinger MJ. Heat shock RNA levels in brain and other tissues after hyperthermia and transient ischemia. *J Neurochem* 1990;54:451–458.
25. Brown IR, Rush S, Ivy GO. Induction of a heat shock gene at the site of tissue injury in the rat brain. *Neuron* 1989;2:1559–1564.
26. Dwyer BE, Nishimura RN, Brown IR. Synthesis of the major inducible heat shock protein in rat hippocampus after neonatal hypoxia–ischemia. *Exp Neurol* 1989;104:28–31.
27. Nishimura RN, Dwyer BE, Cole R, de Vellis J, Picard K. Induction of the major inducible 68-kDa heat-shock protein after rapid changes in extracellular pH in cultured rat astrocytes. *Exp Cell Res* 1989;180:276–280.
28. Gonzalez MF, Lowenstein DH, Hisanaga K, Simon RP, Sagar SM, Sharp FR. Induction of heat shock protein 72-like immunoreactivity in the hippocampal formation following transient global ischemia. *Brain Res Bull* 1991;26:241–250.
29. Lowenstein DH, Simon RP, Sharp FR. The pattern of 72-kDa heat shock protein-like immunoreactivity in the rat brain following fluorothyl-induced status epilepticus. *Brain Res* 1990;531:173–182.
30. Craig EA. The heat shock response. *CRC Crit Rev Biochem* 1985;18:239–280.
31. Deshaies RJ, Koch BD, Schenkman R. The role of stress proteins in membrane biogenesis. *Trends Biol Sci* 1989;13:384–388.
32. Lindquist S. The heat shock response. *Annu Rev Biochem* 1986;55:1151–1191.
33. Schlesinger MJ, Ashburner M, Tissieres A (eds). *Heat shock: from bacteria to man.* Cold Spring Harbor, NY: Cold Spring Harbor Laboratory; 1982.
34. Pelham HRB. Speculations on the functions of the major heat shock and glucose-regulated proteins. *Cell* 1986;46:959–961.
35. Chappell T, Welch W, Schlossmann D, Plater K, Schlesinger M, Rothman J. Uncoating ATPase is a member of the 70kD family of stress proteins. *Cell* 1986;45:3–13.
36. Cheng MY, Hartl F-U, Martin J, et al. Mitochondrial heat shock protein *hsp60* is essential for assembly of proteins imported into yeast mitochondria. *Nature* 1989;337:620–625.
37. Chiang H-L, Terlecky SR, Plant CP, Dice JF. A role for a 70-kilodalton heat shock protein in lysosomal degredation of intracellular proteins. *Science* 1989;246:382–385.
38. Chirico WJ, Waters MG, Blobel G. 70kD heat shock related proteins stimulate protein translocation into microsomes. *Nature* 1988;332:805–810.
39. Beckmann RP, Mizzen LA, Welch WJ. Interaction of HSP70 with newly synthesized proteins: Implications for protein folding and assembly. *Science* 1990;248:850–854.
40. Dienel GA, Cruz NF, Rosenfeld SJ. Temporal profiles of proteins responsive to ischemia. *J Neurochem* 1985;44:600–610.
41. Dienel GA, Kiessling M, Jacewicz M, Pulsinelli WA. Synthesis of heat shock proteins in rat brain cortex after transient ischemia. *J Cereb Blood Flow Metab* 1986;6:505–510.
42. Kiessling M, Dienel GA, Jacewicz M, Pulsinelli WA. Protein synthesis in postischemic rat brain: A two-dimensional electrophoretic analysis. *J Cereb Blood Flow Metab* 1986;6:642–649.
43. Vass K, Welch WH, Nowak TS Jr. Localization of

70kD stress protein induction in gerbil rat brain after ischemia. *Acta Neuropathol* 1988;77:128–135.
44. Vass K, Berger ML, Nowak TS Jr, Welch WJ, Lassmann H. Induction of stress protein *hsp70* in nerve cells after status epilepticus in the rat. *Neurosci Lett* 1989;100:259–264.
45. Nishimura RN, Dwyer BE, Welch W, Cole R, de Vellis J, Liotta K. The induction of the major heat-stress protein in purified rat glial cells. *J Neurosci Res* 1988;20:12–18.
46. Marini AM, Kozuka M, Lipsky RH, Nowak TS Jr. 70-kD heat shock protein induction in cerebellar astrocytes and cerebellar granule cells *in vitro:* Comparison with immunocytochemical localization after hyperthermia *in vivo.* *J Neurochem* 1990;54:1509–1516.
47. Swanson RA, Sharp FR. Zinc toxicity and induction of the 72kD heat shock protein in primary astrocyte culture. *Glia* [*in press*].
48. Olney JW, Labruyere J, Price MT. Pathological changes induced in cerebrocortical neurons by phencyclidine and related drugs. *Science* 1989; 244:1360–1362.
49. Sharp FR, Jasper P, Hall J, Noble L, Sagar SM. MK801 and ketamine induce heat shock protein HSP72 in injured neurons in posterior cingulate and retrosplenial cortex. *Ann Neurol* 1991;30:801–809.
50. Johnston RN, Kucey BF. Competitive inhibition of *hsp70* gene expression causes thermosensitivity. *Science* 1988;242:1551–1553.
51. Barbe MF, Tytell M, Gower DJ, Welch WJ. Hyperthermia protects against light damage in the rat retina. *Science* 1988;241:1817–1820.
52. Chopp M, Chen H, Ho K-L, et al. Transient hyperthermia protects against subsequent forebrain ischemic cell damage in the rat. *Neurology* 1989; 39:1396–1398.

Advances in Neurology, Vol. 59, edited by
Fredrick J. Seil. Raven Press, Ltd.,
New York © 1993.

23

The Role of Immediate Early Genes in the Regeneration of the Central Nervous System

C. de Felipe, R. Jenkins, R. O'Shea, T. S. C. Williams, and S. P. Hunt

Molecular Neurobiology Unit, MRC Centre, Cambridge CB2 2QH, England

Immediate early genes (IEGs) were originally identified as a class of genes that were rapidly and transiently expressed in cells following stimulation by growth factors but were not themselves dependent on new protein synthesis for their induction (1). Many of these IEGs, such as *fos* and *jun,* were subsequently shown to be transcription factors (2,3) binding to DNA, and their expression within the nervous system has led to speculation that they may well be involved in establishing longer-term changes in neurons that follow particular patterns of stimulation (4).

It had been shown, for example, that IEGs were expressed in PC-12 cells following electrical or chemical depolarization (5) and that various programs of IEG expression could be seen within the central nervous system following seizure (6–8), sensory stimulation (9,10), or pharmacologically (11) induced neurotransmitter receptor activation. It has also become clear that this class of genes cannot simply be regarded as "activity markers" but that their presence may signal long-term consequences for the neuron. For example, the induction of long-term potentiation within the dentate gyrus of the hippocampus following perforant path stimulation is associated with the expression of only the gene *ngfi-a* (also known as *egr1* and *zif268*) within dentate granule cells (12). Similarly, the activation of *fos* and *jun* in the suprachiasmatic nucleus by light only occurs in situations in which light induces a physiological effect (13).

THE TRANSIENT POSTSYNAPTIC ACTIVATION OF IEGS IN THE SPINAL CORD

We previously described the rapid induction of *fos* and a wide range of other IEGs in a subset of spinal cord neurons as a result of sensory stimulation (9,14). Most of our initial analysis was made with antibodies to Fos protein. We found that the type of stimulation was crucial for a change in gene expression within postsynaptic neurons of the dorsal horn. Brief (5- to 20-sec) stimulation of high-threshold C or Aδ sensory fibers, but not of low-threshold A fibers, in the rat results in substantial long-term changes in spinal cord physiology. A similar brief noxious stimulus results, within 1 hr, in the induction of Fos protein and in the mRNA and protein for a large number of other IEGs within superficial and deep neurons of the ipsilateral dorsal horn. Activation of nonnociceptive low-threshold afferents results in the appearance of Fos in a subset of neurons in the intermediate layers of the dorsal horn that are not generally positive following noxious stimulation (9). Induction of IEGs was never seen within sensory neurons in the dorsal root ganglion, even following direct electrical stimulation. Similarly, we have rarely seen Fos immunoreactivity within neurons in areas of termination of large-diameter (low-threshold) primary sensory fibers, including the dorsal column nuclei and the ventral horn.

These observations highlight the specificity of the gene induction within the spinal cord.

Expression of IEGs within the dorsal horn following sensory stimulation is generally a transient event, with levels of mRNA for *c-fos, c-jun* (Fig. 1A), and *ngfi-a* returning to basal levels within 4 to 6 hr. However, recent studies have suggested that for other products of the gene class, Jun D and Fos B, peak expression of protein is between 4 and 8 hr following a brief noxious stimulation (15). We have also described a pattern of Fos staining that changes over time following either 20 sec of noxious stimulation or crush of the sciatic nerve (16; unpublished observations). At 2 hr following stimulation, we see the familiar ipsilateral pattern of stained neurons within the most superficial layers of the spinal cord and within neurons scattered in the deeper layers of the dorsal horn. By 24 hr, this pattern has changed radically, and positive neurons are now seen bilaterally but predominantly within deeper layers of the dorsal horn. This observation emphasizes the dynamic, changing pattern of IEG expression set up within the spinal cord following a brief but highly relevant stimulus.

What could be the function of these changes in gene expression? The most plausible suggestion is that the appearance of Fos and Jun together, presumably in the same neurons, could lead to a change in expression

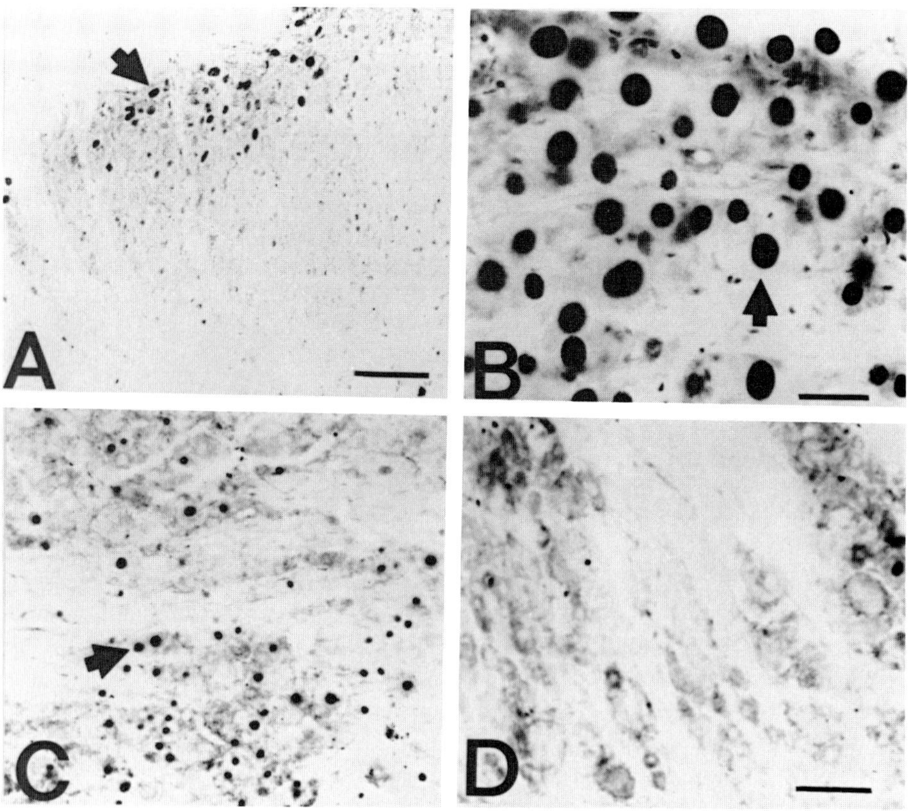

FIG. 1. (**A**) Jun-positive neurons in the superficial layers of the spinal cord (*arrow*). The animal was deeply anesthetized with Equithesin, and the stimulus was immersion of the hind paw in water at 52°C for 20 sec. The poststimulus survival period was 2 hr. Scale bar, 170 μm. (**B**) Jun-positive sensory neurons (*arrow*) in L-4 DRG at 24 hr post-section of the sciatic nerve. Scale bar, 50 μm. (**C**) Jun-positive sensory neurons (*arrow*) in L-3 DRG at 21 days post-section and ligation of the sciatic nerve. (**D**) Jun-negative sensory neurons in L-3 DRG contralateral to a sciatic nerve lesion. Scale bar in **C,D,** 80 μm.

of the neuropeptide genes for dynorphin and enkephalin, both of which possess AP1 or AP1-like Fos–Jun binding sequences on their promoters (17–20). The expression of both of these neuropeptide genes is massively increased following a peripheral inflammatory lesion or in an adjuvant model of arthritis, and with a time course compatible with an initial Fos–Jun activation. It has been argued that the increased production of these peptides could serve to reduce excessive activity in chronic pain conditions (18). Alternatively, it has been suggested that the long-term physiological sequelae within the spinal cord of a brief C-fiber volley, including changing sizes of receptive field and reduced reflex thresholds (21), could be underpinned by changes at the molecular and structural levels.

THE INDUCTION OF JUN FOLLOWING AXOTOMY

Activation of *c-jun* Following Peripheral Nerve Damage

One of the most intriguing recent observations has been the demonstration that axon

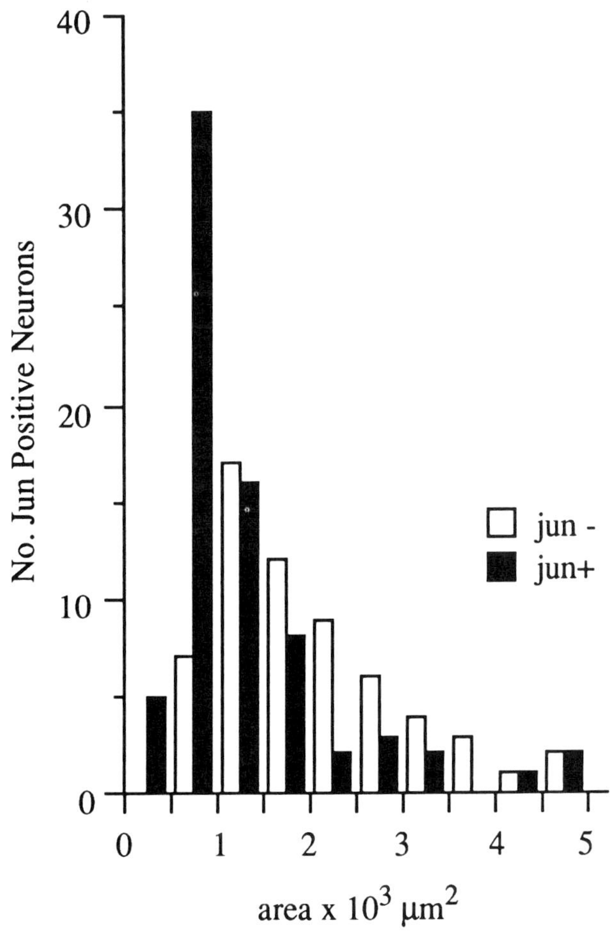

FIG. 2. The histogram demonstrates that 24 hr following capsaicin application to one sciatic nerve there is a preferential appearance of Jun protein in smaller-diameter sensory neurons of ipsilateral L-4 and L-5 ganglia.

damage is accompanied by a delayed, long-term increase of expression of *c-jun* within the cell body (22,23) (Figs. 1B,D). This increase is maintained if regeneration is prevented or returns to basal levels if regeneration is allowed. This is not accompanied by any substantial increase in the expression of *fos* or any other IEG studied to date. Thus, at 24 hr, but not 2 hr, after crush or section (with or without ligation) of the sciatic nerve, there was a greater than fivefold increase in mRNA for *c-jun* (using *in situ* hybridization) and a substantial increase in protein immunoreactivity levels in dorsal root ganglia (DRG) (using immunocytochemistry). Increased labeling was seen in both large- and small-diameter DRG cells. Application of the drug capsaicin (33 mM) (Fig. 2) to the sciatic nerve resulted by 24 hr in the appearance of Jun in small-diameter DRG cells, whereas with colchicine application to the nerve, Jun was found in both large- and small-diameter DRG cells (data not shown). Capsaicin has been shown to cause a selective "axotomy" of small-diameter axons, whereas colchicine causes a nonspecific block in axonal transport.

This unique change in *c-jun* gene expression was also seen in many of the motor neurons damaged by sciatic nerve lesion (Fig.

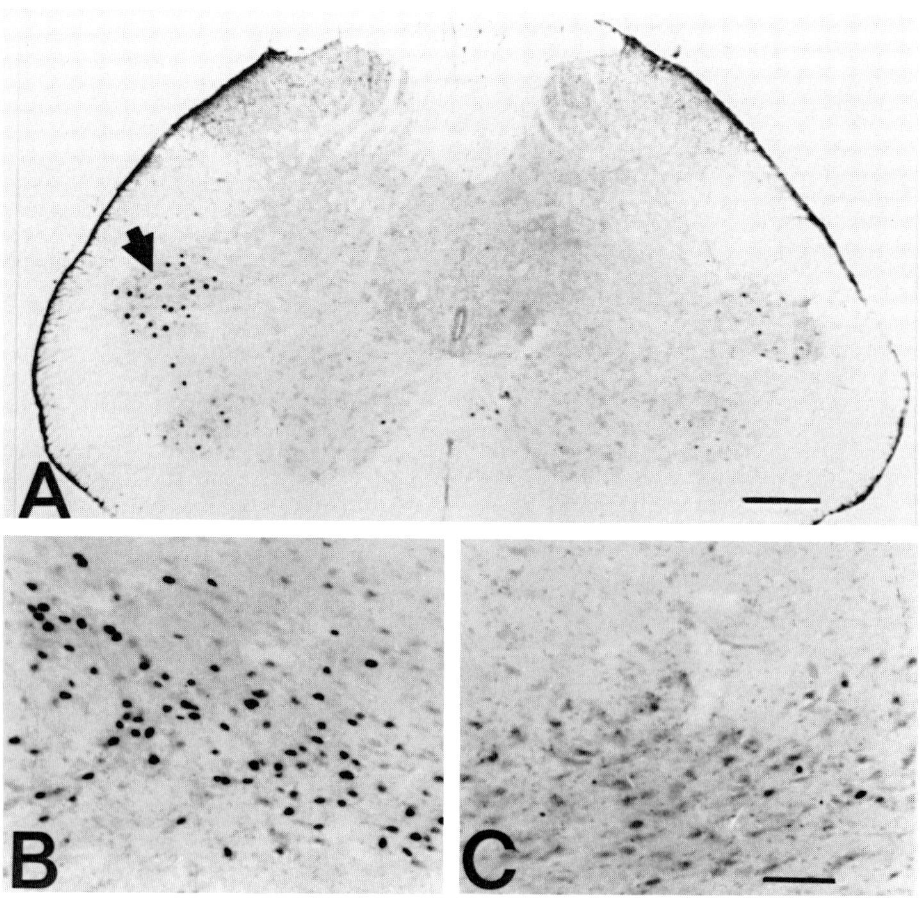

FIG. 3. (**A**) Lumbar spinal cord with a unilaterally increased staining of motor neurons for Jun protein (*arrow*) 1 day following section of the sciatic nerve on the same side. Scale bar, 400 μm. (**B**) Substantia nigra pars compacta neurons positive for Jun protein 4 days following injection of the dopamine-specific neurotoxin 6-OHDA into the striatum of the same side. (**C**) The substantia nigra of the contralateral side with few positive neurons. Scale bar in **B,C,** 80 μm.

3A). Silver grain counting suggested a greater than fourfold increase in mRNA levels after axon damage. Expression also remained high at 21 days following nerve ligation but returned to basal levels by 8 weeks post-crush, when regeneration would be expected to be complete. No changes were seen in sham-operated animals.

We also wanted to know if the Jun response was dependent on damage to the axon or whether any axonal growth was associated with increased levels of Jun protein and mRNA. Previous studies have demonstrated that following sciatic nerve section and ligation, there is a sprouting of the adjacent undamaged saphenous nerve into peripheral territory vacated by the sciatic nerve fibers (16) (see Discussion). This new growth peaks at around 24 days post-lesion. Axons from DRG L-4 and L-5, with a smaller component from L-6, make up the bulk of the sciatic nerve. The L-3 DRG sends no axons into the sciatic nerve trunk but forms a large component of the saphenous nerve. At 1 day following sciatic nerve lesion there were large numbers of Jun-positive neurons in L-4 and L-5 DRG and the occasional positive cell in the L-3 ganglion. By 7 days and 21 days post-

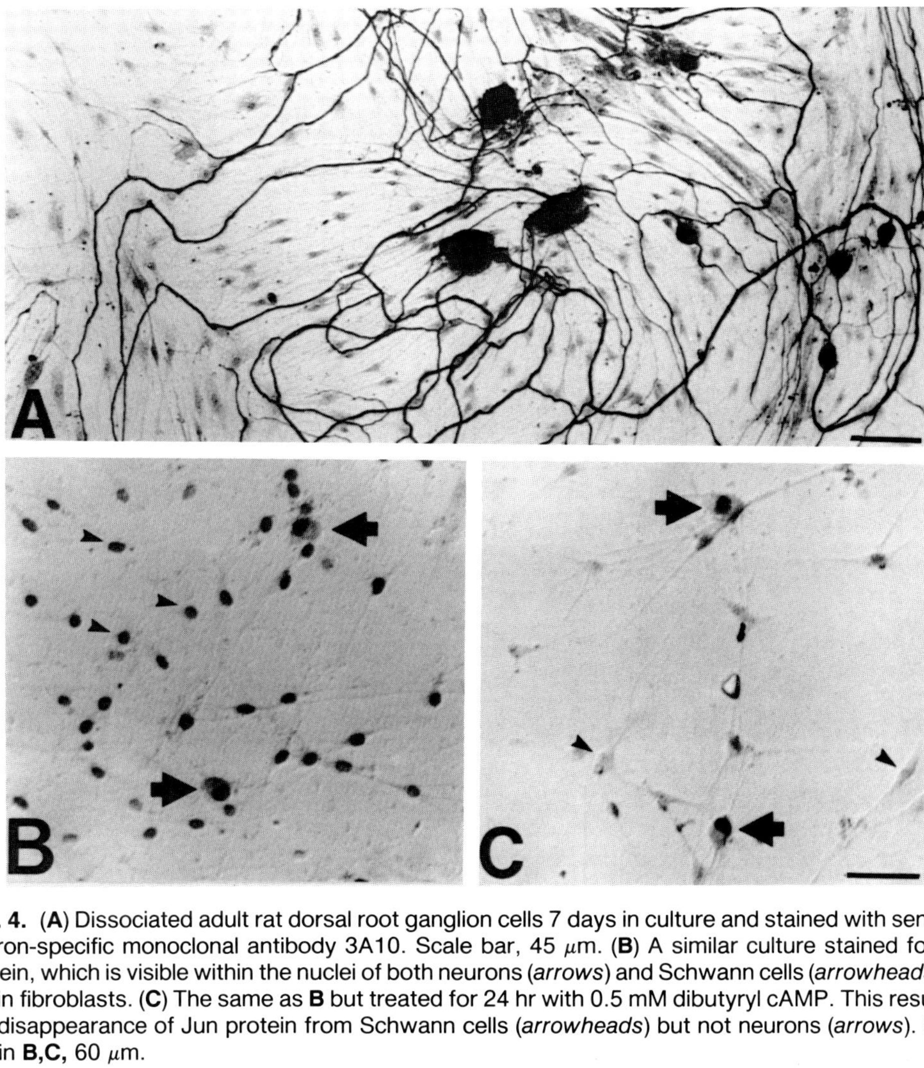

FIG. 4. (**A**) Dissociated adult rat dorsal root ganglion cells 7 days in culture and stained with sensory-neuron-specific monoclonal antibody 3A10. Scale bar, 45 μm. (**B**) A similar culture stained for Jun protein, which is visible within the nuclei of both neurons (*arrows*) and Schwann cells (*arrowheads*) but not in fibroblasts. (**C**) The same as **B** but treated for 24 hr with 0.5 mM dibutyryl cAMP. This results in the disappearance of Jun protein from Schwann cells (*arrowheads*) but not neurons (*arrows*). Scale bar in **B,C,** 60 μm.

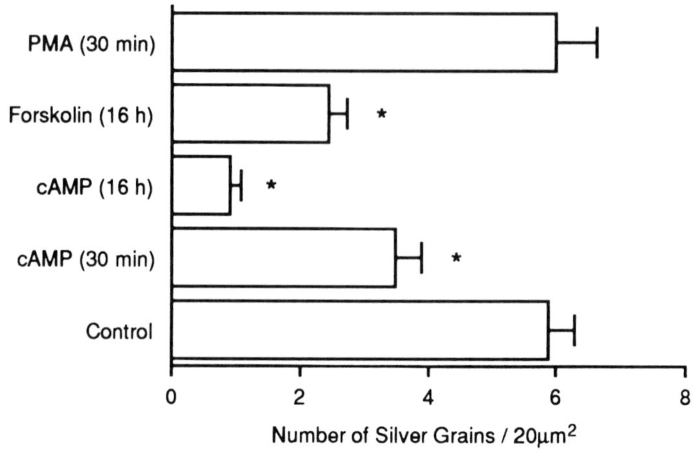

FIG. 5. Bar chart quantifying the change in *c-jun* mRNA levels in cultured Schwann cells following a variety of treatments. Cultures of adult Schwann cells and dorsal root ganglia were treated for periods of time indicated. Cultures were then fixed and hybridized to a *c-jun* antisense oligonucleotide labeled with ^{35}S-dATP and dipped in photographic emulsion. Silver grains were quantified by grain counting or densitometry of individual cells.

sciatic-lesion, there were a substantial number of Jun-positive neurons within L-3 (Fig. 1C). This suggested that neurons with axons within the saphenous nerve that grow as a response to damage to the neighboring sciatic nerve also express high levels of Jun. Thus, Jun expression may not simply occur as a response to axon damage but may be related to the underlying phenomenon of axonal growth.

The Expression of Jun in Primary Cultures of Sensory Neurons

The increase in *c-jun* expression in sensory neurons following axotomy may have resulted from (a) growth factor "starvation" as a result of the loss of axonally transported factors from the periphery, (b) the production or increased production of factors by the damaged nerve or its supporting cells, or (c) the loss of an inhibitory factor that maintains the cell in a quiescent state. In order to test some of these possibilities, we cultured adult DRG cells (24) and their supporting Schwann cells in serum-free defined medium for 1 to 7 days and added growth factors. High levels of Jun protein and *c-jun* mRNA were found constitutively in both neurons and glial cells at all time points. Addition of nerve growth factor (NGF) (50 ng/ml), basic or acidic fibroblast growth factor (FGF) (200 ng/ml), transforming growth factor b (TGFb) (1 ng/ml), platelet-derived growth factor (PDGF) (200 ng/ml), or epidermal growth factor (EGF) (100 ng/ml) had no effect on Jun levels. Although the addition of phorbol 12-myristate 13-acetate (PMA) (200 nM) was without effect, the addition of dibutyryl cAMP (0.5 mM) caused a rapid and substantial decline in *c-jun* mRNA and Jun protein immunoreactivity, but only in Schwann cells and not in neurons (Figs. 4 and 5). Cyclic AMP has been shown to have an indirect mitogenic effect on Schwann cells, possibly by initially inducing growth factor receptor genes, resulting in a greater response to growth factors present in serum (25). The inhibition of Jun expression may well play a role in this change in receptor gene induction in Schwann cells. However, the control of expression of Jun in neurons is clearly more complex.

The Expression of Jun in Central Neurons Following Axotomy

It was important to know if the appearance of Jun following axon damage was a general phenomenon shared by neurons with peripheral axons and central neurons with axons entirely confined to the central nervous system. Damage to a peripheral nerve, such as the sciatic nerve, which contains the axons of both sensory and motor neurons, is followed by a complex series of events finally leading to the regeneration of damaged axons. The extent of the regenerative response is dependent on the initial degree of damage but is virtually complete following simple crush of the nerve. In contrast, damage to the axons of neurons wholly contained within the central nervous system is followed by a brief period in which an attempted regenerative response is mounted, only to finally abort. The damaged neurons will atrophy or, more rarely, die (26–28). The failure of central neurons to regenerate is not thought to imply that neurons of different origins have a different intrinsic capacity to regrow but to reflect the presence of a nonpermissive glial environment, which exists within the adult brain (26,29). That is, adult central and peripheral neurons are both capable of regenerating, given a favorable environment to do so. Indeed, a number of studies have suggested that central neurons can regenerate into peripheral nerve grafts and that the program of gene responses that follows axon damage is initially similar in central and peripheral neurons and only begins to diverge at relatively long intervals following the initial insult.

We therefore examined the effects of axotomy in two systems: the nigrostriatal dopaminergic pathway and the rubrospinal pathway. The time course of Jun expression was similar in both pathways. For example, 6-OHDA injection into the striatum, which selectively lesions dopaminergic terminals, results in a massive increase in Jun levels within nigral neurons at 4 to 8 days post-treatment (Fig. 3B,C). However, Jun levels have virtually returned to basal levels by 15 days post-injection. A similar time course of Jun appearance was seen in rubral neurons following spinal cord hemisection (W. Tetzlaff and S. P. Hunt, unpublished observations). Tetzlaff et al. (27) found that the response of rubrospinal neurons to cervical cord hemisection was followed by (a) the up-regulation of two developmentally regulated gene products, GAP43 and a tubulin isoform $T_{\alpha 1}$, and (b) the elevation of adult forms of tubulin and of actin and the down-regulation of neurofilament gene expression. This was very similar to the changes observed in facial motor neurons and in DRG cells following axotomy. However, although these changes in mRNA levels persisted in facial and sensory neurons even when the axons were prevented from regenerating by ligation, this was not the case for damaged central neurons. Within 2 weeks, levels of actin and adult tubulin mRNA fell to basal levels, apparently in concert with an atrophy of the axotomized rubrospinal neurons. However, levels of GAP43 and $T_{\alpha 1}$ remained high. The authors thus conclude that the failure of rubrospinal neurons to regenerate is not caused by a failure to initiate gene expression changes characteristic of regenerating peripheral neurons. It is reflected in the failure to maintain tubulin and actin synthesis at a level comensurate with the demands of a regenerating process.

DISCUSSION

We have demonstrated that IEGs can be induced within the central nervous system either with early-onset characteristics or, in the case of Jun, with a slower onset and with maintained expression. Both Jun and Fos and other members of these gene families code for transcription factors that form homo- or heterodimers either with similar proteins or with other proteins containing the so-called "leucine zipper" motif. This greatly increases the possible number of combinations of proteins that could be formed that bind to DNA. In many cases these protein dimers bind to AP1 or AP1-like sequences, but with an affinity that is in part determined by the flanking regions of DNA, and whose activity is determined by the presence of other transcription factors (30–33). Thus, it would be extremely difficult to predict the change in gene expression that could follow a change in the pattern of Fos or Jun expression within the central nervous system. However, there are some possible outcomes that should be considered.

(a) Direct action of Fos and Jun on downstream gene expression (20). There is evidence that enkephalin and dynorphin gene expression can be directly altered following activation of Fos and Jun and binding to AP1 or AP1-like sites present on the promoters of these peptide genes.

(b) Fos and Jun can act as selectors of responsiveness (33,34). It has been demonstrated that single factors can evoke opposite regulatory effects from a specific DNA sequence. In the presence of Jun, glucocorticoid receptor (GR) activates proliferin gene expression. However, if both Fos and Jun are present, GR shows a negative hormone-dependent transcriptional effect. In the absence of Jun, GR is inactive (33). This type of mechanism may be reflected in the persistent Jun expression seen in neurons following axotomy. Activation of the *c-jun* gene may make the neuron more responsive to hormones or locally produced cytokines and growth factors. These in turn would stimulate neuronal growth.

What Controls the Expression of *c-jun*?

From the observations described above and a number of other published reports, *c-jun* has been shown to be developmentally regulated, constitutively high in some cells such as motor neurons, transiently expressed following various forms of stimulation, and expressed at high levels and over long periods of time in regenerating neurons (14,22,34, 35). This suggests that there are a variety of mechanisms regulating *c-jun* expression. Transient expression is largely under the control of neurotransmitters and perhaps growth factors. However the association of Jun expression with regeneration could be mediated by either the production of a factor by damaged or denervated tissue or the loss of some diffusible inhibitory substance from the environment of the cell. In the central nervous system, the loss of Jun expression from damaged neurons may be associated with the failure of central neurons to regenerate, and strategies to increase Jun levels may enhance the regenerative ability of central neurons.

REFERENCES

1. Cochran BH, Reffel AC, Stiles CD. Molecular cloning of gene sequences regulated by platelet-derived growth factor. *Cell* 1983;33:939–947.
2. Gentz R, Rauscher FJ, Abate C, Curran T. Fos and Jun dimerize through a parallel leucine zipper that juxtaposes DNA-binding domains. *Science* 1989; 243:1695–1699.
3. Rauscher FJ III, Voulaslas PJ, Franza BR Jr, Curran T. Fos and Jun bind cooperatively to AP-1 site: reconstitution *in vitro. Genes Dev* 1988;2:1687–1699.
4. Berridge MJ. Secondary messenger dualism in neuromodulation and memory. *Nature* 1986;323: 294–295.
5. Greenberg ME, Ziff EB, Greene LE. Stimulation of neuronal acetylcholine receptor induces rapid gene expression. *Science* 1986;234:80–83.
6. Morgan JI, Cohen DR, Hempstead JL, Curran T. Mapping patterns of *c-fos* expression in the central nervous system after seizure. *Science* 1987; 237:192–197.
7. Saffen DW, Cole AJ, Worley PF, Christy BA, Ryder K, Baraban JM. Convulsant-induced increase in transcription factor messenger RNAs in rat brain. *Proc Natl Acad Sci USA* 1988;85:7795–7799.
8. Sagar SM, Sharp FR, Curran T. Expression of *c-fos* protein in brain: metabolic mapping at the cellular level. *Science* 1988;240:1328–1331.
9. Hunt SP, Pini A, Evan G. Induction of *c-fos* like protein in spinal cord neurons following sensory stimulation. *Nature* 1987;328:632–634.
10. Menetrey D, Gannon A, Levine JD, Basbaum AI. Expression of *c-fos* protein in interneurons and projection neurons of the rat spinal cord in response to noxious somatic, articular, and visceral stimulation. *J Comp Neurol* 1989;285:177–195.
11. Graybiel AM, Moratalla R, Robertson HA. Amphetamine and cocaine induced drug specific activation of the *c-fos* gene in striosome–matrix compartments and limbic subdivisions of the striatum. *Proc Natl Acad Sci USA* 1990;87:6912–6916.
12. Cole AJ, Saffen DW, Baraban JM, Worley PF. Rapid increase of an immediate early gene messenger RNA in hippocampal neurons by synaptic NMDA receptor activation. *Nature* 1989;340: 474–476.
13. Rusak B, Robertson HA, Wisden W, Hunt SP. Light pulses that shift rythms induce gene expression in the suprachiasmatic nucleus. *Science* 1990;248: 1237–1240.
14. Wisden W, Errington ML, Williams S, et al. Differential expression of immediate early genes in the hippocampus and spinal cord. *Neuron* 1990;4: 603–614.
15. Herdegen T, Tolle TR, Bravo R, Zieglgansberger W. Sequential expression of Jun B, Jun D and Fos B

proteins in rat spinal neurons: a cascade of transcriptional operations during nociception. *Neurosci Lett* 1991;129:221–224.

16. Williams S, Evan GI, Hunt SP. Changing patterns of *c-fos* induction in spinal neurons following thermal cutaneous stimulation in the rat. *Neuroscience* 1990;36:73–81.
17. Noguchi K, Dubner R, Ruda MA. Preproenkephalin mRNA in spinal dorsal horn neurons is induced by peripheral inflammation and is colocalized with Fos and Fos-related proteins. *Neuroscience* 1992; 46:561–570.
18. Noguchi K, Kowalski K, Traub R, Solodkin A, Iadarola MJ, Ruda MA. Dynorphin depression and Fos-like immunoreactivity following inflammation induced hyperalgesia are colocalized in spinal cord neurons. *Mol Brain Res* 1991;10:229–234.
19. Sonnenberg JL, Macgregor-Leon PF, Curran T, Morgan JI. Dynamic alterations occur in the levels and composition of transcription factor AP-1 complexes after seizure. *Neuron* 1989;3:359–365.
20. Sonnenberg JL, Rauscher FJ III, Morgan JI, Curran T. Regulation of proenkephalin by Fos and Jun. *Science* 1989;246:1622–1625.
21. Woolf CJ, Wall PD. Relative effectiveness of C primary afferent fibers of different origins in evoking a prolonged facilitation of the flexor reflex in the rat. *J Neurosci* 1986;6:1433–1442.
22. Jenkins R, Hunt SP. Long term increases in the levels of *c-jun* mRNA and Jun protein like immunoreactivity in motor and sensory neurons following axon damage. *Neurosci Lett* 1991;129:107–111.
23. Leah JD, Herdegen T, Bravo R. Selective expression of Jun proteins following axotomy and axonal transport block in peripheral nerves in the rat; evidence for a role in the regeneration process. *Brain Res* 1991;566:198–207.
24. Lindsay RM, Harmar AJ. Nerve growth factor regulates expression of neuropeptide genes in adult sensory neurons. *Nature* 1989;337:362–364.
25. Lemke G. Glial growth factors. *Semin Neurosci* 1990;2:437–443.
26. Fawcett JW. Intrinsic neuronal determinants of regeneration. *Trends Neurosci* 1992;15:5–8.
27. Tetzlaff W, Alexander S, Miller FD, Bisby MA. Response of facial and rubrospinal neurons to axotomy: changes in mRNA expression for cytoskeletal proteins and GAP-43. *J Neurosci* 1991;11: 2528–2544.
28. Tetzlaff W, Bisby MA. Cytoskeletal protein synthesis and regulation of nerve regeneration in PNS and CNS neurons of the rat. *Restor Neurol Neurosci* 1990;1:189–196.
29. Schwab ME. Myelin associated inhibitors of neurite growth and regeneration in the CNS. *Trends Neurosci* 1990;13:452–456.
30. Halazonetis TD, Georgopoulos K, Greenberg ME, Leder P. *c-jun* dimerises with itself and with *c-fos,* forming complexes of different DNA binding affinities. *Cell* 1989;55:917–924.
31. Lamb P, McKnight SL. Diversity and specificity in transcriptional regulation: the benefits of heterotypic dimerization. *Trends Biochem Sci* 1991; 16:417–422.
32. Ryseck R-P, Bravo R. *c-jun, jun B* and *jun D* differ in their binding affinities to AP-1 and CRE consensus sequences: effect of FOS proteins. *Oncogene* 1991;6:533–542.
33. Schule R, Evans RM. Cross-coupling of signal transduction pathways: zinc finger meets leucine zipper. *Trends Genet Sci* 1991;7:377–381.
34. Diamond MI, Miner JN, Yoshinaga SK, Yamamoto KR. Transcription factor interactions: selectors of a negative or positive regulation from a single DNA element. *Science* 1990;249:1266–1272.
35. Wilkinson DG, Bhatt S, Ryseck RP, Bravo R. Tissue-specific expression of *c-jun* and *jun-B* during organogenesis in the mouse. *Development* 1989; 106:465–471.

Advances in Neurology, Vol. 59, edited by
Fredrick J. Seil. Raven Press, Ltd.,
New York © 1993.

24

Early Response Genes as Markers of Neuronal Activity and Growth Factor Action

Stephen M. Sagar and Frank R. Sharp

Department of Neurology, Veterans Affairs Medical Center and University of California, San Francisco, California 94143

The study of early response genes is of interest from several perspectives. Some early response genes, including *c-fos, c-jun,* and *c-myc,* are proto-oncogenes and are consequently involved in mechanisms of carcinogenesis and regulation of the cell cycle (1). Many early response gene products are transcription factors and hence are of interest in the study of the regulation of gene expression (2). In addition, early response gene products have evolved a modular organization that employs structural motifs for protein–protein and protein–nucleic acid binding that are of importance to structural biochemistry (3).

In this chapter we discuss the anatomic localization of early response gene expression in the nervous system as a neuroanatomic tool (4–7). The goal, although not fully realizable, is to develop methods of functional neuroanatomic mapping to identify individual neurons that are activated by specific experimental manipulations. Such methods would allow the demonstration of the total population of neurons that participate in a given nervous system function.

The most successful method of functional mapping has been 2-deoxyglucose (2-DG) autoradiography (8). The power of the 2-DG technique is its ability to demonstrate metabolic activity of populations of neurons. It is assumed that this metabolic activity correlates with electrical activity and the consequent metabolic work required for membrane ion pumps. Equivalent information concerning the activity of neuronal populations can be obtained from electrophysiological recordings only with much greater effort.

A major limitation of the 2-DG technique is its lack of cellular resolution. Glucose utilization is primarily a marker of neuropil function, reflecting ion pumping in synaptic terminals. In spite of many efforts, some heroic in extent, the method has generally been unsuccessful in identifying activated cell bodies. The limitation lies not in autoradiographic technique but in the basic biology of neuronal glucose metabolism. Immunocytochemical staining of Fos, the protein encoded by the proto-oncogene *c-fos,* may provide a method to perform functional neuroanatomic mapping at the cellular level (4–7).

In addition to neuronal activity, it is useful to map cells in the nervous system that respond to trophic factors and injury. Many trophic factors are present in the mammalian central nervous system (CNS), but, since these factors act over long time periods, experiments that measure long-term biological effects are technically demanding. The use of early response gene expression in short-term experiments to identify putative target cells of growth and differentiation factors greatly facilitates their study.

EARLY RESPONSE GENES

Early response genes, also called cellular immediate-early genes, are expressed rapidly after serum-deprived nondividing cells are stimulated to enter the cell cycle. Some investigators include in the definition that early response genes are expressed (i.e., their mRNA is synthesized) independently of new protein synthesis. Many early response genes code for transcription factors that regulate the expression of target genes. Known early response genes include the *fos* and *jun* families, NGFI-A (also called *egr-1, zif268,* and *Krox* 24), and *c-myc.* The best studied of these is *c-fos.*

c-fos is the normal cellular homolog of the retroviral oncogene *v-fos,* which causes osteogenic sarcomas in mice (1). The product of the *c-fos* gene, Fos, is a DNA-binding protein that is localized to the nucleus by immunocytochemistry (Fig. 1) (9). It regulates the expression of target genes by forming a complex with members of the Jun family and perhaps other proteins. The Fos–Jun complex, which is also referred to as AP-1, binds to a relatively specific sequence in many target genes to regulate their transcription.

Because *c-fos* is a proto-oncogene, initial studies focused on its role in regulating cell division: c-*fos* is rapidly and transiently expressed *in vitro* when quiescent cells are exposed to mitogens (reviewed in ref. 1). Many growth factors, including epidermal growth factor (EGF), platelet-derived growth factor, fibroblast growth factor (FGF), and interleukins, stimulate Fos synthesis in quiescent cells on their entry into the cell cycle. Moreover, blockade of *c-fos* action with antisense RNA or the intracellular injection of anti-Fos or anti-Jun antisera inhibits DNA synthesis following serum stimulation (10–12). Although *c-fos* is not expressed at high levels in exponentially growing cells, the injection of anti-Fos antibodies can inhibit DNA synthesis in asynchronously cycling fibroblasts (11). Therefore, Fos and Jun may be directly involved in the regulation of the cell cycle.

The work on the *c-fos* response to growth factors led to the study of neurons. PC-12 cells, which are derived from a rat pheochromocytoma, express *c-fos* mRNA in response to nerve growth factor (NGF), EGF, and FGF (13,14). Importantly, NGF and FGF are not mitogenic for PC-12 cells; rather, they induce cessation of cell division and differen-

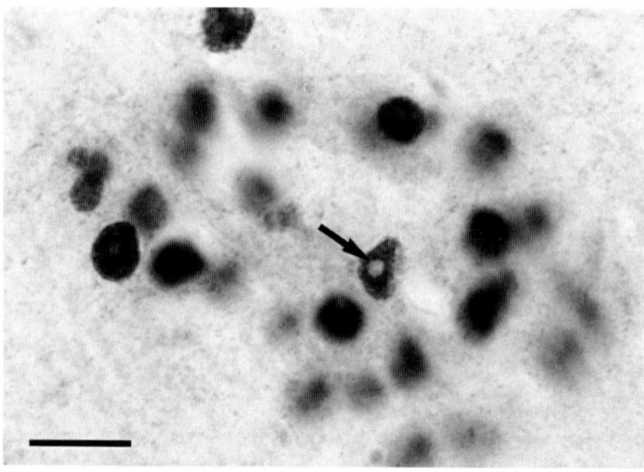

FIG. 1. Fos-immunostained accessory magnocellular neurons of the rat hypothalamus 1 hr following the systemic administration of hypertonic saline. A monoclonal anti-Fos antibody was used that is thought to be specific for Fos and not to cross-react with Fos-related antigens. The intensity of immunostaining varies from cell to cell. The reaction product is confined to the cell nucleus, and in less intensely stained nuclei, the characteristic granular distribution of reaction product and the failure of the nucleolus (*arrow*) to stain are apparent. Scale bar, 20 μm.

tiation into a neuronal phenotype. Similarly, in F9 teratocarcinoma cells, *c-fos* expression is correlated with differentiation rather than cell division (15). These observations led to an expansion of the concept of the role of nuclear proto-oncogenes. Whereas they had previously been considered to have a specialized role in regulating cell division, it became clear that they had a more generalized role in intracellular signal transduction mechanisms.

A key observation was that membrane depolarization can also stimulate *c-fos* expression in PC-12 cells. Ba^{2+}, nicotinic agonists, and high extracellular K^+ all evoke synthesis of *c-fos* mRNA (16–18). Therefore, early response gene expression in PC-12 cells is a quite general response to many types of stimuli acting through multiple second messenger systems. As a rule, the early genetic response is associated with major, rapid changes in the functional activity of cells, whether it is the transition from G_0 to the cell cycle, differentiation, or persistent neuronal depolarization.

In cell culture, the *c-fos* gene can be induced in brain neurons and astrocytes by manipulations similar to those effective in PC-12 cells. Cortical neurons in primary cell culture demonstrate nuclear immunostaining for Fos or a Fos-related antigen in response to depolarization with high extracellular K^+ and the application of glutamate agonists, cAMP, vasoactive intestinal peptide (VIP), phorbol esters, and basic FGF (bFGF) (19). Neither NGF nor EGF is effective. Cerebellar granule cells, like cerebral cortical neurons, express the *c-fos* gene in response to glutamate and NMDA agonists (20). Astrocytes in cell culture express *c-fos* in response to EGF, bFGF, cAMP, and phorbol esters (21–23). Therefore, the basic mechanisms of regulation of *c-fos* gene expression appear to be general throughout the nervous system.

The intracellular mechanisms that lead to *c-fos* gene transcription are known only in outline (24). The activation of many second messenger pathways leads to early response gene expression, including stimulation of adenylate cyclase, protein kinase C, and tyrosine kinases; Ca^{2+} entry into cells; and mobilization of intracellular Ca^{2+}. The detailed biochemical events that couple these second messenger systems to early response gene expression remain unknown, although, as discussed below, intracellular Ca^{2+} appears to be important in coupling neuronal depolarization to *c-fos* expression (24–27).

On a genetic level the situation is clearer. There are at least two sequences in the upstream regulatory region of the *c-fos* gene that are required for normal transcriptional regulation: the serum response element (SRE) and the cAMP response element (CRE) (25). Both sequences bind proteins that are constitutively expressed. There is evidence that growth factor signals, cAMP, and increased intracellular Ca^{2+} concentrations activate kinases and, perhaps, phosphorylases that alter the phosphorylation state of the serum response factor (SRF) and CRE binding protein (CREB), thereby converting them into active transcription factors for *c-fos* (26,28). In the case of neuronal depolarization, Ca^{2+} entry through voltage-activated Ca^{2+} channels and resultant activation of a calmodulin-dependent protein kinase, or a similar enzyme, and phosphorylation of CREB have been strongly implicated (16,17,24–28).

The same manipulations that induce *c-fos* in neurons and glia induce other early response genes, although some follow more protracted time courses; *c-fos* expression is typically followed by the expression of related genes, including *fos B,* whose products are termed Fos-related antigens (29). (*Fra-1,* the first Fos-related antigen identified, which was cloned from fibroblasts, is not expressed in the CNS.) In general the basal expression of *c-jun* in the CNS is higher than that of Fos, and *c-jun* tends to be expressed for a longer time following a stimulus than *c-fos* (30,31); *jun B* expression typically parallels *c-jun,* whereas *jun D* tends to be constitutively expressed and often does not respond acutely to stimuli; NGFI-A tends to behave like *c-fos.*

A major question about early response genes is how such a general cellular mechanism can lead to specific responses. In PC-12 cells, for example, why is a similar early genetic response associated with such diverse cellular processes as mitosis, differentiation, and depolarization? One would expect a much different set of target genes to be involved in these processes. One hypothesis, known as the "combinatorial" model of gene regulation, is that a different set of early response genes is induced in response to each stimulus (32,33). There is a limited amount of evidence for this hypothesis in the nervous system. In PC-12 cells, the pattern of early response gene expression in response to depolarization is at least quantitatively different from that to growth factors (34). In astrocytes, different patterns of early response gene expression occur after different growth factors (35). Moreover, axotomy induces the expression of the *jun* family of genes in the parent neuron to a much greater degree than *c-fos* (36).

An extremely difficult problem is to determine the function of the early response genes *in vivo*. Assuming they act as transcription factors, it is technically challenging to rigorously identify their target genes. Using a combination of *in vitro* and *in vivo* approaches, there is good, although still circumstantial, evidence that the Fos/Jun complex induces prodynorphin (37,38) and proenkephalin (38,39) gene expression in spinal cord neurons and tyrosine hydroxylase (40) and NGF (41) gene expression in other cells. However, in the vast majority of experiments in which early response genes have been studied *in vivo* in the CNS, the target genes are unknown. It is apparent, however, that a neuron suddenly stimulated to intense electrical activity needs to increase the expression of many genes, including those coding for neuropeptides, neurotransmitter synthetic enzymes, and synaptic vesicle proteins. Many such genes have appropriate sequences in their regulatory regions to bind Fos/Jun and NGFI-A. Therefore, it is plausible that the early response genes regulate their expression.

In summary, there are three features of the regulation of early response gene expression that are of importance in interpreting studies in the nervous system *in vivo*. The first is the generality of the early genetic response. It occurs in neurons and glia after many types of stimulation, including depolarization and trophic factors. Second, the response appears to occur only after a relatively quiescent cell is subjected to a powerful or novel stimulus. Early response genes can be considered to signal a major "life-style" change for the cell. They tell the cell that either its overall function, in the case of cell division or differentiation, or the level of its activity, in the case of depolarized neurons, has undergone a fundamental change. And finally, until the detailed biochemistry of the coupling between second messenger systems and early response gene expression is known, and until the target genes are identified, it will be difficult to interpret the expression of a particular early response gene in precise physiological terms.

FUNCTIONAL NEUROANATOMIC MAPPING

Knowing that PC-12 cells express *c-fos* in response to depolarization, Morgan et al. (4) asked whether electrical activity of CNS neurons causes the gene to be expressed. They induced generalized seizures in mice with pentylenetetrazol. Following seizures, the mice expressed *c-fos* mRNA, demonstrated by Northern blotting, and Fos protein, demonstrated by immunocytochemistry, in an anatomically specific pattern. Neurons displayed intense nuclear Fos immunostaining in the dentate gyrus and hippocampal pyramidal cells, cerebral neocortex, and pyriform cortex. The expression of both mRNA and protein was rapid and transient, with the protein response fading 6 hr after the seizures. This experiment suggested that the expression of the *c-fos* gene might be a marker of synaptically activated neurons, at least in circumstances in which they receive intense stimulation.

Subsequent studies documented the anatomic specificity of the CNS Fos response. Hunt et al. (7) reported Fos nuclear immunostaining of spinal cord dorsal horn neurons in response to various forms of cutaneous stimulation in rats. The pattern is specific for each modality of stimulation (brushing the fur, intradermal injection of chemical irritants, or heating the extremity). This line of research, which is reviewed by de Felipe et al. in this volume, has produced a series of excellent studies from several laboratories (43).

Sagar et al. (5) demonstrated that electrical stimulation of rat sensory/motor cortex induces Fos nuclear immunostaining in structures known to connect to motor/sensory cortex by monosynaptic or polysynaptic pathways, including ipsilateral thalamus and pons and contralateral cerebellum. The expression of Fos immunostaining in cerebellar "microzones" that correspond closely to 2-DG autoradiographs clearly demonstrated the induction of the *c-fos* gene by synaptic activity as well as the anatomic specificity of the response (5,42).

An additional experiment demonstrated that Fos is expressed in response to physiological stimuli as well as to unphysiological levels of stimulation. Rats that are water deprived overnight display nuclear Fos immunostaining in magnocellular neurons of hypothalamus, the cell bodies of origin of the hypothalamo–neurohypophyseal system (5). These neurons are known to undergo dramatic changes in electrical activity in response to osmotic stimuli (46). Although it is a minor point in this context, the Fos-like immunoreactivity demonstrated in this study represents Fos-related antigens rather than authentic Fos, since an antibody specific for Fos fails to demonstrate immunostaining of magnocellular neurons after 24 hr of water deprivation (S. M. Sagar, unpublished data).

The anatomic differences between Fos immunocytochemistry and 2-DG autoradiographs are instructive. Electrical stimulation of motor/sensory cortex activates glucose metabolism but not *c-fos* expression at the site of stimulation. There is no current explanation for the failure of neurons at the site of electrical stimulation to express Fos. These neurons are repeatedly depolarized by the stimulus, so that depolarization alone is not sufficient to induce Fos synthesis in CNS neurons as it is in PC-12 cells. Secondly, salt-loaded rats have dramatically increased 2-DG retention in posterior pituitary gland, the site of nerve terminals of the hypothalamo–neurohypophyseal tract, but led to only modest increases in the hypothalamic magnocellular nuclei, which contain the cell bodies. This reflects the sensitivity of the 2-DG method to activity in nerve terminals, whereas Fos immunocytochemistry labels cell bodies.

Although synaptic input stimulates neuronal Fos expression, experiments in the retina have shown that not all activated cells express Fos (44). Dark-adapted rabbit retinas have little or no detectable nuclear Fos immunostaining. After exposure to bright 3/sec flashing white light for 1 hr, Fos immunostaining appears in only a minority of neurons of the inner nuclear and ganglion cell layers. Since flashing light is known from electrophysiological studies to activate virtually all retinal neurons, Fos expression is not an invariant accompaniment of synaptic activation. It is possible that a certain strength or type of input must occur or that Fos is expressed in response to certain neurotransmitters and not others.

Another possibility is that not all neuronal electrical activity has a marked effect on the Ca^{2+} concentration in the soma. The processes of retinal amacrine and horizontal cells are electrically isolated from the cell body (45). If the Ca^{2+} concentration in the cell body is indeed what couples depolarization to early response gene expression, all neuronal activity would not be effective. Moreover, there is evidence that Ca^{2+} entry through L-type voltage-activated Ca^{2+} channels is especially important in regulating *c-fos* expression after neuronal depolarization (17,27). Therefore, the distribution of L-type channels over the surface of the neuron may be of importance. An additional possibility is that the temporal pattern of electrical activity, which may also play an important role in regulating intracellular Ca^{2+}, may be an important determinant of early response gene expression. In magnocellular neurons of the hypothalamus, where osmotic stimuli induce dramatic levels of *c-fos* expression, the major electrophysiological correlate is the change from a tonic to a phasic firing pattern (46). One would expect the phasic pattern of firing to greatly increase Ca^{2+} entry (47).

Finally, it is not known whether all CNS neurons are able to express early response genes when physiologically stimulated. Cells that are tonically active may not undergo an early genetic response to increased electrical activity. There is no evidence that inhibition, in particular stimulation of $GABA_A$ receptors, induces early response genes. In some brain regions, particularly thalamus and cerebellum, inhibition is the predominant mechanism of information processing. In fact, many experimental manipulations, including generalized seizures, fail to induce *c-fos* expression in thalmus or cerebellum. Finally, there are mechanisms of regulating gene expression other than early response genes; some neurons may preferentially employ those other mechanisms.

Fos expression in the CNS may also result from stimuli other than synaptic input. Growth factors and injury, as discussed below, may also induce *c-fos* gene expression. Therefore, one cannot equate neuronal Fos expression with electrical or synaptic activity.

FUNCTIONAL MAPPING OF THE NEUROENDOCRINE SYSTEM

The neuroendocrine system provides an illustration of the potential uses of Fos immunocytochemistry in functional neuroanatomic mapping. Osmotic stimuli, including dehydration and the administration of hypertonic saline or mannitol, induce *c-fos* gene expression in a specific anatomic pattern in brainstem and forebrain (5,48,49) (Figs. 2 and 3). Fos nuclear immunostaining is stimulated in the circumventricular organs, including the organum vasculosum of the lamina terminalis (OVLT), the subfornical organ (SFO), and the area postrema, in the median nucleus of the preoptic area, in the hypothalamic magnocellular neurons, in parvocellular neurons of the paraventricular nucleus (PVN), and in the nucleus of the solitary tract. These are all regions that are known from electrophysiological studies to participate in osmotic regulation.

The nuclear localization of Fos immunostaining (Fig. 1) permits double-label immunocytochemical procedures to be used to identify individual neurons that express the *c-fos* gene. Both oxytocin- and vasopressin-immunoreactive magnocellular neurons of the hypothalamus express *c-fos* after the systemic administration of hypertonic saline. In the nucleus of the solitary tract, both tyrosine-hydroxylase-positive and -negative neurons display Fos nuclear immunostaining, whereas in the ventrolateral medulla, all Fos-positive cells are tyrosine hydroxylase-positive.

The systemic administration of bacterial lipopolysaccharide (LPS, endotoxin) provokes the febrile response in rats (50). It provides an instructive comparison to osmotic stimuli, because LPS induces Fos nuclear immunostaining in a regional pattern similar to hypertonic saline, but with important differences on a cellular level. In particular, in the magnocellular hypothalamic neurons, far more oxytocin than vasopressin neurons express *c-fos* in response to LPS, although both groups of neurons respond to hypertonic saline (51). In addition, in catecholaminergic neurons of the ventrolateral medulla, the A1 cell group, many more neurons exhibit Fos immunostaining in response to LPS than to hypertonic saline. These differences highlight the ability of *c-fos* expression to identify individual neurons and subdivisions of anatomic nuclei that are activated by an experimental stimulus.

Another productive line of neuroendocrine investigation has been to exploit *c-fos* expression in the study of circadian rhythms. The suprachiasmatic nucleus (SCN) of the hypothalamus is thought to contain the major circadian pacemaker of mammalian brain. In the SCN of rats, *c-fos* expression is low during the night and high during the day (52–56). In rodents maintained in constant dark-

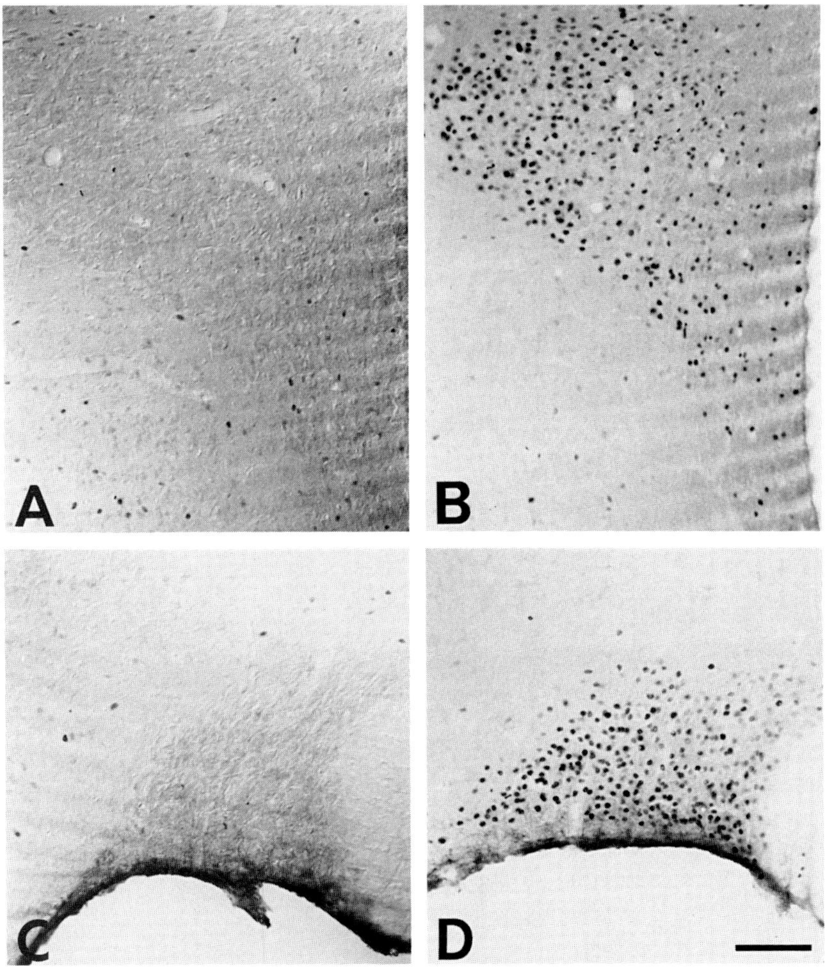

FIG. 2. Rat magnocellular hypothalamic regions immunostained for Fos 1 hr after the intraperitoneal administration of 4 ml 0.15 M saline (**A, C**) or 4 ml 1.5 M saline (**B, D**). **A** and **B** show the paraventricular nucleus (PVN), and **C** and **D** show the supraoptic nucleus (SON). Whereas there is very little Fos immunostaining of the PVN and SON in controls, virtually all the magnocellular neurons display Fos nuclear immunostaining after hypertonic saline. There is also Fos immunostaining induced in parvocellular neurons of the PVN after hypertonic saline. Scale bar, 50 μm.

ness, light pulses administered during the subjective night, but not during subjective day, induce *c-fos* expression in the nucleus. Hence, *c-fos* expression in the SCN correlates with the ability of stimuli to affect the circadian rhythm of animals and suggests that early response genes may mediate setting the circadian clock.

Another line of investigation has been the relationship between steroid hormones and early response gene expression. One might hypothesize that since receptors for steroid hormones are themselves transcription factors, these hormones might bypass the early response gene mechanism. In general, this appears to be the case, in that dexamethasone, testosterone, and estrogen administered at high dose levels fail to induce early response gene expression in the brain regions known to have appropriate receptors. However, in some circumstances *c-fos* expression is correlated with steroid hormone actions.

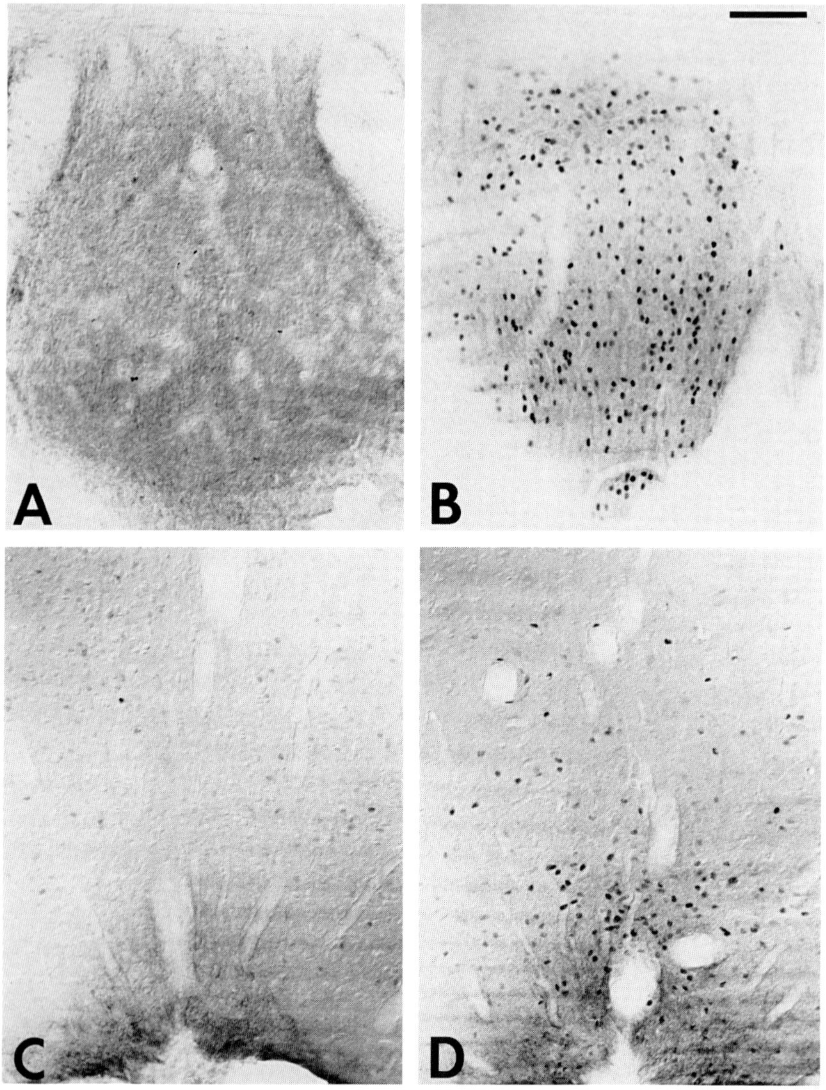

FIG. 3. Circumventricular organs display Fos nuclear immunostaining after the administration of hypertonic saline. The subfornical organ (**A**) and organum vasculosum of the lamina terminalis (**C**) of control rats injected with normal saline display little or no Fos immunostaining. One hour after the administration of hypertonic saline, these structures contain many Fos-immunoreactive nuclei (**B** and **D**). Scale bar, 50 μm.

Estradiol induces *c-fos* gene expression in certain hypothalamic neurons (57), *c-fos* is expressed during the proestrous surge of luteinizing hormone in luteinizing hormone-releasing hormone-immunoreactive neurons (58), and glucocorticoids induce *c-fos* in corticotropin-releasing hormone cells of the PVN of adrenalectomized rats (59). In none of these experiments, however, is it shown that a steroid hormone acts directly on a neuron to induce early response gene expression.

These studies demonstrate that Fos immunocytochemistry and *c-fos in situ* hybridization histochemistry permit the detailed cellular mapping of neuroendocrine function in the brain. The success of the method in the neuroendocrine system is probably related to several factors. It is possible to suddenly excite relatively quiescent neurons with powerful stimuli. In other systems, such as somatosensory or motor systems, it is sometimes difficult to design experiments to obtain physiological inactivity prior to stimulation. In addition, much of the information processing in neuroendocrine circuits is mediated by excitatory synaptic activity rather than inhibitory modulation of tonically active neurons.

TROPHIC FACTOR ACTIONS

Since the expression of early response genes is the most rapid genetic response to growth factor action, it is a convenient measure of growth factor action in cell culture. Many investigators have used early response genes to study the biochemical mechanisms of the initial actions of trophic factors (60–62). In addition, it is of note that the overexpression of *c-fos* (63) or *fra-1* (64) can block the NGF- and FGF-induced differentiation of PC-12 cells. Although several hypotheses can explain these latter observations, they provide additional evidence for the involvement of early response genes in neuronal differentiation.

Early response gene expression can also serve as a measure of trophic factor action *in vivo.* We have shown that EGF and transforming growth factor-α (TGF-α), which act at the same receptor, induce *c-fos* gene expression selectively in retinal Müller cells after intravitreal injection in the rabbit (Fig. 4) (65). This observation demonstrates that adult glia are targets, although perhaps indirectly, of EGF or TGF-α. This effect is specific to EGF and TGF-α, since other growth factors, including bFGF and NGF, fail to induce *c-fos* in the neural retina *in vivo.* The failure of bFGF is puzzling, since it induces Fos immunostaining in cortical neurons in cell culture (19) and has biological activity in retina (66).

An early paper (67) reporting the widespread induction of Fos immunostaining in rat forebrain after the intracerebroventricular injection of NGF was misleading. The effect shown was not a specific effect of NGF but rather was a nonspecific effect of the injections, perhaps spreading depression (68). We and others have seen the same pattern of Fos immunostaining in the forebrain after the in-

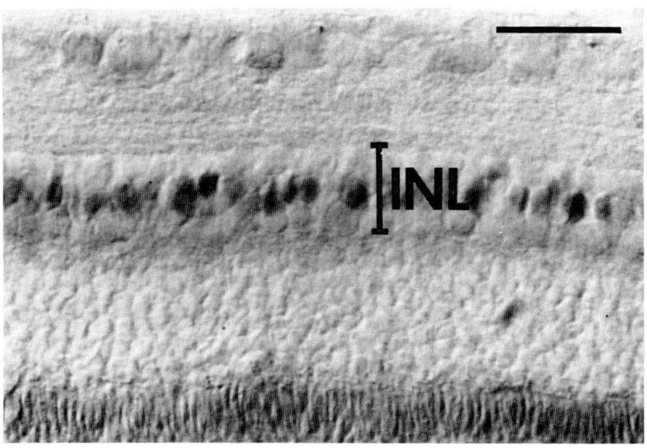

FIG. 4. Cross section of a rabbit retina immunostained for Fos-like immunoreactivity 3 hr after an intravitreal injection of 50 μg EGF. The ganglion cell layer is at the top of the photograph, and the photoreceptors are at the bottom. The row of Fos-immunoreactive nuclei in the inner nuclear layer (INL) belong to Müller cells, as can be verified by double labeling for vimentin. Control retinas stained after the intravitreal injection of saline vehicle failed to demonstrate Fos immunostaining of Müller cell nuclei. The staining of photoreceptor outer segments is nonspecific. Scale bar, 50 μm.

tracerebroventricular injection of a number of substances, including normal saline, and after cortical injury (67,69–74).

The importance of growth factor induction of *c-fos* and other early response genes is that it potentially allows early response gene expression to be used to dissect the action of trophic factors after nervous system injury. The expression of *c-fos* or *c-jun* has been demonstrated in neurons and glia after a variety of nervous system insults, including brain ischemia (69,70,73,75), axotomy (36,76–78), and neurotoxins (75). If an antibody or antagonist to a growth factor or cytokine could be shown to block the early response gene induction following injury, that factor would be strongly implicated in the response. An analogous approach has demonstrated that NMDA antagonists can inhibit *c-fos* expression after neuronal injury, including ischemia and spreading depression (68,70,71,74).

CONCLUSIONS

Despite reservations, many of which are generic to all methods of metabolic mapping, the localization of early response gene expression represents a major advance in neuroanatomic methodology. It allows the identification of individual neurons that are activated by an experimental procedure. In order to fully exploit the technique, many questions concerning the regulation of early response gene expression by neurotransmitters and growth factors must still be answered. In addition, although the *c-fos* gene is the best studied, it is only one of a group of cellular immediate-early genes, each of which might map a restricted group of metabolic functions or second messenger systems. Study of these proteins may provide an armamentarium of techniques for the mapping of neuronal and glial activities in a wide range of experimental circumstances.

ACKNOWLEDGMENTS

The authors thank Kristen Price for preparing the figures. The following people made valuable contributions to the work performed in the authors' laboratories: Karen Baner, Robert Edwards, Katy Hicks, Kinya Hisanaga, Mary Pat Jasper, Jari Koistinaho, Matthew Morton, and Kristen Price. The work was supported by the VA Merit Review Program and by the NIH (NS27864, NS27488).

REFERENCES

1. Curran T. The *fos* oncogene. In: Reddy EP, Skalka AM, Curran T, eds. *The oncogene handbook.* Amsterdam: Elsevier; 1988:307–325.
2. Mitchell PJ, Tjian R. Transcriptional regulation in mammalian cells by sequence-specific DNA binding proteins. *Science* 1989;245:371–378.
3. Kouzarides T, Ziff E. Behind the Fos and Jun leucine zipper. *Cancer Cells* 1989;1:71–76.
4. Morgan JI, Cohen DR, Hempstead JL, Curran T. Mapping patterns of c-*fos* expression in the central nervous system after seizure. *Science* 1987;237: 192–197.
5. Sagar SM, Sharp FR, Curran T. Expression of c-*fos* protein in brain: metabolic mapping at the cellular level. *Science* 1988;240:1328–1331.
6. Dragunow M, Faull R. The use of c-*fos* as a metabolic marker in neuronal pathway tracing. *J Neurosci Methods* 1989;29:261–265.
7. Hunt SP, Pini A, Evan G. Induction of c-*fos*-like protein in spinal cord neurons following sensory stimulation. *Nature* 1987;328:632–634.
8. Sokoloff L, Reivich M, Kennedy C, et al. The [^{14}C]deoxyglucose method for the measurement of local cerebral glucose utilization: theory, procedure, and normal values in the conscious and anesthetized albino rat. *J Neurochem* 1977;28:897–916.
9. Mugnaini E, Berrebi AS, Morgan JI, Curran T. Fos-like immunoreactivity induced by seizure in mice is specifically associated with euchromatin in neurons. *Eur J Neurosci* 1989;1:46–52.
10. Holt JT, Venkat Gopal T, Moulton AD, Nienhuis AW. Inducible production of *c-fos* antisense RNA inhibits 3T3 cell proliferation. *Proc Natl Acad Sci USA* 1986;83:4794–4798.
11. Riabowal KT, Vosatka RJ, Ziff EB, Lamb NJ, Feramisco JR. Microinjection of *fos*-specific antibodies blocks DNA synthesis in fibroblast cells. *Mol Cell Biol* 1988;8:1670–1676.
12. Kovary K, Bravo R. The Jun and Fos protein families are both required for cell cycle progression in fibroblasts. *Mol Cell Biol* 1991;11:4466–4472.
13. Kruijer W, Schubert D, Verma I. Induction of the proto-oncogene *fos* by nerve growth factor. *Proc Natl Acad Sci USA* 1985;82:7330–7334.
14. Greenberg ME, Greene LA, Ziff EB. Nerve growth factor and epidermal growth factor induce rapid transient changes in proto-oncogene transcription in PC12 cells. *J Biol Chem* 1985;260:14101–14110.
15. Muller R, Wagner EF. Differentiation of F9 teratocarcinoma stem cells after transfer of c-*fos* proto-oncogene. *Nature* 1984;311:438–442.
16. Curran T, Morgan JI. Barium modulates c-*fos* ex-

pression and post-translational modification. *Proc Natl Acad Sci USA* 1986;83:8521–8524.
17. Morgan JI, Curran T. Role of ion flux in the control of c-*fos* expression. *Nature* 1986;322:552–555.
18. Greenberg ME, Ziff EB, Greene LA. Stimulation of neuronal acetylcholine receptors induces rapid gene transcription. *Science* 1986;234:80–83.
19. Hisanaga K, Sagar SM, Sharp FR. N-Methyl-D-aspartate antagonists block Fos-like protein expression induced via multiple signalling pathways in cultured cortical neurons. *J Neurochem* 1992;58: 1836–1844.
20. Szekely AM, Barbaccia ML, Alho H, Costa E. In primary cultures of cerebellar granule cells the activation of N-methyl-D-aspartate-sensitive glutamate receptors induces *c-fos* mRNA expression. *Mol Pharmacol* 1989;35:401–408.
21. Hisanaga K, Sagar SM, Hicks KJ, Swanson RA, Sharp FR. C-*fos* proto-oncogene expression in astrocytes associated with differentiation or proliferation but not depolarization. *Mol Brain Res* 1990;8: 69–75.
22. Condorelli DF, Kaczmarek L, Nicoletti F, et al. Induction of proto-oncogene *fos* by extracellular signals in primary glial cell cultures. *J Neurosci Res* 1989;23:234–239.
23. Arenander AT, de Vellis J, Herschman HR. Induction of *c-fos* and *TIS* genes in cultured rat astrocytes by neurotransmitters. *J Neurosci Res* 1989;24: 107–114.
24. Sheng M, Greenberg ME. The regulation and function of c-*fos* and other immediate early genes in the nervous system. *Neuron* 1990;4:477–485.
25. Sheng M, Dougan ST, McFadden G, Greenberg ME. Calcium and growth factor pathways of c-*fos* transcriptional activation require distinct upstream regulatory sequences. *Mol Cell Biol* 1988;8:2787–2796.
26. Sheng M, McFadden G, Greenberg ME. Membrane depolarization and calcium induce c-*fos* transcription via phosphorylation of transcription factor CREB. *Neuron* 1990;4:571–582.
27. Murphy TH, Worley PF, Baraban JM. L-Type voltage-sensitive calcium channels mediate synaptic activation of immediate early genes. *Neuron* 1991; 7:625–635.
28. Misra RP, Rivera VM, Wang JM, Fan P-D, Greenberg ME. The serum response factor is extensively modified by phosphorylation following its synthesis in serum-stimulated fibroblasts. *Mol Cell Biol* 1991;11:4545–4554.
29. Sonnenberg JL, Macgregor-Leon PF, Curran T, Morgan JI. Dynamic alterations occur in levels and composition of transcription factor AP-1 complexes after seizure. *Neuron* 1989;3:359–365.
30. Wisden W, Errington ML, William S, et al. Differential expression of immediate early genes in the hippocampus and spinal cord. *Neuron* 1990;4: 603–614.
31. Herdegen T, Tolle TR, Bravo R, Zieglansberger W, Zimmermann M. Sequential expression of JUN B, JUN D and FOS B proteins in rat spinal neurons: cascade of transcriptional operations during nociception. *Neurosci Lett* 1991;129:221–224.
32. Struhl K. Mechanisms for diversity in gene expression patterns. *Neuron* 1991;7:177–181.
33. He X, Rosenfeld MG. Mechanisms of complex transcriptional regulation: implications for brain development. *Neuron* 1991;7:183–196.
34. Bartel DP, Sheng M, Lau LF, Greenberg ME. Growth factors and membrane depolarization activate distinct programs of early response gene expression: dissociation of *fos* and *jun* induction. *Genes Dev* 1989;3:304–313.
35. Arenander AT, Lim RW, Varnum BC, Cole R, de Vellis J, Herschman HR. *TIS* gene expression in cultured rat astrocytes: multiple pathways of induction by mitogens. *J Neurosci Res* 1989;23:257–265.
36. Herdegen T, Kummer W, Fiallos CE, Leah J, Bravo R. Expression of c-Jun, Jun B and Jun D proteins in rat nervous system following transection of vagus nerve and cervical sympathetic trunk. *Neuroscience* 1991;45:413–422.
37. Naranjo JR, Mellstrom B, Achaval M, Sassone-Corsi P. Molecular pathways of pain: Fos/Jun-mediated activation of a noncanonical AP-1 site in the prodynorphin gene. *Neuron* 1991;6:607–617.
38. Draisci G, Iadarola MJ. Temporal analysis of increases in c-*fos*, preprodynorphin and preproenkephalin mRNAs in rat spinal cord. *Mol Brain Res* 1989;6:31–37.
39. Sonnenberg JL, Rauscher FJ, Morgan JI, Curran T. Regulation of proenkephalin by Fos and Jun. *Science* 1989;246:1622–1625.
40. Gizang-Ginsberg E, Ziff EB. Nerve growth factor regulates tyrosine hydroxylase gene transcription through a nucleoprotein complex that contains c-Fos. *Genes Dev* 1990;4:477–491.
41. Hengerer B, Lindholm D, Heumann R, Ruther U, Wagner EF, Thoenen H. Lesion-induced increase in nerve growth factor mRNA is mediated by c-*fos*. *Proc Natl Acad Sci USA* 1990;87:3899–3903.
42. Sharp FR, Gonzalez MF, Sharp JW, Sagar SM. c-*fos* expression and (^{14}C)2-deoxyglucose uptake in the caudal cerebellum of the rat during motor/sensory cortex stimulation. *J Comp Neurol* 1989;284: 621–636.
43. Menetrey D, Gannon D, Levine JD, Basbaum AI. Expression of c-*fos* protein in interneurons and projection neurons of the rat spinal cord in response to noxious somatic, articular, and visceral stimulation. *J Comp Neurol* 1989;285:177–195.
44. Sagar SM, Sharp FR. Light induces a Fos-like nuclear antigen in retinal neurons. *Mol Brain Res* 1990;7:17–21.
45. Ellias SA, Stevens JK. The dendritic varicosity: a mechanism for electrically isolating the dendrites of cat retinal amacrine cells? *Brain Res* 1980;196: 365–372.
46. Renaud LP, Bourque CW. Neurophysiology and neuropharmacology of hypothalamic neurons secreting vasopressin and oxytocin. *Prog Neurobiol* 1991;36:131–169.
47. Slesinger PA, Lansman JB. Reopening of Ca^{2+} channels in mouse cerebellar neurons at resting membrane potentials during recovery from inactivation. *Neuron* 1991;7:755–762.
48. Sharp FR, Sagar SM, Hicks K, Lowenstein D, Hisanaga K. c-*fos* mRNA, Fos, and Fos-related antigen induction by hypertonic saline and stress. *J Neurosci* 1991;11:2321–2331.
49. Carter DA, Murphy D. Regulation of *c-fos* and *c-jun*

expression in the rat supraoptic nucleus. *Cell Mol Neurobiol* 1990;10:435–445.
50. Sagar SM, Price KJ. Fos immunostaining in rat brain following endotoxin administration. *Soc Neurosci Abstr* 1991;17:1122.
51. Giovannelli L, Shiromani PJ, Jirikowski GF, Bloom FE. Oxytocin neurons in the rat hypothalamus exhibit c-*fos* immunoreactivity upon osmotic stress. *Brain Res* 1990;531:299–303.
52. Aronin N, Sagar SM, Sharp FR, Schwartz WJ. Light regulates expression of a Fos-related protein in rat suprachiasmatic nuclei. *Proc Natl Acad Sci USA* 1990;87:5959–5962.
53. Rea MA. Light increases Fos-related protein immunoreactivity in the rat suprachiasmatic nuclei. *Brain Res Bull* 1989;23:577–581.
54. Rusak B, Robertson HA, Wisden W, Hunt SP. Light pulses that shift rhythms induce gene expression in the suprachiasmatic nucleus. *Science* 1990;248: 1237–1240.
55. Kornhauser JM, Nelson DE, Mayo KE, Takahashi JS. Photic and circadian regulation of c-*fos* gene expression in the hamster suprachiasmatic nucleus. *Neuron* 1990;5:127–134.
56. Earnest DJ, Iadarola M, Yeh HH, Olschowka JA. Photic regulation of c-*fos* expression in neural components governing the entrainment of circadian rhythms. *Exp Neurol* 1990;109:353–361.
57. Insel TR. Regional induction of c-*fos*-like protein in rat brain after estradiol administration. *Endocrinology* 1990;126:1849–1853.
58. Lee W-S, Smith MS, Hoffman GE. Luteinizing hormone-releasing hormone neurons express Fos protein during the proestrus surge of luteinizing hormone. *Proc Natl Acad Sci USA* 1990:87:5163–5167.
59. Jacobson L, Sharp FR, Dallman MF. Induction of *fos*-like immunoreactivity in hypothalamic corticotropin-releasing factor neurons after adrenalectomy in the rat. *Endocrinology* 1990;126:1709–1719.
60. Sigmund O, Naor Z, Anderson DJ, Stein R. Effect of nerve growth factor and fibroblast growth factor on SCG10 and c-*fos* expression and neurite outgrowth in protein kinase C-depleted PC12 cells. *J Biol Chem* 1990;265:2257–2261.
61. Thomson TM, Green SH, Trotta RJ, Burstein DE, Pellicer A. Oncogene N-*ras* mediates selective inhibition of c-*fos* induction by nerve growth factor and basic fibroblast growth factor in a PC12 cell line. *Mol Cell Biol* 1990;10:1556–1563.
62. Altin JG, Kujubu DA, Raffioni S, Eveleth DD, Herschman HR, Bradshaw RA. Differential induction of primary-response (*TIS*) genes in PC12 pheochromocytoma cells and the unresponsive variant PC12nnr5. *J Biol Chem* 1991;266:5401–5406.
63. Ito E, Sonnenberg JL, Narayanan R. Nerve growth factor-induced differentiation in PC-12 cells is blocked by *fos* oncogene. *Oncogene* 1989;4:1193–1199.
64. Ito E, Sweterlisch LA, Tran PB, Rauscher FJ, Narayanan R. Inhibition of PC-12 cell differentiation by the immediate early gene *fra*-1. *Oncogene* 1990;5:1755–1760.
65. Sagar SM, Edwards RH, Sharp FR. Epidermal growth factor and transforming growth factor-α induce c-*fos* gene expression in retinal Müller cells *in vivo*. *J Neurosci Res* 1991;29:549–559.
66. Faktorovich EG, Steinberg RH, Yasumura D, Matthes MT, LaVail MM. Photoreceptor degeneration in inherited retinal dystrophy delayed by basic fibroblast growth factor. *Nature* 1990;347:83–86.
67. Sharp FR, Gonzalez MF, Hisanaga K, Mobley WC, Sagar SM. Induction of the c-*fos* gene product in rat forebrain following cortical lesions and NGF injections. *Neurosci Lett* 1989;100:117–122.
68. Herrera DG, Robertson HA. Application of potassium chloride to the brain surface induces the *c-fos* proto-oncogene: reversal by MK-801. *Brain Res* 1990;510:166–170.
69. Herrera DG, Robertson HA. Unilateral induction of c-*fos* protein in cortex following cortical devascularization. *Brain Res* 1989;503:205–213.
70. Herrera DG, Robertson HA. N-Methyl-D-aspartate receptors mediate activation of the *c-fos* proto-oncogene in a model of brain injury. *Neuroscience* 1990;35:273–281.
71. Dragunow M, Faull RLM, Jansen KLR. MK-801, an antagonist of NMDA receptors, inhibits injury-induced *c-fos* protein accumulation in rat brain. *Neurosci Lett* 1990;109:128–133.
72. Sharp JW, Sagar SM, Hisanaga K, Jasper P, Sharp FR. The NMDA receptor mediates cortical induction of *fos* and *fos*-related antigens following cortical injury. *Exp Neurol* 1990;109:323–332.
73. Onodera H, Kogure K, Ono Y, Igarashi K, Kiyota, Nagaoka A. Proto-oncogene *c-fos* is transiently induced in the rat cerebral cortex after forebrain ischemia. *Neurosci Lett* 1989;98:101–104.
74. Dragunow M, Goulding M, Faull RLM, Ralph R, Mee E, Frith R. Induction of *c-fos* mRNA and protein in neurons and glia after traumatic brain injury: pharmacological characterization. *Exp Neurol* 1990;107:236–248.
75. Popovici T, Represa A, Crepel V, Barbin G, Beaudoin M, Ben-Ari Y. Effects of kainic acid-induced seizures and ischemia on c-*fos*-like proteins in rat brain. *Brain Res* 1990;536:183–194.
76. Sharp FR, Griffith J, Gonzalez MF, Sagar SM. Trigeminal nerve section induces Fos-like immunoreactivity (FLI) in brainstem and decreases FLI in sensory cortex. *Mol Brain Res* 1989;6:217–220.
77. Roivainen R, Koistinaho J. Decentralization induces long-term *c-fos* protein-like immunoreactivity in non-neuronal cells in the rat superior cervical ganglion. *Neurosci Lett* 1991;119:105–108.
78. Pyykonen I, Koistinaho J. c-*fos* protein like immunoreactivity in non-neuronal cells of rat peripheral nerve after transection. *Acta Neuropathol* 1991;82: 66–71.

Advances in Neurology, Vol. 59, edited by
Fredrick J. Seil. Raven Press, Ltd.,
New York © 1993.

25

A *fos–lac* Z Transgenic Mouse That Can Be Used for Neuroanatomic Mapping

Richard J. Smeyne, Karl Schilling, John Oberdick, *Linda Robertson, *Daniel Luk, *Tom Curran, and James I. Morgan

*Departments of Neuroscience and *Molecular Oncology and Virology, Roche Institute of Molecular Biology, Roche Research Center, Nutley, New Jersey 07110*

A basic issue in biology is how a brief period of stimulation can lead to a protracted alteration in the phenotype of a particular cell. Although this question is not unique to the neurosciences, it is of especial relevance to the nervous system, since transient periods of neuronal activation can result in long-lasting alterations in the behavior of neural circuits that may persist for the lifetime of the organism.

Many studies have shown that stimulation of cells results in alterations in gene transcription. Furthermore, several studies have established that protein synthesis is essential for the acquisition of a number of long-lasting responses (reviewed in ref. 1). Therefore, mechanisms must exist to couple extracellular stimuli to intracellular transcriptional machinery. It has been suggested that activation of cells results in a coordinated transcriptional response via cellular immediate-early genes (1–5). This notion emanated from discoveries first made in the field of oncology. It was recognized that several proto-oncogenes (the normal cellular counterparts of cancer-causing oncogenes) were rapidly induced following stimulation of fibroblasts with serum or serum-derived growth factors. At that time, the best characterized examples of inducible proto-oncogenes were *c-fos* and *c-myc*. Since both *c-fos* and *c-myc* were known to encode nuclear proteins (Fos and Myc, respectively) it was postulated that they were inducible transcription factors that controlled the expression of further, target, genes whose products contributed to the altered phenotype (2–4).

THE CELLULAR IMMEDIATE-EARLY RESPONSE

The induction of *c-fos* and *c-myc* mRNAs was known to occur even if protein synthesis was inhibited, establishing that this was one of the earliest transcriptional consequences of cell activation and that all the machinery necessary for this induction was already present in the unstimulated cell. Since these characteristics are shared by the immediate-early genes of viruses, which control subsequent stages of viral replication, the term cellular (to distinguish them from viral) immediate-early (cIE) gene was coined (2,3). Again by analogy, it was suggested that the cIE genes should control downstream events that contribute to the long-term response of a particular cell to a specific stimulus. Subsequently, many other inducible genes were identified, which permitted the scheme to be extended beyond that of a simple stimulus–transcription coupling cascade. For example, although many of the cIE genes encoded nuclear proteins, some clearly did not (5). Indeed, some cIE gene products bore significant homologies to secreted cytokines. Thus, it was supposed that the cellular immediate-early response not only coordinated transcriptional responses within a given cell but could also integrate or transmit it to other cells and organs via autocrine or paracrine mediators (3). Furthermore, it was recognized that some cIE gene products appeared with a delay, and their profiles of appearance and disappearance were sometimes staggered, suggesting a temporal integration of the cIE response (6). An additional aspect of regulation involved feedback inhibition. Some of the cIE genes showed a refractory period whereby they could not be reinduced for hours or even days following some types of stimulation (7). Although the precise basis for the refractory period is not understood, there is evidence to suggest that Fos is an autorepressor of its own transcription (reviewed in ref. 8). This would account for the finding, typical among cIE genes, that *c-fos* is induced within 5 min of stimulation but repressed about 15 to 20 min later (9), presumably by the synthesis and translocation of its own product to the nucleus. However, the precise details of this interaction are a matter of active research at present.

Taken together, the present view of the cellular immediate-early response is one in which cell stimulation leads to the rapid, usually transient, activation of immediate-early genes. The products of these genes initiate, among other things, further transcriptional events that culminate in an alteration in the phenotype of the cell. These alterations might involve changes in the transcription rate of target genes encoding elements of the cell's stimulus–signal transduction and stimulus–response machinery. This could provide, for example, more or fewer receptors, G proteins, second messenger metabolizing enzymes, kinases, and ion channels or secretory products as well as structural proteins involved in growth responses. Since some of the long-term alterations take some time to become apparent, we feel that this response may need to be integrated over time. For example, the staggered induction of some cIE genes may provide a way to sequentially induce and then repress a set of genes or, alternatively, to activate different sets of genes in a specific order. Refractory periods may also be critical in this regard, precluding reinitiation of the response before it has been completed. As also noted above, further levels of regulation may be obtained by the release of cIE gene products to act on neighboring or distant cells, providing for integration at an organismal level.

Although several classes of transcription factors (e.g., leucine zipper, zinc finger, and steroid receptor superfamily) and some cytokines are represented among the cIE gene products, as yet no other proteins with known biological properties have been identified among this class of inducible genes. However, this is likely to change in the future, since cIE genes whose proteins conform to no known motif have been found (reviewed in ref. 5). Therefore, it is predicted that cIE gene products will be identified in the future that represent other elements within the signal transduction cascade, such as kinases, phosphatases, and guanosine triphosphate binding proteins. This will provide a mechanism whereby the coupling efficiency of the signal transduction cascade can be modulated, resulting in changes in both short-term responses and long-term phenotype.

FOS, JUN, AND AP-1 IN THE NERVOUS SYSTEM

A considerable literature has accumulated concerning the expression of *c-fos* in the nervous system (5). To place these studies in perspective a brief review is given here of the molecular biology of Fos.

The products of the inducible proto-oncogenes, *c-fos* and *c-jun,* encode nuclear proteins (Fos and Jun, respectively) that form heterodimers (Fos–Jun) with one another (8). These heterodimeric complexes exhibit cooperative binding to the DNA consensus sequence TGATGCA, identified independently as the recognition sequence for transcription factor AP-1 (activator protein 1) (reviewed in ref. 10). Subsequently, AP-1 was shown to consist of Fos and Jun as well as several Fos- and Jun-related proteins. These related proteins [FosB, Fra-1, Fra-2 (for Fos-related antigens) JunB, and JunD] also form dimeric complexes that interact at AP-1 sites (reviewed in ref. 11). In addition, both Fos and Jun were found to associate with nuclear proteins (e.g., CRE binding protein/1 and activating transcription factors) that bound to the DNA sequence TGAGCTCA, which confers responsiveness to cAMP (the cAMP-responsive element or CRE) (11,12). Thus, Fos and Jun, depending on their partners, can behave as transcription factors acting via AP-1 or CRE sites.

All of the Fos- and Jun-related proteins, as well as many of the ATF and CREB proteins, are now known to belong to a larger gene family (the basic-zipper family) that is characterized by the presence of two structural motifs: a basic DNA-binding domain and a leucine-zipper dimerization domain (11). Each of the family members possesses a single leucine-zipper domain. This is a region of α-helix that contains a heptad repeat of leucine residues that interacts with the same domain in a partner to generate a coiled-coil-like structure that provides for stable dimerization. DNA binding occurs through a domain containing an abundance of basic amino acids. Each partner in the dimeric complex provides a half site for binding, and two half sites are essential for binding to occur. This region shows a high level of sequence conservation among family members and was fortuitously the region to which many of the initial Fos antisera were raised. This resulted in the discovery of Fos-related antigens on immunoblots and in immunoprecipitates as well as their subsequent cloning from expression libraries. However, it also meant that these antibodies detected many Fos-like proteins in immunohistochemical studies, leading to an ambiguity in precise identification of Fos (reviewed in ref. 5).

In the CNS various types of seizures were shown to induce *c-fos* and *c-jun* as determined by Northern blot, *in situ* hybridization, immunohistochemistry, immunoblotting, and AP-1 gel shift analysis (reviewed in ref. 5). Although Fos and Jun contribute to AP-1, it could be established *in vivo* for the first time that the precise molecular composition of AP-1 varied with time after seizure in the brain (6). Whereas *fos* mRNA and protein rose rapidly and declined soon thereafter, AP-1 DNA binding activity rose rapidly but remained elevated for many hours following a seizure. Furthermore, it remained elevated when no further Fos was present in brain. It was recognized that following the induction of Fos, other Fos-related proteins appeared in the brain, and their expression was more protracted than Fos. It was these Fra that maintained the elevated AP-1 DNA binding activity. Since these proteins appeared and disappeared in a staggered manner, it was assumed that this dynamic state in AP-1 complex composition resulted in alterations in function and/or specificity. However, this all begged the question of the precise functions that AP-1 subserves in brain during seizures.

Besides the practical use of mapping the sites of expression of immediate-early gene products as a way of identifying neurons activated during particular responses, two general types of conclusions have been drawn concerning AP-1 function in the nervous system. First, a temporal and spatial correlation has been made between the sites of *fos* induction and the increased expression of proenkephalin in dentate gyrus granule cells and prodynorphin in spinal cord neurons (e.g., 5,13,14). In addition, proenkephalin can be cooperatively transactivated by Fos and Jun in transient transfection assays, leading us to suggest that stimulus–secretion coupling and stimulus–transcription coupling are themselves integrated cellular functions (13,14). The suggestion is that basal expression from the proenkephalin gene is appropriate for maintaining enkephalin protein levels under normal conditions of neural activity. However, on abnormal excitation, such as occurs in hippocampus during seizures, release would outstrip synthesis, and thus the cellular immediate-early response is recruited to supplement proenkephalin biosynthesis.

A second general type of observation concerning cIE gene involvement in neurobiological processes involves growth responses in adult CNS (reviewed in ref. 14). Like proenkephalin, mRNA levels for the neurotrophic factors NGF, BDNF and NT3 have been observed to rise in the dentate gyrus following seizures (15–18). These increases appear to be preceded by a rise in *fos* and *jun* transcription and an increase in AP-1-like DNA-binding activity. Furthermore, Fos and Jun have been suggested to directly regulate NGF transcription (19). Subsequent to these changes, Sutula and colleagues (20,21) have established that seizure-like excitation results in a growth response in the hippocampus (and other brain regions) that is characterized by axonal sprouting. The following scenario has been suggested to link these various events (reviewed in ref. 14). First, seizure activity induces a cellular immediate-early response in the dentate gyrus. Second, cellular immediate-early transcription factors, such as Fos and Jun, then transactivate growth factor genes such as those encoding NGF and BDNF. In turn, the neurotrophic factors are released, interact with their receptors, and induce transcription of target genes (perhaps via cIE genes) that encode proteins required for axonal sprouting. These target genes might encode cytoskeletal proteins, synaptic proteins, receptors and ion channels, etc. Because some cIE genes appear to encode cytokines, it cannot be formally ruled out that neurotrophic factors are themselves cIE genes with slower kinetics of induction. Recently the details of this hypothetical scheme have been reviewed (14). If this proposal bears any truth, then it is likely that the cIE gene response may be involved in other growth responses in the nervous system, such as regeneration.

To pursue the issue of cIE gene expression *in vivo,* we have developed a novel inducible *fos–lac* Z construct that functions in transgenic mice (22,23; Fig. 1). We have fused bacterial β-galactosidase in frame into exon 4 of *c-fos.* The *fos* genomic fragment contains all of the known upstream and intragenic regulatory elements (22). Furthermore, the fusion protein conserves many of the motifs in Fos, including those that target it to the nucleus. Therefore, induction of this transgene should result in β-galactosidase activity in the nucleus. This construct is inducible, as predicted, in stably transfected cells lines (22), cultured cells from transgenic mice (23), and in the transgenic mice themselves (23). The kinetics of induction and repression of the transgene are essentially the same as for cognate *fos,* as is the repertoire of agents that induce it (22,23).

The distributions of constitutive and induced *fos–lac* Z have been mapped in adult (23; Fig. 1) and developing transgenic mice. Constitutive expression has been noted in several tissues, notably skin and hair follicle, cartilage, and bone. These sites of expression involve cells that are undergoing terminal differentiation leading to death. This led us to examine other tissues and cell types that have these properties. Two other sites of constitutive expression were identified, follicular cells in the degenerating corpus luteum of the ovary and cells in the thymic medulla, both of which undergo cell death. In the CNS, expression could be observed in a few regions, notably the raphe. Since it is unlikely that this is associated with cell death, we presume expression is being induced in this structure, perhaps as a function of arousal. In development, constitutive expression of *fos–lac* Z is seen in mitral cells of the olfactory bulb, CA1 pyramidal neurons, and neurons of the parafascicular nucleus from the day of birth to about day 10. Additional sites of transient ex-

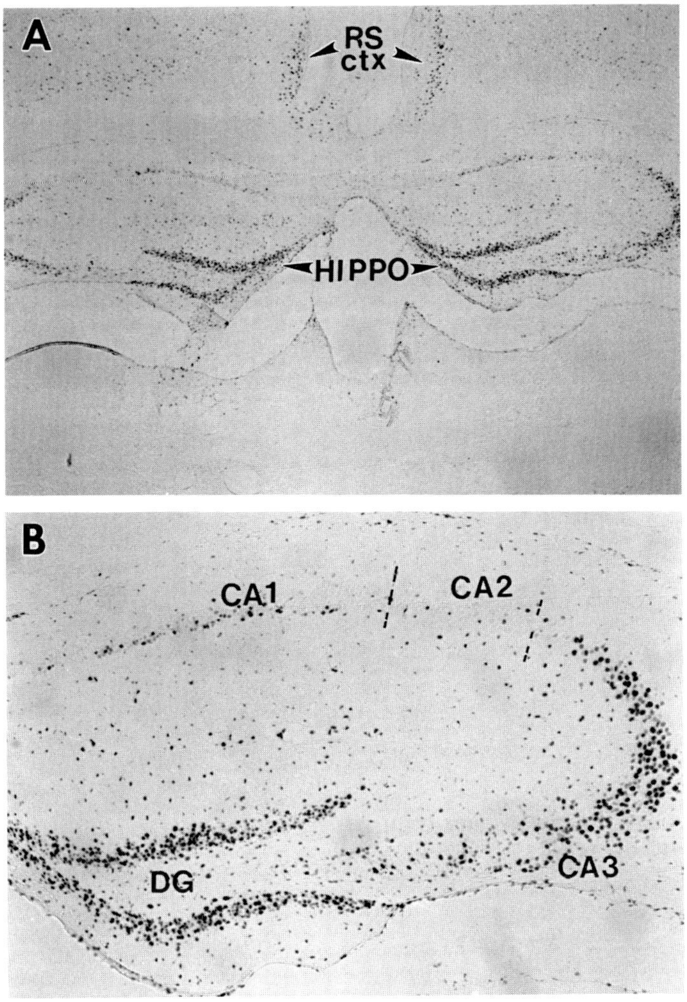

FIG. 1. Induction of *fos–lac* Z after seizure. (**A**) Two hours after kainic acid (KA) seizure, the majority of cells in the hippocampus (HIPPO) express *fos–lac* Z. Scattered *fos–lac* Z-positive cells are also noted in the cerebral and retrosplenial (RS ctx) cortices. (**B**) Higher-power photomicrograph of **A.** In the hippocampus, almost all cells of the dentate gyrus (DG) express the transgene. In the pyramidal cell layer, CA3 and CA1 contain *fos–lac* Z-positive neurons, whereas those in CA2 are *fos–lac* Z-negative. This pattern mirrors the known neurotoxicity profile of KA in hippocampus and presumably reflects the distribution of kainate-type glutamate receptors. Magnification: (**A**) ×45; (**B**) ×105.

pression are seen, particularly in the developing cerebellum, where cells within the inner granular layer express the transgene.

Different types of stimuli resulted in transient but distinct patterns of transgene expression in the CNS. In general these patterns agreed with those reported on the basis of immunohistochemistry (see Fig. 1). However, some differences were observed, which we attribute to the detection of Fras by the antisera (23). In addition to chemoconvulsant seizures, induction of the transgene can be elicited with amphetamines and cocaine as well as by photic stimulation (23) in the nighttime; i.e., physiological stimuli as well as pharmacological ones can induce the gene. We are now extending this study by constructing transgenic mice that have point mutations in the promoter elements of the transgene. Since individual elements seem to confer inducibility by particular second messenger pathways, this may provide a means to obtain some indication of the signaling cascades operating in particular neurons in a specific response. For example, what second messengers are involved in coupling photic stimulation to *fos* expression in the suprachiasmatic nucleus?

Finally, we have made primary neuronal cultures and stable cell lines from the transgenic mice. These can be used to gain insights into which growth factors or neurotransmitters are acting on a particular cell type in culture. It also provides a means to analyze the interaction of other genes with the cIE gene response by transfecting them into stable cell lines from these mice.

SUMMARY

Cellular immediate-early genes are rapidly induced by a diverse range of agents and conditions. Since many cIE genes encode known or potential transcription factors, they are believed to couple extracellular stimuli to long-lasting alterations in cellular phenotype through the regulation of gene transcription. In addition, the localization of the products of cIE genes has been used as a method for determining the cellular sites of action of particular agents in the nervous system. However, the methods of analysis are tedious, and the results may be ambiguous because of cross-reaction of reagents with related proteins. To further the utility of this approach, a bacterial gene encoding β-galactosidase (*lac* Z) has been fused, in frame, into the fourth exon of *c-fos*, and this *fos–lac* Z fusion gene has been introduced into the germ line of mice. We have analyzed the expression of β-galactosidase (under the control of the *c-fos* promoter) in the developing and adult nervous systems of these transgenic mice. As far as can be determined, the constitutive and stimulated expression of the transgene accurately reflects the expression of cognate *c-fos* in both cultured cells and the intact animal. This study has also revealed novel sites of constitutive and induced expression of *c-fos* that were overlooked using conventional analysis. In particular, constitutive expression of *c-fos* is associated with cells that are entering terminal differentiation and are destined to die. In addition, induced expression of the transgene in adult brain mirrors the pattern of neurotoxicity elicited by kainic acid.

In the future, we hope to construct transgenic mice that have a dominant-negative supressor of Fos action driven by the c-*fos* promoter. It is hoped that such mice can lead to an unambiguous understanding of the role Fos fulfills *in vivo*.

REFERENCES

1. Hayward M, Curran T, Morgan JI. Immediate-early genes: their involvement in physiological and pathological responses in the nervous system. *NIDA Tech Rev* [*in press*].
2. Lau LF, Nathans D. Expression of a set of growth-related immediate-early genes in BALB/c 3T3 cells: coordinate regulation with c-*fos* or c-*myc*. *Proc Natl Acad Sci USA* 1987;84:1182–1186.
3. Curran T, Morgan JI. Memories of *fos*. *BioEssays* 1987;7:255–258.
4. Morgan JI, Curran T. Stimulus–transcription coupling in neurons; role of cellular immediate-early genes. *Trends Neurosci* 1989;12:459–462.
5. Morgan JI, Curran T. Stimulus–transcription coupling in the nervous system: involvement of the inducible proto-oncogenes *fos* and *jun*. *Annu Rev Neurosci* 1991;14:421–451.
6. Sonnenberg JL, Macgregor-Leon PF, Curran T, Morgan JI. Dynamic alterations occur in the levels and composition of transcription factor AP-1 complexes after seizure. *Neuron* 1989;3:359–365.
7. Morgan JI, Cohen DR, Hempstead JL, Curran T. Mapping patterns of c-*fos* expression in the central nervous system after seizure. *Science* 1987;237: 192–197.
8. Curran T. The *fos* oncogene. In: Reddy EP, Skalka AM, eds. *The oncogene handbook*. Amsterdam: Elsevier; 1988:307–325.
9. Greenberg ME, Greene LA, Ziff EB. Nerve growth factor and epidermal growth factor induce rapid transient changes in proto-oncogene transcription in PC12 cells. *J Biol Chem* 1985;260:14101–14110.
10. Curran T, Franza BR Jr. Fos and Jun: the AP-1 connection. *Cell* 1988;55:395–397.
11. Kerppola TK, Curran T. Transcription factor inter-

actions: basics on zippers. *Curr Opin Struct Biol* 1991;1:71–79.
12. Hai T, Curran T. Cross-family dimerization of transcription factors Fos/Jun and ATF/CREB alters DNA binding specificity. *Proc Natl Acad Sci USA* 1991;88:1–5.
13. Sonnenberg JL, Rauscher FJ III, Morgan JI, Curran T. Regulation of proenkephalin by proto-oncogenes *fos* and *jun*. *Science* 1989;246:1622–1625.
14. Morgan JI, Curran T. Proto-oncogene transcription factors and epilepsy. *Trends Pharmacol Sci* 1991;12:343–349.
15. Gall CM, Isackson PJ. Limbic seizures increase neuronal production of messenger RNA for nerve growth factor. *Science* 1989;245:758–761.
16. Zafra F, Hengerer B, Leibrock J, et al. Activity-dependent regulation of BDNF and NGF mRNAs in the rat hippocampus is mediated by non-NMDA glutamate receptors. *EMBO J* 1990;9:3545–3550.
17. Ernfors P, Bengzon J, Kokaia Z, et al. Increased levels of messenger RNAs for neurotrophic factors in the brain during kindling epileptogenesis. *Neuron* 1991;7:165–176.
18. Gall CM, Murray K, Isackson PJ. Kainic acid-induced seizures stimulate increased expression of nerve growth factor mRNA in rat hippocampus. *Mol Brain Res* 1991;9:113–123.
19. Hengerer B, Lindholm D, Heumann R, et al. Lesion-induced increase in nerve growth factor mRNA is mediated by c-*fos*. *Proc Natl Acad Sci USA* 1990;87:3899–3903.
20. Sutula T, He XX, Cavasos J, Scott G. Synaptic reorganization in the hippocampus induced by abnormal functional activity. *Science* 1988;239:1147–1150.
21. Sutula T, Cascino G, Cavazos J, et al. Mossy fiber synaptic reorganization in the epileptic human temporal lobe. *Ann Neurol* 1989;26:321–330.
22. Schilling K, Luk D, Morgan JI, Curran T. Regulation of a *fos–lac* Z fusion gene: a paradigm for quantitative analysis of stimulus–transcription coupling. *Proc Natl Acad Sci USA* 1991;88:5665–5669.
23. Smeyne RJ, Schilling K, Robertson L, et al. *fos–lac* Z transgenic mice: mapping sites of gene expression in the central nervous system. *Neuron* 1992; 8:13–23.

Advances in Neurology, Vol. 59, edited by
Fredrick J. Seil. Raven Press, Ltd.,
New York © 1993.

26

Stress (Heat Shock) Protein Accumulation in the Central Nervous System

Its Relationship to Cell Stress and Damage

*Michael Tytell, †M. F. Barbe, and ‡I. R. Brown

**Department of Neurobiology and Anatomy, Bowman Gray School of Medicine, Wake Forest University, Winston-Salem, North Carolina 27157-1010; †Department of Physical Therapy, Temple University, Philadelphia, Pennsylvania 19140; and ‡Department of Zoology, University of Toronto, Toronto, Ontario MIC 1A4, Canada*

Ritossa (1), working with polytene chromosomes of salivary glands from *Drosophila* larvae, observed that puffs, reflecting mRNA transcription in specific regions of the chromosomes, could be reproducibly induced by exposing the tissue to a few minutes of elevated temperature. Ritossa also found that those chromosomal puffs could be induced by a variety of other metabolic stressors such as anoxia, 2,4-dinitrophenol, sodium salicylate, and sodium azide, so even from these first observations, it was clear that the response was to metabolic stress in general and not specific to hyperthermia. For some time, this phenomenon was used as a tool by *Drosophila* geneticists to investigate the factors involved in the turning on of stress genes. It was not until about a decade later that Tissières (2) related the appearance of those puffs to the production of a small family of proteins, which were named heat shock proteins (hsps). Within just a few more years, the heat shock response was found to occur in a wide variety of organisms (3), and, most significantly, the new proteins induced by the heat and other metabolic stressors in all the organisms studied appeared to have an unusually high degree of homology (4). Even the proteins induced in *E. coli* and mammalian cells had about 50% overlap in their amino acid sequences (5). Thus, the heat shock protein response is highly conserved across divergent species and appears to be quite old phylogenetically.

Once it became clear that hyperthermia and many other kinds of metabolic stressors could elicit similar kinds of changes in gene expression and protein synthesis in the treated cells, the study of the hsp response expanded rapidly to include many types of prokaryotic and eukaryotic cells (6). Presently, hsps can be divided into about six different classes based on apparent denatured molecular weights, ranging from the small hsps at 20 to 30 kD to the large hsp at about 110 kD (7). Of these, the 70-kD hsps have been the most extensively studied, in part because the high level of homology of the nucleotide sequence of the genes and corresponding homology of the proteins have simplified the application of cDNA, riboprobe, and antibody probes across species. Additionally, the 70-kD hsp has been easier to purify from tissues than the others, in part because of its high affinity for ATP (8).

The hsp70 can be found in many normal

cells and tissues as the so-called constitutive form, frequently referred to as hsp73 to reflect its apparent denatured molecular weight (9). The form of hsp70 that is markedly induced in stressed cells has been designated hsp72, to reflect the fact that it is the product of a different gene than hsp73 and that it has a slightly lower apparent molecular weight (9). This nomenclature has become confusing, however, because the reported molecular weights for these proteins can vary by a few thousand between organisms and as a function of differences in gel electrophoretic conditions. Therefore, in the rest of this chapter, where it is necessary to distinguish between the two forms, hsp70c will refer to the constitutive form and hsp70i to the inducible one.

The presence of hsp70 in normal, unstressed cells and tissues suggested that it had a role in normal cell metabolism in addition to its activity during metabolic stress. Two normal functions have been implicated. First, hsp70 appears to serve as the clathrin-uncoating ATPase; that is, it catalyzes the disassembly of the clathrin coats from coated vesicles in an ATP-dependent manner (10,11). Second, for proteins that are synthesized on free polysomes and then imported into the mitochondrion or the endoplasmic reticulum posttranslationally, hsp70 serves as a "chaperone," binding to them from the time that they are synthesized until they reach their destinations within the organelle lumen. This function also requires ATP and has generated another name for the hsp70 family, the chaperonins (12–14).

Though initially the clathrin-uncoating and chaperone functions of hsp70 seemed more puzzling than helpful in suggesting what the protein might do to help cells under metabolic stress, some additional work revealed a common thread. Many types of metabolic stress lead to the formation of proteins with abnormal structures and to denaturation of many preexisting proteins. The hsp70 is able somehow to recognize such abnormal proteins and bind to them (15,16). *In vitro* experiments with cytosolic proteins and individual model enzymes subjected to heat showed that added hsp70 made them more resistant to heat denaturation and could even restore the activity of an enzyme that was partially denatured (17–19); the latter required the presence of ATP. The general theme one can extract from these observations is that hsp70 can bind to both normal and abnormal cellular proteins in a way that influences the tertiary structure of the target protein. In a stressed cell, perhaps this activity of hsp70 can prevent the inactivation of vital cellular enzymes from reaching catastrophic levels, rendering the cell stress tolerant.

The central nervous system (CNS) is especially sensitive to metabolic stress because of its high rate of energy consumption. Thus, it is not surprising that hsp70c is relatively abundant there, constituting about 1% of the total protein found in axons (20). Observations made during the last decade have shown clearly that the increased transcription of hsp70 mRNA and accumulation of the protein itself are fundamental aspects of the CNS response to injury, whether the injury is physical trauma, ischemia, or chemical toxicity (21). We have proposed that hsp70 may be important in preventing the death of injured neural cells, and our work has been aimed at understanding how to promote the CNS stress protein response in order to reduce posttraumatic neuron loss.

We have chosen the retina as the model system for this work for a number of reasons. First, it is the most easily accessed part of the CNS and includes most of the same variety of cell types as the brain, such as glia (Müller cells and some astrocytes), neurons with short axons (amacrine, bipolar, and horizontal cells), and neurons with long axons (retinal ganglion cells). Second, damage of graded severity can be produced easily in the albino rat retina by exposing the animal to various intensities of light for variable periods of time. Third, the extent of damage is relatively easy to measure: the irreversibly damaged photoreceptor cells (PRCs) are cleared from the retina within 2 weeks after light damage, and the number of surviving PRCs can be determined from standard histological sec-

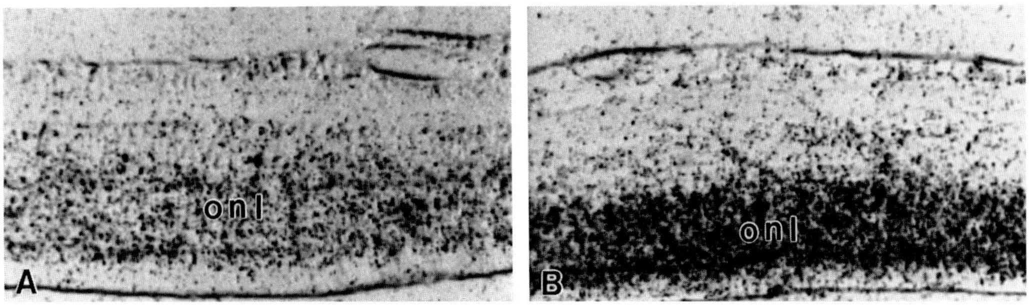

FIG. 1. Autoradiography of retinal sections from a control rat (**A**) and another 18 hr after heat stress (**B**) after *in situ* hybridization using an α-^{35}S-uridine triphosphate-labeled riboprobe for hsp70 mRNA. The silver grains (*black dots*) reflect the distribution and relative abundance of the message in the various layers of the retinas. Most of the message is found in the layer containing mainly the photoreceptor cells, the outer nuclear layer (onl) in both the control and heat-stressed retinas. Photographed at about ×200 magnification.

tions by manual or computer-assisted measurements of the thickness or area of the PRC layer. Finally, the administration of agents designed to alter the hsp response is simplified by the fact that the retina is enclosed within the eyeball.

OBSERVATIONS

Induction of hsp70 mRNA

The distribution of hsp70 mRNA in the retina was examined by *in situ* hybridization as a function of time after the hyperthermic stress. The *in situ* hybridization procedure and characteristics of the probe were as described previously (22–24), and hyperthermia was produced by placing each pentobarbital-anesthetized rat in a 42°C chamber until its rectal temperature reached 41 to 42°C and remained there for 15 min (25). Figure 1 illustrates the patterns of silver grains reflecting mRNA localization after *in situ* hybridization in a control retina and one collected from a rat 18 hr after hyperthermia. The probe used binds to both the constitutive and inducible mRNAs and so reflects the changes in both forms. There was a relatively low level of message present in the control retina, and this increased dramatically after

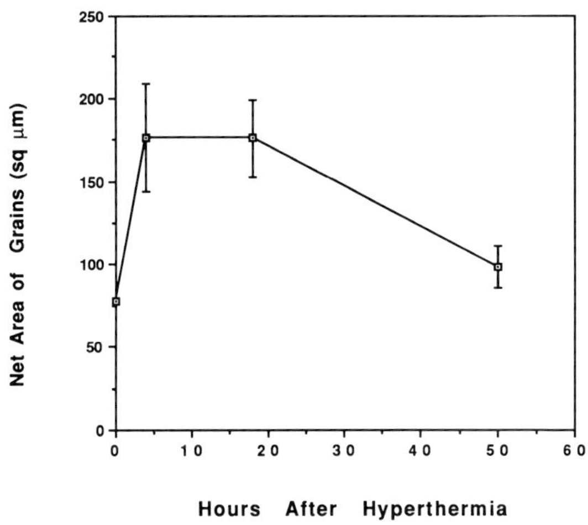

FIG. 2. Quantification of the numbers of silver grains overlying the photoreceptor cell layer in retinas from rats at increasing times after heat stress. Each point in the graph represents the mean (±S.E.M.) of the number of silver grains above background at three regions in one retina at each time. The amount of hsp70 mRNA approximately doubled within 4 hr of the heat stress and remained at that level through at least 18 hr. By 48 hr after the stress, the mRNA level had returned to the control level. The *in situ* hybridization was replicated in a second set of rats treated in the same manner; these demonstrated a very similar distribution of hsp70 mRNA but were not quantitatively analyzed.

hyperthermia. However, the distribution of mRNA in the various retinal layers did not change in response to the hyperthermia. In both the control and heat-stressed retinas, the major proportion of the mRNA was located in the photoreceptor cell (PRC) layer. Nonspecific mRNA binding and the background level of silver grains were evaluated in additional retinal sections reacted with the sense form of the riboprobe and were insignificant (data not shown).

The relative changes in posthyperthermia hsp70 mRNA of the PRC layer were quantified by counting silver grains per unit area using a computer and video-based morphometry system. The results are depicted in Fig. 2. The hsp70 mRNA increased rapidly to about twofold above control in 4 hr after the heat stress and remained that high through 18 hr. By 50 hr, the hsp70 mRNA level had declined back to that of the control. None of the other layers of the retina demonstrated a significant induction of hsp70 mRNA (data not shown).

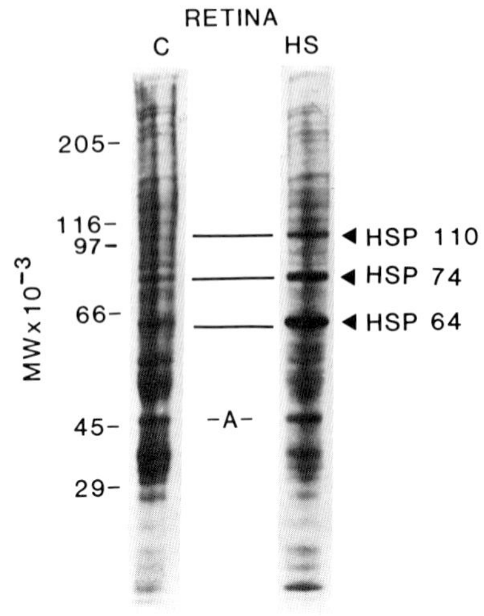

FIG. 3. The pattern of newly synthesized ^{35}S-methionine-labeled polypeptides from a control rat retina (C) and another at 2 hr after heat stress (HS). The numbers along the left indicate the positions and sizes of molecular weight standards. In the HS retina, three bands corresponding to expected positions of known hsps were much more highly labeled than in the C retina. The number designations of the hsp bands are the approximate molecular weights. Additional analyses confirmed that hsp64 was a member of the hsp70 family (see text). The 45-kD band indicated by A is actin and is an example of a protein whose synthesis was not greatly altered by heat stress. This comparison of C and HS retinas is based on loading equal amounts of ^{35}S-methionine-labeled protein from each sample, and the samples were run on the same gel.

Synthesis of hsp70

The synthesis of hsp70 was monitored by labeling newly synthesized retinal proteins via an intravitreal microinjection of ^{35}S-methionine at increasing intervals after the hyperthermic stress, as described (25). The retinas were prepared for SDS-PAGE at 2 or 4 hr after the radioisotope injection, and the labeled proteins were visualized by fluorography. An example of such fluorographs is shown in Fig. 3, illustrating retinal labeled proteins from a control rat and one that was given an intravitreal injection of isotope at 2 hr after hyperthermia and sacrificed 4 hr later, thus reflecting protein synthesis during the 2- to 6-hr period after heat stress. Three polypeptide bands, designated hsp64, -74, and -110, were much more radioactive in the retina from the heat-stressed rat than in that of the control. Subsequent analysis of the labeled retinas with the antibody specific for hsp70i confirmed that the 64-kD band in Fig. 3 was immunologically equivalent to hsp70 (data not shown). Its lower apparent molecular weight was at least in part a result of the electrophoresis sample buffer used (unpublished observations).

To examine the time course of the changes in retinal hsp70 synthesis, retinas were labeled and subjected to gel electrophoresis at 0 to 50 hr after the hyperthermia. The density of the hsp70 band on each fluorograph was measured using an LKB Ultrascan laser densitometer. The results are summarized in Fig. 4 and demonstrate that hsp70 synthesis was significantly elevated at 2 and 4 hr after hyperthermia. Because the time between the intravitreal injection of radioisotope and collec-

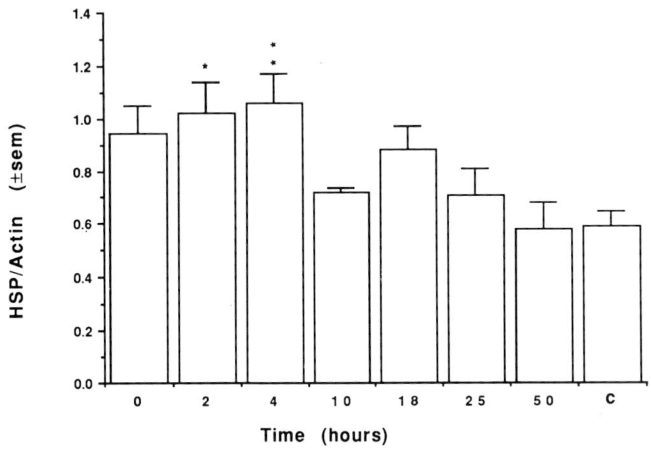

FIG. 4. Relative changes in retinal hsp70 synthesis with time after heat stress. The patterns of labeled polypeptides synthesized in retinas collected from rats at increasing times after heat stress were quantified by scanning laser densitometry of the fluorographs. The density of the hsp70 band was divided by that of the actin band in the same sample to obtain the relative change in hsp70 synthesis (HSP/Actin). Significant increases in hsp70 synthesis were observed at 2 and 4 hr after heat stress ($^*p < 0.05$; $^{**}p < 0.01$) compared to control retinas (C, the last bar in the series). $N = 4$ to 5 for each time.

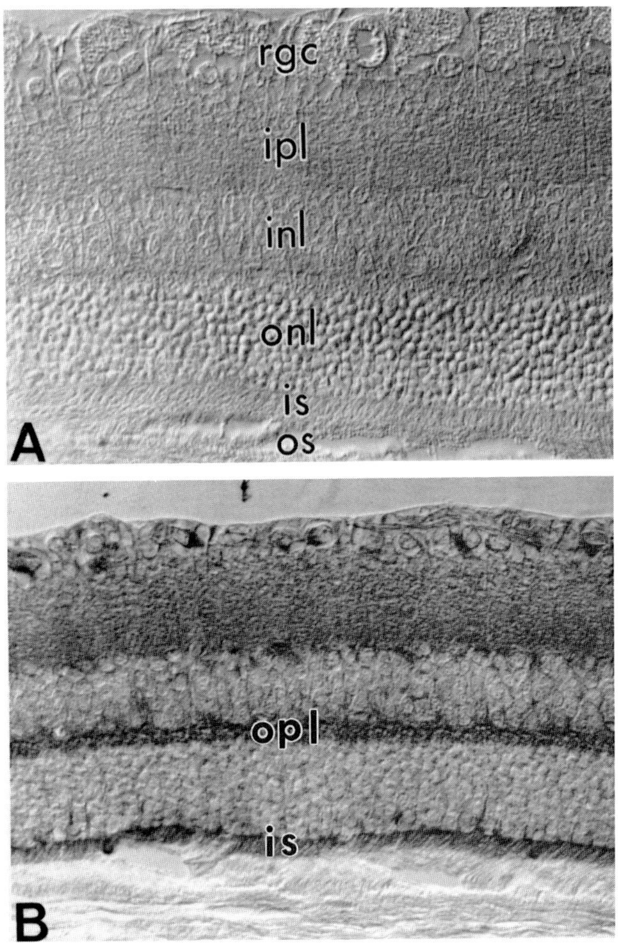

FIG. 5. Micrographs of the immune reaction product reflecting the distribution of hsp70i in a control retina and one from a rat heat stressed 18 hr earlier. Compared to the control (**A**), the heat-stressed retina (**B**) shows a much greater amount of hsp70i immunoreaction product in all layers, especially the inner segment (is) and outer plexiform layer (opl). Note that even after heat stress, neither of the two major nuclear layers of the retina, the outer nuclear layer (onl) containing the photoreceptor nuclei or the inner nuclear layer (inl) containing the nuclei of retinal interneurons, accumulates very much hsp70i relative to the cytoplasmic layers [is, opl, and inner plexiform layer (ipl)]. Other layers shown are the outer segment (os) and the retinal ganglion cell layer (rgc). Photographed at a magnification of about ×200 using differential interference contrast optics.

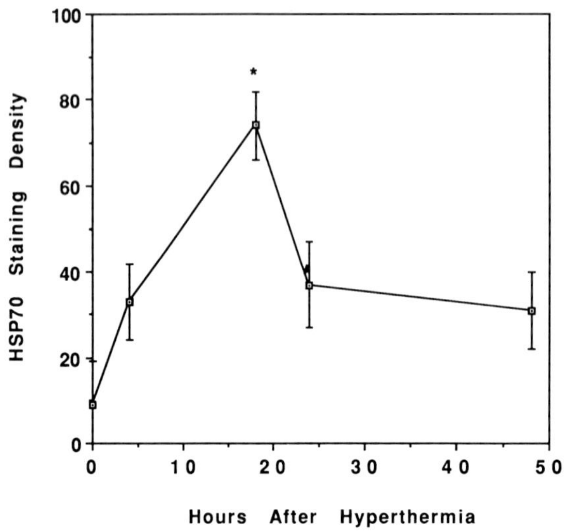

FIG. 6. Mean density (±S.E.M.) of hsp70i immunoreaction product in the inner segment layer of retinas collected at increasing times after heat stress. The accumulation of hsp70i peaked at 18 hr after heat stress ($p <$ 0.01) and then declined at 24 hr to a level not significantly greater than control. The 0-hr group was comprised of unheated control rats. N = 4 or 5 rats per interval.

tion of the retinas was 2 hr, the actual time of elevated hsp70 synthesis was through at least 6 hr after hyperthermia.

Accumulation of hsp70

To determine if the increased synthesis of hsp70 was occurring in the PRC layer where most of the elevated mRNA was located, we probed retinas from control and heat-stressed rats with an anti-hsp70i monoclonal antibody (24,25). The bound antibody was detected with a horseradish peroxidase secondary antibody system. This immunohistochemical analysis revealed that there was a very low basal level of hsp70i present in several layers of the retina (Fig. 5): photoreceptor inner segments, outer plexiform layer (opl), inner plexiform layer (ipl), and in the cell bodies of some retinal ganglion cells (rgc). When the procedure was repeated on a retinal section from a rat that had been heat stressed 18 hr earlier, an increase in immunoreactive hsp70i was detected in all retinal layers (Fig. 5) but was particularly pronounced in the inner segments and opl, which are the two layers on either side of the photoreceptor nuclear layer (onl), where much of the cytoplasm of the photoreceptors is located. Quantification of the density of immunoreaction product in the inner segment layer was performed using the Bioquant image analysis system. In retinas collected at increasing intervals after heat stress, we found that hsp70 accumulated to maximal levels by 18 hr and then declined back toward the control level by 50 hr (Fig. 6).

Photoreceptor Stress Tolerance

In the albino rat, graded destruction of PRCs can be produced by a single 24-hr exposure to light brighter than the level to which it is acclimated (26–29). The biochemical basis for such light-induced PRC death is not completely understood, but it is clear that it involves photooxidation and the generation of free radicals; the effects of the light are exacerbated by elimination of the dark period, during which repair can occur. We used a 24-hr exposure to 250 foot-candles of illuminance, which is roughly equivalent to a bright, sunny day, as the test stress to determine if the heat-induced elevation in retinal hsp70 correlated with increased resistance of the PRCs to light damage. Groups of rats were first heat stressed and then exposed to the light at intervals ranging from 0 to 50 hr later, the same time course during which retinal hsp70 content rose and fell (Fig. 6). The

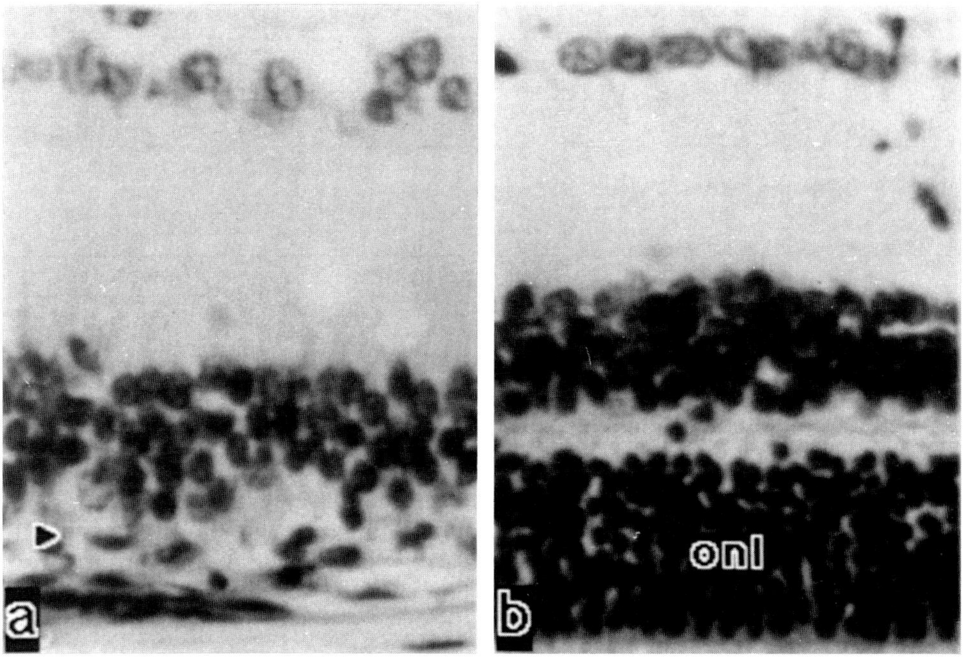

FIG. 7. (**a**) Retina of a rat heat stressed and exposed to light simultaneously. (**b**) Retina from a rat heat stressed 18 hr prior to light exposure. Similar regions of the superior retinas from each rat are shown. Most of the photoreceptor cell nuclei that make up the onl were destroyed in the rat subjected to heat and light together (**a;** the *arrowhead* at the lower left edge shows where that layer had been), whereas the onl from the rat with an 18-hr interval between the heat and light is close to normal thickness (**b**). Shown are 7-μm sections of hematoxylin and eosin-stained retinas photographed at about ×200 magnification. (Modified from Barbe et al., ref. 25; copyright 1988 by the AAAS.)

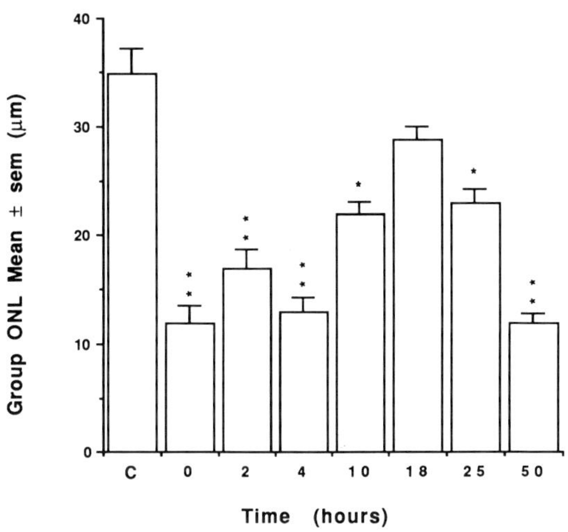

FIG. 8. Mean thickness (±S.E.M.) of the onl in retinas from control rats (C) and those that were heat stressed at various intervals prior to light exposure (250 foot-candles for 24 hr). ONL thickness is a function of the number of surviving PRCs, and it is clear that the greatest resistance of PRCs to light damage occurred when the interval between heat stress and light exposure was 10 to 25 hr. All of the light-exposed onl thickness measurements were compared statistically to those of the control group, and this comparison showed that the onl of the 18-hr post-heat-stress group had as many surviving PRCs as the control (*$p < 0.05$; **$p < 0.01$; $n = 4$ per group). (Reproduced from Barbe et al., ref. 25; copyright 1988 by the AAAS.)

rats were returned to standard housing and cyclic illumination for 2 weeks to allow the PRCs killed by the light to be cleared from the retina, after which the eyes were prepared for routine light microscopy. The light micrographs shown in Fig. 7 illustrate that there was a marked increase in PRC survival when the interval between heat stress and light exposure was 18 hr. This protective effect was quantified by measuring the thickness of the PRC layer (onl) at multiple points along the superior–inferior plane and plotting the mean values as a function of time between heat stress and light exposure. As shown in Fig. 8, PRC survival was greatest when the hyperthermia–light exposure interval was 18 hr and, in fact, was not significantly different from the PRC layer thickness in rats not exposed to the damaging light. At either shorter or longer hyperthermia–light exposure intervals, PRC survival was reduced.

Administration of Exogenous hsp70

The similarity of the time course of posthyperthermic protection of the PRCs against light damage with that of hsp70 mRNA induction and the synthesis and accumulation of hsp70 suggests, but does not confirm, that hsp70 was responsible for increasing PRC stress tolerance. However, whole-body hyperthermia causes many other physiological changes that might also influence PRC stress tolerance. To obtain direct evidence for the role of hsp70 in PRC survival, we considered various ways in which retinal hsp70 might be increased without altering the physiology of the rest of the animal. From work done in another system, we suspected that cells might be able to take up hsp70 from the extracellular environment (30). To test this possibility in the retina, we used purified hsp70 provided by D. J. Gower (University of Okla-

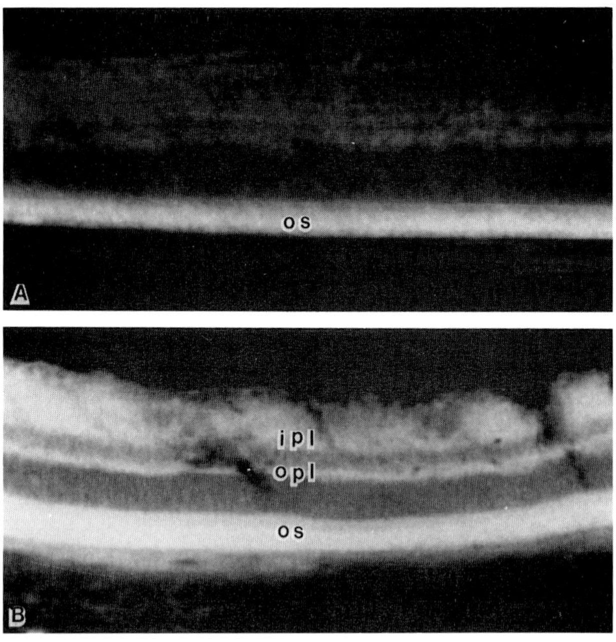

FIG. 9. Epifluorescence micrographs illustrating retinal uptake of fluorescent material after an intravitreal injection of fluorescently tagged hsp70. In the control retina (**A**), autofluorescence of the outer segments (os) of the photoreceptors can be seen, probably a consequence of the photopigments present there. The lower panel (**B**) shows the fluorescence visible in the inner (ipl) and outer plexiform (opl) layers of the retina 4 hr after the injection of fluorescent hsp70. Photographed at about ×100 magnification.

homa Health Science Center, Oklahoma City, OK), who prepared it from bovine brain according to Schlossman et al. (31) and Schmidt and Rothman (32). The protein was fluorescently tagged using 7-amino-4-methy-coumarin-3-acetate succinimidyl ester following recommendations of the manufacturer (Molecular Probes, Inc., Eugene, OR). This tagged hsp70 was microinjected into the vitreal chamber of the eye, and, 4 hr later, the eyes were collected and prepared for frozen sectioning, and 20-μm sections were examined by epifluorescence microscopy (354 nm excitation, 442 nm emission). Figure 9 shows that fluorescent material was indeed taken up by the retina.

If material taken up by the retina was biologically active hsp70, then the PRCs should show increased resistance to light damage. This point was examined in the following way. Three groups of rats were given intravitreal injections of solutions of 2, 10, or 20 μg of unlabeled, purified hsp70 in one eye and either the buffered saline vehicle or 20 μg of bovine serum albumin (BSA) in the other eye. To control for any nonspecific effects of injecting bovine protein into the eye, another group was given 20 μg of BSA in one eye and saline in the other. One additional control group received no intravitreal injections. Four hours after the injections, each group was exposed to about 175 foot-candles of light for 24 hr. Two weeks later, the retinas were prepared for light microscopy, and the PRC layer in each eye was measured. To determine if the injected hsp70 or BSA increased PRC survival, the difference in PRC layer areas between the two eyes was calculated. Thus, a protective effect would yield a significant positive number, and no effect would yield a number not significantly different from zero. The results are shown in Fig. 10. Only the group that received 10 μg of hsp70 in one eye showed a significant increase in PRC survival. Surprisingly, the 20-μg dose of hsp70 was ineffective, suggesting that a higher concentration of hsp70 may negate its cytoprotective effects.

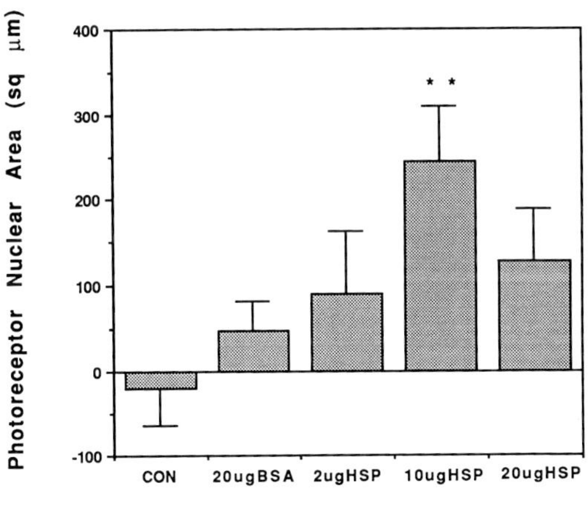

FIG. 10. Effects of intravitreal injections of BSA or hsp70 on PRC survival after light exposure. Since in each rat one eye served as a control and the other as the experimental eye, the data are reported as the mean differences (±S.E.M.) in onl area between the eyes. BSA had no effect on PRC survival, whereas 10 μg hsp70 increased survival significantly (**$p < 0.01$). Twenty micrograms of hsp70 did not significantly improve PRC survival (see Discussion). The number of rats in each group was as follows: CON, 2; 20 μg BSA, 4; 2 μg hsp70, 3; 10 μg hsp70, 3; 20 μg hsp70, 4.

DISCUSSION

Our results show that a brief period of elevated body temperature, within the range of that possible in fever produced by infection, is sufficient to elicit the full repertoire of the stress protein response in the retina, beginning with the rise in hsp70 mRNA and leading to increased synthesis and accumulation of the protein in a concordant fashion. That these changes are more than just epiphenomena of metabolically stressed tissue is supported by the close correlation of increased PRC resistance to light damage with the peak in accumulation of retinal hsp70. Similar experiments using a conditioning heat or ischemic stress prior to a more severe stress also have demonstrated increased cellular stress tolerance in the heart (33) and brain (34,35). All of these results implicate the induction of the hsp70 response as an important element in the ability of cells to survive injury or abnormal conditions, but the evidence remains indirect because of all the other physiological changes that occur in an animal subjected to hyperthermic or ischemic stress. To obtain direct proof of the role of hsp70 in the survival of neurons and/or glia after CNS injury will require a means of locally and specifically elevating cellular hsp70 content. That requirement is the reason we have begun to explore the possibility that exogenous hsp70 administered to a tissue can be taken up and utilized by the cells in the same way as the endogenously produced protein. The initial results reported here on the protective effect of intravitreally injected hsp70 are promising, but much more work remains to be done to determine how the exogenous hsp70 is functioning. We are encouraged by other work on cultured smooth muscle cells that also indicates that they can take up exogenous hsp70 and exhibit increased stress tolerance (36,37).

A better understanding of the contribution of hsp70 and the other members of the hsp family to the survival of damaged neurons may make it possible to manipulate this response at the genetic or protein level to promote neuron survival and regeneration after trauma or disease.

ACKNOWLEDGMENTS

The authors thank C. R. Hollman for help in preparing the figures included in this chapter and D. J. Gower, M.D., for supplying the purified hsp70 needed for some of the experiments. The work was supported by NEI grant EY-07616 to M. Tytell and a grant from the Medical Council of Canada to I. R. Brown.

REFERENCES

1. Ritossa FM. A new puffing system induced by temperature shock and DNP in *Drosophila*. *Experientia* 1962;18:571–573.
2. Tissières A, Mitchell HK, Tracy UM. Protein synthesis in salivary glands of *Drosophila melanogaster*. *J Mol Biol* 1974;84:389–398.
3. Schlesinger MJ, Ashburner M, Tissières A, eds. *Heat shock—from bacteria to man*. Cold Spring Harbor, NY: Cold Spring Harbor Laboratory; 1982.
4. Morimoto RI, Milarski KL. Expression and function of vertebrate hsp70 genes. In: Morimoto RI, Tissières A, Georgopoulos C, eds. *Stress proteins in biology and medicine*. Cold Spring Harbor, NY: Cold Spring Harbor Laboratory; 1990:323–359.
5. Lindquist S, Craig EA. The heat-shock proteins. *Annu Rev Genet* 1988;22:631–677.
6. Nover L, ed. *Heat shock response*, Boca Raton, FL: CRC Press; 1991.
7. Morimoto RI, Tissières A, Georgopoulos C. The stress response, function of the proteins, and perspectives. In: Morimoto RI, Tissières A, Georgopoulos C, eds. *Stress proteins in biology and medicine*. Cold Spring Harbor, NY: Cold Spring Harbor Laboratory, 1990:1–36.
8. Welch WJ, Feramisco JR. Rapid purification of mammalian 70,000-dalton stress proteins: affinity of the proteins for nucleotides. *Mol Cell Biol* 1985;5:1229–1237.
9. Welch WJ, Garrels GP, Thomas GP, et al. Biochemical characterization of the mammalian stress proteins and identification of two stress proteins as glucose and Ca^{2+} ionophore regulated proteins. *J Biol Chem* 1983;258:7102–7111.
10. Ungewickell E. The 70-kD mammalian heat shock proteins are structurally and functionally related to the uncoating protein that releases clathrin triskelia from coated vesicles. *EMBO J* 1985;4:3385–3391.
11. Chappell TG, Welch WJ, Schlossman DM, et al. Uncoating ATPase is a member of the 70 kilodalton family of stress proteins. *Cell* 1986,45:3–13.
12. Hooper C. Origami enzymes: hints of a new preoccupation for molecular chaperones. *J NIH Res* 1990;2:63–66.
13. Flynn GC, Chappell TG, Rothman JE. Peptide binding and release by proteins implicated as catalysts of protein assembly. *Science* 1989;245:385–390.
14. Hartl F-U, Neupert W. Protein sorting to mitochondria: evolutionary conservations of folding and assembly. *Science* 1990;247:930–938.
15. Welch WJ, Mizzen LA, Arrigo A-P. Structure and function of mammalian stress proteins. In: Pardue ML, Feramisco JR, Lindquist S, eds. *Stress-induced proteins*. New York: Alan R. Liss; 1989:187–202.
16. Palleros DR, Welch WJ, Fink AL. Interaction of hsp70 with unfolded proteins: effects of temperature and nucleotides on the kinetics of binding. *Proc Natl Acad Sci USA* 1991;88:5719–5723.
17. Stevens FA, Gower DJ. *In vitro* protection of bovine brain supernate proteins by exogenous heat shock protein-70. *Soc Neurosci Abstr* 1991;17:164.
18. Goloubinoff P, Christeller JT, Gatenby AA, et al. Reconstruction of active dimeric ribulose bisphosphate carboxylase from an unfolded state depends on two chaperonin proteins and Mg-ATP. *Nature* 1989;342:884–888.
19. Skowyra D, Georgopoulos C, Zylicz M. The *E. coli* dnaK gene product, the hsp70 homolog, can reactivate heat-inactivated RNA polymerase in an ATP hydrolysis-dependent manner. *Cell* 1990;62: 939–944.
20. de Waegh S, Brady ST. Axonal transport of a

clathrin uncoating ATPase (HSC70): a role for HSC70 in the modulation of coated vesicle assembly *in vivo*. *J Neurosci Res* 1989;23:433–440.
21. Brown IR. Induction of heat shock (stress) genes in the mammalian brain by hyperthermia and other traumatic events: a current perspective. *J Neurosci Res* 1990;27:247–255.
22. Perry MD, Moran LA. Isolation of a mouse heat shock gene (hsp68) by recombinational screening. *Gene* 1987;51:227–236.
23. Sprang GK, Brown IR. Selective induction of a heat shock gene in fibre tracts and cerebellar neurons of the rabbit brain detected by *in situ* hybridization. *Mol Brain Res* 1987;3:89–93.
24. Yamaguchi K, Barbe MF, Brown IR, et al. Induction of stress (heat shock) protein 70 and its mRNA in rat corneal epithelium hyperthermia. *Curr Eye Res* 1990;9:913–918.
25. Barbe MF, Tytell M, Gower DJ, et al. Hyperthermia protects against light damage in the rat retina. *Science* 1988;241:1817–1820.
26. Noell WK, Walker VS, Bok SK, et al. Retinal damage by light in rats. *Invest Ophthalmol Vis Sci* 1966;5:450–473.
27. O'Steen WK, Anderson KV, Shear CR. Photoreceptor degeneration in albino rats: dependency on age. *Invest Ophthalmol Vis Sci* 1974;13:334–339.
28. O'Steen WK, Donnelly JE. Antagonistic effects of adrenalectomy and ether/surgical stress on light-induced photoreceptor damage. *Invest Ophthalmol Vis Sci* 1982;22:1–7.
29. Duncan TE, O'Steen WK. The diurnal susceptibility of rat retinal photoreceptors to light-induced damage. *Exp Eye Res* 1985;41:497–507.
30. Tytell M, Greenberg SG, Lasek RJ. Heat shock-like protein is transferred from glia to axon. *Brain Res* 1986;363:161–164.
31. Schlossman DM, Schmid SL, Braell WA, et al. An enzyme that removes clathrin coats: purification of an uncoating ATPase. *J Cell Biol* 1984;99:723–733.
32. Schmid SL, Rothman JE. Two classes of binding sites for uncoating protein in clathrin triskelions. *J Biol Chem* 1985;260:10050–10056.
33. Currie RW, Karmazyn M, Kloc M, et al. Heat shock response is associated with enhanced post-ischemic ventricular recovery. *Circ Res* 1988;63:543–549.
34. Chopp M, Chen H, Ho K-L, et al. Transient hyperthermia protects against subsequent forebrain ischemic cell damage in the rat. *Neurology* 1989;39:1396–1398.
35. Chopp M, Tidwell CD, Lee YJ, et al. Reduction of hyperthermic ischemic acidosis by a conditioning event in cats. *Stroke* 1989;20:1357–1360.
36. Johnson AD, Tytell M, Berberian PA. Exogenous 70kD heat shock protein (HSP70) is cytoprotective for oxysterol stressed aortic smooth muscle cells. *J Cell Biol* 1991;115:405a.
37. Johnson AD, Tytell M. Cytoprotective effects of 70kD heat shock protein (HSP70) on oxysterol toxicity in aortic smooth muscle cells. *FASEB J* 1992;6:A1042.

Advances in Neurology, Vol. 59, edited by
Fredrick J. Seil. Raven Press, Ltd.,
New York © 1993.

27
The Function of Phagocytic Cells in the Nervous System

Marion E. Smith

Department of Neurology, Veterans Administration Medical Center, Palo Alto, California 94304 and Stanford University School of Medicine, Stanford, California 94305

The presence of resident migratory cells with phagocytic capability has long been suspected in the central nervous system (CNS). These were described by various authors as early as 1874 as derived from the mesoderm and capable of ameboid movements. Cajal included these cells under his "third element of the central nervous system" and defined them as "small adendritic corpuscles, probably of mesodermal origin, and different from neurons and neuroglia" (1). In 1919 and the years following, one of Cajal's students, Del Rio-Hortega, undertook a thorough study of these cells. He found the "third element" of Cajal to consist of two components, one of which he named oligodendroglia and the other microglia. His conclusions were summarized in a well-known review (2), where he described microglia as motile cells that represent the reticulo-endothelial system in the CNS and showed that they could phagocytize erythrocytes and cellular remnants. He wrote that the microglia "actively intervenes in all inflammatory and necrotizing processes of the nervous tissue and it adopts, as a result of its motility and macrophagic role, elongated forms (rod cells), [and] lamellar and roundish aspects (fat granule cells)." These cells were said to arise from embryonic cells of the meninges during late stages of development and to disseminate themselves throughout the nervous system for a few days after birth and become resting microglia. Del Rio-Hortega extensively investigated microglia in their various forms in a variety of normal and pathological situations with the use of silver stains.

Much disagreement and controversy over the findings of Del Rio-Hortega arose over the ensuing years. A substantial amount of the opposition to the concept of CNS resident macrophages was related to pathological situations where the blood–brain barrier was damaged, thus allowing migration of peripheral monocytes and macrophages into the CNS parenchyma. Del Rio-Hortega showed that damage to the nervous system caused resting microglia to become activated and move toward the injury, where they phagocytized the cell debris. Some investigators were particularly critical of the stab wound experiments, concluding that the inflammatory cells were derived from the peripheral cells in the blood with little or no contribution of endogenous cells to the phagocytic population (3). Similar conclusions followed from experiments with Japanese encephalitis and retrograde degeneration of the facial nucleus after cutting the facial nerve, where the phagocytic cells appeared to be exclusively blood derived. The so-called microglioblasts were said to be precursors of three kinds of neuroglia: oligodendroglia, astrocytes, and resting microglia. The microglia were considered to be a kind of neuroglia of ectodermal origin that do not become phagocytes (4).

In recent years, the study of microglia has undergone a renaissance, largely because of the development of methods for isolating these cells from newborn rats (5). Microglia have been shown to contain nonspecific esterase activity, a property common to most macrophages, to express Fc and type 3 complement receptors and the surface antigens common to macrophages, such as Mac-1, and to phagocytize latex beads. For the most part, the findings of Del Rio-Hortega have been confirmed. Four of the remaining chapters in this volume are authored by investigators who have made major contributions to the recent explosion of new findings about these cells. The toxic properties of microglia (Giulian and Corpuz, this volume), their activation and possible priming capacity of the CNS prior to inflammation (Molleston et al., this volume), the capability of these cells to produce reactive oxygen species in the CNS (Colton and Gilbert, this volume), and their growth factors and receptors (Brosnan et al., this volume) are important new aspects of microglial function.

The possibility that resident macrophages exist in the peripheral nervous system (PNS) has received less attention. It is well established that after peripheral nerve injury the damaged segment quickly degenerates, and a new nerve regenerates. In the CNS, however, under similar circumstances, degeneration is very slow, and little if any regeneration occurs. Two of the following chapters address the mechanisms of peripheral nerve demyelination and the contributions of macrophages to nerve degeneration, demyelination, and the growth of new axons. Perry et al. compare CNS and PNS degeneration and regeneration and show evidence that macrophages play a decisive role in these processes. Friede and Brück discuss the requirements for phagocytosis of PNS myelin in Wallerian degeneration, concluding that macrophages show a spectrum of functions in the disease process.

MACROPHAGES, MICROGLIA, AND MYELIN PHAGOCYTOSIS

When Lampert and Carpenter (6) first showed that phagocytic cells are responsible for destruction of the CNS myelin sheath in experimental allergic encephalomyelitis (later a similar process was shown in multiple sclerosis), it was assumed that the macrophages were derived from the bloodstream. With the breakdown of the blood–brain barrier, monocytes were shown migrating into the CNS parenchyma. At present, the relative participation of the blood-derived macrophages and the resident microglia in the phagocytic attack is not known. In our investigations of factors affecting myelin phagocytosis, we have established an *in vitro* system in which radioactive myelin containing ^{14}C-labeled lipids is incubated with macrophages. Phagocytosis and myelin digestion are assessed by the appearance of radioactive myelin cholesterol ester (7). Very little cholesterol ester appears when rat peritoneal macrophages are incubated with untreated myelin, but if the myelin is preincubated with certain antibodies to myelin constituents and then presented to macrophages, very much more labeled cholesterol ester is produced. Preimmune serum is not nearly as active in promoting the appearance of labeled cholesterol ester. Antisera causing stimulation of cholesterol ester production include those to myelin basic protein, galactocerebroside, CNS myelin, and PNS myelin. On the other hand, antisera to proteolipid protein or to myelin-associated glycoprotein show no activity. Immunoglobulin G (IgG) prepared from the active antisera also shows stimulation of cholesterol ester production equivalent to that of the parent serum (Fig. 1). Antisera heated to destroy complement are also active, thus implicating the IgG as the ligand between the myelin and the macrophage Fc receptor. Peripheral nerve myelin appears to be phagocytized by a similar mechanism in this *in vitro* system (8). On the other hand, in their chapter Friede and Brück describe pe-

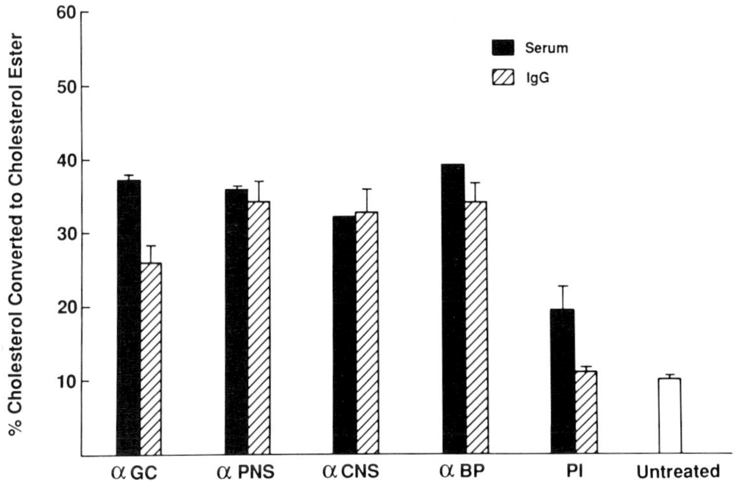

FIG. 1. Percentage of myelin cholesterol converted to cholesterol ester by cultured macrophages. Radioactive myelin is opsonized with designated antisera and applied to macrophage cultures. After 30 hr the cells plus the incubation mixture are removed, and the labeled lipids are extracted and separated by thin-layer chromatography. The cholesterol and cholesterol ester spots are recovered, and their radioactivity determined. Antisera: GC, galactocerebroside; PNS, peripheral nerve myelin; CNS, central nerve myelin; BP, myelin basic protein; PI, preimmune.

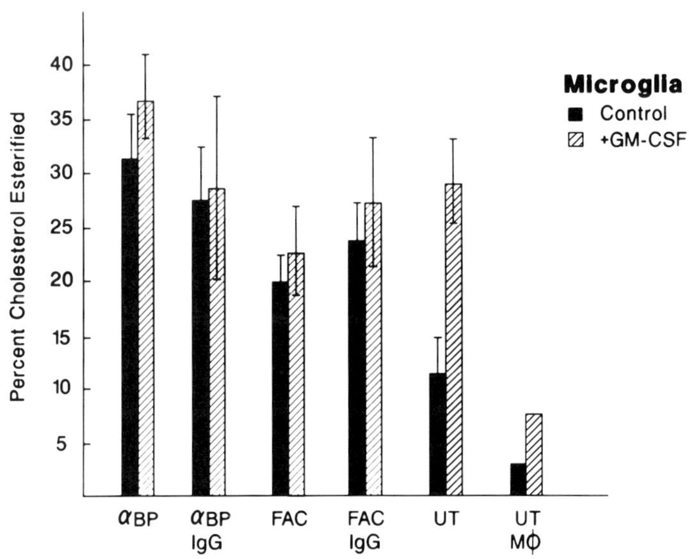

FIG. 2. Percentage of myelin cholesterol converted to cholesterol ester by microglia in culture with and without pretreatment with GM-CSF. Radioactive myelin is opsonized with sera or IgG to myelin basic protein (BP), Freund's adjuvant control serum (FAC), or left untreated (UT). Mϕ, macrophage. Values for untreated myelin incubated with peritoneal macrophages are shown for comparison.

ripheral nerve demyelination as complement dependent, with no involvement of the Fc receptor. Different demyelinative mechanisms are obviously possible according to the pathological state of the animal and the demyelinative model used.

Whether microglia are also involved in demyelinative disease where damage to the blood–brain barrier occurs is difficult to determine. In his chapter in this section Hickey indicates a role for microglia in conferring susceptibility to experimental allergic encephalomyelitis, most likely by activation for antigen presentation. It is not known, however, whether they also become phagocytic.

In our laboratory, microglia prepared from primary cultures of newborn rats appear to be somewhat more active in phagocytizing myelin *in vitro* than are rat thioglycollate-elicited macrophages, but on the whole, the two kinds of phagocytes behave quite similarly. The microglial uptake of radioactive myelin and production of radioactive cholesterol ester are somewhat enhanced by antibody, but larger amounts of untreated myelin are also phagocytized. The exposure of freshly prepared microglia to granulocyte–macrophage colony-stimulating factor (GM-CSF) overnight before presentation of myelin, although not increasing the antibody mediated phagocytosis, greatly increases phagocytosis of untreated myelin to levels attained by microglia ingesting the myelin–antibody complex (Fig. 2). The GM-CSF had no such effect on peritoneal macrophages. Microglia, therefore, when sufficiently activated, show the capacity to phagocytize myelin in large amounts without participation of antibody and presumably the Fc receptor. Nor are complement receptors involved, since the microglia are cultured in defined medium. Clearly, much remains to be learned about microglia, the receptors involved in phagocytosis, their function in demyelinative diseases, and the mechanism of activation from the resting state.

REFERENCES

1. Ramón y Cajal S. Contribucion al conocimiento de la neuroglia del cerebro humano. *Trab Lab Invest Biol Univ Madrid* 1913;11:255–315.
2. Del Rio-Hortega P. Microglia. In: Penfield W, ed. *Cytology and cellular pathology of the nervous system,* vol 2. New York: Paul B. Hoeber; 1932:482–534.
3. Fujita S, Kitamura T. Origin of brain macrophages and the nature of the so-called microglia. *Acta Neuropathol* 1975;Suppl VI:291–296.
4. Fujita S, Kitamura T. Origin of brain macrophages and the nature of microglia. In: Zimmerman HM, ed. *Progress in neuropathology,* vol 3. New York: Grune & Stratton; 1976;1–50.
5. Giulian D, Baker TJ. Characterization of ameboid microglia isolated from the developing mammalian brain. *J Neurosci* 1986;6:2163–2178.
6. Lampert P, Carpenter S. Electron microscopic studies on the vascular permeability and the mechanism of demyelination in experimental allergic encephalomyelitis. *J Neuropathol Exp Neurol* 1965;24:11–24.
7. Trotter J, DeJong LA, Smith ME. Opsonization with antimyelin antibody increases the uptake and intracellular metabolism of myelin in inflammatory macrophages. *J Neurochem* 1986;47:779–789.
8. Smith ME, Sadler RH, Dyer C, Benjamins JA, Yu ACH. Phagocytosis of peripheral nerve myelin *in vitro:* effect of antibody. *J Neurosci Res* 1990;27: 298–306.

Advances in Neurology, Vol. 59, edited by
Fredrick J. Seil. Raven Press, Ltd.,
New York © 1993.

28

Macrophage Responses to Central and Peripheral Nerve Injury

*V. Hugh Perry, †Michael C. Brown, and *Peter-Brian Andersson

**Department of Pharmacology, University of Oxford, Oxford OX1 3QT, England; and †University Laboratory of Physiology, University of Oxford, Oxford OX1 3PT, England*

Nerve degeneration and regeneration have been intimately linked since the beginning of studies on nerve injury (1). It is well known that following injury to a peripheral nerve the distal segment undergoes rapid degeneration, so-called Wallerian degeneration. The cell body reacts by initiating the molecular machinery for axonal regeneration. In contrast, axonal injury in the central nervous system (CNS) is followed by slow Wallerian degeneration and an abortive attempt at regeneration before the neuron undergoes retrograde degeneration.

In the peripheral nervous system (PNS), rapid degeneration of the distal segment has long been thought to be an important element in providing a favorable environment for axonal regeneration. The degeneration of the axon is rapidly followed by the disintegration and phagocytosis of the myelin. It was believed for many years that the major, if not the exclusive, cell type involved in removal of degeneration products was the Schwann cell (2), which then proliferated and provided growth factors for the regenerating axons (3). The work of Beuche and Friede (4) suggested that macrophages may be an important and largely ignored cellular component of Wallerian degeneration in the PNS. Subsequently it was shown by immunocytochemical techniques that macrophages do indeed invade the distal segment of a degenerating nerve with a time course compatible with their playing a part in the removal of debris from the distal segment and providing factors that may promote Schwann cell division (5,6). We also found, using macrophage-specific markers, that the appearance of macrophages in degenerating optic nerve, a CNS tract, was slower and involved many fewer cells than are seen in the PNS. We suggested that the dramatic difference in the rate of clearance of debris from CNS and PNS may be a consequence of the differences in macrophage recruitment and, furthermore, that macrophages might play a role in the successful regeneration of peripheral nerves. An obvious corollary of this is that the poor regeneration in the CNS may be related to the slow removal of debris. Recent work showing that a protein in CNS myelin is inhibitor for axonal growth (7,8) adds some weight to this notion. In addition, recent studies in lower vertebrates, where CNS fibers retain the capacity to regenerate, have revealed a vigorous mononuclear phagocyte response to nerve injury more akin to that seen in the mammalian PNS (9,10).

One of our goals over the last few years has been to try to establish what role cells of the mononuclear phagocyte lineage may play in nerve regeneration. In nonneuronal tissues there is evidence that macrophages play an important, if not essential, role in tissue repair after injury (11). Not only are the recruited cells involved in removal of debris, they secrete a plethora of factors that may be important for successful cellular repair (12,13). In this chapter we review some of our recent studies on the macrophage response to PNS and CNS injury.

INJURY IN THE PERIPHERAL NERVOUS SYSTEM

To investigate the possible role of macrophages in PNS regeneration after a crush lesion, we sought a method by which we could prevent or reduce macrophage recruitment to the distal segment. This would allow us to investigate the role of macrophages in the processes of degeneration and regeneration. However, most of the available methods that prevent myelomonocytic recruitment, for example, whole-body irradiation or treatment with glucocorticoids, have many undesired side effects. Treatment with silica dust intraperitoneally reduces the number of macrophages but does not abrogate their recruitment (14).

In light of these difficulties, we were fortunate to discover in our own animal facility a strain of C57BL mice with a most useful mutation. On transection of a nerve the axons in the distal segment undergo very slow Wallerian degeneration compared to other mice (15). Not only do many axons in the distal segment appear morphologically intact for several weeks, but many retain the capacity to conduct action potentials for up to 2 weeks or more. In the absence of axonal degeneration, monocytes are not recruited to the distal segment; thus, we are able to address the issue of how the absence of degeneration and paucity of macrophages influence peripheral nerve regeneration.

The absence of degeneration and little monocyte recruitment in the distal segment beg the question as to which comes first: does the nerve fail to degenerate because monocytes are unable to be recruited, or do the monocytes not appear because the nerve is not degenerating and the signals that result in monocyte recruitment are not generated? In essence, is the mutation in the circulating monocyte population or in the nerve itself? To answer this issue we made chimeric mice in which C57BL/Ola mice were given whole-body irradiation and reconstituted with histocompatible bone marrow from C57BL/6J mice (16). Several months after reconstitution, one sciatic nerve was sectioned, and we looked to see whether the rate of nerve degeneration was dependent on the host or the donor bone marrow. The rate of degeneration was dependent on the host; chimeric C57BL/6J mice with rapidly degenerating nerves were found to have many macrophages in the distal segment. Since the macrophages were derived from C57BL/Ola bone marrow, this showed that these macrophages will readily respond to signals from a degenerating nerve, whatever they may be. In contrast, nerves from C57BL/Ola mice still degenerated slowly despite the presence of C57BL/6J-derived monocytes.

Other evidence that the mutation was intrinsic to the nerve came from *in vitro* studies (16). Pieces of sciatic nerve from C57BL/Ola mice were placed in culture, as were nerves from wild-type mice. The nerves from C57BL/Ola mice survived several days longer than those from wild-type mice. The slow Wallerian degeneration of optic nerve fibers in C57BL/Ola (17) also suggests that the mutation affects nerve fibers and not Schwann cells. From a genetic analysis we have found that this mutation is inherited in a single autosomal dominant fashion (18), and studies are in progress to map the location of the gene.

The discovery of the C57BL/Ola mice has allowed us to study how motor and sensory axons are able to regenerate along a territory where the distal fibers have not degenerated and there are virtually no recruited macrophages. We found that motor axons regenerate well (15), but sensory axons regenerate poorly (19,20). However, it should be further recognized that among the sensory axons there is considerable heterogeneity in the response to nerve injury (20). The reasons for this dramatic difference in the regenerative behavior of the motor and sensory axons is unclear. The motor axons regenerate in association with bundles of unmyelinated axons and nonmyelinating Schwann cells (21). Despite this unusual route of regeneration, the motor axons appear to find their appropriate targets (21). It is possible that the adhesion molecules expressed on nonmyelinating Schwann cells (22) and the presence of ciliary neurotrophic factor (CNTF), a growth factor for motor neurons (23), within the Schwann cells of the adult nerve (24) are sufficient to provide a favorable environment for regenerating motor axons. In contrast, the sensory nerves regenerate very slowly, and a large number of unmyelinated axons degenerate after the initial injury (20,21). One possible reason for the failure of sensory axon regeneration that we have studied lies in the absence or paucity of nerve growth factor (NGF) (20). Unlike CNTF, which is constitutively expressed in the peripheral nerve, the synthesis of NGF is up-regulated in the degenerating peripheral nerve, probably as a consequence of interleukin-1 secretion from invading macrophages (25,26). In the C57BL/Ola mouse, NGF levels in the distal sciatic nerve rise much more slowly after injury and to a lesser extent than in other mice (20). Although this provides a pointer to a role for NGF in sensory nerve regeneration, its precise contribution is unclear. Local injections of NGF into the nerves of C57BL/Ola mice after injury cannot reinstate normal sensory nerve regeneration (20).

Studies on the C57BL/Ola mouse have shown that sensory nerves regenerate poorly along territory that has intact axons and intact myelin sheaths and few macrophages. However, the role of the macrophage in PNS regeneration beyond that of removing the debris is by no means certain. It should be remembered that the myelomonocytic response in the distal segment of an injured nerve is unlike the response to cellular degeneration seen in other tissues. First, there are very few polymorphonuclear cells recruited, and second, there is a delay of several days before monocytes enter the tissue (5,20). The delay in monocyte recruitment to the distal segment is possibly not surprising when we take into account the fact that even in wild-type mice many axons will conduct action potentials for at least 24 hr after a cut or crush injury (15). However, what is surprising is that even at the crush site there is a delay in the monocyte recruitment despite the fact that the tissue has been directly traumatized and the blood–nerve barrier wholly disrupted. The paucity of polymorphonuclear cells seen in the distal segment is also apparent at the crush site, even when survival times of less than 24 hr are examined (unpublished observations). The unusual kinetics of the myelomonocytic response to peripheral nerve injury is similar in many respects to the myelomonocytic response to CNS injury (see below).

INJURY IN THE CENTRAL NERVOUS SYSTEM

It has been known for many years that debris from degenerating CNS axons will persist for a very long time in comparison to that seen in the PNS (27). The nature of the cells involved in the removal of the debris has also been much debated. Since we now know that macrophages are recruited to the peripheral nerves undergoing Wallerian degeneration and that they play a major role in the removal of debris (see above), we might ask whether macrophages play a similar role in CNS Wallerian degeneration.

The use of immunocytochemical markers for mononuclear phagocytes in CNS and PNS tracts undergoing Wallerian degeneration quickly revealed that there were important differences. In the PNS, large numbers of macrophages were recruited, albeit with a delay, but in the CNS, recruitment or increase in number was much more modest and followed a clear delay (5,28). The slow recruitment of monocytes to a degenerating optic nerve could in part be explained by the fact that CNS axons will conduct action potentials for several days longer than PNS axons and that within a fiber tract different axon populations degenerate with different time courses (e.g., ref. 17). Thus, we might imagine that the slowly evolving nature of the degeneration fails to generate a large recruitment signal. However, another important feature of macrophages in the degenerating optic nerve is that the cells labeled with plasma membrane markers for mononuclear phagocytes have the morphology of microglia rather than the rounded or stellate phagocytic cells in a degenerating peripheral nerve. Microglia morphology in the CNS is associated with a macrophage phenotype that is in general more down-regulated and less phagocytic than macrophages elsewhere (29). Thus, we might imagine the following scenario: monocytes are slowly recruited to a degenerating optic nerve, but on entering the nerve where the architecture is still relatively intact, they bind to an endogenous ligand. This hypothetical ligand induces microglial morphology and a weakly phagocytic phenotype. The persistence of cellular debris in CNS Wallerian degeneration would be a consequence of this weak phagocytic response.

The delay in monocyte recruitment is an intriguing feature of CNS degeneration. To investigate whether this was only present in Wallerian degeneration, we examined the mononuclear phagocyte response to kainic acid injection into the hippocampus (30). The reason for using kainic acid is that this glutamate agonist produces very rapid degeneration of the pyramidal cells in the hippocampus; the vast majority degenerate within 12 hr of injection. We thus have a "pulse" of cell degeneration rather than the slowly evolving Wallerian or retrograde degeneration. Following a kainic acid lesion there is no significant monocyte recruitment until the third day, and there is virtually no polymorphonuclear recruitment at any stage. Despite the rapid onset of the degeneration and the presence of degeneration products for at least 48 hr, the mononuclear phagocytes do not enter the tissue. The absence of recruitment during this time should not be confused with the permeability of the blood–brain barrier to solutes. In the first 24 hr after the lesion, when there is no recruitment, the blood–brain barrier in the hippocampus is permeable to intravenously delivered horseradish peroxidase (HRP), but when the mononuclear phagocyte numbers are rising on the third day, the barrier is no longer permeable to HRP (30).

The mononuclear phagocytes restricted recruitment, and the delay could be caused, however unlikely this may seem, by the nature of the inflammatory stimulus. It was conceivable that the signals elicited by degenerating CNS neurons are in some way unique and only poorly proinflammatory. We thus explored whether intrahippocampal injection of LPS (endotoxin), a very potent inflammogen, would give rise to a more typical myelmonocytic reaction similar to that seen in other tissues (31). To our considerable surprise, 20 ng of LPS injected into the hippocampus elicited almost no myelomonocytic response within the parenchyma but did elicit a response in the choroid plexus and ventricles. A 200-ng injection of LPS produced recruitment of mononuclear phagocytes on the third day, but prior to this time very few polymorphonuclear cells or monocytes were recruited. At pharmacological doses (2 μg) of LPS, the virtual absence of a myelomonocytic reaction in the CNS parenchyma in the first 24 to 48 hr was dramatically contrasted with a vigorous response in the choroid plexus and ventricles. The delay in mononuclear phagocyte recruitment, first quantified after kainic-acid-induced neuronal death, appears to be a general property of the CNS even in the presence of a potent inflammogen such as LPS and also in the presence of several proinflammatory cytokines and chemotaxins (unpublished observations).

The reasons for the unusual kinetics of the CNS inflammatory response are not known, but there are a number of obvious possibilities. The initiation of an inflammatory response requires activation of the endothelium, and it could be that (a) the resident macrophages are so down-regulated that they do not produce the appropriate monokines or (b) the CNS endothelium is relatively refractory to various monokines. The virtual absence of polymorphonuclear cells in the first few hours may also contribute to the delayed monocyte recruitment, since polymorphonuclear cells secrete a large number of proinflammatory molecules, which would be expected to rapidly amplify the inflammatory signal. In the lung it has been shown that polymorphonuclear recruitment precedes and is necessary for monocyte recruitment in response to infusion of fragments of the fifth component of complement (32), but this is a highly specific situation. The role of polymorphonuclear cells in amplifying the recruitment of monocytes deserves further investigation.

CONCLUSION

Wallerian degeneration in both PNS and CNS provokes a highly modified inflammatory response. The distinction between other tissues and the nervous system is more marked for the CNS than PNS. In contrast to other tissues, where polymorphonuclear cells are recruited within a few hours accompanied by or rapidly followed by monocytes (33), few polymorphonuclear cells appear in PNS or CNS tracts. The monocytes appear after a delay of a few days. In the PNS, recruited monocytes rapidly phagocytize degenerating axons and myelin and may also contribute to regeneration. In the CNS, recruited monocytes are fewer in number and differentiate to adopt a microglial morphology. The factors that result in this differentiation to a microglial form may contribute to the relatively poor phagocytic activity of microglia and thus to the persistence of debris in CNS Wallerian degeneration. The slow removal of CNS debris may be of consequence for axonal regeneration, given the presence of a myelin protein inhibitory for axonal elongation. Understanding the factors that control the influx of myelomonocytic cells into the fiber tracts of the nervous system may be of considerable therapeutic value.

ACKNOWLEDGMENTS

We would like to thank all our colleagues who have joined with us in the experimental work described here. This work was supported by the Wellcome Trust. V. H. Perry is a Wellcome Trust Senior Research Fellow; P.-B. Andersson is a Rhodes Scholar.

REFERENCES

1. Ramón y Cajal S. *Degeneration and regeneration of the nervous system.* London: Oxford University Press; 1928. May RN, translator.
2. Sunderland S. *Nerves and nerve injuries,* 2nd ed. London: Churchill Livingston; 1978.
3. Politis JJ, Ederle K, Spencer PS. Tropism in nerve cell regeneration *in vivo.* Attraction of regenerating axons by diffusible factors derived from cells in distal nerve stumps of transected peripheral nerves. *Brain Res* 1982;253:1–12.
4. Beuche W, Friede RL. The role of non-resident cells in Wallerian degeneration. *J Neurocytol* 1984;13: 767–796.
5. Perry VH, Brown MC, Gordon S. The macrophage response to central and peripheral nerve injury. A possible role for macrophages in regeneration. *J Exp Med* 1987;165:1218–1223.
6. Stoll G, Griffin JW, Li CY, Trapp BB. Wallerian degeneration in the peripheral nervous system: participation of both Schwann cells and macrophages in myelin degradation. *J Neurocytol* 1989;18: 671–683.
7. Schwab ME, Caroni P. Oligodendrocytes and CNS myelin are nonpermissive substrates for neurite growth and fibroblast spreading *in vitro. J Neurosci* 1988;8:2381–2393.
8. Schnell L, Schwab ME. Axonal regeneration in the rat spinal cord produced by an antibody against myelin-associated neurite growth inhibitors. *Nature* 1990;343:269–272.
9. Goodbrand IA, Gaze RM. Microglia in tadpoles of *Xenopus laevis:* normal distribution and response to optic nerve injury. *Anat Embryol* 1991;184:71–82.
10. Dowding AJ, Maggs A, Scholes J. Diversity amongst the microglia in growing and regenerating fish CNS: immunohistochemical characterization using FL.1, an antimacrophage monoclonal antibody. *Glia* 1991;4:345–364.
11. Leibovich SJ, Ross R. The role of the macrophage in wound repair. *Am J Pathol* 1975;78:71–91.
12. Nathan CF. Secretory products of macrophages. *J Clin Invest* 1987;79:319–326.
13. Rappolee DA, Werb Z. mRNA phenotyping for studying gene expression in small numbers of cells: Platelet derived growth factor and other growth factors in wound derived macrophages. *Am J Respir Cell Mol Biol* 1990;2:3–10.
14. Beuche W, Friede RL. Myelin phagocytosis in Wallerian degeneration of peripheral nerves depends on

silica sensitive, bg/bg-negative and Fc-positive monocytes. *Brain Res* 1986;378:97–106.
15. Lunn ER, Perry VH, Brown MC, Rosen H, Gordon S. Absence of Wallerian degeneration does not hinder regeneration in peripheral nerve. *Eur J Neurosci* 1989;1:27–33.
16. Perry VH, Brown MC, Lunn ER, Tree P, Gordon S. Evidence that the rate of Wallerian degeneration is an intrinsic property of the peripheral nerve. *Eur J Neurosci* 1990;2:802–808.
17. Perry VH, Brown MC, Lunn ER. Very slow retrograde and Wallerian degeneration in the CNS of C57BL/Ola mice. *Eur J Neurosci* 1991;3:102–105.
18. Perry VH, Lunn ER, Brown MC, Cahusac S, Gordon S. Evidence that the rate of Wallerian degeneration is controlled by a single autosomal dominant gene. *Eur J Neurosci* 1990;2:408–413.
19. Bisby MA, Chen S. Delayed Wallerian degeneration in sciatic nerves of C57BL/Ola mice is associated with impaired regeneration of sensory axons. *Brain Res* 1990;530:117–120.
20. Brown MC, Perry VH, Lunn ER, Gordon S, Heumann R. Macrophage dependence of peripheral sensory nerve regeneration: possible involvement of nerve growth factor. *Neuron* 1991;6:359–370.
21. Brown MC, Lunn ER, Perry VH. Consequences of slow Wallerian degeneration for regenerating motor and sensory axons. *J Neurobiol* 1992;[in press].
22. Martini R, Schachner M. Immunoelectronmicroscopic localization of neural cell adhesion molecules (L1, N-CAM, and myelin-associated glycoprotein) in regenerating adult mouse sciatic nerve. *J Cell Biol* 1988,106.1735–1744.
23. Sendtner M, Kreutzberg GW, Thoenen H. Ciliary neurotrophic factor prevents the degeneration of motor neurons after axotomy. *Nature* 1990;345: 440–441.
24. Stockli KA, Lottspeich F, Sendtner M, et al. Molecular cloning, expression and regional distribution of rat ciliary neurotrophic factor. *Nature* 1989;342: 920–923.
25. Heumann R, Lindholm D, Bandtlow C, et al. Differential regulation of mRNA encoding nerve growth factor and its receptor in rat sciatic nerve during development, degeneration and regeneration, role of macrophages. *Proc Natl Acad Sci USA* 1987;84:8735–8739.
26. Lindholm D, Heumann R, Meyer M, Thoenen H. Interleukin-1 regulates synthesis of nerve growth factor in nonneuronal cells of the rat sciatic nerve. *Nature* 1987;330:658–659.
27. Cook RD, Wisniewski HM. The role of oligodendroglia and astroglia in Wallerian degeneration of the optic nerve. *Brain Res* 1973;61:191–206.
28. Stoll G, Trapp BD, Griffin JW. Macrophage function during Wallerian degeneration of rat optic nerve: clearance of degenerating myelin and Ia expression. *J Neurosci* 1989;9:2327–2335.
29. Perry VH, Gordon S. Macrophages and the nervous system. *Int Rev Cytol* 1991;125:203–244.
30. Andersson P-B, Perry VH, Gordon S. The kinetics and morphological characteristics of the macrophage–microglial response to kainic acid-induced neuronal degeneration. *Neuroscience* 1991; 42:201–214.
31. Andersson P-B, Perry VH, Gordon S. The acute inflammatory response to lipopolysaccaride in CNS parenchyma differs from that of other body tissues. *Neuroscience* 1992;48:169–186.
32. Doherty DE, Downey GP, Worthen GS, Haslett C, Henson PM. Monocyte retention and migration in pulmonary inflammation. Requirement for neutrophils. *Lab Invest* 1988;59:200–213.
33. Movat HZ. *The inflammatory reaction.* Amsterdam: Elsevier; 1985.

Advances in Neurology, Vol. 59, edited by
Fredrick J. Seil. Raven Press, Ltd.,
New York © 1993.

29

Microglial Secretion Products and Their Impact on the Nervous System

Dana Giulian and Margaret Corpuz

Department of Neurology, Baylor College of Medicine, Houston, Texas 77031

It has long been recognized that the onset of microglial reactivity is one of the first cellular responses to central nervous system (CNS) injury (1). This rapid inflammatory process, marked by changes in glial shapes and cell surface receptors, occurs within hours after trauma and stroke (2). The hypothesis put forth here is that these microglia release factors that determine in part the structural and functional consequences of brain damage (Fig. 1).

Study of microglial secretion products began in 1985 (3) with the ability to isolate and grow homogeneous populations of cells in culture (4). Application of these culture techniques made it possible to compare factors released specifically by astroglia, microglia, and oligodendroglia. As described, microglia have now been discovered to be the principal source of brain cytokines, vasoregulators, and cytotoxins.

MICROGLIA AND IMMUNOREGULATORY MOLECULES

Cytokines are molecules released by the immune system that help regulate the growth or function of immune cells. Over the past 5 years there has been increasing interest in the production and actions of cytokines after damage to neural tissues. One of the first immunoregulatory molecules to be examined closely in the CNS was interleukin 1 (IL-1; 5,6). Interleukin 1 is a pluripotent molecule with functions that include activation of T cells, production of fever, and growth effects on fibroblasts and hepatocytes (7). During investigation of glial growth factors, we found that IL-1 was a mitogen for cultured astroglia (6). Furthermore, *in vivo* studies demonstrate that recombinant IL-1, but not interleukin-2 or interferon γ, elicited a reactive astrogliosis at the site of cerebral infusion (8). Importantly, released IL-1 was detected in tissues during development of rat brain (9) or at sites of injury following stroke or trauma (10).

To better understand events that drive IL-1 production in the CNS, it became necessary to determine its cellular sources. Several brain cell types have been reported to release IL-1, including astroglia (11), neurons (12), and microglia (13). Careful comparisons using cultured cells showed that only microglia produced significant quantities of this cytokine (Fig. 2A). Work by Hetier et al. (14) using probes for mRNA has confirmed that microglia, but not astroglia, were the principal source of IL-1 in cultured brain cells. Moreover, Higgins and Olschowka (15) demonstrated by immunohistochemistry significant amounts of IL-1 in reactive microglia but not in neurons.

Tumor necrosis factor α (TNF-α) is another pluripotent cytokine found in the brain that acts as a cytotoxin, a growth factor, or an

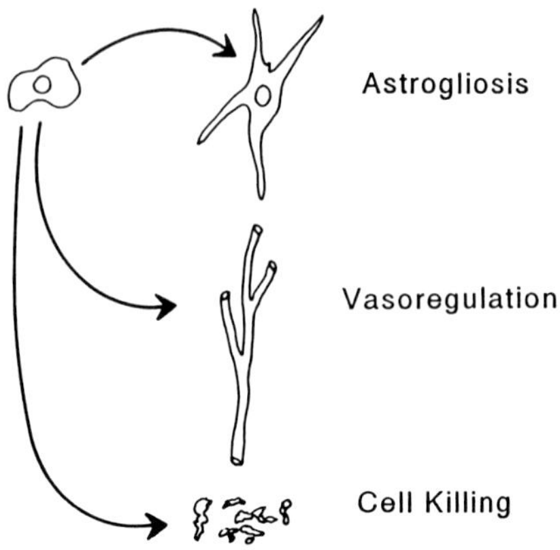

FIG. 1. The putative role of microglial secretion products on damaged neural tissues. Activated microglia release factors including cytokines that stimulate wound healing with astrogliosis. Short-lived substances such as eicosanoids act on the brain vasculature to control capillary permeability and blood flow. In addition, microglia release cytotoxins, some of which are neurotoxic molecules that may account for the progressive loss of neurons seen after acute CNS injury. Inflammatory cell release of soluble factors constitutes a significant pathogenic event common to a variety of CNS insults including stroke and trauma.

immunoactivator (16). Brain TNF-α is thought to serve as an endogenous pyrogen (16) as well as an agent that expedites myelin destruction (17). As in the case of IL-1, TNF-α has been reported to be produced by astrocytes (18) and by microglia (13). In our experience, a careful comparison of microglial and astroglial cultures show that TNF-α is only produced by activated microglia (Fig. 2B). The controversy regarding the glial sources of brain cytokines stems from shortcomings in cell culture techniques. For example, microglia readily grow among beds of astroglia, and, unless special precautions are taken to eliminate microglial elements in the "astroglia-pure" culture, microglia remain a significant contaminant. Unfortunately, many investigators do not yet use appropriate markers (3) to identify or appropriate techniques to eliminate microglia from cultures of astrocytes. When such precautions are taken, cytokine release is detected only in populations of microglia (Fig. 2).

The morphological consequences of brain cytokine release have been suggested by the close association among inflammatory cells, the production of IL-1, and the subsequent appearance of astrogliosis (13). Following a stab wound to the cerebral cortex of rat (2), both reactive microglia and invading macrophages appeared within hours after injury. These cells provided the bulk of the inflammatory response, with peak numbers noted at around 2 days after injury. At this same time, a peak in IL-1 production was observed (2) that subsequently declined as the inflammatory response dissipated. Immediately following this secretory phase of inflammation,

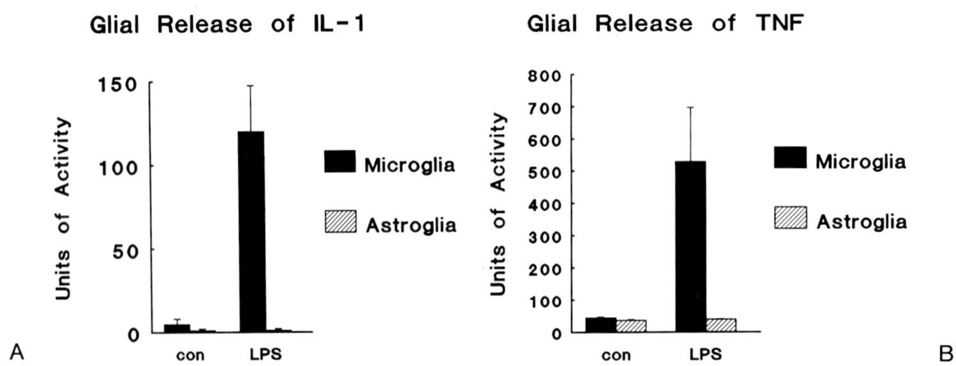

FIG. 2. Production of cytokines by brain glia. Both cytokines IL-1 and TNF-α are produced in injured brain. Study of isolated glia stimulated by various activators, including the lipopolysacchraride (LPS), shows that only microglia release detectable amounts of IL-1 (**A**) and TNF-α (**B**) when compared with identical preparations of astroglia. Cytokine levels in untreated controls (con) are also indicated.

there was the appearance of reactive astrocytes (2). Importantly, drug suppression of inflammation blocked both the production of IL-1 and astroglial reactivity (2).

At the present time it is not clear what net benefits microglial cytokines offer the diseased nervous system. TNF-α, for example, has been implicated in the neurological complications of cerebral malaria (19) as well as in the pathogenesis of multiple sclerosis (17). The IL-1-mediated astrogliosis may have a negative impact by reducing axonal remyelination. Alternatively, animal studies clearly show that IL-1 accelerates wound healing, which in turn may provide an environment to protect injured neurons from further insult (13). Further work, using more specific agents such as IL-1 receptor antagonists, will be necessary to sort out the specific actions of brain cytokines in damaged neural tissues.

MICROGLIAL RELEASE OF VASOREGULATORS

The eicosanoids (a class of molecules that include leukotrienes, prostaglandins, and thromboxanes) are thought to influence the nervous system in a variety of ways through modulation of synaptic transmission and regulation of vascular flow and permeability (20,21). One eicosanoid in particular, thromboxane A_2 (TxA_2), has received much attention as a potent vasoconstrictor and as a stimulant of platelet aggregation (21). Because TxA_2 concentrations are thought to be elevated after insult to the CNS, this eicosanoid has been implicated as an important mediator of tissue injury in cerebrovascular disease (21,22).

The TxA_2 produced in brain tissues was thought to come from astroglia (23). This conclusion, however, was based on study of "enriched" cultures of astrocytes, which, as noted earlier, usually have significant numbers of contaminating microglia. In view of the fact that mononuclear phagocytes outside the CNS were a major source of Tx, we considered the possibility that TxA_2 was also produced by mononuclear phagocytes of the brain. To determine which types of brain cells synthesize and release TxA_2, we measured the appearance of its stable metabolite, thromboxane B_2 (TxB_2), in medium conditioned by highly enriched cultures of astroglia or microglia. A comparison of various culture preparations clearly demonstrated (Fig. 3) that microglia were the principal source of brain thromboxane. Western blots also showed that the requisite synthetic enzyme, thromboxane synthase, was only present in isolated microglia and not in astroglia. Cell-mixing experiments indicated, moreover, that Tx produced in heterogeneous astroglial cultures could be accounted for by the presence of microglial cells (Fig. 3). The calcium ionophore A23187, zymosan A particles, fixed *S. aureus,* and endotoxin were potent activators of microglia to release thromboxane with a much shorter response time than that noted for the cytokines.

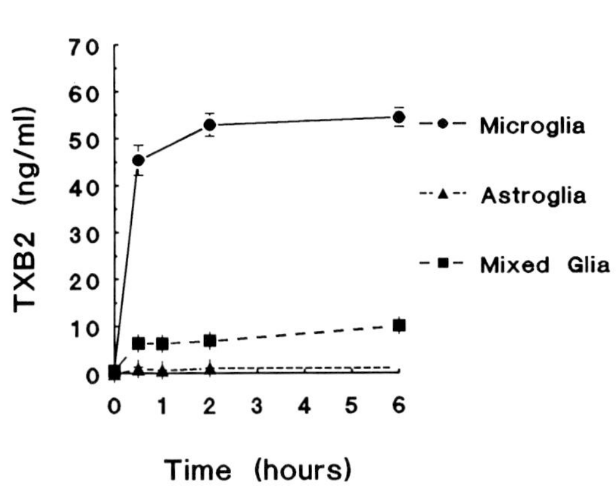

FIG. 3. Production of thromboxane B_2 by brain glia. Cells were exposed to the calcium ionophore A23187 to elicit release of TxB_2. As shown, only microglia are a source of significant eicosanoid production. Homogeneous populations of astroglia are free of TxB_2, whereas astroglia containing microglial contaminants (mixed glia) show an intermediate level of TxB_2 release.

Large Molecules	Small Molecules
cytokines	eicosanoids
lipases	superoxide anion
proteases	nitric oxide

FIG. 4. Cytotoxins produced by macrophages. Mononuclear phagocytes are known to release a variety of cytotoxic agents including large proteinaceous molecules (>10 kD) as well as small, short-lived factors like free radicals (<1 kD). In contrast, the microglia-derived neurotoxins as described here are small, heat-stable, protease-resistant molecules that can be recovered from inflamed neural tissues.

The significance of microglial Tx in the CNS remains unclear. Although investigators have reported increased brain concentrations of TxB_2 within minutes after injury (21,22), this rapid appearance occurs too quickly to be the product of microglial activation. Perhaps elevations of Tx seen at the time of ischemia come from vascular sources, including platelets (21), whereas Tx observed at later stages of injury may arise from microglia (24).

MICROGLIA AS A SOURCE OF ENDOGENOUS BRAIN CELL POISONS

It has long been recognized that macrophages have the capacity to release cytotoxic factors (Fig. 4), which in turn may be important mediators of immune surveillance and tissue remodeling (25). Over the past several years, microglia have also been noted to produce such putative cell poisons as proteases and free radicals (26). These observations implicate microglia as brokers of brain cell death (Fig. 1).

To ascertain the glial capacity to produce neurotoxic factors, we developed a cell culture system in which astroglia (>99% homogeneous population) or microglia (>98% homogeneity) were seeded into MilliCell-CM chambers and placed into wells with chick ciliary neurons grown on glass coverslips. Under such conditions, glia had no direct contact with neurons. Factors released by astroglia actually increased survival of neurons (Fig. 5) and stimulated neuritic outgrowth. In contrast, activated microglia released neuron killing factors. The effects of these microglial poisons were noted within hours with loss of nucleolar morphology and cytoplasmic vacuolation, and cell death within 24 to 48 hr after exposure. Comparisons between the growth factors produced by astroglia and the cell poisons released by microglia showed the two classes of molecules to be strikingly different. For example, ultrafiltration demonstrated the growth-promoting factors from astroglia to be large molecules (>10 kD) that were heat-inactivated, protease-sensitive molecules and probably included such molecules as ciliary neuronotrophic factor (27). In contrast, the neurotoxins from microglia were

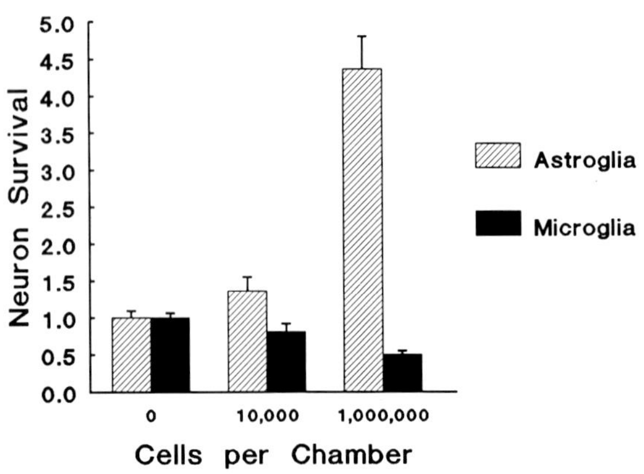

FIG. 5. Microglia secrete neurotoxins, and astroglia release neuron survival-promoting factors. Isolated microglia (>98% homogeneity) or astroglia (>99% homogeneous population) were seeded at the densities indicated and placed in MilliCell-CM chambers. The chambers were then placed into wells (12-well plates; 3.8 cm^2 per well) and cocultured for 48 hr with approximately 8,000 chick ciliary neurons per well grown on poly-L-lysine-coated glass coverslips. Significant differences among controls and microglia or astroglia cocultures were noted at 1,000,000 cells/chamber concentrations using Student's *t*-test.

small (<500 D), heat-stable, protease-resistant molecules with biological activities blocked by N-methyl-D-aspartate (NMDA) receptor antagonists. These toxic factors can be distinguished from cytokines, from free radical intermediates, from the excitatory amino acids glutamate and aspartate, and from the NMDA-receptor-mediated toxin quinolinic acid (13).

We suggest that potent neurotoxic factors are produced by activated microglia during the acute phases of injury. The release of these neurotoxins, in turn, expands the boundaries of tissue damage. In the case of both stab wound and ischemic injury, we obtain a good correlation between the appearance of inflammatory cells and the release of neurotoxic substances (13).

CONCLUSIONS

The inflammatory response to acute CNS injury is marked by the secretion of factors that promote wound healing, regulate blood flow, and kill neurons. The production of these factors is a significant pathogenic event common to a variety of CNS insults, including stroke, trauma (13), and human immunodeficiency virus 1 infection (28). Microglia-derived neurotoxins may account for the progressive loss of neurons seen after stroke (29). Support for this view comes from the observation that suppression of CNS inflammation prevents delayed deterioration in hindlimb motor function after ischemic injury to the spinal cord (30). Further study of mechanisms that direct microglial release of immunoregulatory, vasoregulatory, and cytotoxic molecules may offer new strategies to treat neurological disease.

ACKNOWLEDGMENTS

This work was supported in part by program project P01 NS23327 and R01 NS23113 from NINDS and from the American Paralysis Association.

REFERENCES

1. Del Rio-Hortega P. Microglia. In: Penfield W, ed. *Cytology and cellular pathology of the nervous system,* Vol 2. New York: Paul P. Hoeber; 1932:482–534.
2. Giulian D, Chen J, Ingeman JE, George J, Noponen M. The role of mononuclear phagocytes in wound healing after traumatic injury to adult mammalian brain. *J Neurosci* 1989;9:4416–4429.
3. Giulian D, Baker TJ. Peptides released by ameboid microglia regulate astroglial proliferation. *J Cell Biol* 1985;101:2411–2415.
4. Giulian D, Baker TJ. Characterization of ameboid microglia isolated from developing mammalian brain. *J Neurosci* 1986;6:2163–2178.
5. Giulian D, Lachman LB. Interleukin-1 stimulation of astroglial proliferation after brain injury. *Science* 1985;228:497–499.
6. Giulian D, Baker TJ, Shin L-N, Lachman LB. Interleukin-1 of the central nervous system is produced by ameboid microglia. *J Exp Med* 1986;164: 594–604.
7. Dinarello CA. Interleukin-1. *Rev Infect Dis* 1984;6:51–95.
8. Giulian D, Woodward J, Young D, Krebs JF, Lachman LB. Interleukin-1 injected into mammalian brain stimulates astrogliosis and neovascularization. *J Neurosci* 1988;8:2485–2490.
9. Giulian D, Young DG, Woodward J, Brown DC, Lachman LB. Interleukin-1 is an astroglial growth factor in the developing brain. *J Neurosci* 1988;8:709–714.
10. Giulian D. Microglia, cytokines, and cytotoxins: modulators of cellular responses after injury to the central nervous system. *EOS J Immunol Immunopharmacol* 1990;10:15–21.
11. Fontana A, Kristensen F, Dubs R. Production of prostaglandin E and interleukin-1 like factor by cultures of astrocytes and C6 glioma cells. *J Immunol* 1982;129:2413–2415.
12. Breder CD, Dinarello CA, Saper CB. Interleukin-1 immunoreactive innervation of the human hypothalamus. *Science* 1988;240:321–324.
13. Giulian D. Microglia and disease of the nervous system. *Curr Top Neurol* 1992;12:23–54.
14. Hetier E, Ayala J, Denefle A, et al. Brain macrophages synthesize interleukin-1 and interleukin-1 mRNAs *in vitro. J Neurosci Res* 1988;21:391–397.
15. Higgins GA, Olschowka JA. Induction of interleukin-1β in adult rat brain. *Mol Brain Res* 1991;9:143–148.
16. Le J, Vilcek J. Tumor necrosis factor and interleukin-1: cytokines with multiple overlapping activities. *Lab Invest* 1987;56:234–248.
17. Selmaj KW, Raine CS. Tumor necrosis factor mediates myelin and oligodendrocyte damage *in vitro. Ann Neurol* 1988;23:339–346.
18. Sawada M, Kondo N, Suzumura A, Marunouchi T. Production of tumor necrosis factor-alpha by microglia and astrocytes in culture. *Brain Res* 1989;491:394–397.
19. Grau GF, Fajardo LF, Piguet F-P, Allet B, Lamber

P-H, Vassalli P. Tumor necrosis factor (cachectin) as an essential mediator in murine cerebral malaria. *Science* 1987;237:1210–1212.
20. Wolfe LS, Pellerin K, Rostworowski K, Pappius HM. Synthesis and functions of cyclooxygenase and lipoxygenase products in brain; new findings and an appraisal. In Wong PY-K, Sun EF, eds. *Advances in prostaglandin, thromboxane, and leukotriene research,* Vol 19. New York: Raven Press; 1989:387–393.
21. Chen ST, Hsu CY, Hogan EL, et al. Thromboxane, prostacyclin, and leukotrienes in cerebral ischemia. *Neurology* 1986;36:466–470.
22. Yergey JA, Heyer MP. Brain eicosanoid formation following acute penetration injury as studied by *in vivo* microdialysis. *J Cereb Blood Flow* 1990;10: 143–146.
23. Murphy S, Pearce B, Jeremy J, Dandona P. Astrocytes as eicosanoid producing cells. *Glia* 1988;1:241–245.
24. Jacobs TP, Shohami E, Baze W, et al. Deteriorating stroke model: histopathology, edema, and eicosanoid changes following spinal cord ischemia in rabbits. *Stroke* 1982;18:741–750.
25. Cameron DJ, Churchill WH. Macrophage mediated cytotoxicity in man. *Int J Immunopharmacol* 1981;3:77–85.
26. Giulian D. Ameboid microglia as effectors of inflammation in the central nervous system. *J Neurosci Res* 1987;18:155–171.
27. Manthorpe M, Ray J, Pettmann B, Varon S. Ciliary neuronotrophic factors. In: Rush RA, ed. *Nerve growth factors.* New York: John Wiley & Sons; 1989:31–56.
28. Giulian D, Vaca K, Noonan C. Secretion of neurotoxins by mononuclear phagocytes infected with HIV-1. *Science* 1990;250:1593–1596.
29. Pulsinelli WA, Brierly JB, Plum F. Temporal profile of neuronal damage in a model of transient forebrain ischemia. *Ann Neurol* 1982;11:491–498.
30. Giulian D, Robertson C. Inhibition of mononuclear phagocytes reduces ischemic injury in the spinal cord. *Ann Neurol* 1990;27:33–42.

Advances in Neurology, Vol. 59, edited by
Fredrick J. Seil. Raven Press, Ltd.,
New York © 1993.

30

Microglia, an *In Vivo* Source of Reactive Oxygen Species in the Brain

*Carol A. Colton and †Daniel L. Gilbert

**Department of Physiology and Biophysics, Georgetown University Medical School, Washington, D.C. 20007; and †Laboratory of Biophysics, NINDS, National Institutes of Health, Bethesda, Maryland 20892*

Since the theory proposed in 1954 by Gerschman et al. (1) that oxygen free radicals were likely mediators of tissue damage during hyperoxia and the discovery of the functional role of superoxide dismutase by McCord and Fridovich (2) in 1969, the effects of reactive oxygen species (ROS) on cellular function have been intensively studied. Exposure of cells to ROS can result in oxidation of sulfhydryl-containing molecules such as coenzyme A and glutathione, oxidation of enzymes and structural proteins, oxidation of membrane phospholipids, and damage to DNA (3). The ROS include the single-electron reduction products of oxygen, that is, the superoxide radical anion ($O_2^-\cdot$), hydrogen peroxide (H_2O_2), and the hydroxyl free radical ($OH\cdot$). The reactions that are considered to be the most important in generating ROS are shown in Fig. 1. It is generally believed that the $OH\cdot$ is the final mediator of tissue damage. This highly reactive molecule is produced primarily via the metal-catalyzed Haber–Weiss reaction, although other sources of $OH\cdot$ such as the decomposition of nitric-oxide-derived radicals (4,5) are known.

All tissues in the body are susceptible to oxidative damage by ROS. Under normal conditions both enzymatic and nonenzymatic antioxidant protective mechanisms (Table 1) exist that limit ROS-induced damage (3,6,7). In fact, without antioxidants, life in an oxygen environment would not be possible. Changes in the balance between prooxidant and antioxidant factors can occur, however, resulting in oxidative stress to the tissue. Disruption of the normal oxidative balance has been linked to a variety of pathological conditions including Parkinson disease, Down syndrome, Alzheimer disease, and aging (3,8–10). Table 2 lists some of the pathological conditions in which ROS-induced damage may be a factor.

The CNS is no exception and is especially susceptible to oxidative damage because of the presence of high levels of iron in many regions and the presence of fatty acids, which are easily peroxidized (11–14). Although it is clear that oxidative damage can occur in the CNS, what is not clear is the source of the reactive oxygen species mediating the changes. Table 3 provides a list of potential sources and includes the mitochondrial electron transport chain, the production of superoxide anion by the interaction of xanthine with xanthine oxidase, an enzyme located in cerebral endothelial cells (15) as well as in other cells, and the production of H_2O_2 via the action of monoamine oxidase. The amount and importance of the reactive oxygen species produced by these mechanisms

Dedication: This chapter is dedicated to the memory of the late Rebeca Gerschman.

$$M^{(n+)} + O_2^{\cdot -} \rightarrow M^{(n+)-1} + O_2 \quad (1)$$

$$M^{(n+)-1} + H_2O_2 \rightarrow M^{(n+)} + OH^{\cdot} + OH^- \quad (2)$$

$$O_2^{\cdot -} + H_2O_2 \rightarrow O_2 + OH^{\cdot} + OH^- \quad (3)$$

$$M^{(n+)-1} + O_2^{\cdot -} + 2\,H^+ \rightarrow M^{(n+)} + H_2O_2 \quad (4)$$

$$2\,O_2^{\cdot -} + 2\,H^+ \rightarrow O_2 + H_2O_2 \quad (5)$$

Reaction (3) = Reaction (1) + Reaction (2).
Reaction (5) = Reaction (1) + Reaction (4).

Reaction (2) = FENTON REACTION.
Reaction (3) = HABER-WEISS REACTION.
Reaction (5) = DISMUTATION REACTION.

FIG. 1. Generation of reactive oxygen species via metal-catalyzed reactions.

has been disputed. Recent evidence provided originally by Giulian and Baker (16) and subsequently from our laboratory (17), however, indicates that a potent source of oxyradicals is present in the CNS. We have shown that the resident macrophages of the CNS, i.e., the microglia, produce superoxide anion and the OH·.

Microglia have been shown by a variety of investigators to share morphological, biochemical, and functional characteristics with other tissue macrophages (16–19). These multifunctional cells play a role in many aspects of CNS development as well as in the response of the CNS to injury and infection (20,21). Part of the ability of microglia to perform these functions is dependent on the production of ROS. Phagocytic cells have been known since 1933 to increase oxygen consumption during phagocytosis (22,23). In 1973 Babior et al. (24) demonstrated that this increase was a result of the production of $O_2^-\cdot$. In monocytes, neutrophils, and other tissue macrophages, $O_2^-\cdot$ is produced by the action of a membrane-localized NADPH-dependent oxidase (24,25). Our studies indicate that a similar mechanism is present in microglia. A hypothetical view of the pathways involved in microglial $O_2^-\cdot$ production is shown in Fig. 2.

TABLE 1. *Some natural antioxidants*

Metal chelators (flavonoids)
Salicylic acid
Ubiquinone
Uric acid
Enzymes
Catalase
Glutathione peroxidase
Superoxide dismutase
Vitamins
Vitamin A (β-carotene)
Vitamin C (ascorbic acid)
Vitamin E (α-tocopherol)

TABLE 2. *Diseases in which reactive oxygen species may be involved*

Alzheimer disease
Down syndrome
Autoimmune diseases (rheumatoid arthritis)
Ischemia–reperfusion injury
Stroke
Multiple sclerosis
Parkinson disease
Retinopathy of prematurity
Cataract formation
Spinal cord injury
Normal aging

METHODS

We have studied the production of superoxide anion in microglia cultured from neonatal rat cerebral cortices. Essentially, a primary mixed glial culture was prepared as described previously (17) and grown for 12 to 14 days in a 5% CO_2, 95% air atmosphere. With a procedure based on their differential adherence properties, microglia were separated from the underlying astrocytes by shaking and purified through a series of adherence and washing steps. The microglia were then

TABLE 3. *Potential CNS sources of reactive oxygen species*

Autooxidation of catecholamines
Enzymatic processes
Mitochondrial electron transport chain
Xanthine/xanthine oxidase
Monoamine oxidase
Arachidonic acid/lipoxygenase cascade
Cytochrome P450
Cellular
CNS macrophage, the microglia

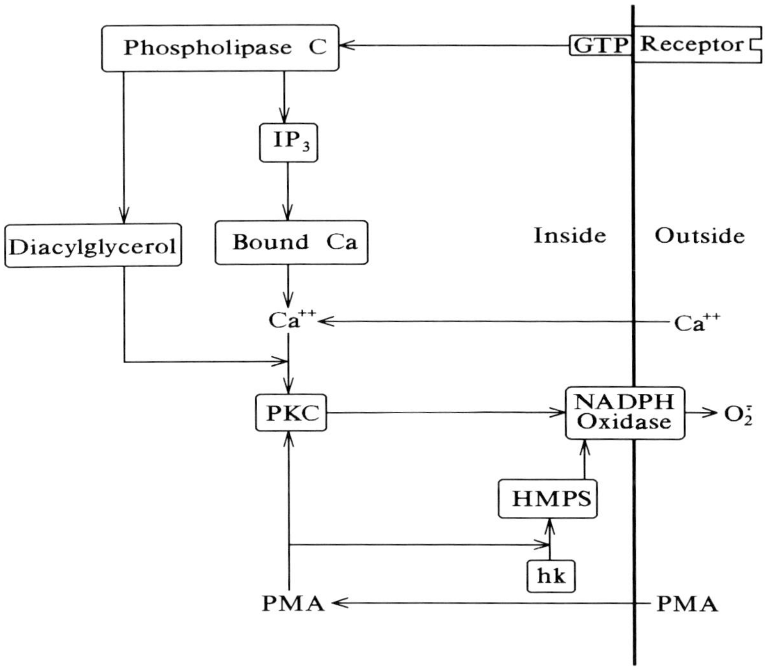

GTP = Guanosine triphosphate-binding protein
IP_3 = Inositol 1, 4, 5-triphosphate
PKC = Protein kinase C
HMPS = Hexose monophate shunt
hk = Hexokinase
PMA = Phorbol 12-myristate 13-acetate

FIG. 2. Hypothetical scheme for generation of superoxide anion in microglia.

stimulated to produce superoxide anion under a variety of conditions, and the amount of superoxide released was measured by a ferricytochrome c assay (17).

RESULTS AND DISCUSSION

We have shown that a variety of agents stimulate production of superoxide anion by cultured microglia. These agents include opsonized zymosan (OPZ), concanavalin A (a plant lectin), phorbol myristate acetate (PMA), and the calcium ionophore A23187. Typical superoxide production curves over a 2-hr stimulation period for PMA, OPZ, and A23187 are shown in Fig. 3. Each of these agents has been commonly used to induce superoxide anion release from other tissue macrophages, neutrophils, and monocytes (24). Certain known stimulators of superoxide anion release from other monocytic lineage cells do not, however, affect cultured neonatal rat microglia. For example, lipopolysaccharide (LPS) and N-met-leu-phe, both bacterial products, do not increase rat microglial superoxide anion production. Exposure to LPS will increase production of the cytokine interleukin 1 (IL-1) from rat microglia (26). These data suggest, then, that the release of ROS is not necessarily coupled to the release of other microglial secretory products.

We have also demonstrated that microglial superoxide anion production can be enhanced by certain potentiating factors. As in other tissue macrophages, microglia exist in various stages of activation, ranging from a relatively quiescent, resting state to an amoeboid, phagocytic form to a primed and activated state (27). One of the characteristics of

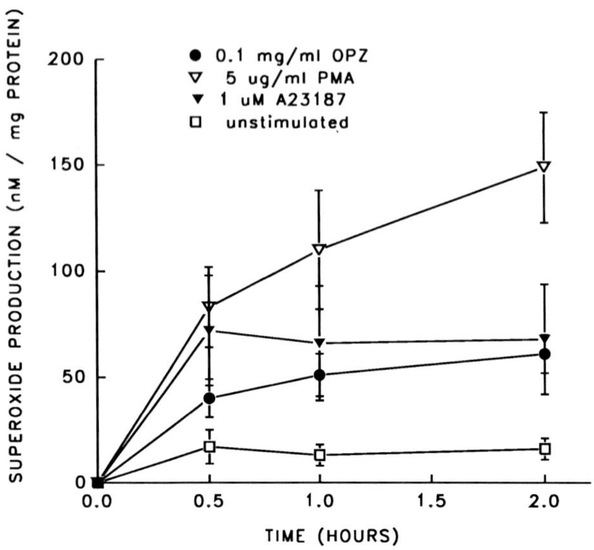

FIG. 3. Stimulated superoxide anion production in cultured neonatal rat microglia. Microglia were cultured for 12 to 14 days and then assayed for superoxide production using a cytochrome c reduction assay with and without superoxide dismutase. Values are presented as nanomoles superoxide produced per milligram protein (mean ± S.E.M.), where the amount of protein was determined using a Lowry assay. A minimum of three wells were assayed for each of at least three different culture groups.

the primed and activated state is an increase in the release of ROS above that seen in other states (28,29). The enhancement of oxyradical production is thought to contribute to the cytotoxicity of this state. Certain agents, particularly the lymphokines, are known to promote formation of a primed and activated macrophage (29,30). γ-Interferon (γ-IFN) is the most potent priming agent, although α/β-interferon (α/β-IFN) can perform a similar function. Typical values of superoxide anion production in microglia pretreated with 1,000 U/ml γ-IFN or 1,000 U/ml α/β-IFN for 48 hr and then stimulated to release superoxide anion with 5 μg/ml PMA are shown in Fig. 4. Under these conditions, superoxide anion production was increased by 51 ± 12% for γ-IFN and 67 ± 23% for α/β-IFN compared to untreated, PMA-stimulated controls.

Exposure to Earle's basic salt solution (EBSS) containing 55 mM potassium produced a similar potentiation of PMA-stimulated microglia superoxide anion production. For these experiments, isoosmotic

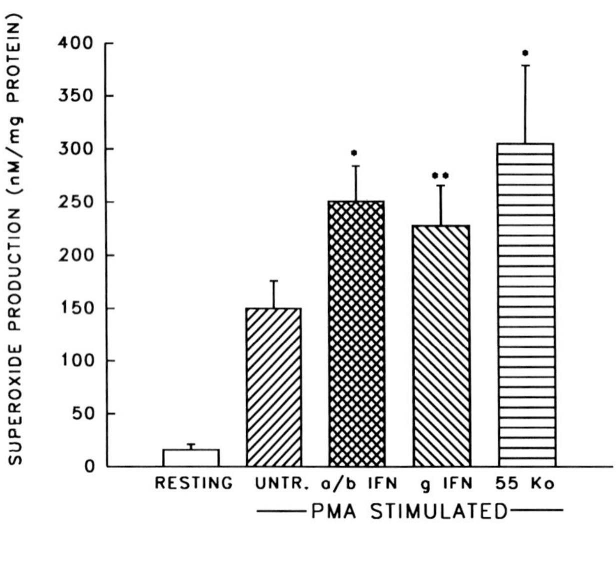

FIG. 4. Potentiation of stimulated microglial superoxide production. Microglia were stimulated to produce superoxide anion by 5 μg/ml PMA after pretreatment for 48 hr with 1,000 U/ml of either α/β-IFN or γ-IFN or in the presence of media containing 55 mM K^+. Values are presented as the average amount of superoxide (nM/mg protein) ± S.E.M. and were obtained at 2 hr of stimulation with PMA. Statistical analysis was done using an unpaired Student's *t* test. *Significantly different from untreated PMA stimulated microglia ($p < 0.01$); ** $p < 0.05$. A minimum of three wells were assayed for each of at least three different culture groups.

conditions were maintained by replacing sodium chloride with potassium chloride in the EBSS. Microglia were placed into the high-extracellular-potassium medium and then assayed for superoxide production under unstimulated conditions and when stimulated with 5 μg/ml PMA. Like the IFNs, high extracellular K^+ had no effect on superoxide production by itself (data not shown), but in the presence of an initiator of release, K^+ potentiated the production of superoxide anion. Superoxide anion levels increased by 159 ± 51% from the values obtained in normal EBSS. Since this level of extracellular potassium will depolarize the membrane potential, some of the potentiation may be linked, at least in part, to a change in membrane potential. Alternatively, the depolarization may allow increased calcium entry via plasma membrane calcium channels. Using patch-clamp techniques, we have recently shown the presence of a voltage-dependent calcium-permeable channel on microglial membrane. Bay K 8644, a dihydropyridine agonist for calcium channels, increased the current through this channel (unpublished observations). Although calcium is clearly linked to superoxide production in microglia, the exact manner in which it regulates release is unknown.

The production of ROS by monocytic cells has been shown to be an important aspect of the body's defense against injury and infection (24,25). The same is probably true in the CNS. A variety of investigators have demonstrated an accumulation of microglia and circulating monocytes (depending on the type of injury) at wound sites (31,32). The presence of inflammatory mediators and lymphokines as well as an increase in the local concentration of potassium from damaged cells would provide the signals necessary to promote release of microglial reactive oxygen species. These reactive molecules, in turn, would kill any invading organisms and would provide a beneficial service to the CNS. However, macrophages are notorious as indiscriminate killers (24), and their inappropriate activity has been linked to various pathological states such as rheumatoid arthritis (3). In the CNS, abnormal activation of the microglia has been seen in a mouse model for Down syndrome, the trisomy 16 mouse (33). Cultured microglia from the Ts16 mouse produce significantly greater amounts of superoxide anion on stimulation than their normal littermates. Microglial ROS, thus, may be deleterious to nearby neurons and other glia. How much damage is done will depend on the amount of ROS produced and the level of antioxidant defenses available for protection.

ACKNOWLEDGMENTS

We acknowledge the following individuals who participated in these studies: Drs. Jibin Yao, Jonette Keri, Mary Lou Oster-Granite, and Min Jia. This work is supported, in part, by a contract from the Office of Naval Research to C. Colton.

REFERENCES

1. Gerschman R, Gilbert DL, Nye SW, et al. Oxygen poisoning and X-irradiation: a mechanism in common. *Science* 1954;119:623–626.
2. McCord J, Fridovich I. Superoxide dismutase: an enzymatic function for erythrocuprein. *J Biol Chem.* 1969;244:6049–6055.
3. Halliwell B, Gutteridge JMC. *Free radicals in biology and medicine,* 2nd ed. New York: Oxford University Press; 1989.
4. Beckman JS, Beckman TW, Chen J, et al. Apparent hydroxyl radical production by peroxynitrite: Implication for endothelial injury from nitric oxide and superoxide. *Proc Natl Acad Sci USA* 1990;87: 1620–1624.
5. Mincada S, Palmer RMJ, Higgs EA. Nitric oxide: physiology, pathophysiology and pharmacology. *Pharmacol Rev* 1991;43:109–142.
6. Foreman HJ, Fisher A. Antioxidant defenses. In: Gilbert D, ed. *Oxygen and living processes: an interdisciplinary approach.* New York: Springer; 1981:235–249.
7. Boxer LA. The role of antioxidants in modulating neutrophil functional responses. In: Bendich A, Phillips M, Tengerdy RP, eds. *Antioxidant nutrients and immune functions.* New York: Plenum Press; 1988:19–33.
8. Sinet PM. Metabolism of oxygen derivatives in Down's syndrome. *Ann NY Acad Sci* 1982;396: 83–94.
9. Bannister WH. Superoxide dismutase and disease. In: Bannister JV, Bannister WH, eds. *The biology*

and chemistry of active oxygen. New York: Elsevier; 1984:208–236.
10. Stadtman ER. Metal ion catalyzed oxidation of proteins: biochemical mechanisms and biological consequences. *Free Radical Biol Med* 1990;9:315–25.
11. Subbarao KV, Richardson JS. Iron dependent peroxidation of rat brain: a regional study. *J Neurosci Res* 1990;26:224–232.
12. Floyd RA. Role of oxygen free radicals in carcinogenesis and brain ischemia. *FASEB J* 1990;4: 2587–2597.
13. Oliver CN, Starke-Reed PE, Stadtman ER, et al. Oxidative damage to brain proteins, loss of glutamine synthetase activity and production of free radicals during ischemia/reperfusion mediated injury to gerbil brain. *Proc Natl Acad Sci USA* 1990;87: 5144–5147.
14. Zaleska MM, Floyd RA. Regional lipid peroxidation in rat brain *in vitro:* possible role of endogenous iron. *Neurochem Res* 1985;10:397–410.
15. Betz L. Identification of hypoxanthine transport and xanthine oxidase activity in brain capillaries. *J Neurochem* 1985;44:574–580.
16. Giulian D, Baker TL. Characterization of ameboid microglia isolated from developing mammalian brain. *J Neurosci* 1986;6:2163–2178.
17. Colton C, Gilbert D. Production of superoxide anions by a CNS macrophage, the microglia. *FEBS Lett* 1987;223:284–288.
18. Perry VH, Gordon S. Macrophages and microglia in the nervous system. *Trends Neurosci* 1988;11: 273–277.
19. Yao J, Harvath L, Gilbert D, Colton C. Chemotaxis by a CNS macrophage, the microglia. *J Neurosci Res* 1990;27:36–42.
20. Ashwell K. The distribution of microglia and cell death in the fetal rat forebrain. *Dev Brain Res* 1991;58:1–15.
21. Giulian D. Ameboid microglia as effectors of inflammation in the central nervous system. *J Neurosci Res* 1987;18:155–171.
22. Ado A. Über den Verlauf der oxydativen und glykolytischen Prozesse in den Leukocyten des entzundeten Gewebes wahrend der Phagocytose. *Z Ges Exp Med* 1933;87:473–480.
23. Baldridge C, Gerard R. The extra respiration of phagocytosis. *Am J Physiol* 1933;103:235–236.
24. Babior B, Kipnes R, Curnutte J. Biological defense mechanisms: the production by leucocytes of superoxide, a potential bactericidal agent. *J Clin Invest* 1973;52:741–751.
25. Roos D, Lutter R, Bolscher BG. The respiratory burst and the NADPH oxidase of phagocytic leukocytes. In: Sbarra AJ, Strauss RR, eds. *The respiratory burst and its physiological significance.* New York: Plenum Press; 1988:53–76.
26. Colton C, Yao J, Keri J, et al. Regulation of microglial function by interferons. *J Neuroimmunol,* [*in press*].
27. Streit W, Graeber M, Kreutzberg G. Functional plasticity of microglia. *Glia* 1988;1:301–308.
28. Johnston RB, Kitagawa S. Molecular basis for the enhanced respiratory burst of activated macrophages. *Fed Proc* 1985;44:2927–2932.
29. Adams D, Hamilton TA. The cell biology of macrophage activation. *Annu Rev Immunol* 1984;2: 283–318.
30. Murray H. Interferon gamma, the activated macrophage and host defense against microbial challenge. *Ann Intern Med* 1988;108:595–608.
31. Streit W, Kreutzberg G. Lectin binding by resting and reactive microglia. *J Neurocytol* 1987;16: 249–261.
32. Giulian D, Johnson B, Krebs JF, et al. Microglial mitogens are produced in the developing and injured mammalian brain. *J Cell Biol* 1991;112: 323–333.
33. Colton C, Yao J, Gilbert D, Oster-Granite ML. Enhanced production of superoxide anion by microglia from trisomy 16 mice. *Brain Res* 1990;519: 236–242.

Advances in Neurology, Vol. 59, edited by Fredrick J. Seil. Raven Press, Ltd., New York © 1993.

31

Macrophage Functional Properties During Myelin Degradation

*Reinhard L. Friede and †Wolfgang Brück

*Departments of *Neuropathology and †Pathology, University of Göttingen, D-3400 Göttingen, Germany*

Wallerian degeneration may be seen as the most elementary type of myelin degradation in diseased tissue. Both the macrophage and the Schwann cell have been shown to possess the capacity to ingest myelin particles. Yet, the brunt of myelin digestive activity during Wallerian degeneration seems to be borne by the macrophage, at least under the conditions existing *in situ* or in an organ culture. The present review focuses on the functional properties of macrophages during Wallerian degeneration of mouse and rat peripheral nerves. These studies aim at a base-line understanding of how macrophages recognize myelin as a target to ingest and how they distinguish it from Schwann cells and other tissue structures not subject to phagocytosis. A clear concept of this relatively uncomplicated situation—when other cells of the immune system are not known to be engaged—may help to understand the role played by the macrophage during more complex interactions with other immune cells, as in demyelination.

In the following text we review the results obtained in our laboratories during the past 10 years. These data represent a coherent series of tests done under identical laboratory conditions in which the positive results gain weight against the background of a multitude of negative tests. The investigations can be divided into three phases. The first phase concerns studies aimed at documenting the involvement of monocytes/macrophages in Wallerian degeneration of peripheral nerves. The second phase is directed at an understanding of how the macrophage identifies and targets myelin as an object of phagocytosis. The third, just beginning, aims at an understanding of the interplay between macrophages and other cells of the immune system in more complex disease processes such as tissue rejection or demyelination.

THE INVOLVEMENT OF MONOCYTES/MACROPHAGES IN WALLERIAN DEGENERATION OF PERIPHERAL NERVE

The Diffusion Chamber Method

A rigid exclusion of nonresident cells from nerves undergoing Wallerian degeneration is possible by sealing nerve segments within chambers made of a ring and two Millipore membranes (1,2) and implanting these chambers into the peritoneal cavity of a host animal of the same strain (3). In such chambers, Wallerian degeneration takes a very different course depending on the pore size of the membranes. Chambers having membranes of 5- to 8-μm pore size ("large pore") are subject to massive invasion by macrophages (and granulocytes). The enclosed nerve segments undergo Wallerian degeneration indistinguishable from that occurring *in situ*. Chambers of 0.21-μm pore size ("small pore") are accessible to all body fluids, but their membranes are impermeable to migrating cells. Nerve segments sealed in such chambers show no evidence of myelin phagocytosis. The myelin sheaths may become ballooned or collapsed, but they persist in that state for many weeks, subject to only a very slow thermal decay. Corresponding to these morphological findings, there is rapid decrease of myelin proteins, with their almost complete disappearance within 28 days, in large-pore chambers compared to minimal decay in small-pore chambers (4). This behavior of tissue in small-pore chambers is not from tissue necrosis. The fine structure of Schwann cells and their organelles are well preserved even after several weeks in the chambers. In chambers invaded by macrophages, the Schwann cells undergo transformation into typical bands of Hanken-Bünger on complete removal of myelin debris.

Identification of Phagocytic Cells

The cell population invading the large-pore chambers was identified as monocytes/macrophages by the immunohistochemical demonstration of the Fc and the Mac-1 markers, corroborating the conclusions derived from strictly morphological criteria in earlier investigations (5–7). The reactions were positive both in the cells trapped within the meshwork of the Millipore membrane and also in those that had invaded organ cultures. The expression of Ia was more variable (8,9). There were also granulocytes invading the chambers, but the lymphocyte population was virtually excluded. Lymphocytes seemed to be incapable of traversing the Millipore membrane. As a consequence of this separation of cell populations, there was no tissue rejection when allogeneic nerves were placed inside large-pore chambers, even though phagocytosis of the foreign myelin by the host animals' macrophages proceeded undisturbed (10).

Sheath Rejection as an Initial Event of Wallerian Degeneration

One important benefit of the small-pore chamber is the opportunity to study the initial events taking place in the Schwann cells and in their myelin sheaths in the absence of intervention by nonresident cells. Schwann cells were found to reject their sheaths by about the second to third day (3,11). The perikarya and cytoplasmic processes of the Schwann cells then lie within the basement membranes side by side along the rejected myelin sheaths. Their plasma membranes have no continuity.

This phenomenon of myelin sheath rejection is not as evident in the presence of a substantial population of active phagocytes (*in situ* or in large-pore chambers) because phagocytes rapidly invade the basement membrane tubes, interposing themselves tightly between the Schwann cells and their rejected sheaths. It is important to realize that the critical initial events of Wallerian degeneration take place in the Schwann cell, leading to the rejection of its sheath. There is probably no initial attack by the phagocyte on a Schwann cell that has its sheath still undisturbed. The C57BL/Ola mice, characterized by very slow Wallerian degeneration, may serve as a paradigm. The retardation of degeneration results from a property of the nerve tissue and not of the circulatory monocytes (12,13). A down-regulation of the P_0 gene is involved in this phenomenon (14).

One may interject at this point that there are situations in which the invasion of a diseased nerve by macrophages has functional significance quite different from their role in myelin degradation. In demyelinated fibers, their apposition to the axon may improve the fibers' cable properties (15).

Macrophages During *in Situ* Wallerian Degeneration

The observations made in diffusion chambers are readily extrapolated to Wallerian degeneration *in situ*. Degenerating nerves were heavily invaded by cells bearing the Fc and Mac-1 markers or the F4180 antibody (16). The rate of myelin removal, moreover, was retarded on nonspecific damage to the macrophage population with silica (8,17). This is comparable to the effect of silica on lysolecithin- or virus-induced demyelination (18,19). Also, slow or sparse leukocyte invasion of degenerating nerves in C57BL/Ola mice correlates with an extremely slow removal of myelin and very slow axon degeneration (20). An understanding of these mechanisms during Wallerian degeneration may help to evaluate the role of macrophages during demyelinative neuropathies, where they also play a central role (21–23), even though the nature of their interplay with other immune-competent cells still awaits clarification (see below).

Limitations of the Millipore Chamber Model

The Millipore chamber model is an efficient method for excluding nonresident cells. However, it is not suitable for quantitative studies of the invading cell population; the Millipore membrane itself is a target of monocytes even in empty chambers (9). The cells invading the tissue inside the large-pore chambers, therefore, are only that fraction of the migratory cell population that managed to cross the membrane. These shortcomings

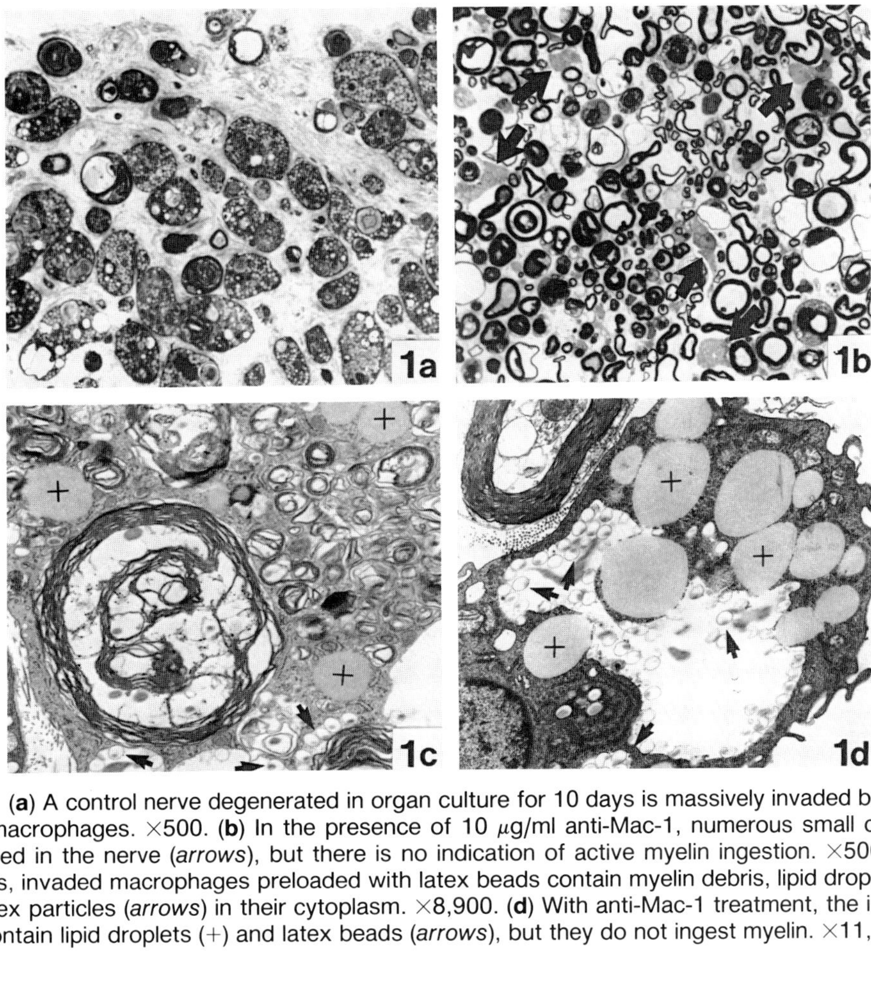

FIG. 1. (**a**) A control nerve degenerated in organ culture for 10 days is massively invaded by cocultured macrophages. ×500. (**b**) In the presence of 10 μg/ml anti-Mac-1, numerous small cells are dispersed in the nerve (*arrows*), but there is no indication of active myelin ingestion. ×500. (**c**) In controls, invaded macrophages preloaded with latex beads contain myelin debris, lipid droplets (+), and latex particles (*arrows*) in their cytoplasm. ×8,900. (**d**) With anti-Mac-1 treatment, the invading cells contain lipid droplets (+) and latex beads (*arrows*), but they do not ingest myelin. ×11,000.

were eliminated with the organ culture model, described next.

FUNCTIONAL PROPERTIES OF MACROPHAGES IN RECOGNIZING MYELIN AS A TARGET FOR PHAGOCYTOSIS

The Organ Culture Model

The organ culture model was developed to obviate the difficulties set forth in the preceding paragraph (24). In this model, segments of fascicles of peripheral nerves were exposed to cultured macrophages *in vitro*. Cultured macrophages are obtained by peritoneal lavage 4 days after intraperitoneal injection of thioglycolate; a constant number of 2×10^6 cells per milliliter was added to the organ cultures. Nerve segments were about 3 mm in length and were desheathed before being placed into the culture vessels. Both nerves and macrophages were from the same strain of mice; cultures were maintained with cytosine arabinoside (see below) for standard periods of 10 days. A method of line sampling allows semiquantitative assessment of the degree of macrophage invasion of the culture. Point sampling can be used to quantify sheath degradation.

The degenerating nerves in the organ culture model are rapidly invaded by macrophages, which engage in active myelin phagocytosis similar (Fig. 1a,c) to that in large-pore chambers or in nerves *in situ*. These macrophages are identified by their Fc or Mac-1 markers. Schwann cells persist with intact fine structure; they may form typical bands of Hanken-Büngner after complete myelin removal by macrophages.

The functional integrity of this residual Schwann cell population was tested by reimplanting the organ cultures after 10 days into a host animal between the proximal and distal stumps of a transected sciatic nerve. The transplant was secured within a silicon tube. Sprouting axons invaded the cell population of the organ culture and underwent myelination.

Role of Cell Proliferation

All of the experiments described in the following section were done with the addition of 10 mmol cytosine arabinoside to the culture medium. This ensures that the culture model contains only the cell populations entered at the beginning of the experiment, unaltered by proliferation of subpopulations. This point is important: in the absence of cytosine arabinoside, one does not obtain negative controls when no macrophages are added; there is a considerable proliferative capacity of resident endoneurial macrophages in the organ culture. Beyond that, proliferating Schwann cells may differ from nonproliferating Schwann cells in terms of their capacity for myelin uptake, as discussed below. Proliferation and outgrowth of resident macrophages, producing apolipoprotein E, were found in explant cultures of nerves by Goodrum and Novicki (25).

METABOLIC ACTIVATION

The role of metabolic activation to produce a respiratory burst was studied using recombinant interferon-γ, one of the most potent modulators of the mononuclear phagocyte system. Cultured macrophages were activated to produce luminol-dependent chemiluminescence by interferon-γ in a dose-dependent manner from 10 to 1,000 U/ml (26). Adding macrophages to organ cultures did not cause a metabolic burst; conversely, a metabolic burst could be elicited by interferon-γ at any phase of exposure of the macrophages to the organ culture. These experiments gave no indication of a dependence of myelin phagocytosis on metabolic activation of the macrophages, and they are consistent with the data presented below on the role of complement in our system. CBG complement-mediated phagocytosis of erythrocytes was shown to fail to induce an oxidative burst, whereas ingestion of IgG-opsonized erythrocytes gave a chemiluminescent response (27). Also, treatment of microglia or peritoneal monocytes with interferon resulted in increased expression of Fc receptors and production of superoxide anions.

Role of Carbohydrate Receptors

The potential involvement of carbohydrate receptors, e.g., mannose, fucose, or sialic receptors, in myelin phagocytosis was explored by exposing organ cultures to a panel of 14 simple or complex sugars at concentrations between 1 and 100 mM or to eight sugar-splitting enzymes (28). Some of the sugars were toxic to the macrophages, depending on concentration. None of the tested sugars had a clear-cut inhibitory effect on myelin phagocytosis by macrophages. Negative data were also obtained with most of the sugar-splitting enzymes except for a dramatic blocking of myelin phagocytosis by L-fucosidase in a 10 mU/ml concentration. This effect was highly specific: macrophages cultured in the presence of L-fucosidase were still quite capable of ingesting carbon particles or latex microspheres. If such prelabeled macrophages were then added to organ cultures (in continued presence of L-fucosidase), they were capable of invading the cultures, but they had lost their potential for ingesting myelin. This striking and specific effect of L-fucosidase is probably caused by an interaction between L-fucosidase and a fucose-bearing macrophage surface receptor for the lymphokine that activates the macrophage's C3 receptor for phagocytosis (29), consistent with the results described below.

Role of the Fc Receptor

The immunohistochemical demonstration of the Fc receptor served as a standard marker in our organ cultures. Hence, it was logical to explore whether this receptor served merely as a marker or whether the Fc receptor played an active role in myelin phagocytosis. We found no evidence for an *in vivo* role of the Fc receptor in Wallerian degeneration in two parallel series of experiments (30). In one we used chickens with total elimination of immunoglobulin production by bursectomy. In the other experiment we used mice injected after birth with antibodies against IgM, causing a selective severe reduction of immunoglobulin M levels. The sciatic nerve was transected in both series, and the rate of myelin degradation was determined by morphometry. No difference was detectable between the immunoglobulin-depleted animals and the controls. Further evidence for the noninvolvement of the Fc receptor in myelin phagocytosis was obtained *in vitro* in the organ culture model by exposing the cultures to antibodies against the Fc receptor. This had no effect on the macrophages' capacity to ingest myelin (31).

Role of Complement and Complement Receptor

In view of the dramatic inhibition of myelin phagocytosis by L-fucosidase, we investigated the potential role of complement and complement receptors (32) in myelin phagocytosis. The myelin phagocytic capacity of the invading macrophages was dramatically abolished by treating organ cultures and macrophages with a monoclonal antibody against the complement receptor type 3 (CR3) (31). This effect was highly specific. Similar to the experiments with L-fucosidase, blocking of the complement receptor did not impair the macrophages' capacity to ingest latex microspheres. If macrophages prelabeled *in vitro* with latex beads were added to organ cultures with continued blocking of CR3, the macrophages were capable of undisturbed invasion of the cultures; their cytoplasm contained only lipid droplets and latex beads but no myelin particles (Fig. 1b,d). Inhibition of myelin phagocytosis was also obtained by depletion of serum complement with cobra venom factor. In the various experiments done earlier, the complement content of the tissue culture medium had obviously been sufficient to provide opsonization and to maintain an unimpaired myelin phagocytic system.

Further evidence for the role of the complement receptor in Wallerian degeneration was obtained in *in vivo* experiments in which the rate of myelin removal from transected nerve was studied in animals receiving a monoclonal antibody to the macrophage CR3 (33). This caused a significant reduction in the rate of myelin removal in the living animal. The presence of complement on the decaying myelin sheaths was shown with immunoelectron microscopy, consistent with its location on sheaths in patients with neuropathy (34) or the activation of serum complement by myelin membranes (35,36). The capacity of normal human serum to demyelinate mouse cerebellum cultures (37) forms a bridge between the present data and demyelinating lesions, where complement also plays an important role (38).

Role of Inhibition of Macrophage Invasion

Myelin phagocytosis was tested in the above experiments in terms of the ingestion of myelin after the macrophages had entered the organ cultures, positioning themselves in the immediate proximity of the degenerating fibers. Some of these experiments also gave evidence of an indirect inhibition of myelin phagocytosis as a result of a diminished capacity of macrophages to invade organ cultures. The most dramatic effect was observed on metabolic activation with recombinant interferon-γ (26). Metabolic activation correlated with marked inhibition of macrophage invasion; hence, the removal of myelin from the cultures was reduced by a paucity of phagocytes in the tissue. This effect was not evident if metabolic activation was induced a few days after starting the cultures, allowing the nonactivated macrophages to invade the tissue before their activation.

Many of the various sugars tested also showed some degree of inhibition of cell invasion; for instance, there was a medium grade of inhibition with L-mannose, D-galactose, N-acetylglucosamine, L-acetylgalactosamine, xylose, L-fucose, and D-mannose-6-phosphate at different concentrations. Diminished invasion was also seen with sialidase, α-galactosidase, and sulfatase (28). None of these sugars or enzymes, however, diminished invasion as dramatically as metabolic activation by interferon-γ.

Role of the Phagocytic Activity and Proliferation of Schwann Cells

The functional parameter used throughout these experiments was the transformation of cells into macrophages with enlarged cytoplasmic bodies filled with fat and myelin debris. There was no indication in our experiments for the transformation of Schwann cells into macrophages either in small-pore chambers or in organ cultures without added macrophages, particularly in the presence of cytosine arabinoside. If the latter was omitted, there was active cell proliferation in organ cultures, including formation of macrophages, but most if not all of these macrophages were derived from a resident monocyte population, as evident from their Fc or Mac-1 markers.

Uptake of latex particles or myobacteria was observed in a rat Schwannoma cell line (39,40). Cultured Schwann cells were also found to phagocytose myelin membranes, and they did so slower than macrophages but more quickly than fibroblasts (41,42). However, at least in thickly myelinated fibers, most myelin degradation was accomplished by macrophages identified by the monoclonal antibody ED1 for rat monocytes/macrophages (43).

Although these data do not affect the interpretation of macrophage capacities described in the preceding text, they indicate a potential interaction between invading macrophages and the proliferative capacity of resident cell populations and probably also between the proliferative capacity and the phagocytic capacity of Schwann cells under various experimental conditions.

A striking effect of macrophage invasion on the proliferation of fibroblasts was seen in Millipore diffusion chambers, where the massive proliferation of fibroblasts in small-pore chambers did not occur in large-pore chambers accessible to the macrophages (3). Wallerian degeneration elicits an initial burst of Schwann cell proliferation (44), which is substantially greater in myelinated than in unmyelinated nerves (45). Its concurrence with macrophage recruitment may imply Schwann cell mitogens derived from the latter. Conversely, myelin (on ingestion) and axolemma (on transduction to the Schwann cell surface) represent mitogenic signals to the Schwann cell (41). In nerve explants presumably devoid of macrophages, Schwann cells were seen to proliferate, escaping from the basal lamina tube (11,46).

If one attempts to correlate such diverse observations with the behavior of macrophages during myelin phagocytosis, one needs to consider at least two points. First, the functional properties of a proliferating Schwann cell population or of Schwann cells in culture are not necessarily a valid paradigm for the properties of a Schwannian internode at the onset of phagocytic invasion; cultured Schwann cells are known to lose myelin-associated markers (47–49). Second, the opsonin-dependent targeted myelin ingestion by macrophages (which occurs when a phagocyte invades the basal lamina envelope of a degenerating nerve fiber) differs from the behavior of macrophages toward homogenized myelin particles. Ingestion of the latter (like that of latex beads) is not complement dependent (31).

MODULATION OF MACROPHAGES BY LYMPHOKINES

The role of macrophages during the immune response might go beyond phagocytosis, including the secretion of numerous products. Tumor necrosis factor-alpha (TNF-α) is a cytokine released mainly by monocytes and macrophages. It affects a variety of cell types in quite different ways (50,51); macrophages themselves have been shown to be its targets.

In a series of experiments, we attempted to define the role of cytokines, especially TNF-α and interleukin 1, in myelin removal. Treatment of cultured nerves and macrophages with 1,000 U/ml TNF-α resulted in a significant reduction of the loss of myelin profiles compared with controls. This effect was reversible with anti-TNF-α and also with sulfasalazine, which inhibits the binding of TNF-α to its cell membrane receptor.

The mechanisms by which TNF-α modulates the macrophage's myelin phagocytic capacity were defined by examining macrophage cell surface receptor expression. Since macrophages were shown to ingest myelin via their CR3 (31), we determined CR3 expression by immunofluorescence and by immunoelectron microscopy. Immunofluorescence indicated a reduced CR3 expression during TNF-α treatment. Immunoelectron microscopy confirmed these results: TNF-α-treated macrophages were much less CR3-positive than control cells. These observations indicated that the TNF-α-induced suppression of myelin ingestion by macrophages involved a down-regulation of their CR3 expression.

Similar functional properties of macrophages probably also come into play during the more complex events of demyelinating diseases. In experiments of this type, TNF-α treatment had minimal effects on inflammation, but it dramatically reduced demyelination (52). This selective TNF-α effect resembles the results obtained in our *in vitro* model of myelin ingestion.

A SYNOPSIS OF THE FUNCTIONAL PROPERTIES OF MACROPHAGES IN MYELIN PHAGOCYTOSIS IN WALLERIAN DEGENERATION

Mandatory Requirements

- Complement receptor C3
- Opsonization by serum complement

Modulating Factors

- Ca^{2+}
- Tumor necrosis factor
- L-Fucosidase-sensitive structures

Independent Of

- Metabolic activation
- Interaction with T or B lymphocytes
- Immunoglobulins or Fc receptor
- Receptors for mannose, fucose, sialic acid, and many other components of glycocalix

Specific Features

- Uptake of myelin by means of CR3 differs from uptake of particular material (latex beads) that does not require opsonization.
- The mechanism by which the macrophage distinguishes between the decaying myelin and the surviving Schwann cell is still unknown.

INTERACTION OF MACROPHAGES WITH OTHER IMMUNE-COMPETENT CELLS DURING TISSUE REJECTION

An *in vitro* system of peripheral nervous tissue rejection was established to analyze lymphocyte–macrophage interactions. Homogenized rat peripheral nerve was injected intraperitoneally in C57BL/6J mice. The sensitized cell population obtained, composed of lymphocytes and macrophages, was then exposed to degenerating rat peripheral nerves *in vitro.*

The sensitized mouse macrophages massively attacked the peripheral rat nerves in a manner similar to organ rejection. Preliminary data reveal a massive myelin phagocytosis combined with a cytotoxic attack on Schwann cells. The phagocytic part of tissue rejection can be blocked by adding antibodies to the macrophage CR3 to the cultures. Under these conditions, cytotoxic phenomena persist. Lymphocyte depletion experiments indicate that phagocytes need a permanent lymphocyte activation to maintain rejection.

Further experiments should clarify more exactly the role of cell-to-cell interactions as well as that of interleukins in this situation.

OUTLOOK

One may speculate that the near future will open up a new classification of the roles played by macrophages in neuropathology. No longer will they be seen as the indolent scavengers that clean up the litter left by disease. Rather, they evidently utilize their complex repertoire of functional capacities in very different ways, depending on the nature of the process. Phagocytosis of particular material, e.g., foreign bodies, can occur without opsonization or metabolic activation. Perhaps the organization of an infarct—filled by an abundance of macrophages—also falls into that class. In Wallerian degeneration there is invasion of the neural tubes followed by phagocytosis of the sheaths without disturbing the surviving Schwann cells. This targeting requires opsonization of myelin by serum complement and engagement of the CR3 without metabolic activation. Myelin ingestion in autoimmune diseases may well differ, involving opsonization by immunoglobulins with engagement of the Fc receptor and probably with a consequent metabolic burst. This in turn may induce a bystander demyelination (53). Enhanced myelin phagocytosis by macrophages was found on opsonization with IgG from antisera to myelin or to myelin components (54–56). Finally, at the most complex level, the capacities of the macrophage will be utilized in interaction with other cells of the immune system.

EPILOGUE

Ramón y Cajal (57) showed his remarkable facility for sound judgment when he wrote in 1928 (p. 94): "The careful examination of many preparations of the peripheral nerve stump has convinced us that all the independent spherical cells that are present in the nerve tube and contain fat droplets are in reality migrated leukocytes."

REFERENCES

1. Algire GH, Weaver JM, Prehn RT. Growth of cells *in vivo* in diffusion chambers. I. Survival of homo-

grafts in immunized mice. *J Natl Cancer Inst* 1954;15:493–507.
2. Benestad HB. Formation of granulocytes and macrophages in diffusion chamber cultures of mouse blood leucocytes. *Scand J Haematol* 1970;7: 279–288.
3. Beuche W, Friede RL. The role of non-resident cells in Wallerian degeneration. *J Neurocytol* 1984;13: 767–796.
4. Scheidt P, Waehneldt TV, Beuche W, Friede RL. Changes of myelin proteins during Wallerian degeneration *in situ* and in Millipore diffusion chambers preventing active phagocytosis. *Brain Res* 1986; 379:380–384.
5. Liu HM. Schwann cell properties. II. The identity of phagocytes in the degenerating nerve. *Am J Pathol* 1974;75:395–416.
6. Gibson JD. The origin of the neural macrophage: a quantitative ultrastructural study of cell population changes during Wallerian degeneration. *J Anat* 1979;129:1–19.
7. Schubert T, Friede RL. The role of endoneural fibroblasts in myelin degradation. *J Neuropathol Exp Neurol* 1981;40:134–154.
8. Beuche W, Friede RL. Myelin phagocytosis in Wallerian degeneration of peripheral nerves depends on silica-sensitive, bg/bg-negative and Fc-positive monocytes. *Brain Res* 1986;378:97–106.
9. Scheidt P, Friede RL. Myelin phagocytosis in Wallerian degeneration. Properties of Millipore diffusion chambers and immunohistochemical identification of cell populations. *Acta Neuropathol* 1987;75:77–84.
10. Beuche W, Friede RL. A new approach toward analyzing peripheral nerve fiber populations. II. Foreshortening of regenerated internodes corresponds to reduced sheath thickness. *J Neuropathol Exp Neurol* 1985;44:73–84.
11. Crang AJ, Blakemore WF. Observations on Wallerian degeneration in explant cultures of cat sciatic nerve. *J Neurocytol* 1986;15:471–482.
12. Perry VH, Brown MC, Lunn ER, Tree P, Gordon S. Evidence that very slow Wallerian degeneration in C57BL/Ola mice is an intrinsic property of the peripheral nerve. *Eur J Neurosci* 1990;2:802–808.
13. Perry VH, Brown MC, Lunn ER. Very slow retrograde and Wallerian degeneration in the CNS of C57BL/Ola mice. *Eur J Neurosci* 1991;3:102–105.
14. Thomson CE, Mitchell LS, Griffiths IR, Morrison S. Retarded Wallerian degeneration following peripheral nerve transection in C57BL/6/Ola mice is associated with delayed down-regulation of the P_o gene. *Brain Res* 1991;538:157–160.
15. Shrager P, Rubinstein CT. Optical measurement of conduction in single demyelinated axons. *J Gen Physiol* 1990;95:867–890.
16. Perry VH, Brown MC, Gordon S. The macrophage response to central and peripheral nerve injury. A possible role for macrophages in regeneration. *J Exp Med* 1987;165:1218–1223.
17. Müller HW, Minwegen P. Nonresident macrophages in peripheral nerve of rat: effect of silica on migration, myelin phagocytosis, and apolipoprotein E expression during Wallerian degeneration. *J Neurosci Res* 1987;18:222–229.
18. Triarhou LC, Herndon RM. Effect of macrophage inactivation on the neuropathology of lysolecithin-induced demyelination. *Br J Exp Pathol* 1985; 66:293–301.
19. Rodriguez M, Quddus J. Effect of cyclosporin A, silica quartz dust, and protease inhibitors on virus-induced demyelination. *J Neuroimmunol* 1986; 13:159–174.
20. Lunn ER, Perry VH, Brown MC, Rosen H, Gordon S. Absence of Wallerian degeneration does not hinder regeneration in peripheral nerve. *Eur J Neurosci* 1989;1:27–33.
21. Heininger K, Schäfer B, Hartung H-P, Fierz W, Linington C, Toyka KV. The role of macrophages in experimental autoimmune neuritis induced by a P_2-specific T-cell line. *Ann Neurol* 1988;23: 326–331.
22. Griffin JW, Stoll G, Li CY, Tyor W, Cornblath DR. Macrophage responses in inflammatory demyelinating neuropathies. *Ann Neurol* 1990;27:S64–S68.
23. Schmidt B, Stoll G, Hartung H-P, Heininger K, Schäfer B, Toyka KV. Macrophages but not Schwann cells express Ia antigen in experimental autoimmune neuritis. *Ann Neurol* 1990;28:70–77.
24. Hann Bonnekoh PG, Scheidt P, Friede RL. Myelin phagocytosis by peritoneal macrophages in organ cultures of mouse peripheral nerve. A new model for studying myelin phagocytosis *in vitro*. *J Neuropathol Exp Neurol* 1989;48:140–153.
25. Goodrum JF, Novicki DL. Macrophage-like cells from explant cultures of rat sciatic nerve produce apolipoprotein E. *J Neurosci Res* 1988;20:457–462.
26. Brück W, Friede RL. Activation of macrophages by recombinant interferon-gamma has no effect on myelin phagocytosis but hinders invasion of nerves in organ culture. *J Neuroimmunol* 1989;25:47–55.
27. Büscher K-H, Klimetzek V, Opferkuch W. Influence of antibody and complement components on phagocytosis and chemiluminescence of macrophages. *Immunobiology* 1985;170:390–401.
28. Brück W, Friede RL. L-Fucosidase treatment blocks myelin phagocytosis by macrophages *in vitro*. *J Neuroimmunol* 1990;27:217–227.
29. Griffin FM Jr, Mullinax PJ. Augmentation of macrophage complement receptor function *in vitro*. IV. The lymphokine that activates macrophage C3 receptors for phagocytosis binds to a fucose-bearing glycoprotein on the macrophage plasma membrane. *J Exp Med* 1984;160:1206–1218.
30. Hann PG, Beuche W, Neumann U, Friede RL. The rate of Wallerian degeneration in the absence of immunoglobulins. A study in chick and mouse peripheral nerve. *Brain Res* 1988;451:126–132.
31. Brück W, Friede RL. Anti-macrophage CR3 antibody blocks myelin phagocytosis by macrophages *in vitro*. *Acta Neuropathol* 1990;80:415–418.
32. Alex Law SK. C3 receptors on macrophages. *J Cell Sci Suppl* 1988;9:67–97.
33. Brück W, Friede RL. The role of complement in myelin phagocytosis during PNS Wallerian degeneration. *J Neurol Sci* 1991;103:182–187.
34. Hays AP, Lee SSL, Latov N. Immune reactive C3d on the surface of myelin sheaths in neuropathy. *J Neuroimmunol* 1988;18:231–244.
35. Silverman BA, Carney DF, Johnston CA, Vanguri

P, Shin ML. Isolation of membrane attack complex of complement from myelin membranes treated with serum complement. *J Neurochem* 1984;42: 1024–1029.
36. Koski CL, Vanguri P, Shin ML. Activation of the alternative pathway of complement by human peripheral nerve myelin. *J Immunol* 1985;134: 1810–1814.
37. Silberberg DH, Manning MC, Schreiber AD. Tissue culture demyelination by normal human serum. *Ann Neurol* 1984;15:575–580.
38. Linington C, Morgan BP, Scolding NJ, Wilkins P, Piddlesden S, Compston DAS. The role of complement in the pathogenesis of experimental allergic encephalomyelitis. *Brain* 1989;112:895–911.
39. Band H, Talwar GP. Effect of macrophage activators on the phagocytosis of mycobacteria by Schwann cells. *J Neuroimmunol* 1986;13:109–113.
40. Band H, Bhattacharya A, Talwar GP. Mechanism of phagocytosis by Schwann cells. *J Neurol Sci* 1986;75:113–119.
41. Meador-Woodruff JH, Yoshino JE, Bigbee JW, Lewis BL, De Vries GH. Differential proliferative responses of cultured Schwann cells to axolemma and myelin-enriched fractions. II. Morphological studies. *J Neurocytol* 1985;14:619–635.
42. Bigbee JW, Yoshino JE, De Vries GH. Morphological and proliferative responses of cultured Schwann cells following rapid phagocytosis of a myelin-enriched fraction. *J Neurocytol* 1987;16:487–496.
43. Stoll G, Griffin JW, Li CY, Trapp BD. Wallerian degeneration in the peripheral nervous system: participation of both Schwann cells and macrophages in myelin degradation. *J Neurocytol* 1989;18: 671–683.
44. Salzer JL, Bunge RP. Studies of Schwann cell proliferation. I. An analysis in tissue culture of proliferation during development, Wallerian degeneration, and direct injury. *J Cell Biol* 1980;84:739–752.
45. Clemence A, Mirsky R, Jessen KR. Non-myelin-forming Schwann cells proliferate rapidly during Wallerian degeneration in the rat sciatic nerve. *J Neurocytol* 1989;18:185–192.
46. Crang AJ, Blakemore WF. Observations on the migratory behaviour of Schwann cells from adult peripheral nerve explant cultures. *J Neurocytol* 1987;16:423–431.
47. Raff MC, Fields KL, Hakomori S-I, Mirsky R, Preuss RM, Winter J. Cell-type-specific markers for distinguishing and studying neurons and the major classes of glial cells in culture. *Brain Res* 1979;174:283–308.
48. Mirsky R, Winter J, Abney ER, Pruss RM, Gavrilovic J, Raff MC. Myelin-specific proteins and glycolipids in rat Schwann cells and oligodendrocytes in culture. *J Cell Biol* 1980;84:483–494.
49. Kreider BQ, Messing A, Doan H, Kim SU, Lisak RP, Pleasure DE. Enrichment of Schwann cell cultures from neonatal rat sciatic nerve by differential adhesion. *Brain Res* 1981;207:433–444.
50. Patton JS, Rice GC, Ranges GE, Palladino MA Jr. Biology of the tumor necrosis factors. In: Sorg C, ed. *Macrophage-derived cell regulatory factors. Cytokines. Vol 1.* Basel: S Karger; 1989:89–104.
51. Gordon C, Wofsy D. Effects of recombinant murine tumor necrosis factor-α on immune function. *J Immunol* 1990;144:1753–1758.
52. Paya CV, Leibson PJ, Patick AK, Rodriguez M. Inhibition of Theiler's virus-induced demyelination *in vivo* by tumor necrosis factor alpha. *Int Immunol* 1990;2:909–913.
53. Griot C, Bürge T, Vandevelde M, Peterhans E. Antibody-induced generation of reactive oxygen radicals by brain macrophages in canine distemper encephalitis: a mechanism for bystander demyelination. *Acta Neuropathol* 1989;78:396–403.
54. Trotter J, DeJong LJ, Smith ME. Opsonization with antimyelin antibody increases the uptake and intracellular metabolism of myelin in inflammatory macrophages. *J Neurochem* 1986;47:779–789.
55. Goldenberg PZ, Kwon EE, Benjamins JA, Whitaker JN, Quarles RH, Prineas JW. Opsonization of normal myelin by anti-myelin antibodies and normal serum. *J Neuroimmunol* 1989;23:157–166.
56. Smith ME, Sadler RH, Dyer C, Benjamins JA, Yu ACH. Phagocytosis of peripheral nerve myelin *in vitro:* effect of antibody. *J Neurosci Res* 1990;27: 298–306.
57. Ramón y Cajal S. *Degeneration and regeneration of the nervous system,* Vol 1. New York: Hafner Publishing; 1928.

Advances in Neurology, Vol. 59, edited by
Fredrick J. Seil. Raven Press, Ltd.,
New York © 1993.

32

Novel Major Histocompatibility Complex Expression by Microglia and Site-specific Experimental Allergic Encephalomyelitis Lesions in the Rat Central Nervous System After Optic Nerve Transection

*Michael C. Molleston, †Matthew L. Thomas, and †William F. Hickey

*Departments of *Neurosurgery and †Pathology, Washington University School of Medicine, Saint Louis, Missouri 63110*

In the mammalian central nervous system (CNS) regeneration of an axonal process, once separated from its neuron, is extremely limited. Thus, accidental or iatrogenic axotomy is a significant cause of permanent disability as a result of this fundamental property of the CNS. Extensive characterizations of injured neural systems have been carried out from structural (1,2), ultrastructural (3–5), and molecular (6,7) perspectives, but only recently have these investigations begun to include immunologically important phenomena (8–11).

Historically the CNS has been considered an "immunologically privileged" site (12). One reason for this is that the expression of major histocompatibility complex (MHC) molecules and other accessory molecules, both important participants in T-cell-mediated immune reactions (13,14), are virtually absent within the healthy CNS. MHC class I gene products, generally thought to be present on all somatic cells (14), as well as MHC class II molecules, are normally undetectable by immunohistochemistry in the CNS (15–19). Nevertheless, in certain disease states these molecules become readily detectable on selected cells of the CNS, most prominently on microglia (18,19) and perivascular cells (20,21).

Microglia are bone-marrow-derived mononuclear cells that reside in the CNS (20,22). Their function as the antigen-presenting cell of the CNS is well characterized (20,23). However, their role in CNS injury, and specifically in Wallerian degeneration, is less well defined. Rao and Lund, using a rat optic nerve model of Wallerian degeneration, found increased expression of MHC on microglial cells in the zones of termination of the optic nerve (8). Konno et al. reported class II induction on microglial cells in a variety of models of Wallerian degeneration in the CNS (24). Moreover, we, as well as Konno and co-workers, have reported that microglial activation is associated with susceptibility to inflammation (10,11). Yet, the exact time course and relationship to inflammation sensitivity for these induced MHC molecules appearing on microglial cells is unknown.

In the present study we employ a model of Wallerian degeneration produced by transection of an optic nerve, which is comprised of the axons of retinal ganglion cells (RGC). Decussation of the axonal projections of the

RGCs in the albino rat optic nerve is almost complete (95%) (25–27). The ipsilateral fibers (5%) are restricted to a visual field corresponding to a small area of the superior temporal retina (anteromedial superior colliculus) (27). The major axonal output of the rat retina is to the superior colliculus, with only about one-third of the RGC projecting to the lateral geniculate nucleus (1). As a result, the optic nerve can be transected outside the cranium, and the effects of denervation examined in the contralateral terminal optic tract and superior colliculus. The intact structures of the undamaged visual pathway present in each histological section serve as an internal negative control. In this model the cerebral blood–brain barrier is not mechanically disrupted, nor is there direct trauma to the tectum itself.

Using this system of optic nerve transection in the rat, which has been well characterized from neuroanatomic (25,27), functional (26), and regenerative perspectives (28), we have studied the time course and distribution in the superior colliculus of the novel expression of MHC antigens, accessory molecules of antigen presentation, leukocyte common antigen (29) (CD45/LCA), and susceptibility to the development of inflammation.

MATERIALS AND METHODS

Optic Nerve Transection

Adult Lewis rats (150 to 200 g, Charles River) were anesthetized with sodium pentobarbital. The right optic nerve was cauterized and divided at an intraorbital location after being exposed by incising the conjunctiva and superior extraocular muscles. The wound was closed by a tarsorraphy of the right eye.

Tissue Preparation

Rats were sacrificed at specified times following surgery. Two groups were created for immunohistochemistry: one group was perfused with a mixture of 4% paraformaldehyde in 0.1 M phosphate buffer, pH 7.4, and the brain was removed. The coronal section containing the superior colliculi was placed in 0.2 M phosphate buffer until use. The second group was perfused with Dulbecco's phosphate-buffered saline (PBS), and the coronal slice of the brain containing the superior colliculi was snap frozen in OCT compound (Miles Laboratories) for fresh frozen sections.

Under deep anesthesia, rats were perfused via the aorta with 50 to 100 ml of Dulbecco's PBS. Brains to be examined in the unfixed state were immediately removed, and the coronal section containing the brachium superior colliculus and the superior colliculus was snap frozen in OCT. From these slices, cryostat sections 10 μm thick were cut and fixed in 100% methanol (−20°C) for 30 to 60 sec. These glass-mounted sections were washed in 0.5 M Tris buffer, pH 7.4, plus 1% fetal calf serum (FCS) and incubated with primary antibodies as described below. Brains to be prefixed with paraformaldehyde were initially perfused via the aorta with Dulbecco's PBS, followed by perfusion with 200 ml of a solution containing 4% paraformaldehyde in 0.1 M phosphate buffer, pH 7.4. The brains were then removed, cut into 3- to 5-mm-thick coronal slices and postfixed in 4% paraformaldehyde in 0.1 M phosphate buffer, pH 7.4, for 1 hr. The brain slices were washed repeatedly with 0.2 M phosphate buffer, pH 7.4, for 24 hr and then allowed to equilibrate overnight in 30% sucrose. These tissue blocks were then frozen in OCT, and 10-μm serial sections of the brachium superior colliculus and superior colliculus were cut. These paraformaldehyde-prefixed tissue sections were placed on gelatin/alum-coated slides and allowed to air dry for 1 hr prior to being washed in 0.5 M Tris, pH 7.4, plus 1% FCS. Primary antibodies were then applied.

Immunohistochemistry

Murine monoclonal antibodies against RT-1B/rat MHC class II (OX-6) (30), CD45/

LCA (OX-1) (31), and CD11b/CR3, the C3bi receptor (OX-42) (32), were obtained from Bioproducts for Science (Indianapolis) as ascites and used at a dilution of 1 : 500. Anti-CD4 (W3/25) (33) from the same source was used at a dilution of 1 : 400. Rabbit anti-glial fibrillary acidic protein (GFAP) was obtained from Dako (Sweden) and used at a dilution of 1 : 800. A supernatant containing the monoclonal antibody Il-69 (34), which recognizes Lewis rat MHC class I molecules (RT-1A^1), was a generous gift from Dr. Hiromitsu Kimura.

Immunohistochemistry was performed on fresh frozen tissue sections with the avidin–biotin methodology as previously detailed (35). Sections of paraformaldehyde-fixed tissue were blocked for nonspecific protein binding with 0.5 M Tris, pH 7.4, plus 1% FCS for 1 hr and then incubated with the primary antibody at 4°C overnight. Sections were washed in 0.5 M Tris/1% FCS for 1 hr and incubated overnight at 4°C for a second time with biotinylated antimouse IgG or antirabbit IgG (Vector Laboratories, Burlingame, CA). Next they were washed for 1 hr in 0.5 M Tris/1% FCS and incubated overnight at 4°C a final time with an avidin–horseradish peroxidase complex in solution. The peroxidase labeling was visualized by incubation with a solution of 1% 3,3′-diaminobenzidine tetrahydrochloride (Sigma Chemical, St. Louis), 0.03% hydrogen peroxide, and 10 mM imidazole. This reaction produced dark brown staining. Sections were dehydrated in alcohol and xylene, and coverslips were mounted.

The innervated superior colliculus ipsilateral to the optic nerve section served as a base-line control for the constitutive level of staining for each section. In addition, a section was processed as above but received no primary antibody, to serve as a control for nonspecific staining in secondary steps of the procedure.

Adoptive Transfer of EAE

An encephalitogenic $CD4^+$ rat T-cell line specific for myelin basic protein was produced as previously reported (20,36). Clinical recognizable experimental allergic encephalomyelitis (EAE) consistently developed after adoptive transfer of 10^7 cells/animal to Lewis rats. These rats had had optic nerve transections on specified days prior to or following the injection of myelin basic protein-specific T lymphoblasts. Control animals had no surgical procedure prior to adoptive transfer. The EAE was graded as previously defined (35). In brief, a flaccid tail was graded as 1, hind-limb paralysis as 2, a moribund state as 3, and death as 4. When clinical signs of EAE became fully developed, typically on the fifth day post-infusion of encephalitogenic cells, the rat was sacrificed, and the spinal cord and superior colliculi were assessed histologically for the presence and severity of inflammation.

Determination of Immunohistochemical Findings

To assess the degree of enhanced immunohistochemical positivity between the damaged (denervated) and normal colliculi, a semiquantitative scale was established. Induction of antigen expression was graded as 0 if the strength of staining on CNS parenchymal cells or vessels was similar between the two colliculi. Values of 1+, 2+, and 3+ were assigned according to the strength of the immunoperoxidase staining of the denervated colliculus compared to the innervated colliculus: 1+ was mildly stronger, 2+ was moderately stronger, and 3+ was markedly stronger.

RESULTS

Optic nerve transection produced dramatic changes in both the amount and distribution of MHC class I and II, CD4, CD45 (LCA), and CD11b (CR3) by microglia in the denervated superior colliculus (Fig. 1), as well as changes in GFAP expression by astrocytes. There were two patterns of positivity, with each pattern defined by its own group of

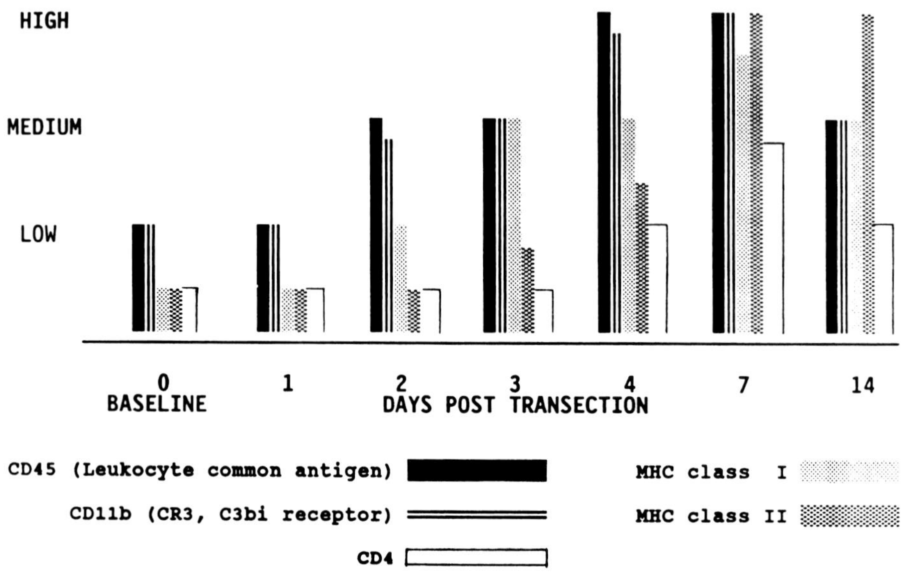

FIG. 1. The time course of elevation of immunologically important molecules on microglial cells following optic nerve transection. MHC class I and II and CD4 are undetectable at base line.

induced markers and its own time course of induced expression (Fig. 2).

The earliest changes involved increased staining for CD45 and CD11b on microglial cells, which became elevated above control (i.e., contralateral colliculus) levels within 48 hr of optic nerve division. The distribution of the positive cells was within the intermediate and superficial layers of the denervated colliculus. In addition to microglial cells, vascular endothelial cells and/or perivascular cells in these same layers of the colliculus were positive for MHC class I by 48 hr. Enhanced astrocytic staining for GFAP was observed in the superficial and intermediate layers of the colliculus by 48 hr.

By 3 days, the staining for CD45, CD11b, and MHC class I on microglial cells (Fig. 1) and that for GFAP in astrocytes were strongly elevated in the deafferented colliculus compared with the control side. The staining intensity for these four antigens reached maximal levels by 7 days and remained at that intensity for all subsequent time points examined.

MHC class II and CD4 expression were de-

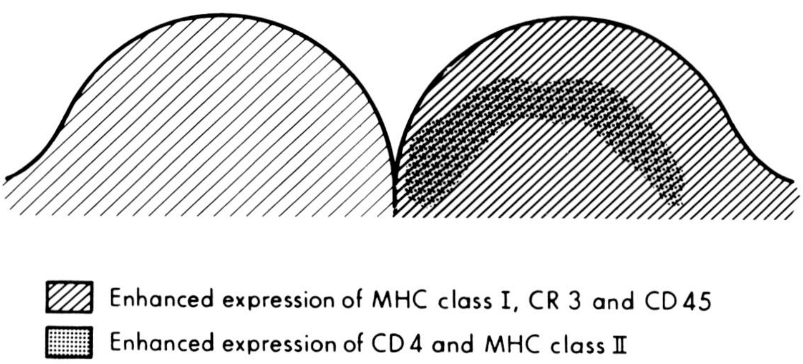

FIG. 2. The pattern of new and enhanced expression of immunologically important molecules in the damaged (right side) colliculus.

layed in onset relative to the other inducible molecules and had a more restricted distribution of expression. Class II became detectable by 4 days and was paralleled in both expression and distribution by CD4. Their pattern of distribution within the injured colliculus was limited to the stratum opticum, the specific collicular layer to which the severed axons of the RGCs project (8,25) (Fig. 2). By 7 days the staining for MHC class II was maximal and strong, whereas the staining for CD4, though easily visible, was less intense than the staining of all the other markers.

Microglial cells within the distal damaged optic tract were strongly positive for LCA, CD11b, and MHC class I and class II, paralleling the changes within the colliculi. Once established, enhanced expression of all molecules positive by 7 days remained strongly expressed well beyond 2 weeks. Their relative positivity and distribution did not change within this time.

Immunohistochemical staining of the fresh frozen tissue and the paraformaldehyde-fixed tissue differed significantly with regard to sensitivity and degree of antigen preservation. Expression of MHC class I, CD45, CD11b, and GFAP was not detectable until 3 days, and MHC class II and CD4 positivity were only weakly present at 4 days in the paraformaldehyde-fixed tissue. This slight disadvantage was counterbalanced by the dramatically enhanced histological detail and tissue integrity produced with paraformaldehyde fixation.

There was only low-level, constitutive expression of CD45 and CD11b on microglial cells of the innervated (uninjured) colliculus, and only rare vascular endothelial cells were positive for MHC class I in these areas. MHC class II and CD4 staining were completely negative on microglial cells in all animals in the uninjured colliculus. At no time were hematogenously derived cells seen, nor were classical inflammatory cell infiltrates present in the deafferented colliculi from animals that had not received encephalitogenic cells.

Animals given encephalitogenic T lympho-

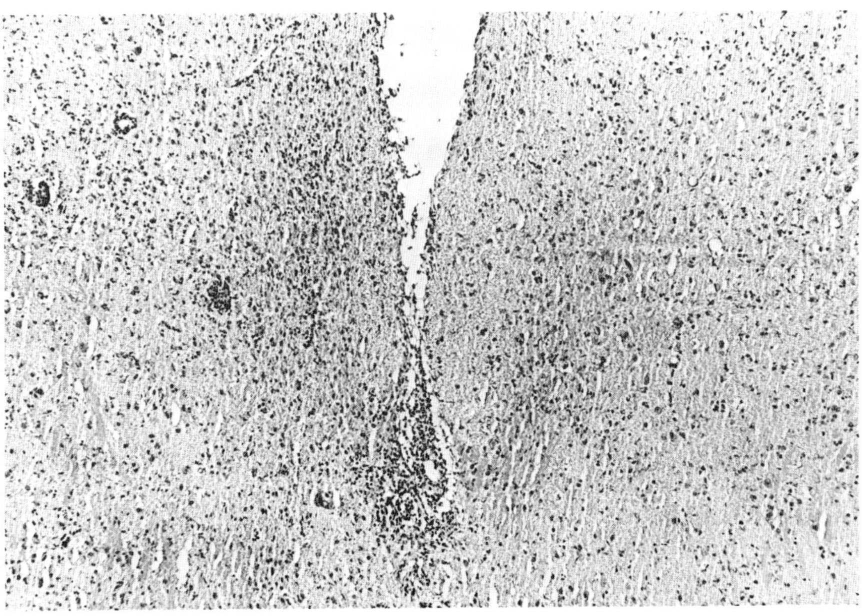

FIG. 3. Adjacent colliculi from a rat given encephalitogenic cells 2 days following optic nerve transection. Note the perivascular inflammatory cells and hypercellular parenchyma on the damaged side (left), whereas the normally innervated side exhibits no evidence of inflammation. Hematoxylin stain, ×125.

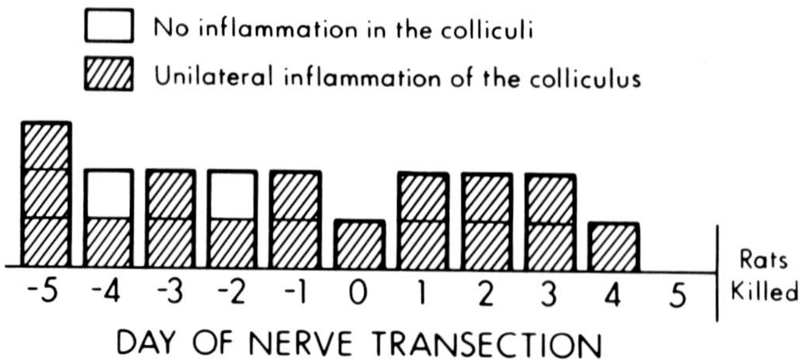

FIG. 4. Relationship between the susceptibility to unilateral collicular inflammation and optic nerve damage.

blasts showed mild signs of EAE on day 4 post-injection and became more severely afflicted on day 5 post-transfer. Animals with previously transected right optic nerves were killed when they exhibited hind-limb paralysis (grade 2 EAE). Histological examination of the superior colliculi revealed that the denervated sides were uniformly infiltrated by inflammatory cells, whereas the uninjured colliculi showed no evidence of infiltrates (Fig. 3). In the superior colliculi exhibiting EAE inflammation, the quantity and distribution of MHC and LCA antigens on microglia markedly exceeded that induced by deafferentation alone. Inflammation of the colliculi was never observed in uninjured rats, even when there was extensive infiltration of the spinal cords and severe clinical disease.

The time of optic nerve transection relative to the injection of the encephalitogenic T lymphocytes did not appear to be a significant factor. Unilateral infiltration by inflammatory cells in the deafferented colliculi developed whether the nerve had been severed 9 days prior to or on the same day as the first evidence of mild clinical signs of EAE (Fig. 4).

DISCUSSION

We have demonstrated that CNS Wallerian degeneration in the superior colliculus, distant from the site of axonal injury, induces novel expression by microglial cells of MHC class I, class II, and CD4 in addition to heightened constitutive expression of CD45 and CD11b by microglia in a distribution confined to the injured nerve and its anatomic target. The time course for these changes is rapid (over a period of days) and precedes by weeks the degeneration and phagocytosis of the myelin sheaths (22,37). There appear to be increased numbers of microglial cells expressing these immunologically relevant molecules. There is not only enhanced expression of these molecules on resident microglia that are normally unstained but also a real increase in the number of microglial cells in the later phases of this reactive process. Proliferation of microglia in response to distant axonal injury is well documented (37–39). Changes occur within the astrocytes in the area of denervation, as they become more strongly positive for GFAP and assume a reactive morphology. This discrete area of microglial and astrocyte activation subsequently is targeted for the inflammatory changes of EAE, a process that typically spares the superior colliculi.

The markedly enhanced expression of CD45 (LCA) by microglial cells in this model of site-specific Wallerian degeneration is especially important in the light of the increased ability of these foci to support antigen-specific, T-cell-mediated immune reactions; LCA is a family of transmembrane protein tyrosine phosphatases uniquely expressed by cells of hematopoietic origin. Although the exact function of these molecules is not understood, it appears that LCA is required for

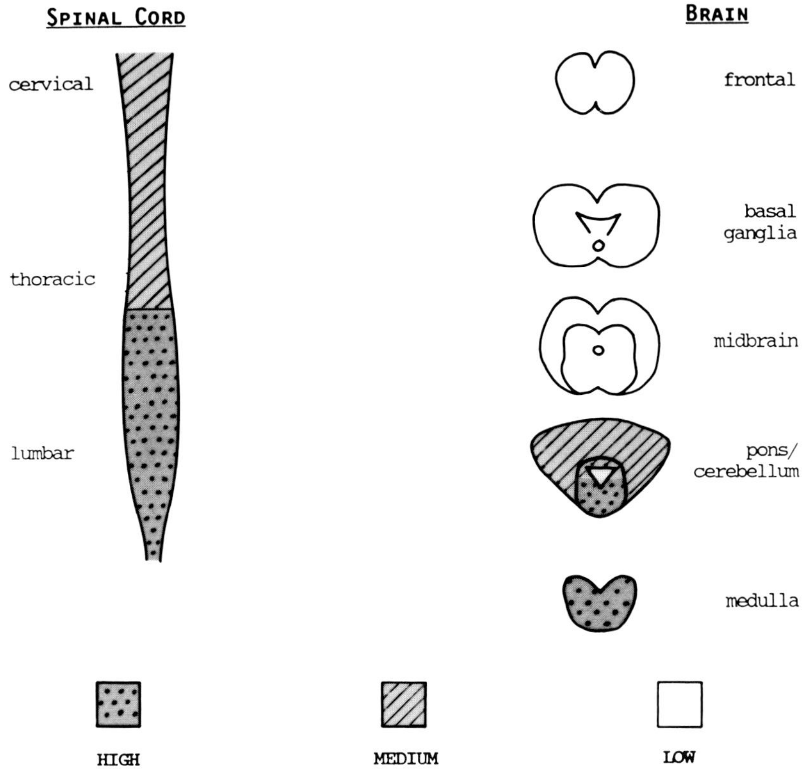

FIG. 5. This figure indicates the areas of high susceptibility versus resistance to developing EAE inflammation during typical EAE in a normal Lewis rat. Note that the colliculi (dorsal surface of the midbrain) are typically EAE resistant.

initial activation of lymphocytes (40–42) and may function to regulate crucial tyrosine kinases (43,44). It is of interest, therefore, that LCA, as well as other transmembrane molecules that may be initial mediators of cellular activation, are expressed at much higher levels on microglial cells at the site of denervation. For CD45 it has previously been shown that expression is increased on granulocytes after activation with various stimuli (45) which supports the conclusion that its expression is increased on microglia at sites subject to inflammation.

The model system used in this study has been employed by others and is very well suited to the investigation of factors controlling CNS immunologic reactivity. Using unilateral enucleation, Rao and Lund (8) first described the induction of MHC expression, both class I and class II molecules, occurring in the optic tract and superior colliculus as a feature of Wallerian degeneration. They found, as we have, that CD4 expression was restricted to areas of MHC class II expression; however, they did not establish with certainty the nature of the cells expressing these molecules. Rao and Lund's investigation was initiated in an attempt to explain their observation that rejection of CNS grafts located near central optic pathways could be induced by removing an eye. They concluded that enucleation-induced MHC expression might serve as an immunologic stimulus for the graft rejection.

Our findings support their conclusion to the extent that the neural parenchyma in such zones is rendered capable of supporting an immune response if T cells of the appropriate antigen specificity enter the zone (11). The demonstration of lymphocytic and macrophage infiltration at the sites of MHC expression in our adoptive encephalomyelitis experiments lends support to the hypothesis that immune-mediated reactions can preferentially affect areas undergoing Wallerian degeneration.

Many zones of the normal CNS do not appear to participate in immune responses. The cellular infiltrates associated with EAE show a distinct hierarchy of area sensitivity (Fig. 5). The colliculi virtually never become inflamed in the Lewis rat, yet there is no suitable explanation for this. The EAE-inducing antigen (myelin basic protein) and antigen-presenting cells (perivascular cells and/or microglia) are present here as in other CNS locations. T lymphocytes are also needed for inflammation to begin. The blood–brain barrier, in combination with the lack of CNS lymphatics, precludes lymphocyte traffic, as we normally define it, in the neural parenchyma (15,16,46,47). Nevertheless, activated T lymphoblasts are known to readily enter all levels of the CNS (11,48) and are of the type able to trigger antigen restricted immune reactions (36,48). Thus, the colliculi would be expected to become inflamed during EAE, but they do not. Nevertheless, within 24 hr of damage to the optic nerve delivered 1 cm to 1.5 cm away, the denervated colliculus is rendered totally susceptible to infiltration. The enhanced expression of the immunologically important molecules that occurs after optic nerve transection may destroy or in some other way diminish the normally "immune-privileged" nature of newly activated areas of Wallerian degeneration. In light of this, it seems that many areas of the healthy CNS are not as much "immunologically privileged" as they are "immunologically incompetent."

It is of great interest that this transformation from an inflammation-resistant to a susceptible area is very rapid. In fact, it occurs more rapidly than the time frame in which there is enhanced expression of the molecules we have investigated. This could indicate that levels of change beyond our level of detection are all that are required. Alternatively, it is equally possible that the critical changes rendering an area prone to inflammation are independent of the molecules we examined. Whether this increased predilection for T-cell-mediated immune reactions results from increased T-cell traffic into the damaged focus, enhanced activity of cells presenting antigen to lymphocytes, or some other mechanism is currently under investigation.

For reasons not clear, denervation creates areas of the CNS that subsequently can support T-cell mediated, antigen-restricted inflammation. But denervation is not alone in this regard. In conditions where a strong systemic immune reaction is ongoing, such as graft-versus-host disease (19), or in idiopathic neurodegenerative conditions of the nervous system (49), significantly elevated levels of CNS MHC expression have been detected. Moreover, graft-versus-host disease has the ability to reactivate encephalomyelitis in rats that have recovered from EAE (50).

The present report is added to prior ones that demonstrate that Wallerian degeneration induces MHC expression on microglial cells in the CNS. Akiyama and associates produced similar changes in a projection-specific manner in microglial cells in the rat thalamus following sterile induction of cortical neuronal death (46). They observed a restricted expression of MHC class II relative to class I, as noted in our study, and observed that microglia in the synaptic zones of termination of the dead axons preferentially expressed MHC class II. They did not investigate accessory molecules of antigen presentation, which accompany MHC class II induction and augment its presence on fully immunocompetent microglia. The time course for the induction of MHC molecular expression in their model was similar to the chronology we report. Konno and coworkers recently described a study very similar to Akiyama's, except that nonspecific cryoinjury to rat cortex was used as the stimulus to Wallerian degeneration instead of kainic acid-induced neuronal death (24). Their results are similar to those of Akiyama et al. (46) and to our findings; however, the extent to which hematogenously derived cells contributed to the observed MHC expression was not addressed, despite the significant disruption of the cerebral blood–brain barrier they describe.

Another form of CNS reaction induced by axonal damage is the axotomy reaction. It appears to cause similar immunologic changes in microglial cells in the CNS. Streit et al. examined degenerating and regenerating facial nerve complexes and reported MHC class I and class II expression on microglial cells in both paradigms (21). They proposed that in the axotomy reaction and in neuronal death, MHC antigens may be performing a nonimmunologic function, perhaps mediating intercellular communication among various subtypes of microglial cells. They did not determine the presence of LCA or CD4. Maehlen et al. have observed novel expression of MHC molecules in models of the axotomy reaction, though that group reported the expression of such molecules on neurons as well as on nonneuronal cells (51,52). It is possible that the MHC antigen expression Maehlen and colleagues observed may actually exist on microglial cell processes closely applied to the neurons, an observation that can not be made at the light microscopic level. Maehlen and co-workers also proposed nonimmunologic roles for MHC molecules and linked nerve regeneration temporally with the appearance and disappearance of MHC expression on neurons and other cells in a facial nerve injury model (51). Additionally, these authors reported increased numbers of lymphocytes in the lumbar spinal cord in areas of enhanced MHC expression following induction of active EAE in rats undergoing sciatic and facial nerve axotomy (9). This last point parallels our findings and may be indicative of a general pattern of enhanced immunoreactivity in damaged CNS tissue. Such a possibility was suggested decades ago by Clark and Bogdanove (53), reviewed by Levine (54), and demonstrated in the superior colliculus denervation model by Konno et al. (10) and by us (11). It is also noteworthy that CNS damage has been suggested to play a role in the development of multiple sclerosis plaques in humans (55).

It is clear from the present study, and from the other work mentioned, that neuronal reaction or death and axonal degeneration change the immunologic substrate in the CNS. Yet we found, as have others, that no lymphocytes or macrophages from the circulation are seen in the CNS following these types of sterile injuries. The absence of these hematogenous cells is particularly important when considering how Wallerian degeneration induces MHC molecules on microglial cells. In both multiple sclerosis and EAE, MHC expression and the expression of the accessory molecules of antigen presentation occur on microglial cells in the inflammatory lesions (18,56). Large numbers of T cells are present in these areas, which could provide a source of γ-interferon to induce these phenotypic changes. This possibility is supported by the findings of the present study, since the strength and distributional area of MHC molecule expression seen in denervated superior colliculus exhibiting the inflammatory changes of EAE exceed by far the MHC expression produced by denervation alone. Yet which factors are responsible for the induction of these important changes on microglia on models of Wallerian degeneration and the axotomy reaction that are devoid of lymphocytes is undefined to date.

In this investigation we noted two patterns of novel molecular expression by microglial cells, with MHC class II and CD4 expression more tightly controlled than CD45, CD11b, and MHC class I. It appears that differential control is determined by the location of the microglia in relation to the degenerating axons and/or deafferented neurons. If the microglia are in the superficial stratum opticum or deep stratum griseum superficiale, where primary retinal myelinated axons are targeted to synapse on first-order collicular cells, then MHC class II and CD4 expression occurs in addition to MHC class I, CD45, and CD11b expression. If the microglia are located in areas more removed from the primary retinal input, then only the latter three molecules are increased. This differential response of microglia might suggest that two factors are responsible for changing their usual molecular expression. Giulian has reported that in injured rat brain, interleukin-1 stimulates astrogliosis (6), a reactive change we also noted in the denervated colliculus. In addition, Giulian has defined two distinct factors derived from injured brain that appear in the wounded area about 2 days following injury, both of which stimulate microglial cells to divide (57). It is tempting to speculate that these factors may be playing distinct roles in microglial activation and/or inflammation susceptibility at sites of Wallerian degeneration and thus could account for our observations.

Transsynaptic changes in neurons similar to the changes produced by axotomy, including transsynaptic neuronal death, occur following deafferentation (1,3,58). As the current study demonstrates, microglial cells become activated and appear to proliferate following the same stimulus. *In vitro* it has been shown that once microglial cells become activated, they can secrete cytokines, stimulating themselves in an autocrine fashion as well as influencing astrocytes and neurons (6,23,59). Assuming a neuron-derived factor, this observation, at least in part, would explain how both Wallerian degeneration (through deafferentation of neurons) and axotomy (through the axotomy reaction) can lead to the novel expression of immune molecules. A recent report showed γ-interferon-like immunoreactivity in the cytoplasm of axotomized motor neurons (60), possibly an important link between neuronal injury and the immune system.

At this time, the possibility that microglial activation relates to reparative and regenerative capabilities in the CNS is unproven. However, it is noteworthy that in the best-studied model of mammalian CNS regeneration, the superior colliculus, the zone of regenerated synapse formation is identical to the area of restricted MHC class II and CD4 expression (8,28). In that system, animals had one colliculus deafferented 2 weeks earlier by optic nerve transection that was to serve as the target for reinnervation by reimplanted regenerating axons. This interval is equivalent to a time in which the expression of these immunologically relevant molecules on microglial cells has become maximal in our model. In addition to studies related to the more general question of communication between the injured nervous system and the immune system, further work specifically addressing the link between induction of microglial immunocompetence and neuronal repair and recovery is warranted.

ACKNOWLEDGMENTS

This study was supported by awards from the National Institutes of Health (NS-27321) and the National Multiple Sclerosis Society (RG-2244).

REFERENCES

1. Matthews MR, Cowan WM, Powell TPS. Trans-neuronal cell degeneration in the lateral geniculate nucleus of the macaque monkey. *J Anat* 1964; 94:145–162.
2. Purves D. Functional and structural changes in mammalian sympathetic neurons following interruption of their axons. *J Physiol* 1975;252: 429–463.
3. Ghetti B, Horoupian DS, Wisniewski HM. Transsynaptic response of the lateral geniculate nucleus and the pattern of degeneration of the nerve terminals in the rheses monkey after eye enucleation. *Brain Res* 1972;45:31–48.
4. Bignami A, Ralston HJ III. The cellular reaction to Wallerian degeneration in the central nervous system of the cat. *Brain Res* 1969;13:444–461.
5. Graeber MB, Streit WJ, Kreutzberg GW. The microglial cytoskeleton: vimentin is localized within activated cells in situ. *J Neurocytol* 1988;17: 573–580.
6. Giulian D, Baker TJ. Peptides released by ameboid microglia regulate astroglial proliferation. *J Cell Biol* 1985;101:2411–2415.
7. Schnell L, Schwab ME. Axonal regeneration in the rat spinal cord produced by an antibody against myelin associated neurite growth inhibitors. *Nature* 1990;343:269–272.
8. Rao K, Lund RD. Degeneration of optic axons induces the expression of major histocompatibility antigens. *Brain Res* 1989;488:332–336.
9. Maehlen J, Olsson T, Zachau A, Lkareskog LK, Kristensson K. Local enhancement of major histocompatibility complex class I and II expression and

cell infiltration in experimental allergic encephalomyelitis around axotomized motor neurons. *J Neuroimmunol* 1989;23:125–132.
10. Konno H, Yamamoto T, Saitoh H, et al. Targeting of adoptively transfered experimental allergic encephalomyelitis lesions at sights of Wallerian degeneration. *Acta Neuropathol* 1990;80:521–528.
11. Hickey WF. Migration of hematogenous cells across the blood brain barrier and the initiation of CNS inflammation. *Brain Pathol* 1991;1:97–105.
12. Barker CF, Billingham RE. Immunologically privileged sites. *Adv Immunol* 1977;25:1–8.
13. Unanue E. Antigen presenting function of the macrophage. *Annu Rev Immunol* 1984;2:395–428.
14. Paul W. *Fundamental immunology.* New York: Raven Press; 1989.
15. Hickey WF, Osborn JP, Kirby WM. Expression of Ia molecules by astrocytes during experimental allergic encephalomyelitis in the Lewis rat. *Cell Immunol* 1985;91:528–532.
16. Hauser SL, Bhan AK, Gilles FH, et al. Immunohistochemical staining of human brain with monoclonal antibodies that identify lymphocytes, monocytes, and Ia antigen. *J Neuroimmunol* 1983;5:197–208.
17. Lampson LA, Hickey WF. Monoclonal antibody analysis of MHC expression in human brain biopsies: tissue ranging from "histologically normal" to that showing different levels of glial tumor involvement. *J Immunol* 1986;136:4054–4062.
18. Matsumoto Y, Hara N, Tanaka R, Fujiwara M. Immunohistochemical analysis of rat central nervous system during EAE with special reference to Ia-positive cells with dendritic morphology. *J Immunol* 1986;136:3668–3675.
19. Hickey WF, Kimura H. Graft-versus-host disease elicits expression of class I and class II histocompatibility antigens and the presence of scattered T lymphocytes in rat central nervous system. *Proc Natl Acad Sci USA* 1987;84:2082–2086.
20. Hickey WF, Kimura H. Perivascular microglial cells of the CNS are bone marrow derived and present antigen *in vivo. Science* 1988;239:290–293.
21. Streit WJ, Graeber MB, Kreutzberg GW. Expression of Ia antigen on perivascular and microglial cells after sublethal and lethal motor neuron injury. *Exp Neurol* 1989;105:115–126.
22. Perry VH, Gordon S. Macrophages and microglia in the nervous system. *Trends Neurosci* 1988;11: 273–278.
23. Frei K, Siepl C, Groscurth P, Bodner S, Schwerdel C, Fontana A. Antigen presentation and tumor cytotoxicity by interferon-G treated microglial cells. *Eur J Immunol* 1987;17:1271–1278.
24. Konno H, Yamamoto T, Iwasaki Y, Suzuki H, Saito T, Terunuma H. Wallerian degeneration induces Ia-antigen expression in the rat brain. *J Neuroimmunol* 1989;25:151–159.
25. Polyak S. *The vertebrate visual system.* Chicago: University of Chicago Press; 1957.
26. Sheridan CS. Memory and visual stimuli in the rat. *J Comp Physiol Psychol* 1965;59:292–310.
27. Lund RD. Uncrossed visual pathways of hooded and albino rats. *Science* 1965;149:1506–1507.
28. Vidal-Sanz M, Bray GM, Villegas-Perez MP, Thanos S, Aguayo AJ. Axonal regeneration and synapse formation in the superior colliculus by retinal ganglion cells in the adult rat. *J Neurosci* 1987;7:2894–2909.
29. Thomas ML. The leukocyte common antigen family. *Annu Rev Immunol* 1989;7:339–370.
30. McMaster WR, Williams AF. Identification of Ia glycoproteins in rat thymus and purification from rat spleen. *Eur J Immunol* 1979;9:426–433.
31. Sunderland CA, McMaster WR, Williams AF. Purification with monoclonal antibody of a predominant leucocyte-common antigen and glycoprotein from rat thymocytes. *Eur J Immunol* 1979;9: 155–159.
32. Robinson AP, White TM, Mason DW. Macrophage heterogeneity in the rat as delineated by two monoclonal antibodies, MRC OX-41 and MRC OX-42, the latter recognizing complement receptor type 3. *Immunology* 1986;57:239–347.
33. Jeffries WA, Green JR, Williams AF. Authentic T helper CD4 (W3/25) antigen on rat peritoneal macrophages. *J Exp Med* 1985;162:117–124.
34. Kimura H, Wilson DB. Anti-idiotypic cytotoxic T cells in rats with graft-versus-host disease. *Nature* 1984;308:463–464.
35. Hickey WF, Gonatas NK, Kimura H, Wilson DB. Identification and quantitation of T lymphocyte subsets found in the spinal cord of the Lewis rat during acute experimental allergic encephalomyelitis. *J Immunol* 1983;131:2805–2809.
36. Hickey WF, Cohen JA, Burns JB. A quantitative immunohistochemical comparison of actively versus adoptively induced experimental allergic encephalomyelitis in the Lewis rat. *Cell Immunol* 1987;109:272–281.
37. Perry VH, Brown MC, Gordon S. The macrophage response to central and peripheral nerve injury. *J Exp Med* 1987;165:1218–1223.
38. Cova JL, Aldskogius H, Arvidsson J, Molander C. Changes in microglial cell numbers in the spinal cord dorsal horn following brachial plexus transection in the adult rat. *Exp Brain Res* 1988;73:61–68.
39. Graeber MB, Tetzlaff W, Streit WJ, Kreutzberg GW. Microglial cells but not astrocytes undergo mitosis following rat facial nerve axotomy. *Neurosci Lett* 1988;85:317–321.
40. Mittler RS, Greenfield RS, Schachter BZ, Richard NF, Hoffman MK. Antibodies to the common leukocyte antigen (T200) inhibit an early phase in the activation of resting human B cells. *J Immunol* 1987;138:3159–3166.
41. Ledbetter JA, Tonks NK, Fischer EH, Clark EA. CD45 regulates signal transduction and lymphocyte activation by specific association with receptor molecules on T and B cells. *Proc Natl Acad Sci USA* 1988;85:8628–8632.
42. Pringel JT, Thomas ML. Evidence that the leukocyte common antigen is required for antigen-induced T lymphocyte proliferation. *Cell* 1989;58: 1055–1065.
43. Mustellin T, Coggeshall KM, Altman A. Rapid activation of the T cell tyrosine protein kinase pp56^{lck} by the CD45 phosphotyrosine phosphatase. *Proc Natl Acad Sci USA* 1989;86:6302–6306.
44. Ostergaard HL, Shackelford DA, Hurley TR, et al. Expression of CD45 alters phosphorylation of the

lck-encoded tyrosine protein kinase in murine lymphoma T cell lines. *Proc Natl Acad Sci USA* 1989;86:8959–8963.
45. Lacal P, Pulido R, Sanchea-Madrid F, Mollinedo F. Intracellular location of T200 and Mol glycoproteins in human neutrophils. *J Biol Chem* 1988;263:9946–9951.
46. Akiyama H, Itagaki S, McGeer PL. Major histocompatibility complex antigen expression on rat microglia following epidural kainic acid lesions. *J Neurosci Res* 1988;20:147–157.
47. Griffin DE, Hess JL, Moktarian F. In: Behan P, Spreafico F, eds. *Neuroimmunology*. New York: Raven Press; 1984:193–206.
48. Hickey WF, Hsu BL, Kimura H. T-lymphocyte entry into the central nervous system. *J Neurosci Res* 1991;28:254–260.
49. McGeer PL, Itagaki S, Boyes BE, McGeer EG. Reactive microglia are positive for HLA-DR in the substantia nigra of Parkinson's and Alzheimer's disease brains. *Neurology* 1988;28:1285–1293.
50. Willenborg DO, Rolinson A, Danta G. Reactivation of allergic encephalomyelitis by means of allogeneic confrontation. *Cell Immunol* 1985;90:614–620.
51. Maehlen J, Nennesmo I, Olsson AB, Olsson T, Schroder HD, Kristensson K. Peripheral nerve injury causes transient expression of MHC class I antigens in rat motor neurons and skeletal muscles. *Brain Res* 1989;481:368–373.
52. Maehlen J, Schroder HD, Klareskog L, Olsson T, Kristensson K. Axotomy induces MHC class I antigen expression on rat nerve cells. *Neurosci Lett* 1988;92:8–13.
53. Clark G, Bagdonave LH. The induction of lesions of allergic meningoencephalomyelitis in a predetermined location. *J Neuropathol Exp Neurol* 1955;14:433–437.
54. Levine S. Hyperacute, neutrophilic, and localized forms of experimental allergic encephalomyelitis. *Acta Neuropathol* 1974;28:179–189.
55. Poser CM. Pathogenesis of multiple sclerosis. *Acta Neuropathol* 1986;71:1–4.
56. Hayes GM, Woodroofe MN, Cruzner ML. Microglia are the major cell type expressing MHC class II antigens in human white matter. *J Neurol Sci* 1987;80:25–31.
57. Giulian D, Johnson B, Krebs JF, George JK, Tapscott M. Microglial mitogens are produced in the developing and injured mammalian brain. *J Cell Biol* 1991;112:323–330.
58. Sunderland S. *Nerves and nerve injuries*. New York: Longman; 1978.
59. Righi M, Mori L, De Libero G, et al. Monokine production by microglial cell clones. *Eur J Immunol* 1987;19:1443–1448.
60. Olsson T, Kristensson K, Ljungdahl A, Maehlen J, Holmdahl R, Klareskog L. Gamma-interferon-like immunoreactivity in axotomized rat motor neurons. *J Neurosci* 1989;9:3870–3875.

Advances in Neurology, Vol. 59, edited by
Fredrick J. Seil. Raven Press, Ltd.,
New York © 1993.

33

Expression of Monocyte/Macrophage Growth Factors and Receptors in the Central Nervous System

*Celia F. Brosnan, *Bridget Shafit-Zagardo, †Dennis A. Aquino, and *Joan W. Berman

**Departments of Pathology (Neuropathology) and †Neurology, Albert Einstein College of Medicine, Bronx, New York 10461*

Cells of the monocyte/phagocyte series play a central role in the host reaction to tissue injury and in the induction and regulation of the immune response. In the central nervous system (CNS) the role of the monocyte/phagocyte cell in tissue remodeling may be mediated by activation and proliferation of the endogenous microglia or by an influx of blood-borne monocytes to sites of tissue injury (reviewed in refs. 1,2). The regulation of these processes in the CNS is not well understood but is thought to reflect the relative levels and distribution of growth and chemotactic factors specific for these cells.

The mediators involved in the stimulation of cells of the monocyte/phagocyte series have been well characterized by their role in hematopoiesis (reviewed in refs. 3–5). A group of four major regulatory glycoproteins has been defined, each of which induces lineage-specific growth of colonies from bone marrow progenitor cells, that are referred to collectively as colony-stimulating factors (CSFs). They include macrophage CSF (CSF-1), which is a dimer of two identical subunits, and granulocyte–macrophage CSF (GM-CSF), granulocyte CSF (G-CSF), and multipotential CSF (multi-CSF or IL-3), all of which consist of a single polypeptide chain (4,5). In addition to their role in the induction of proliferation, these factors are required for the survival and differentiation of each cell type into functionally mature populations. The multiple regulatory effects mediated by the CSFs are considered to be caused by their interaction with specific cell surface receptors that initiate multiple signaling cascades in the responding cells, reflecting in part differences in receptor density, state of maturation of the responding cell, and relative levels of each of the CSFs. Like most other blood cells, monocytes/macrophages must be produced continuously in adult life to maintain appropriate numbers. Whether or not a continuous renewal process also proceeds with the endogenous microglial population has not been defined, although the persistence of microglial progenitor cells in the adult brain has recently been recognized (6).

In addition to the effect of specific growth factors on progenitor cell populations, the accumulation of macrophages at sites of tissue injury involves recruitment and migration of blood-borne cells across the endothelial cell wall and their retention within the perivascular tissues. This process has been shown to involve a complex set of reactions that includes the expression of specific adhesion molecules on the luminal surface of endothelial cells, the release of chemotactic factors that promote transendothelial cell migration, and the expression of cell surface integrins that promote adhesion to components of the extracellular matrix (reviewed in ref. 7). Included in the factors known to be chemotactic specifically for macrophages is monocyte-chemoattractant protein 1 (MCP-1), which was initially isolated from a malignant glioma cell line (8).

MACROPHAGE GROWTH FACTORS IN EXPERIMENTAL ALLERGIC ENCEPHALOMYELITIS

To evaluate the potential role of these factors in the activation and proliferation of endogenous microglia and the influx of blood-borne macrophages to sites of injury within the CNS, we have examined the expression of CSF-1, its receptor encoded by the proto-oncogene *c-fms,* and MCP-1 in animals sensitized to develop experimental allergic encephalomyelitis (EAE), an animal model of multiple sclerosis (9); EAE is an inflammatory demyelinating disease of the CNS that can be induced in susceptible species by sensitization with myelin antigens in complete Freund's adjuvant (CFA). Although the disease has been shown to be dependent on the sensitization of $CD4^+$ T cells (10), macrophages form a major component of the inflammatory infiltrate. Elimination of macrophages through the use of silica quartz dust (11), dichloromethylene-diphosphate-containing mannose liposomes (12), or antibodies that recognize a macrophage-specific leukocyte integrin (13) can suppress both clinical and pathological expression of disease, supporting a pivotal role for these cells in the disease process.

In the Lewis rat, EAE is a monophasic disease with a well defined time course (14). Between 10 and 11 days post sensitization (dps), an abrupt onset of weight loss is detected that is followed during the ensuing days by an ascending paralysis and urinary and fecal incontinence. The rats then recover rapidly, so that by day 20 full function is usually restored. In some females there may be a relapse over the next few days, but most animals remain symptom-free indefinitely (15). The clinical expression of disease is accompanied by an abrupt onset of a perivascular mononuclear inflammatory infiltrate in the CNS and extensive proteinaceous edema commencing 10 dps (16). The extent of these changes generally correlates closely with clinical expression of disease, although residual cellular inflammation in the CNS persists for extended periods of time (17).

The CSF-1 is encoded by a single gene, but alternatively spliced mRNA species of 4.5 kb, 2.3 kb, and 1.6 kb have been shown. All three mRNA species encode for biologically active protein, with the 4.5-kb and 2.3-kb species predominating (18,19). The proto-oncogene *c-fms* encodes the receptor for CSF-1 (20). MCP-1 belongs to a family of cytokines characterized by a low molecular mass (about 10 to 20 kD) and four half-cystines in almost identical locations (reviewed in ref. 21). The MCP-1 attracts monocytes but not neutrophils or lymphocytes. Steady-state mRNA levels for CSF-1, *c-fms,* and MCP-1 expression were determined at various times in the disease process by Northern blot analysis, and biologically active CSF-1 was detected using a bone marrow colony formation assay in semisolid medium. Control animals were sensitized with CFA or ovalbumin (OVA) in CFA.

Northern Blot Analysis of Steady-State mRNA for CSF-1, *c-fms,* and MCP-1 in EAE

The results demonstrated that clinical expression of disease was associated with a dramatic increase in steady-state mRNA for CSF-1, *c-fms,* and MCP-1 as determined by Northern blot analysis (22,23). Total RNA was isolated from the lumbar spinal cord of animals sensitized with guinea pig spinal cord myelin in CFA (EAE animals), OVA (a nonencephalitogenic peptide) in CFA, or CFA alone at varying times post-

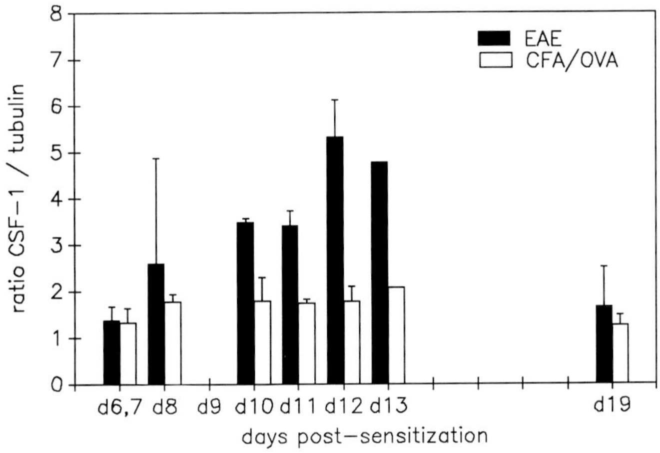

FIG. 1. Total mRNA was extracted from the lumbar spinal cord of control and EAE rats at varying times post-sensitization. Northern blots were sequentially hybridized with probes for CSF-1 and α-tubulin, and the signal quantitated by densitometry. The results are expressed as a ratio of the CSF to tubulin signal. They showed that a significant increase in CSF-1 expression could be detected in the lumbar spinal cord coincident with clinical expression of disease. The clinical index for the EAE rats was +0 on days 6, 7, and 8, +1 on day 10, +2.5 on day 11, +3 on day 12, +2.3 on day 13, and +0 on day 19.

sensitization. The times chosen corresponded to the preclinical period (days 6 and 8), the onset of early clinical signs (days 10 and 11), the height of clinical disease (days 12 and 13), and the recovery period (day 19) in the EAE animals. Filters were probed with murine cDNAs for CSF-1, *c-fms,* and MCP-1. The data were normalized to the signal obtained with the probe for α-tubulin. The results clearly demonstrated that a low endogenous level of CSF-1 was present in all samples (Fig. 1). However, in the animals

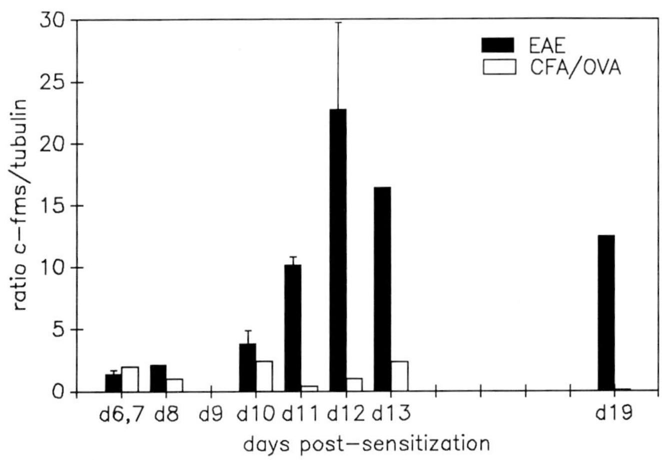

FIG. 2. The filters used for the data shown in Fig. 1 were stripped and rehybridized with the probe for the proto-oncogene *c-fms,* which encodes the CSF-1 receptor. The data are again presented as a ratio of the *c-fms* to tubulin signal. The results showed that a significant increase in the signal for *c-fms* was detected in the EAE animals. In contrast to the results observed for CSF-1, the level of *c-fms* remained elevated at the later time point (day 19).

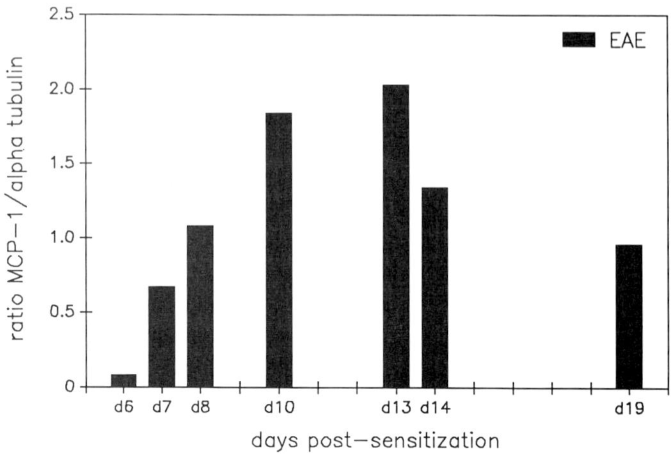

FIG. 3. Northern blots of total mRNA from the lumbar spinal cord of control and EAE animals were sequentially probed for MCP-1 and α-tubulin. The results, calculated as a ratio of the MCP-1 to tubulin signal, showed that no MCP-1 expression could be detected in the control samples. In animals sensitized to develop EAE, however, MCP-1 expression could be detected in the spinal cord early in the course of the disease and peaked at the height of clinical expression of EAE.

sensitized to develop EAE, a marked increase in CSF-1 mRNA was present in samples taken at the early phase and height of clinical disease. On day 12, a 1.5 fold increase in the CSF-1 mRNA level over that present on day 6 was detected. On day 19, when the animals had recovered from clinical signs of disease, the CSF-1 mRNA levels in the EAE animals had returned to control values. In contrast, no change in the CSF-1 mRNA values were noted in the control animals sensitized with OVA in CFA or with CFA alone.

Analysis of the same filters for *c-fms* showed a similar increase in expression in the EAE samples, but with higher levels persisting into the recovery period (Fig. 2). At the height of clinical disease, the levels of *c-fms* mRNA were increased by 8.9-fold over the control values. Low levels of *c-fms* mRNA were present in all of the control samples, and these values did not differ at any of the time points tested from those present in spinal cord samples from control, unsensitized animals.

Analysis of MCP-1 demonstrated that, in contrast to CSF-1 and *c-fms,* no endogenous levels of MCP-1 mRNA were present in any of the control samples. In animals sensitized to develop EAE, however, a prominent signal for MCP-1 mRNA was detected by Northern blot hybridization in samples taken on days 10, 11, 12, 13, and 14 (Fig. 3). In the recovery period, MCP-1 levels were significantly reduced. Protein expression for MCP-1 was assessed by Western blotting using a monoclonal antibody to human MCP-1 that cross-reacts with rat MCP-1. The results demonstrated the presence of MCP-1 immunoreactivity in the EAE animals (data not shown). Thus, expression of MCP in the spinal cord closely correlated with clinical expression of disease and with the influx of macrophages into the CNS (see below).

Determination of Biologically Active CSF-1 Expression in Spinal Cord Homogenates

To confirm that the elevated levels of mRNA for CSF-1 in the spinal cord reflected increased levels of biologically active protein, analysis of spinal cord lysates for colony-stimulating activity was determined. Spinal cord lysates were prepared from EAE animals on days 6, 8, and 12 and from CFA animals on day 12. In a soft-agar culture system of rat bone marrow cells, the results showed a marked increase in the number of colonies in the cultures that used as a source of growth factor spinal cord homogenate from day-12 EAE animals over those cultured in homogenates from days-6 and -8 EAE animals or from day-12 CFA animals. The colony numbers for EAE spinal cord lysate on days 6, 8, and 12 were 12.5 (±1.8), 21.3 (±4.4), and 39.3 (±11.4), respectively. The count for CFA spinal cord lysate on day 12 was 18.3 (±2.1). Heat inactivation of the lysates and morphological analysis of the cultures confirmed that the growth factor had the characteristics of CSF-1 and not of other members of the CSFs. These data also confirmed that low levels of biologically active CSF-1 were present in normal rat brain, consistent with the presence of endogenous CSF-1 mRNA expression.

CSF-1 Expression in Peripheral Lymphoid Organs

The fact that elevated levels of CSF-1 and *c-fms* could be detected in the spinal cord of EAE animals and not in control animals indicated that significant levels of these monocyte/phagocyte-related factors were present in immunologically injured CNS, but they did not address whether this response showed any specificity for the inducing antigen. To analyze this question further, additional total RNA and lysate samples were prepared from the spleen of EAE, CFA, and OVA animals. The results showed that in the spleen, increased expression of both CSF-1 mRNA and biologically active protein was detected in the EAE tissue taken during the acute clinical period over that present in spleen tissue from CFA and OVA animals. The number of colonies responding to growth factors present in EAE spleen lysates for days 8, 10, and 12 were 7.8 (±4.0), 12.2 (±3.8), and 16.4 (±5.6), respectively. The count for CFA spleen lysates on day 12 was 6.5 (±2.4). These data raise the interesting possibility that differences exist in the nature of the antigen-specific T cell response with regard to the expression of CSF-1 in the different groups of animals. Since we and others have shown that clinical and pathological expression of EAE in the rat is dependent on the activation of cells of the monocyte/macrophage series (11–13), this further raises the possibility that expression of CSF-1 by the antigen-specific $CD4^+$ T cell in EAE may be a necessary component of the encephalitogenic potential of these cells.

Immunohistochemical Analysis of Monocytes/Phagocytes Within the CNS in EAE

Immunohistochemistry was performed on sections of lumbar spinal cord using the monoclonal antibody ED1, which stains monocytes/macrophages, and the lectin *Ricinus communis* agglutinin 1 (RCA-1), which stains monocytes/macrophages and activated microglia. The results demonstrated that the number of these cells in the perivascular inflammatory infiltrates closely paralleled the observed increases in the levels of CSF-1, *c-fms,* and MCP-1 and was intimately associated with clinical expression of disease. Quantitation of the immunoreactive cells showed that no immunoreactive cells were present at 8 dps but that significant numbers of these cells could be detected in the spinal cord commencing 10 dps (Table 1). At this time, slightly more immunoreactivity was noted with RCA than with ED1, suggesting

TABLE 1. *Macrophage expression in EAE*[a]

EAE/dps	Clinical index	RCA-1	ED-1
d8	0	0	0
d10	+1	+2	+1
d11	+2.5	+3	+3
d12	+3	+2.8	+3
d13	+2.3	+1	+1
d18	0	+0.5	+0.5

[a] The number of macrophages entering the lumbar spinal cord during the course of EAE was quantitated by immunohistochemistry using the monoclonal antibody ED-1 and the lectin RCA-1, which recognize cells of the monocyte/phagocyte series.

that reactive microglia might contribute to these results in the early stages. At higher magnification, this increased immunostaining was observed throughout the white matter, particularly in specimens harvested 10 dps. It was diffusely distributed and did not appear to be specifically associated with infiltrating macrophages. The cells resembled microglia, but further studies are needed to confirm this transient activation of microglia during the early stages of EAE.

CSF-1 PRODUCTION BY GLIAL CELLS IN CULTURE

The fact that low endogenous levels of CSF-1 and *c-fms* were present in all of the control spinal cord samples indicated that cells within the CNS constitutively expressed these proteins. In addition, the data suggested that products of immune cells could alter this endogenous expression. To examine this issue further, we established cultures of purified populations of glial cells from neonatal rat brain and studied the expression of CSF-1 by Northern blot and biological assay. The results clearly showed that astrocytes endogenously expressed CSF-1 mRNA and biologically active protein (24). Exposure of these cells to the proinflammatory cytokines interleukin 1 (IL-1β) and/or tumor necrosis factor (TNF-α) markedly up-regulated CSF-1 expression in a time- and dose-dependent fashion. To examine the kinetics of IL-1β, TNF-α, and IL-1β + TNFα on steady-state mRNA in rat astrocyte cultures, fresh medium was added to all cultures with or without the addition of 100 U/ml cytokine(s). The filters were then sequentially probed with a random-primed 18S cDNA probe.

The data, when examined as a ratio of the CSF-1 mRNA to 18S RNA densitometric values, demonstrated that maximum CSF-1 mRNA expression was observed at 3 hr following exposure to the cytokines alone or in combination (Fig. 4). To determine the dose response to the cytokines, astrocyte cultures were treated with varying concentrations (25 to 200 U/ml) of TNF or IL-1 for 3 hr. The results, when examined as a ratio of CSF-1/18S for the treated cultures over the ratio of the untreated cultures, demonstrated that 100 U/ml of either IL-1 or TNF yielded maximal stimulation of CSF-1 mRNA and that CSF-1 mRNA levels were highest following treatment with IL-1 (Fig. 5). To determine

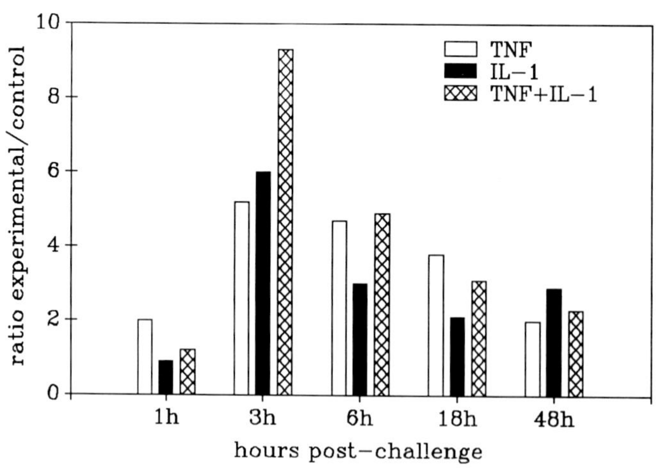

FIG. 4. Primary neonatal rat astrocyte cultures were exposed to 100 U/ml recombinant human TNF, IL-1, or TNF plus IL-1. At varying times post-challenge, total RNA was extracted, and Northern blots were sequentially hybridized with a probe for CSF-1 and ribosomal RNA. The results showed that astrocytes constitutively expressed CSF-1 and that this expression could be significantly up-regulated by exposure to TNF or IL-1. Maximum expression was observed at 3 hr post-challenge, with TNF plus IL-1 showing the greatest stimulatory effect.

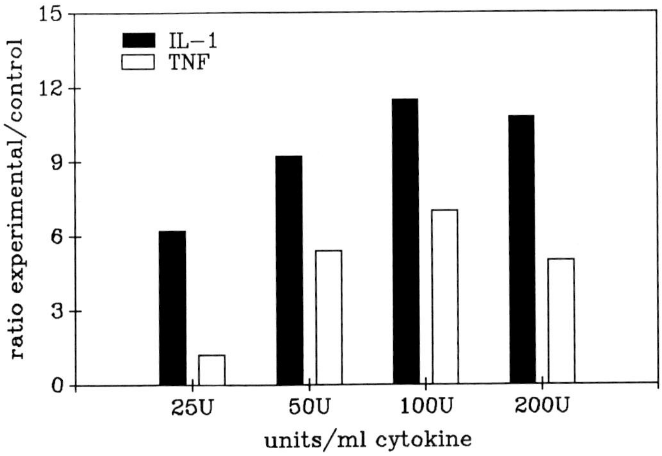

FIG. 5. Primary rat astrocyte cultures were exposed to varying concentrations of IL-1 or TNF for 3 hr. Total RNA was extracted, and Northern blots were sequentially probed for CSF-1 and ribosomal RNA. The data were obtained as a ratio of the CSF-1 to ribosomal RNA signal, and the results expressed as the ratio of the experimental to control values. The data showed that maximal stimulation was obtained with IL-1 at 100 U/ml.

whether biologically active protein was produced in this culture system, rat bone marrow cells were cultured in semisolid medium as before in the presence of supernates from untreated and cytokine-treated astrocyte cultures. The results indicated that supernates from astrocyte cultures contained endogenous CSF-1 activity that was markedly increased in supernates from IL-1-treated cultures and increased to a lesser extent with TNF. With supernates from control cultures, the numbers of colonies formed at 48 hr and 72 hr were 41.3 and 41.8, respectively. Following incubation in supernates from IL-1-treated cultures, the colony counts were 57.3 and 72.3, respectively, and for TNF-treated cultures the counts were 50 and 53.3. The TNF plus IL-1 treatment gave counts of 51.5 and 76.5 at the 48-hr and 72-hr time points.

STUDIES WITH RECOMBINANT CSF-1 IN ORGANOTYPIC CULTURES

The fact that astrocytes constitutively expressed CSF-1 *in vitro* and that this expression could be markedly up-regulated by inflammatory cytokines raised questions regarding the role of CSF-1 in the normal CNS and in conditions of immunologic damage. We therefore assessed the effect of recombinant CSF-1 on glial cell populations *in vitro* (24). Because the recombinant CSF-1 was of mouse origin, we used organotypic cultures of mouse spinal cord as the experimental system (26). In this culture system, all elements (except the vasculature) of the CNS survive, and myelination occurs *de novo*. The effect of the addition of CSF-1 to the medium on microglial numbers and morphology was examined in normal spinal cord explants, and the effect of CSF-1 on immune-mediated damage was addressed in cultures in which demyelination had been induced by the addition of serum from EAE animals.

The Effect of Recombinant CSF-1 on Normal Organotypic Cultures

Cultures were established and then exposed to concentrations of CSF-1 ranging from 100 to 5,000 U/ml. Cultures were examined on a daily basis and, at the end of 2 weeks, were processed for RCA-1 reactivity and electron microscopy. No effect of any of the doses of CSF-1 tested was noted on the extent of myelination or on the structural integrity of the myelin sheath. Occasional areas of myelin vacuolation were noted at the highest dose of CSF-1 used, but other areas appeared normal. The most striking change in these cultures occurred in the morphology of the microglial population. Although the number of microglia was not clearly different between experimental and control cultures stained with RCA-1 using the avidin–biotin technique (Fig. 6), in cultures exposed to CSF-1 in doses greater than 1,000 U/ml for 2 weeks there was a striking increase in the number of RCA-1^+ cells that expressed a ramified rather than amoeboid morphology (Fig. 7). These ramified microglia were present over the explanted cord tissue and in the outgrowth zone. Examination of cultures that had been fixed and stained for RCA-1 reactivity after only 48 hr of exposure to 5,000 U/ml CSF-1 demonstrated that the majority of the labeled cells possessed an amoeboid-type morphology, suggesting that the appearance of the ramified phenotype required more prolonged exposure to CSF-1. To determine the potential role of microglial replication in this phenomenon, cultures were exposed to 5,000 U/ml CSF-1 and to 5-bromodeoxyuridine (BrdU). After 2 weeks of incubation in the continued presence of

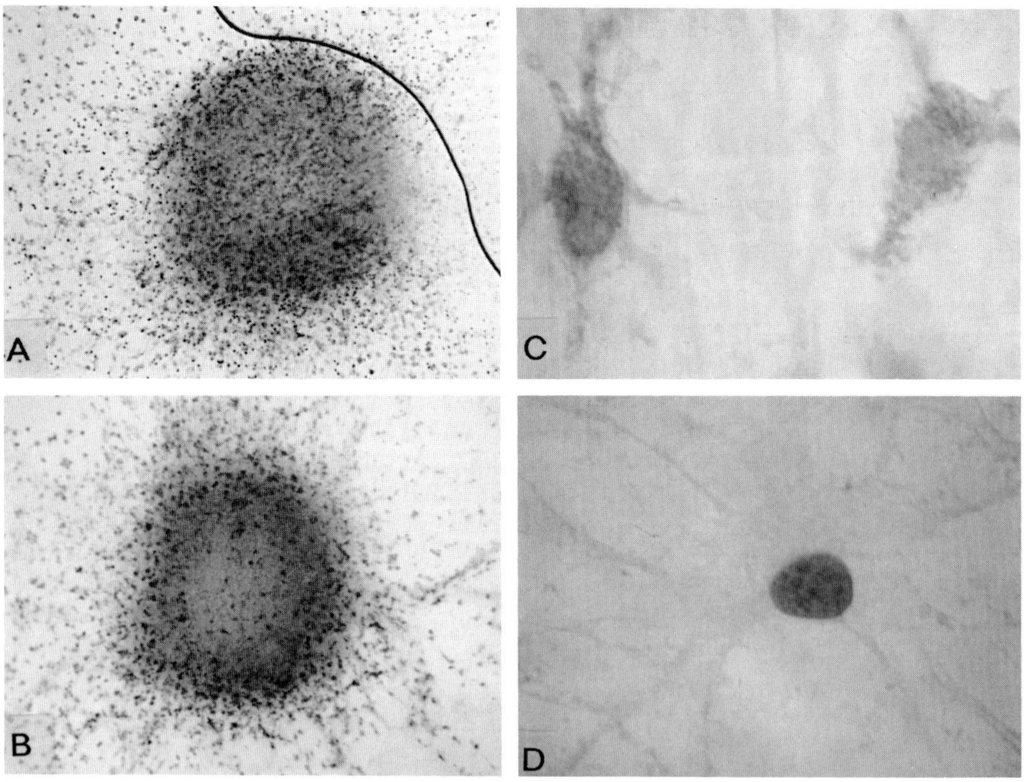

FIG. 6. Organotypic cultures of embryonic mouse spinal cord were exposed to 5,000 U/ml recombinant CSF-1 in medium supplemented with BrdU. After 3 weeks in culture, they were stained with RCA-1 and antibodies to BrdU. A control culture is shown in **A,** and a CSF-1 treated culture in **B** (original magnification ×12). Examination of the cultures at higher magnification demonstrated that cells that were positive for RCA-1 and expressed the ramified phenotype did not show nuclear reactivity for BrdU at a frequency that differed between the experimental cultures (**C**) and control (not shown) cultures. Many of the BrdU-positive cells did not show cytoplasmic staining for RCA-1 and expressed an astrocytic morphology (**D**) (original magnifications for **C** and **D,** ×300).

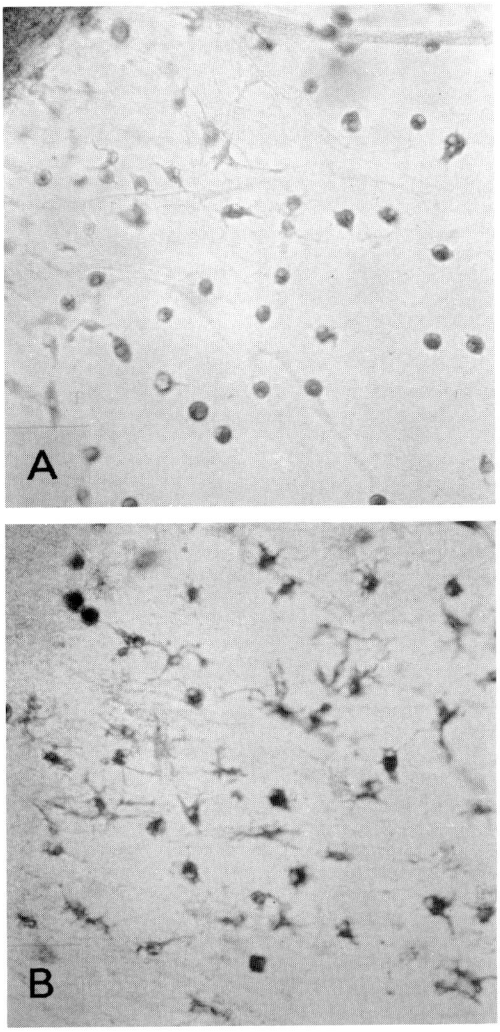

FIG. 7. Organotypic cultures of mouse spinal cord were exposed to CSF-1 as described in Fig. 6. After 3 weeks of exposure they were stained for RCA-1 reactivity. In control cultures most of the RCA-1$^+$ cells displayed an amoeboid-type morphology (**A**), whereas in cultures exposed to CSF-1, RCA-1$^+$ cells expressed a more ramified morphology (**B**) (original magnification ×30).

CSF-1, the cultures were fixed and stained for both BrdU and RCA-1. The results again demonstrated an increase in the appearance of RCA-1$^+$ ramified microglia in the CSF-1-treated cultures, but no obvious increase over that found in control cultures was noted in the colocalization of RCA-1$^+$ cells and immunoreactivity for BrdU (Fig. 6).

The Effect of Recombinant CSF-1 on Immune-Mediated Damage

Organotypic cultures exposed to serum from animals with EAE induced by sensitization with whole CNS tissue or white matter (anti-CNS serum) demonstrate extensive demyelination, loss of oligodendrocytes, and appearance of reactive astrocytes (9). To determine if CSF-1 could alter this pathological change, cultures were exposed to anti-CNS serum and then cultured in the presence or absence of CSF-1. The results demonstrated that 1,000 to 5,000 U/ml did not alter myelin loss or promote remyelination. In addition, reactive astrogliosis was not affected by the presence of CSF-1 in the medium (data not shown).

We conclude from these experiments using organotypic cultures of mouse spinal cord that CSF-1 may play a role in the establishment of ramified microglia. For the paradigms studied here, no morphological effect of CSF-1 was noted on other cells in this culture system.

DISCUSSION

In these studies we have used a combination of *in vivo* and *in vitro* model systems to examine the expression of factors associated with cells of the monocyte/phagocyte series in conditions of immune-mediated damage to CNS tissue. The results have shown that CSF-1, *c-fms,* and MCP-1 can be detected in the CNS. The fact that significant message levels could be quantified by Northern blot analysis in the absence of polymerase chain reaction amplification suggested an abundance of mRNA for these factors in the CNS, and this was confirmed by biological assays. CSF-1 and *c-fms* activity was present in the normal CNS, and these factors were markedly up-regulated in EAE, a T-lymphocyte-dependent primary demyelinating disease.

The central role of T cells sensitized to myelin antigens in the induction of EAE has now been well established; however, studies in which the distribution of these cells in the CNS has been examined have shown that they are few in number and are primarily found in a perivascular location (27). The majority of the infiltrating cells appear not to be antigen specific but to have been called in by inflammatory mediators. The results of the studies presented here support the conclusion that CSF-1 and MCP-1 play a major role in this inflammatory cascade. The CSF-1 levels in the CNS increased immediately before the onset of the acute clinical episode and fell significantly during the recovery period; MCP-1 was not detected in the normal CNS but was markedly elevated coincident with disease expression. These time points correlated with extensive perivascular accumulations of monocytes. The increase in the number of these cells probably accounted for most of the increased expression of *c-fms* in the CNS, and the persistence of elevated levels of *c-fms* even in the recovery period is probably associated with the low levels of inflammation that remain in the CNS for extended periods of time (17). The fact that no change in the levels of any of these factors was detected in the control CFA and OVA animals suggests that the up-regulation of these factors is induced by the entry of T cells into the CNS. That certain activated T cells may express CSF-1 has now been demonstrated (28). However, the extent to which this capability reflects responses to particular antigens and the capacity to elicit disease remains to be determined. In this respect, our observations that similar increases in CSF-1 expression were not detected in the spleen of CFA- and OVA-sensitized animals are intriguing and merit further study.

The source and targets of these factors in the CNS remain to be defined. In addition to the invading inflammatory cells, studies have shown that astrocytes constitutively express CSF-1 (29–31). Our studies have demonstrated that this expression can be markedly up-regulated by IL-1β and TNF-α, suggesting that the influx of inflammatory cells into the CNS may up-regulate the expression of this growth factor in cells endogenous to the CNS (24,25). Similar results have recently been reported by Aloisi et al. (32) and are consistent with the up-regulation of CSFs by interleukins in other cells (33–35). In addition, CSF-1 may be secreted by activated endothelial cells (36). For MCP-1, many cell types *in vitro* have been shown to secrete this monocyte chemoattractant (the human homolog of the mouse JE gene). This factor was originally cloned from a human glioma cell line (8) but has since been shown to be secreted by activated lymphocytes, endothelial cells, and smooth muscle cells (reviewed in ref. 21). *In vivo,* MCP-1 production by macrophages and endothelial cells has been demonstrated by *in situ* hybridization in atherosclerotic lesions (37). Thus, within the inflamed CNS many cell types may be sources of these factors, particularly in the presence of inflammatory mediators.

What are the targets and effects of these factors in the CNS? The *c-fms* proto-oncogene is thought to be almost exclusively expressed on cells of the monocyte/phagocyte series [although recently it has been suggested that certain subpopulations of astrocytes may also express *c-fms* (38)]. Thus, the cell populations that would be expected to be the major targets of these factors include endogenous microglia and blood-borne macrophages. The activation and recruitment of these two cell types in response to tissue damage within the CNS is a reflection of the nature and extent of the tissue damage. When tissue damage is relatively restricted and is present primarily at the cellular level, then activation of microglia is the characteristic response. However, when tissue damage is more extensive and involves disruption of the blood–brain barrier, then influx of circulating blood monocytes occurs. This differential response has come to be known as the "graded response" hypothesis (1). The extent to which this graded response reflects differences in levels of expression in the CNS of monocyte/phagocyte-specific factors such as CSF-1 and

MCP-1 will be an interesting subject to pursue.

The term "microglia" refers to intrinsic or endogenous cells of the CNS with a characteristic morphology and phenotype (1,39). Two major forms are recognized: ramified and amoeboid. [In addition, a perivascular cell that belongs to the macrophage/phagocyte lineage has been identified within the perivascular adventitia of the CNS (40)]. The relationship between the amoeboid and ramified forms of microglia is unresolved, but in the developing brain, evidence suggests that amoeboid microglia evolve into ramified microglia (reviewed in ref. 1). Ramified microglia are usually highly branched and found throughout the neuropil. In some areas they are present as perineuronal satellite cells, particularly in regions rich in cholinergic neurons. Amoeboid microglia usually have fewer processes and a plump cytoplasm. They are relatively rare in the normal adult CNS but are a prominent feature of many inflammatory and immune-mediated encephalitides. In culture, most microglia assume the less differentiated amoeboid form, although recently methods for culturing ramified microglia have been described (41). Little is known about the turnover properties of intrinsic microglia, although these cells clearly retain their capacity to proliferate in response to tissue injury (42). They have been shown to proliferate in response to the CSFs *in vitro* (6,43,44), but the specific role of CSF-1 in this process remains unclear. The results reported here would be consistent with the hypothesis that CSF-1 is primarily a survival and differentiation factor for these cells rather than a proliferation factor, inducing the differentiation of cells from the amoeboid phenotype to the ramified phenotype. However, the possibility that dividing microglia detach from the substrate and are, therefore, not present at the later time points is an issue that needs to be addressed in future experiments (45).

The effect of CSF-1 on monocytes differs according to the maturational state of the cell. In the early stages of monocyte development, CSF-1 has been shown to be a major growth factor. However, at later time points CSF-1 has been considered to induce macrophage differentiation and activation (3–5). CSF-1 is a potent physiological inducer of γ-interferon (IFN-γ), TNF and IL-1, the production of which would implicate CSF-1 as a major activation factor of the immune response (46). However, more recent evidence has brought into question this concept and has suggested that CSF-1 may down-regulate the immune response through the reduced expression of class II major histocompatability complex (MHC) antigens and the secretion of inhibitors of IL-1 (47–50). Our data in animals with EAE that show elevated levels of CSF-1 early in the disease process and rapid down-regulation during the recovery period would be consistent with either hypothesis. Treatment of animals with EAE with recombinant CSF-1 or antibodies to CSF-1 may help to clarify this issue. However, in experiments with microglia of human origin, we have recently found that CSF-1 down-regulates IFN-γ-induced expression of MHC class II molecules (51), in agreement with the data obtained with macrophages.

In conclusion, our results provide additional support for the hypothesis that the CNS expresses a cytokine–cytokine network analogous to that present in the immune system. Maintenance of the normal cytokine balance, including the expression of growth factors specific for cells of the monocyte/phagocyte series, may be important for normal CNS function. Cytokines possess powerful pleiotropic properties, and any alteration in the production of these factors may have widespread effects on normal CNS function. Because CSF-1 is required throughout the life span of the macrophage, it is reasonable to assume that a similar requirement applies to microglia. Microglia secrete factors that are trophic for neurons (52), and macrophage-derived factors are involved in inducing neural development in ectodermal explants (53). In addition, astrocytes proliferate in response to macrophage/microglia-derived cytokines such as TNF (54); thus, cellular signals between astrocytes and microglia may play important functional roles in maintaining the normal glial homeostasis in the CNS (1). Although we did not detect a dramatic effect of CSF-1 on reactive gliosis induced by anti-CNS serum in organotypic cultures, the challenge used in these preliminary experiments was maximal and may have masked more subtle effects. Taken together, the data suggest that alterations in factors specific for cells of the monocyte/phagocyte series may have wide-ranging effects on the process of repair within the CNS and underscore the importance of defining their role in this process.

ACKNOWLEDGMENTS

The work described in this review represents the collaborative efforts of the authors on projects that seek to define the role of cytokines in disorders of the central nervous system. They wish to express their thanks to the students who have contributed to this effort. These include Kathy Hulkower, Nishi Sharma, Davida Rapoport, and Sunita Kulshrestha. We also appreciate the excellent technical support of Michelle Guida and Vince Spada. Supported in part by NIH grants NS 11920, MH 47667, AG 07677, and National Multiple Sclerosis Society Grant 1089.

REFERENCES

1. Dickson DW, Mattiace LA, Kure K, Hutchins K, Lyman WD, Brosnan CF. Microglia in human disease, with an emphasis on acquired immune deficiency syndrome. *Lab Invest* 1991;64:135–156.
2. Giulian D. Ameboid microglia as effectors of inflammation in the central nervous system. *J Neurosci Res* 1987;18:155–171.
3. Stanley ER, Guilbert LJ, Tushinski RJ, Bartelmez SH. CSF-1—a mononuclear phagocyte lineage specific hemopoietic growth factor. *J Cell Biochem* 1983;21:151–159.
4. Clark SC, Kamen R. The human hematopoietic colony stimulating factors. *Science* 1987;236:1229–1237.
5. Metcalf D. Control of granulocytes and macrophages: molecular, cellular and clinical aspects. *Science* 1991;254:529–533.
6. Alliot F, Lecain E, Grima B, Pessac B. Microglial progenitors with a high proliferative potential in the embryonic and adult mouse brain. *Proc Natl Acad Sci USA* 1991;88:1541–1545.
7. Pober JS, Cotran RS. The role of endothelial cells in inflammation. *Transplantation* 1990;50:537–544.
8. Kuratsu J-I, Leonard EJ, Yoshimura T. Production and characterization of human glioma cell-derived monocyte chemotactic factor. *J Natl Cancer Inst* 1989;81:347–351.
9. Raine CS. Biology of disease. Analysis of autoimmune demyelination: its impact upon multiple sclerosis. *Lab Invest* 1984;50:608–635.
10. Swanborg RH, Autoimmune effector cells. V. A monoclonal antibody specific for rat helper T lymphocytes inhibits adoptive transfer of autoimmune encephalomyelitis. *J Immunol* 1983;130: 1503–1505.
11. Brosnan CF, Bornstein MB, Bloom BR. The effects of macrophage depletion on the clinical and pathological expression of experimental allergic encephalomyelitis. *J Immunol* 1981;126:614–620.
12. Huitinga I, van Rooijen N, de Groot CJA, Uitdehaag BMJ, Dijkstra CJ. Suppression of experimental allergic encephalomyelitis in Lewis rats after elimination of macrophages. *J Exp Med* 1990;172:1025–1033.
13. Dijkstra CD, Damoiseaux J, Huitinga I. Suppression of experimental allergic encephalomyelitis by treatment with monoclonal antibody against rat CR3. *J Neuroimmunol* 1991;Suppl 1:49.
14. Paterson PY, Swanborg RH. Demyelinating diseases of the central and peripheral nervous systems. In: Samter M, ed. *Immunological diseases*, 4th ed. Boston: Little Brown; 1988:1877–1916.
15. McFarlin DE, Blank SE, Kibler RF. Recurrent experimental allergic encephalomyelitis in the Lewis rat. *J Immunol* 1974;113:712–715.
16. Brosnan CF, Sacks HR, Goldschmidt RC, Goldmuntz EA, Norton WT. Prazosin treatment during the effector stage f disease suppresses experimental autoimmune encephalomyelitis in the Lewis rat. *J Immunol* 1986;137:3451–3456.
17. Aquino DA, Chiu F-C, Brosnan CF, Norton WT. Glial fibrillary acidic protein increases in the spinal cord of Lewis rats with acute experimental autoimmune encephalomyelitis. *J Neurochem* 1988;51: 1085–1096.
18. Ladner MB, Martin GA, Noble JA, et al. Human CSF-1: gene structure and alternative splicing of mRNA precursers. *EMBO J* 1987;6:2693–2698.
19. Cerretti DP, Wignall J, Anderson D, et al. Human macrophage colony-stimulating factor: alternative RNA and protein processing from a single gene. *Mol Immunol* 1988;25:761–770.
20. Sherr CJ, Rettenmier CW, Sacca R, Roussel MF, Look AT, Stanley ER. The *c-fms* proto-oncogene product is related to the receptor for the mononuclear phagocyte growth factor, CSF-1. *Cell* 1985;41: 665–676.
21. Leonard EJ, Yoshimura T. Human monocyte chemoattractant protein-1 (MCP-1). *Immunol Today* 1990;11:97–101.
22. Hulkower KL, Brosnan CF, Berman JW. Cytokine gene expression in the central nervous system of rats with experimental allergic encephalomyelitis. *FASEB J* 1991;5:A8184.

23. Hulkower KL, Brosnan CF, Berman JW. CSF-1 gene expression and protein levels in the central nervous system and peripheral immune system of rats with experimental autoimmune encephalomyelitis. *J Neuroimmunol* 1991;Suppl 1:147.
24. Sharma N, Berman JW, Brosnan CF, Shafit-Zagardo B. IL-1 and TNF induce CSF-1 in rat astrocyte cultures. *J Neuroimmunol* 1991;Suppl 1:146.
25. Shafit-Zagardo B, Sharma N, Berman JW, Brosnan CF. IL-1 and TNF upregulate CSF-1 expression in rat astrocyte cultures. *J Cell Biol* 1991;115:2450a.
26. Bornstein MB. Immunobiology of demyelination. In: Waxman SG, ed. *Physiology and pathology of axons.* New York: Raven Press; 1978:313–335.
27. Cross AH, Cannella B, Brosnan CF, Raine CS. Homing to central nervous system vasculature by antigen-specific lymphocytes. I. Localization of ^{14}C-labeled cells during acute, chronic and relapsing experimental allergic encephalomyelitis. *Lab Invest* 1990;63:162–170.
28. Hallet M-M, Praloran V, Vie H, et al. Macrophage colony-stimulating factor gene expression in human T-lymphocyte clones. *Blood* 1991;77:780–786.
29. Hao C, Guilbert LJ, Fedoroff S. Production of colony-stimulating factor-1 (CSF-1) by mouse astroglia *in vitro. J Neurosci Res* 1990;27:314–323.
30. Thery C, Hetier E, Evrard C, Mallat M. Expression of macrophage colony stimulating factor gene in the mouse brain during development. *J Neurosci Res* 1990;26:129–133.
31. Giulian D, Johnson B, Krebs JF, George JK, Tapscott M. Microglial mitogens are produced in the developing and injured mammalian brain. *J Cell Biol* 1991;112:323–333.
32. Aloisi F, Borsellino G, Testa U, Care A, Peschle C, Levi G. Cytokine production by normal human astrocytes in culture. *J Neuroimmunol* 1991;Suppl 1:61.
33. Falkenberg JHF, Haarington MA, Walsh WK, Daub R, Broxmeyer H. Gene-expression and release of macrophage-colony stimulating factor in quiescent and proliferating fibroblasts. Effects of serum, fibroblast growth-promoting factors and IL-1. *J Immunol* 1990;144:4657–4662.
34. Tweardy DJ, Mott PL, Glazer EW. Monokine modulation of human astroglial cell production of granulocyte colony-stimulating factor and granulocyte–macrophage colony-stimulating factor. 1. Effects of IL-1α and IL-1β. *J Immunol* 1990;144:2233–2241.
35. Rollins BJ, Pober JS. 1991. Interleukin-4 induces the synthesis and secretion of MCP-1/JE by human endothelial cells. *Am J Pathol* 1991;138:1315–1319.
36. Sieff CA, Niemeyer CM, Mentzer SJ, Faller DD. Interleukin-1, TNF and the production of colony stimulating factor by cultured mesenchymal cells. *Blood* 1988;72:1316–1323.
37. Yla-Herttuala S, Lipton BA, Rosenfeld ME, et al. Expression of monocyte chemoattractant protein 1 in macrophage-rich areas of human and rabbit atherosclerotic lesions. *Proc Natl Acad Sci USA* 1991;88:5252–5256.
38. Fedoroff S, Ahmed I, Young VW, Guilbert L, Antel J. A subpopulation of human astroglia expresses the receptor for colony-stimulating factor-1 which is encoded by *c-fms. J Neuroimmunol* 1991;Suppl 1:100.
39. Perry VH, Hume DA, Gordon S. Immunohistochemical localization of macrophages and microglia in the adult and developing brain. *Brain Res* 1985;15:313–326.
40. Graeber MB, Streit WJ. Perivascular cells defined. *Trends Neurosci* 1990;13:366.
41. Suzumura A, Marunouchi T, Yamamoto H. Morphological transformation of microglia *in vitro. Brain Res* 1991;545:301–306.
42. Graeber MB, Tetzlaff W, Streit WJ, Kreutzberg GW. Microglial cells but not astrocytes undergo mitosis following rat facial nerve axonotomy. *Neurosci Lett* 1988;85:317–321.
43. Sawada K, Suzumura A, Yamamoto H, Marunouchi T. Activation and proliferation of isolated microglia by colony stimulating factor-1 and possible involvement of protein kinase C. *Brain Res* 1990;509:121–124.
44. Giulian D, Ingemann JE. Colony stimulating factors as promoters of ameboid microglia. *J Neurosci* 1988;8:4707–4717.
45. Gebicke-Haerter PJ, Bauer J, Schobert A, Northoff H. Lipopolysaccharide-free conditions in primary astrocyte cultures allow growth and isolation of microglial cells. *J Neurosci* 1989;9:183–194.
46. Warren MK, Ralph P. Macrophage growth factor CSF-1 stimulates human monocyte production of interferon, tumor necrosis factor, and colony stimulating activity. *J Immunol* 1986;137:2281–2285.
47. Calamai EG, Beller DI, Unanue ER. Regulation of macrophage populations. IV. Modulation of Ia expression in bone marrow-derived macrophages. *J Immunol* 1982;128:1692–1694.
48. Falk LA, Wahl LM, Vogel SN. Analysis of Ia antigen expression in macrophages derived from bone marrow cells cultured in granulocyte–macrophage colony stimulating factor or macrophage colony-stimulating factor. *J Immunol* 1988;140: 2652–2660.
49. Willman CL, Stewart CC, Miller V, Yi T-L, Tomasi TB. Regulation of MHC class II gene expression in macrophages by hematopoietic colony stimulating factors. Induction by granulocyte/macrophage CSF and inhibition by CSF-1. *J Exp Med* 1989;170: 1559–1567.
50. Strassmann G, Bertolini DR, Kerby SB, Fong M. Regulation of murine mononuclear phagocyte inflammatory products by macrophage colony-stimulating factor. Lack of IL-1 and prostaglandin E_2 production and generation of a specific IL-1 inhibitor. *J Immunol* 1991;147:1279–1285.
51. Lee SC, Liu W, Roth P, Dickson DW, Berman JW, Brosnan CF. Macrophage colony stimulating factor (CSF-1) in human fetal astrocytes and microglia in culture. Production and function. *J Immunol,* [in press].
52. Mallat M, Houlgatte R, Brachet P, and Prochiantz A. Lipopolysaccharide-stimulated rat brain macrophages release NGF *in vitro. Develop Biol* 1989;133:309–311.
53. Sokol S, Wong GG, Melton DA. A mouse macrophage factor induces head structures and organizes a body axis in *Xenopus. Science* 1990;249:561–564.
54. Selmaj K, Farooq M, Raine CS, Norton WT, Brosnan CF. Proliferation of astrocytes *in vitro* in response to cytokines: a primary role for tumor necrosis factor. *J Immunol* 1990;144:129–135.

Subject Index